# Retina Atlas

# Retina Atlas

**SECOND EDITION**

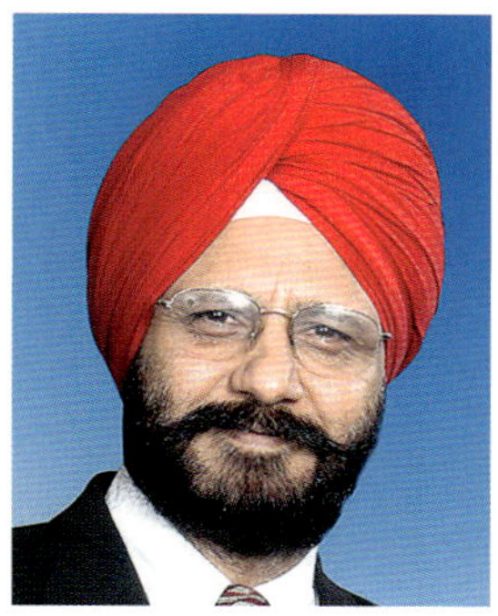

**SPS Grewal** MBBS MD
CEO
Grewal Eye Institute, Chandigarh, India
Adjunct Professor
Department of Ophthalmology
Feinberg School of Medicine
Northwestern University, IL, USA
Fellow
Moorfields Eye Hospital, London, UK
Former Associate Professor
Department of Ophthalmology
Postgraduate Institute of
Medical Education and Research
Chandigarh
*drgrewal@gmail.com*

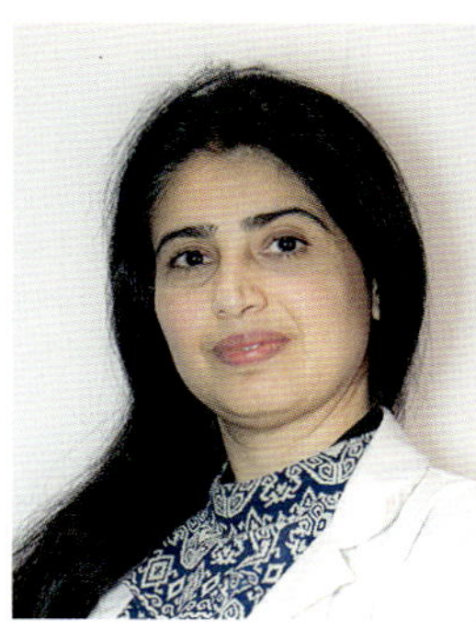

**Manpreet Brar** MBBS MS
Senior Consultant
Department of Vitreoretinal
Diseases and Surgery
Grewal Eye Institute, Chandigarh, India
Fellow in Vitreoretina
University of California, San Diego, USA
Fellow, Moorfields Eye Hospital
Former Consultant
Moorfields Eye Hospital, London, UK
*dr.manpreetbrar@gmail.com*

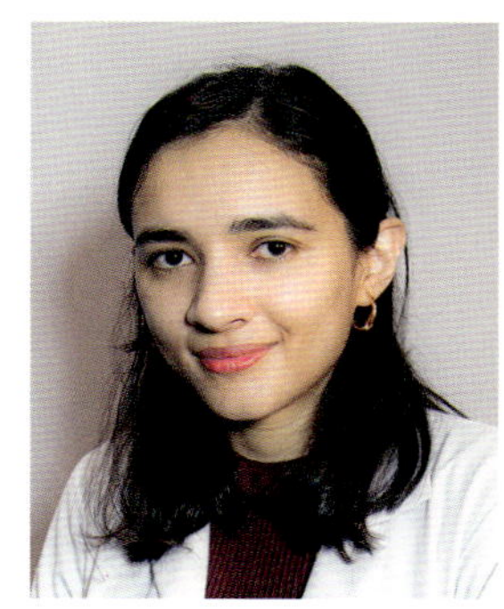

**Mansi Sharma** MBBS DNB FAICO
Consultant
Department of Vitreoretinal Diseases and Surgery
Grewal Eye Institute, Chandigarh, India
Fellowship in Vitreoretinal Surgery
Department of Ophthalmology
Postgraduate Institute of Medical
Education and Research
Chandigarh
Fellowship of the All India Collegium
of Ophthalmology (Vitreoretina)
All India Ophthalmological Society
*dr.mansi.sharma@gmail.com*

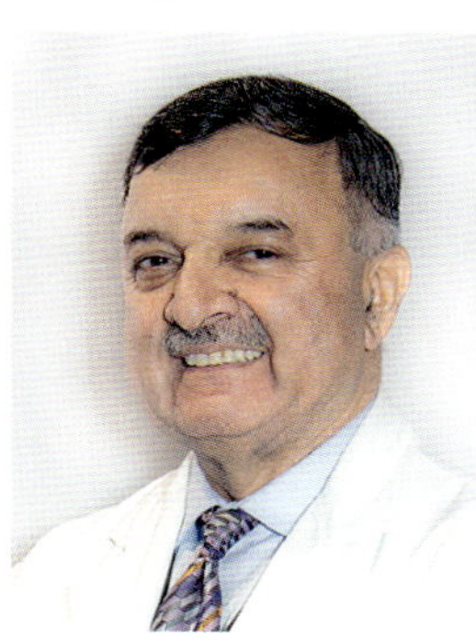

**Mangat R Dogra** MBBS MS
Director
Department of Vitreoretinal
Diseases and Surgery
Grewal Eye Institute, Chandigarh, India
Fellow in Vitreoretina
University of Maryland Hospital
Baltimore, USA
Former Professor and Head
Department of Ophthalmology
Advance Eye Centre
Postgraduate Institute of Medical
Education and Research
Chandigarh
*drmangatdogra@gmail.com*

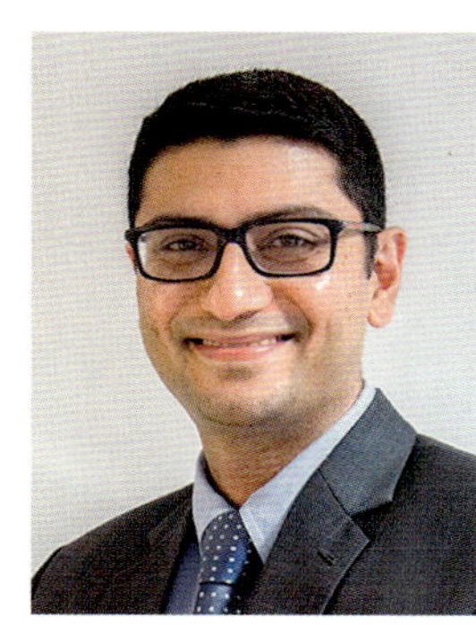

**Dilraj S Grewal** MBBS MD
Associate Professor
Department of Ophthalmology
Vitreoretinal Surgery and Uveitis
Duke Eye Center, Duke University Medical Center
Durham, NC, USA
Fellow, Heed Ophthalmic Foundation
Fellow, Society of Heed Fellows
Ron Michael Fellow, Uveitis Fellow
Moorfields Eye Hospital, London, UK
*dilraj@gmail.com*

JAYPEE

**JAYPEE BROTHERS MEDICAL PUBLISHERS**
*The Health Sciences Publisher*
**New Delhi | London**

**Jaypee Brothers Medical Publishers (P) Ltd**

**Headquarters**
Jaypee Brothers Medical Publishers (P) Ltd
EMCA House, 23/23-B
Ansari Road, Daryaganj
New Delhi 110 002, India
Landline: +91-11-23272143, +91-11-23272703
+91-11-23282021, +91-11-23245672
Email: jaypee@jaypeebrothers.com

**Corporate Office**
Jaypee Brothers Medical Publishers (P) Ltd
4838/24, Ansari Road, Daryaganj
New Delhi 110 002, India
Phone: +91-11-43574357
Fax: +91-11-43574314
Email: jaypee@jaypeebrothers.com

**Overseas Office**
JP Medical Ltd.
83, Victoria Street, London
SW1H 0HW (UK)
Phone: +44 20 3170 8910
Fax: +44 (0)20 3008 6180
Email: info@jpmedpub.com

Website: www.jaypeebrothers.com
Website: www.jaypeedigital.com



**Inquiries for bulk sales may be solicited at:** jaypee@jaypeebrothers.com

***Retina Atlas***

*First Edition: 2020*
*Second Edition:* **2024**

ISBN: 978-93-5696-880-6

*Printed at: Samrat Offset Pvt. Ltd.*

**Dedicated to**

*Sukhbir*

# Preface to the Second Edition

I never expected the first edition of our *Retina Atlas* to be as successful as it has been. The overwhelming response to the first edition has been testimony to the quality of the images and the format of the book. The focus of the book has been to present and highlight the clinical findings on fundus examination, their description, variations, and correlation to the disease. Purposefully, we left out the nitty-gritty of differential diagnoses and treatment, opting instead to delve deep into the clinical landscape to focus on clinical findings and the presentation of a disease.

I have kept the basic structure of the book intact. Since our first dive into the retinal wonders, we have encountered a treasure trove of new cases and amassed a wealth of even better images. Every opportunity to upgrade our visuals has been seized, with the inclusion of newer and rarer entities. Moreover, we have got our hands on images from ultrawide-field fundus imaging systems (Optos), adding a whole new dimension to our exploration.

What's more, we've listened to you, our readers, incorporating your suggestions and feedback to make this edition even more valuable. This book is not just for the seasoned pros; it is a gateway for medical students, residents, and postgraduates to peek into the fascinating world of retinal disorders. For those who might not encounter every spectrum of disease during their training, the *Retina Atlas* offers a window into this captivating realm.

So, here is to hoping that our second edition continues to captivate and educate, serving as an indispensable tool for anyone with a passion for retinal imaging. My sincere thanks to my co-authors and the incredible team at Grewal Eye Institute, Chandigarh, India for their unwavering support in bringing this edition to life. Let us dive in and explore the wonders of the retina together.

**SPS Grewal**

# Preface to the First Edition

Photography has been my passion from college days. I used to enjoy my time in the darkroom created at home for developing and printing black and white photographs way back in 1971. I had never imagined there will be a synergetic and symbiotic fusion of my passion and profession. When I chose ophthalmology as my career, the keen interest in fundus photography was a natural sequence. This not only included taking great pictures but also to train the staff in the skills. Developing the E6 processing for color transparencies and refining black and white prints for fundus fluorescein angiography (FFA) to get right contrast were the next steps. The passion for personal and professional photography never abated.

The era of digitization caught my attention. I modified the Zeiss 450 plus camera to take digital pictures. At that time, there was no proprietary digital camera on the market, and I had to develop a software patch to synchronize the flash and store images. I discussed this with Dr Sohan Singh Hayereh at the annual meeting of Vitreoretinal Society of India at Chandigarh in 2003. He was skeptical and said digital pictures pale in comparison with actual print photographs. However, he agreed to come and see the improvization for a short time, but ended up spending over two hours going through our collections of fundus photographs and fundus fluorescein angiograms. He was awestruck with the details of capillary network in macula and details of foveal avascular zone. The two hours changed his perception about the potential of digital cameras.

My experience with Eidon has been great. Every time I looked at the pictures, there was a keen desire to share them with my colleagues, leading to the germination of an idea to plan an atlas of common retinal disorders and share our collection of retinal imaging. OCT has been added to understand the pathology in a better way.

Being an atlas, a greater space has been allocated to pictures with only minimal necessary text. Enjoy the details in photographs. Look at the details and plethora of lesions visible. A picture shows much more in a shorter time than a fundus examination reveals. It is unmatched documentation to follow the disease progression or recovery. This book is for every ophthalmologist to review the fundus pathologies and great for residents and students.

An indigenously designed software to select cases, design pages and write legends and text came very handy. The software was on the network and each one of us had access to it all the time.

I am thankful to my colleagues accompanying me in this journey. My special thanks to my Co-authors, Drs Manpreet Brar, Mansi Sharma, Mangat R Dogra and Dilraj S Grewal for their efforts, support and guidance for bringing this atlas to the light of day. I thank my wife for her support and understanding in allowing me to devote family time to the atlas.

My special thanks to Mr Parminder Singh, who has been glued to his seat to edit and typeset the artwork for the *Retina Atlas*. Mr Shaurya Bajwa, Research Associate, Grewal Eye Institute, has been a great help in collecting the cases, tabulating them, retrieving the images from machines and select the final frames to be included. My thanks to Mr Swaran Singh, a keen learner, who has been sharing my interest in photography since 1981.

The task to put all data into shape of atlas was far more daunting than we all imagined. I thank all team members at Grewal Eye Institute for their help in turning my vision into reality.

**SPS Grewal**

# Contents

# Abbreviations

| | |
|---|---|
| ACE | Angiotensin-converting Enzyme |
| AD | Autosomal Dominant |
| AMD | Age-related Macular Degeneration |
| ANCA | Anti-Neutrophil Cytoplasmic Antibody |
| Anti-VEGF | Anti-Vascular Endothelial Growth Factor |
| AOVMD | Adult Onset Vitelliform Macular Degeneration |
| AREDS | Age-related Eye Disease Study |
| ARMD | Age-related Macular Degeneration |
| ATT | Anti-Tubercular Therapy |
| AV | Arterio Venous |
| BBG | Brilliant Blue G |
| BCVA | Best Corrected Visual Acuity |
| BRVO | Branch Retinal Vein Occlusion |
| CF | Count Fingers |
| CFCF | Counting Fingers Close to Face |
| CME | Cystoid Macular Edema |
| CNVM | Choroidal Neovascular Membrane |
| CRVO | Central Retinal Vein Occlusion |
| CSCR | Central Serous Chorioretinopathy |
| CSR | Central Serous Retinopathy |
| DCP | Deep Capillary Plexus |
| DM | Diabetes Mellitus |
| DME | Diabetic Macular Edema |
| DRIL | Disorganization of Retinal Inner Layers |
| DRS | Duane Retraction Syndrome |
| EOG | Electro-oculography |
| ESR | Erythrocyte Sedimentation Rate |
| FAF | Fundus Auto-Fluorescence |
| FFA | Fundus Fluorescein Angiography |
| HbA1c | Hemoglobin A1c |
| HM | Hand Motion |
| HMCF | Hand Motion Close to Face |
| HRVO | Hemispheric Retinal Vein Occlusion |
| ICGA | Indocyanine Green Angiography |
| ILM | Internal Limiting Membrane |
| IPCV | Idiopathic Polypoidal Choroidal Vasculopathy |
| IRMA | Intra-retinal Microvascular Abnormalities |
| IS-OS | Inner and Outer Segment |
| IV | Intravenous |
| JXT | Juxtafoveal Telangiectasis |
| MA | Microaneurysm |
| MNFL | Myelinated Nerve Fiber Layer |
| NPDR | Nonproliferative Diabetic Retinopathy |
| NV | Neovascularization |
| NVD | Neovascularization of the Disc |
| NVE | Neovascularization Elsewhere |
| NVG | Neovascular Glaucoma |
| OCT | Optical Coherence Tomography |
| OCTA | Optical Coherence Tomography Angiography |
| OD | Oculus Dextrus |
| OPL | Outer Plexiform Layer |
| ORCC | Outer Retina Choriocapillary Slab |
| OS | Oculus Sinister |
| PCV | Polypoidal Choroidal Vasculopathy |
| PDR | Proliferative Diabetic Retinopathy |
| PDT | Photodynamic Therapy |
| PED | Pigment Epithelial Detachment |
| PEHCR | Peripheral Exudative Hemorrhagic Chorioretinopathy |
| PFT | Parafoveal Telangiectasia |
| PIC | Punctate Inner Choroidopathy |
| PRP | Panretinal Photocoagulation |
| PVD | Posterior Vitreous Detachment |
| PVR | Proliferative Vitreoretinopathy |
| RAM | Retinal Arterial Macroaneurysm |
| RAP | Retinal Angiomatous Proliferation |
| RAPD | Relative Afferent Pupillary Defect |
| RP | Retinitis Pigmentosa |
| RPE | Retinal Pigment Epithelium |
| SD-OCT | Spectral Domain Optical Coherence Tomography |
| SRF | Sub-retinal Fluid |
| SRH | Sub-retinal Hemorrhage |
| SS-OCT | Swept Source Optical Coherence Tomography |
| TB | Tuberculosis |
| VA | Visual Acuity |
| VH | Vitreous Hemorrhage |
| VKH | Vogt-Koyanagi-Harada |

# Introduction

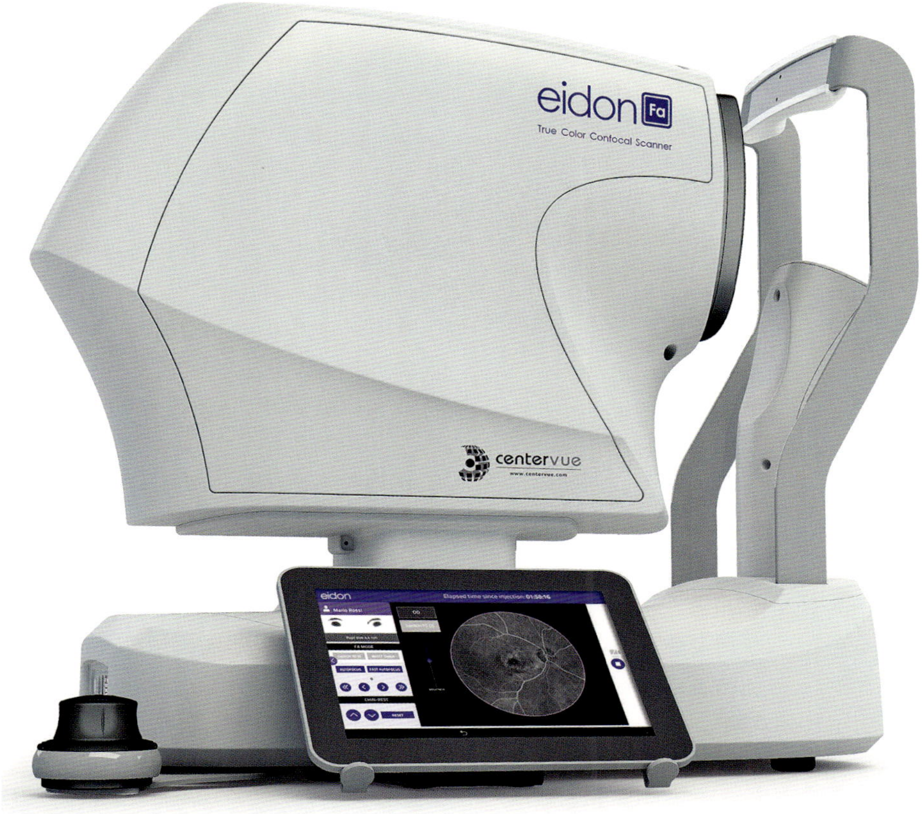


The concept of fundus photography was first introduced in the mid-19th century, after the introduction of photography in 1839. In 1851, Hermann von Helmholtz introduced the Ophthalmoscope, and James Clerk Maxwell presented a color photography method in 1861. In the early 1860s, Henry Noyes and Abner Mulholland Rosebrugh both assembled fundus cameras and tried fundus photography on animals. Early fundus photos were limited by insufficient light, long exposures, eye movement, and prominent corneal reflexes that reduced the clarity detail. It would be several decades before these problems could be rectified.

There has been some controversy regarding the first ever successful human fundus photo. Most accounts credit William Thomas Jackman and JD Webster, since they published their technique, along with a reproduction of a fundus image. These images were published in two photography periodicals in 1886.

Fundus cameras can take a color picture, red-free fundus photograph, angiography including sodium fluorescein angiography (abbreviated FFA, FA or FAG) and indocyanine green angiography (abbreviated ICG), simultaneous stereo-fundus photos, and autofluorescence pictures. Fundus photography has moved from film based to digital images, a wider field of view, collage stitching, low light capability, small pupil and now on to scanning laser-based imaging.

Instead of one photograph taken at one time, the confocal scanning lasers take point-by-point image, which is later combined to make a 2D image.

Confocal microscopy, most frequently called confocal laser scanning microscopy (CLSM) or laser confocal scanning microscopy (LCSM), is an optical imaging technique for increasing optical resolution and contrast of a micrograph by means of using a spatial pinhole to block out-of-focus light in image formation. Confocal laser scanning systems are superior to conventional fundus cameras in many ways, as they exploit a confocal imaging principle which limits the effect of backscattered light from deeper layers and provides enhanced image quality. Another major advantage of SLO systems is that they operate with much smaller pupils than conventional fundus cameras.

The Eidon confocal scanner (Centervue, Padova, Italy) received FDA clearance in December 2014. According to the manufacturer, Eidon is the only wide-view system that combines confocal imaging with natural white-light illumination to provide a true-color image, as opposed to the pseudo-color rendering generated by monochromatic lasers in scanning laser ophthalmoscope-based systems. The merging of color channels in that approach results in a bright orange retinal image, blood having a blue-green hue, and a dark or black optic nerve. Centervue says that white-light illumination reveals greater detail of retinal pathologies and allows a clearer view of the optic nerve.

Eidon, being a confocal optical system, is able to perform high-quality retinal images with increased sharpness, better optical resolution and greater contrast when compared to traditional fundus camera imaging. This technology captures retinal images of preserved quality even in cases of media opacity. Eidon is the first system to combine the advantages of SLO with the fidelity of true-color imaging, setting new performance standards in retinal imaging with super-high resolution and contrast. It provides more-balanced color images, with a wider richness of color content, compared to a conventional flash-fundus camera.

Eidon provides 60° field in a single exposure, a unique, live, confocal view of the retina, three different imaging modalities (True color, red-free and infrared confocal images) and dilation-free operation (minimum pupil 2.5 mm), all integrated in a versatile system that provides new opportunities in retinal diagnostics. Multiple imaging techniques with two different light sources are available—white LED (440–650 nm) and near infrared LED (825–870 nm). LED flash technology offers maximum patient comfort as it uses a low power light source. This in-turn reduces pupil constriction and facilitates the test on non-cooperative subjects. Eidon's optical system operates within the range of –12 D to +15 D. In eyes with a myopic refractive error of more than –12 D, Eidon may be unable to focus on the posterior pole and detect retinal conditions related to pathological myopia.

This fundus camera is operated via a tablet with a multi-touch, high resolution, color display; it works with a dedicated software application and operates as a standalone unit. The ease of use of operating the camera is amazing and unparalleled. The touchscreen tablet makes data entry very easy. The learning curve for a novice user is very short. It requires minimal operator involvement; it automatically aligns with the patient's pupil and focuses on the retina. The alignment, focusing, capturing and storing of images are completely automated. Images are captured from both eyes just by touch of a button. A joystick is provided when manual operation of the device when desired. It has capability to image through cataract and media opacities. Simple networking options are available. The system has built in feature for both remote data review and data backup.

# CHAPTER 1

## NORMAL FUNDUS

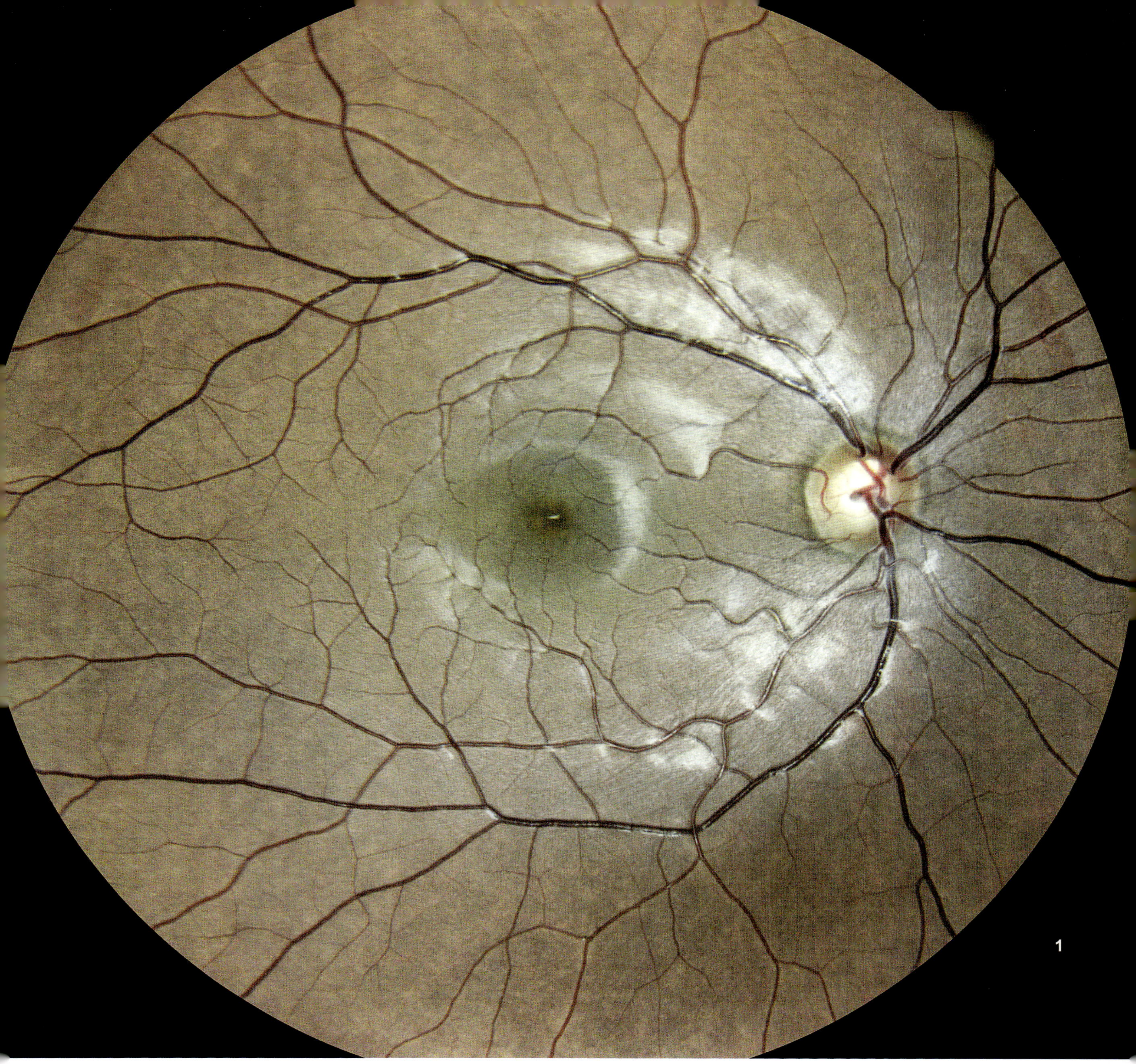


Figure 1 *Color fundus image of normal retina.*

The disk has well-defined sharp margins and peripheral neuroretinal rim is healthy with no thinning and normal in color, i.e., pale pink, with a normal sized central cup. It is 1.5 mm in diameter. Vessels emanate from the optic cup.

Arterioles and venules have normal color, sheen, caliber and course. Venous diameter is normally 1.5 times greater than arterial diameter. Arteriovenous crossing can be seen where the vessels share a common adventitial sheath. Background is in normal color. The fundus receives its uniform bright red coloration from the vessels of the choroid. The macula is enclosed by arching temporal vessels is 3–4 mm temporal to and slightly below the optic disk. The fovea is located by a central pit. Various retinal reflexes can be observed in the fundus photo. They are known as "Water silk" reflexes which are mainly patchy, round, oval and irregular in shape. They are highly mobile and elusive. These can be observed near large vessels as they raise a reflecting surface into a ridge of cylindrical form. They can be seen around macula as a halo coinciding with the outline of macula.

Other special reflexes which deserve a mention include. Gunn's Dot highly glistening colorless spec seen in posterior part of the fundus, seen best in the course of retinal nerve fibers above and below the disk. Weiss's reflex annular reflex concentric with the border of the disk and is mobile. Formed by elevation of internal limiting membrane where the nerve fiber layer is thickened, present at nasal border of the disk.

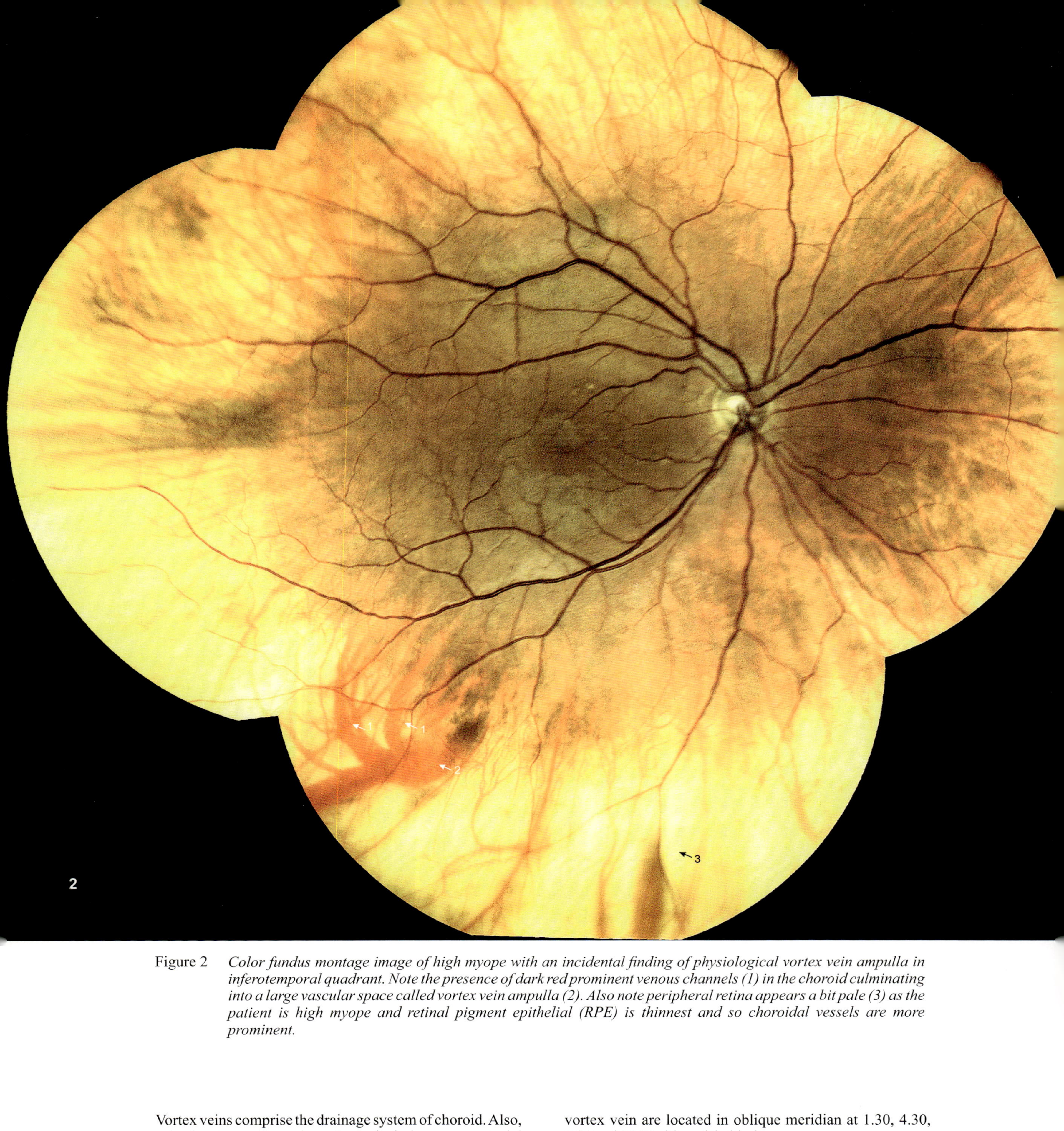


Figure 2 *Color fundus montage image of high myope with an incidental finding of physiological vortex vein ampulla in inferotemporal quadrant. Note the presence of dark red prominent venous channels (1) in the choroid culminating into a large vascular space called vortex vein ampulla (2). Also note peripheral retina appears a bit pale (3) as the patient is high myope and retinal pigment epithelial (RPE) is thinnest and so choroidal vessels are more prominent.*

Vortex veins comprise the drainage system of choroid. Also, scleral entrance to each vortex vein is known equatorial landmark in the fundus. Each eye contains 4–7 (or more) veins. One or more veins are usually located in each quadrant and exit 14–25 mm from the limbus between rectus muscles. The ampulla of vortex vein are 8–9 mm from ora serrata and an imaginary circle connecting these ampulla correspond roughly to the equator and divides central fundus from the peripheral fundus. The ampulla of vortex vein are located in oblique meridian at 1.30, 4.30, 7.30 and 10.30 although behind.

Vortex veins can be easily visualized in patient with lightly pigmented fundus and in myopic subjects who have thin retina. It is important for beginner in retina training course to be familiar with choroidal physiology and appearance and location of vortex vein to avoid any misdiagnosis.□

# CHAPTER 2

## DIABETIC RETINOPATHY

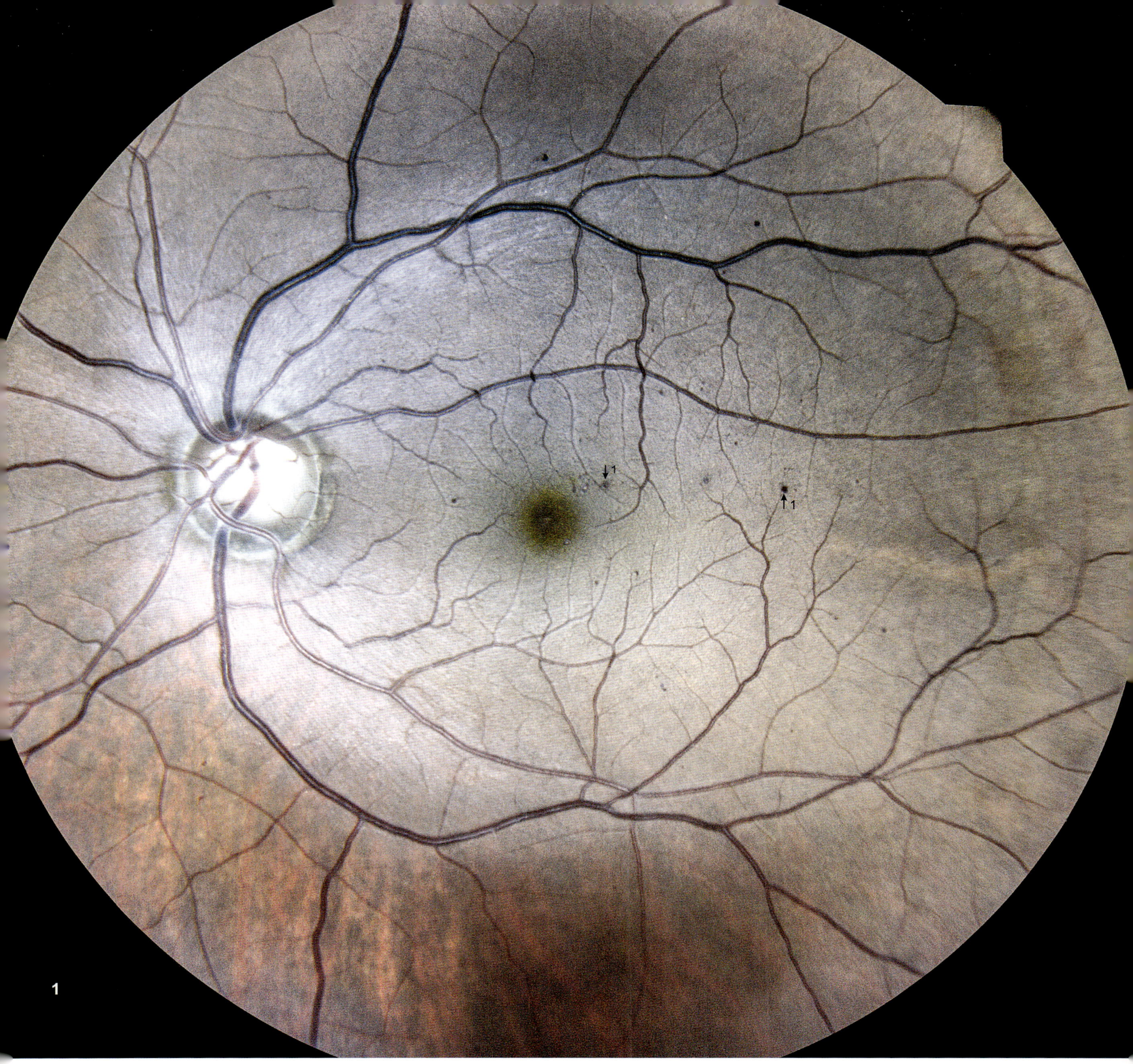


Figure 1 *Color fundus photograph of a patient with mild nonproliferative diabetic retinopathy: note the presence of fine red dot like microaneurysms at the posterior pole (1).*

Retinal capillary microaneurysm is usually the first visible sign of diabetic retinopathy. Microaneurysms are identified clinically by ophthalmoscopy as deep red dots varying from 15 to 60 microns in diameter. They are most common at the posterior pole. Although microaneurysms can be associated with vascular occlusion, they are the hallmark of nonproliferative diabetic retinopathy. As per the diabetic retinopathy severity scale, presence of microaneurysm only classifies into mild nonproliferative diabetic retinopathy. No treatment is indicated at this stage. Annual follow-up is recommended. □

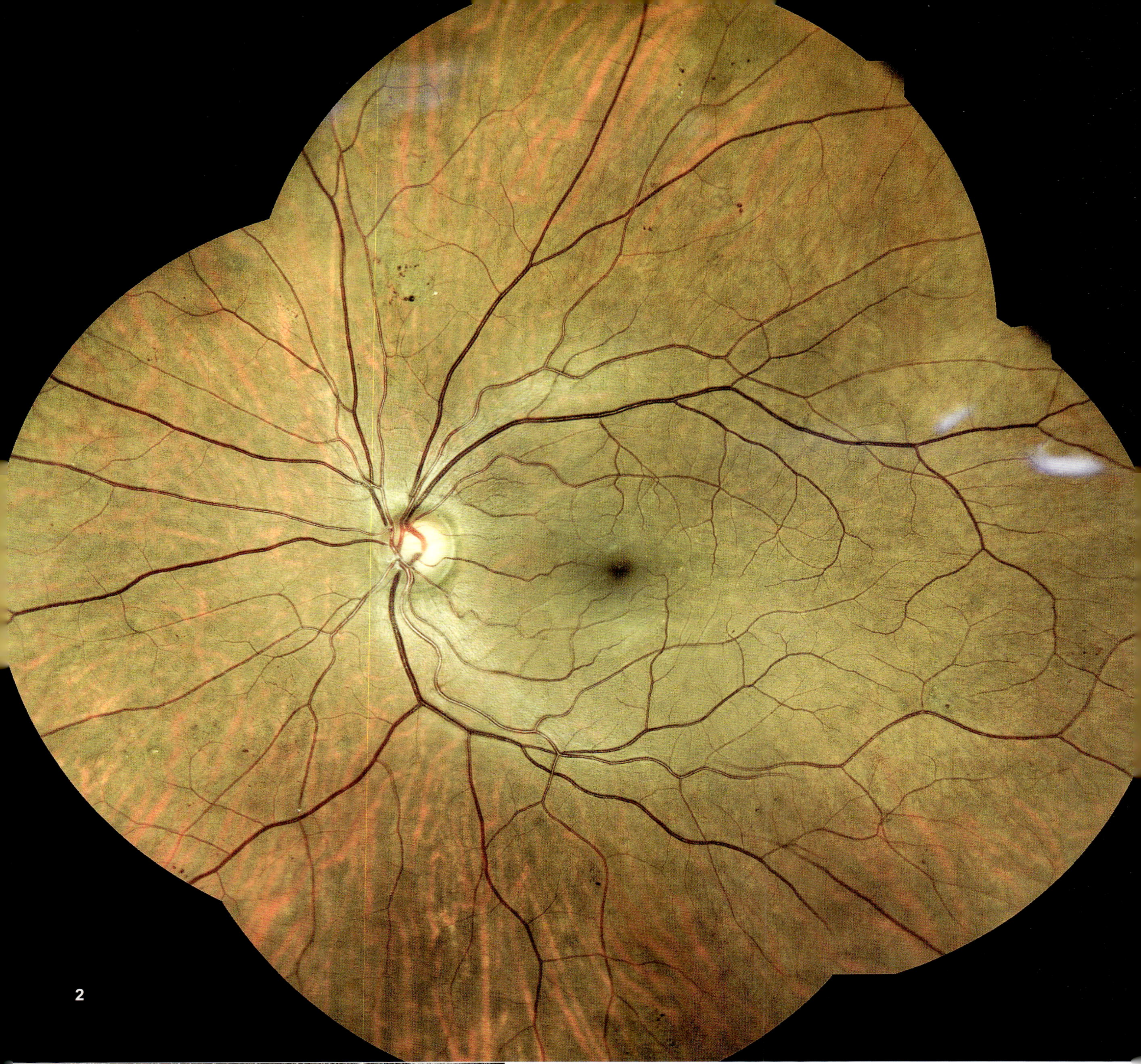

2

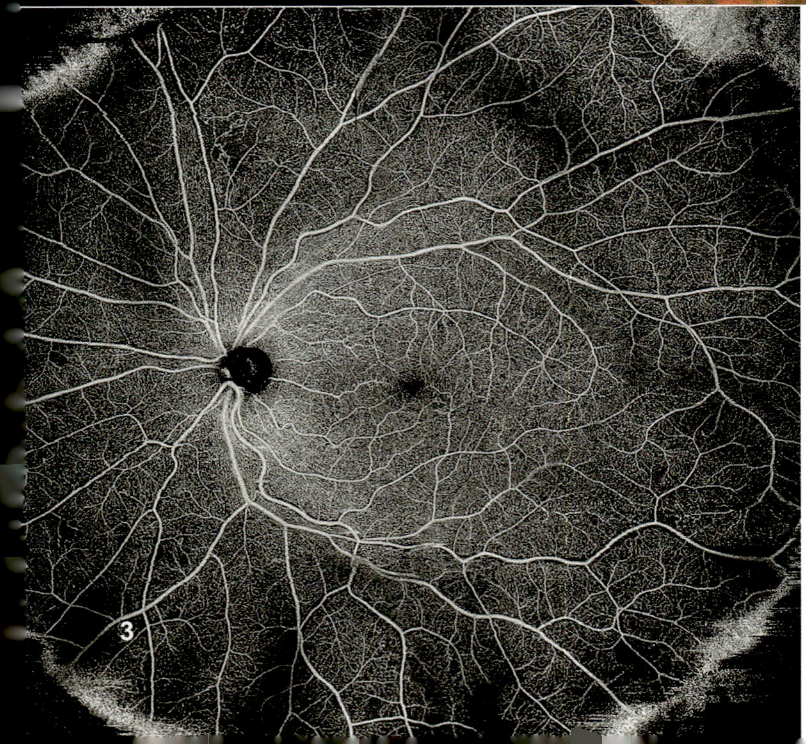

3

Figure 2 *Case of mild nonproliferative diabetic retinopathy without macular edema.*

Color fundus photograph of a case with diabetes mellitus type 2 for the last 10 years. Note the presence of the microaneurysms (pinpoint red dots) only, in the mid-periphery of the retina. No other diabetic changes were seen. Visual acuity was 6/6. Mild nonproliferative diabetic retinopathy is the earliest stage of the disease. No treatment is indicated at this stage. Such cases are recommended a thorough fundus examination once a year.

Figure 3 *12 mm × 12 mm OCT angiography montage photograph of a case of mild nonproliferative diabetic retinopathy: Retina slab demonstrates normal retinal vasculature, except few tiny spots of capillary drop-outs.*□

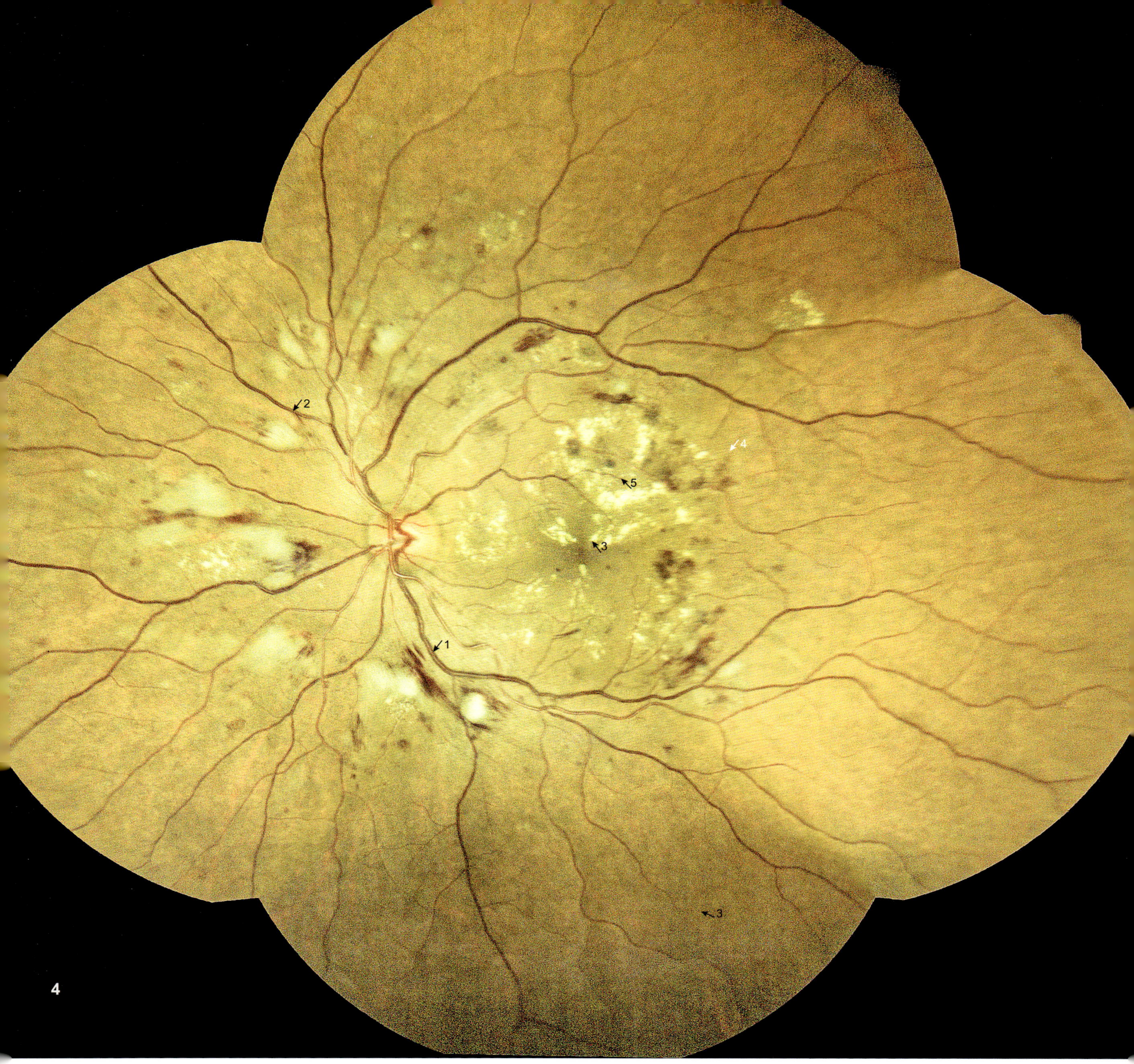


Figure 4 *A case of moderate nonproliferative diabetic retinopathy (NPDR) with diabetic macular edema (DME). Color fundus montage image demonstrating typical feature of moderate NPDR with DME. Note the presence of superficial retinal hemorrhages (1), multiple cotton wool spots (2), microaneurysms (3), dot blot hemorrhages (4) at the posterior pole and mid-peripheral retina. Multiple hard exudates with macular thickening could also be seen (5).*

Moderate NPDR is the third stage of diabetic retinopathy as classified by the international clinical disease severity scale for diabetic retinopathy. This disease severity scale was based upon the findings of the Wisconsin Epidemiologic Study of Diabetic Retinopathy and ETDRS. The third stage is "Moderate NPDR" which is characterized by the presence of microaneurysm, intraretinal hemorrhages or venous beading that do not reach the severity of standard photograph for severe NPDR. This patient has associated moderate diabetic macular edema as well. There is no apparent thickening in center of fovea but hard exudates could be seen threatening the foveal center. □

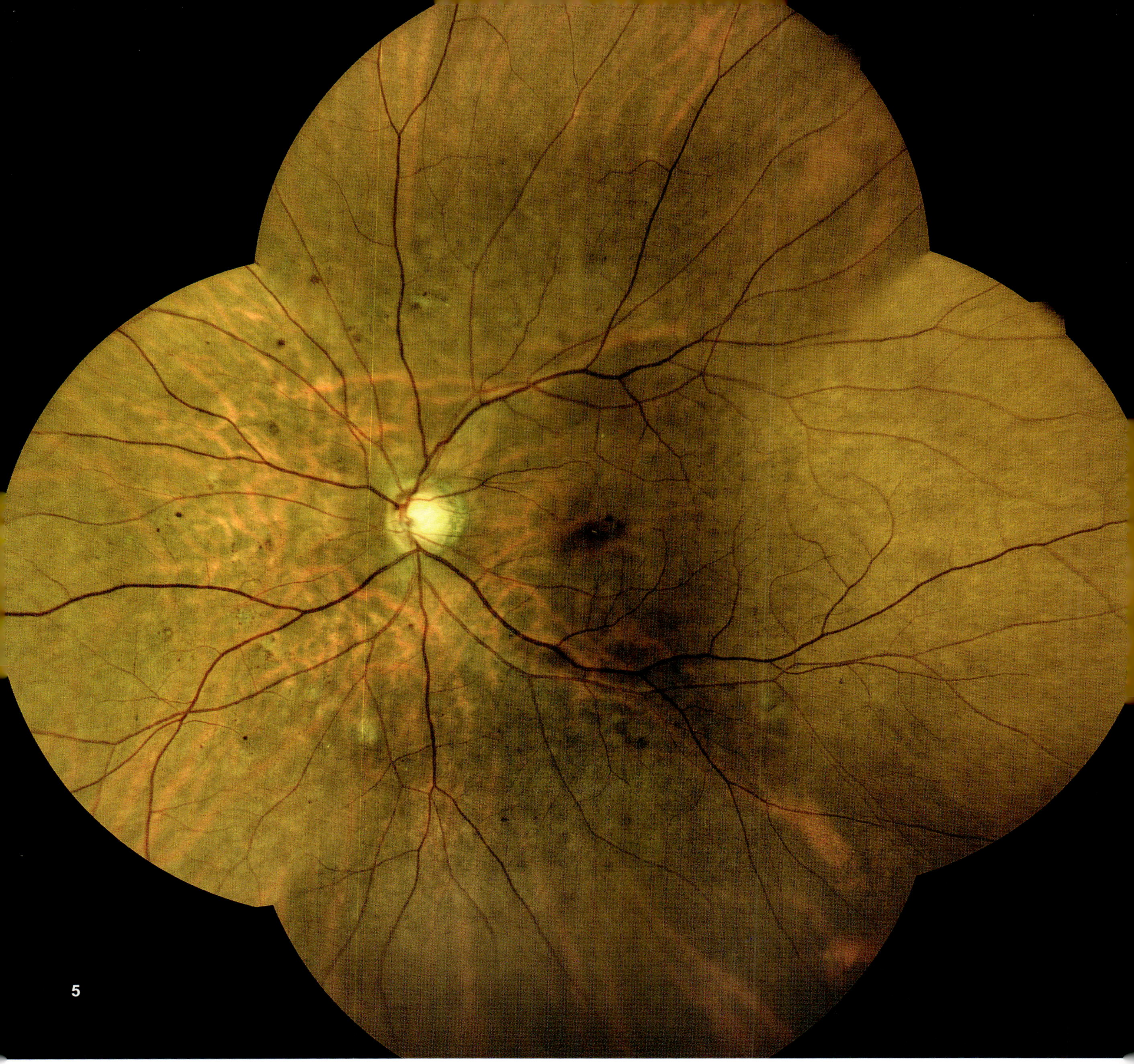


Figure 5 *Color fundus photograph of a case of moderate nonproliferative diabetic retinopathy (NPDR).*

Note the presence of microaneurysms, few hemorrhages and cotton wool spots distributed in macula and peripheral retina. The caliber of retinal vessels is normal.

Moderate NPDR is early stage of the disease. Patient is usually asymptomatic at this stage. Associated development of macular edema however, results in blurring of central vision. There are no evident areas of retinal thickening. There is no retinal neovascularization at the disk or in periphery.

No treatment is indicated at the moderate stage of nonproliferative diabetic retinopathy.

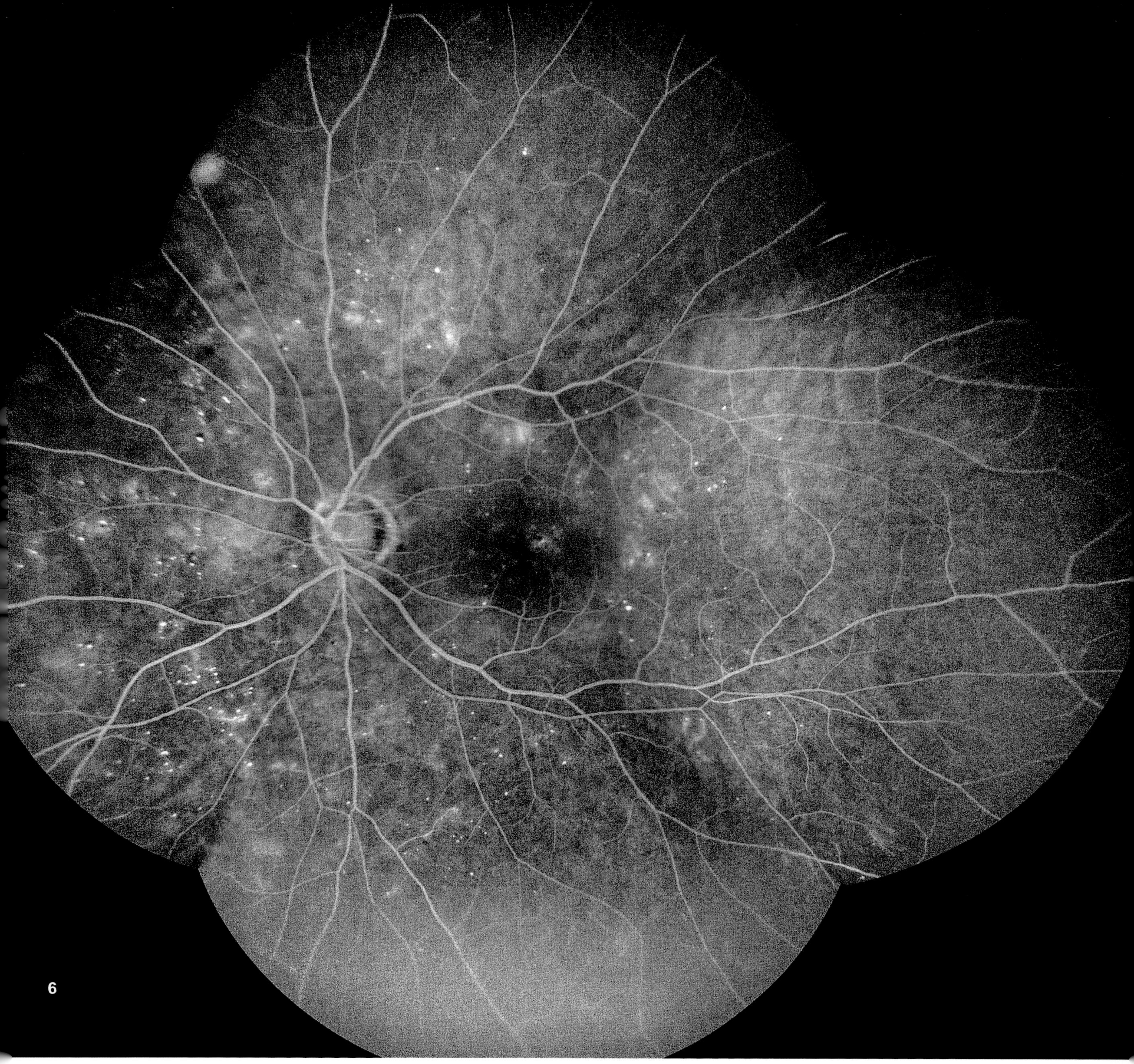

Figure 6 *Fundus fluorescein angiogram montage image shows multiple hyperfluorescent dots. These are more pronounced in the nasal retina. These hyperfluorescent spots correspond to underlying microaneurysms. The hypofluorescent dots correspond to dot-like hemorrhages and cotton wool spots. Note the characteristic absence of IRMA (Intra-Retinal Microvascular Abnormalities), venous beading and nonperfusion. Also note an artifact at the superonasal edge of the image.*

Fluorescein angiography is routinely not indicated in cases with moderate nonproliferative diabetic retinopathy. It should be done only if there is a clinical doubt of the disease being in a preproliferative stage. Fundus fluorescein angiography, being an invasive investigation, has been now slowly replaced with noninvasive dye free OCT angiography. OCT scans are done in patients who present with associated diabetic maculopathy. □

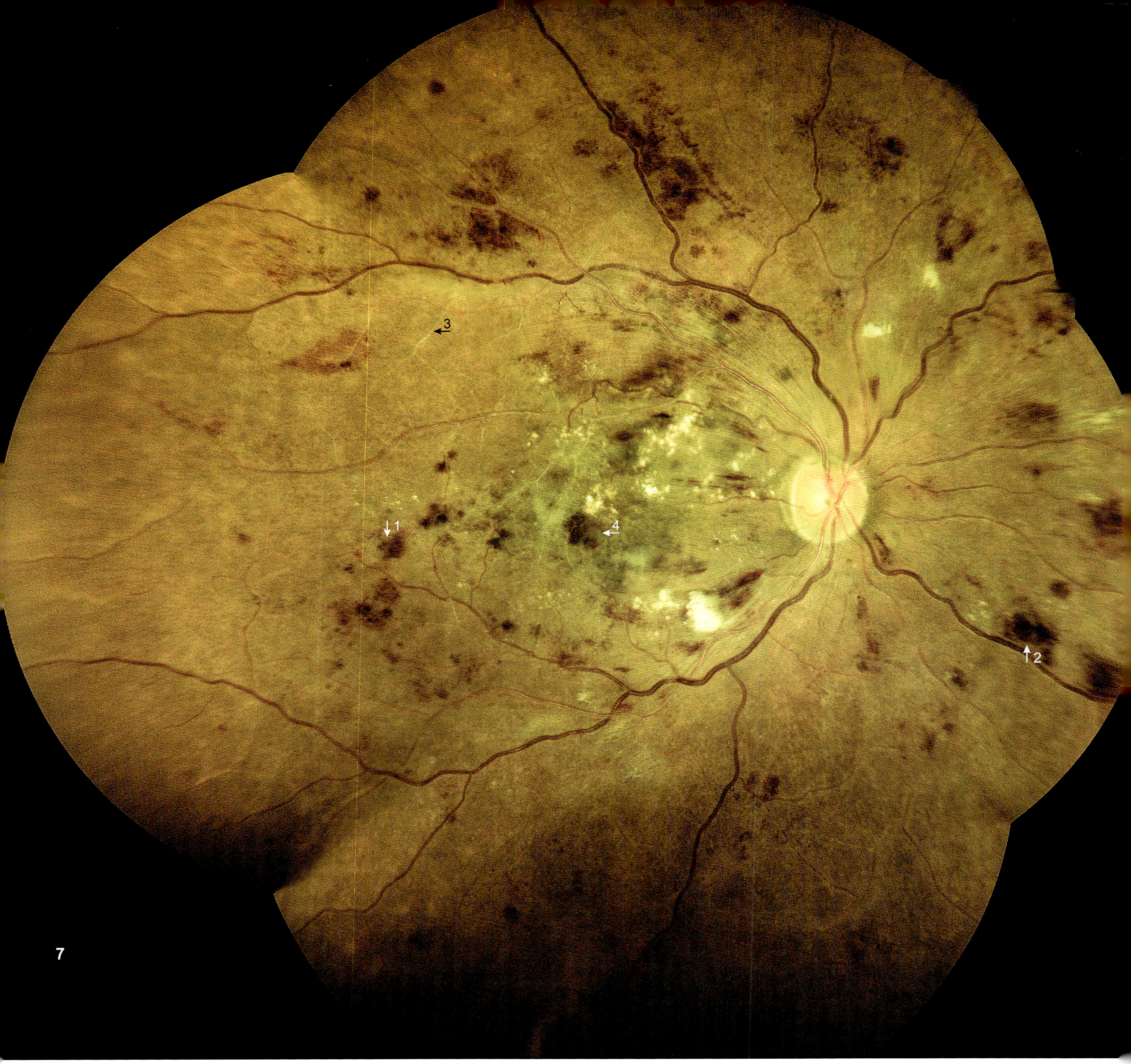


Figure 7 *Clinical fundus photograph of a typical case of severe nonproliferative diabetic retinopathy with macular edema.*

According to the International Diabetic Retinopathy Severity Scale, severe NPDR follows 4:2:1 rule. First rule for diagnosing severe NPDR is the presence of 20 or more intraretinal hemorrhages in each of the 4 quadrants. Color fundus image above shows multiple scattered red dots suggestive of deep retinal hemorrhages (1) and larger superficial splinter retinal hemorrhages in all four quadrants (2). An area of silent featureless retina with sclerosed retinal small vessels is seen in the supero-temporal arcade (3). The sclerosed vessels appear as white thread like lines. Also note presence of gross retinal thickening (4) with the presence of hard exudates and cotton wool spots. Retinal vessels show altered arterio-venous ratio.

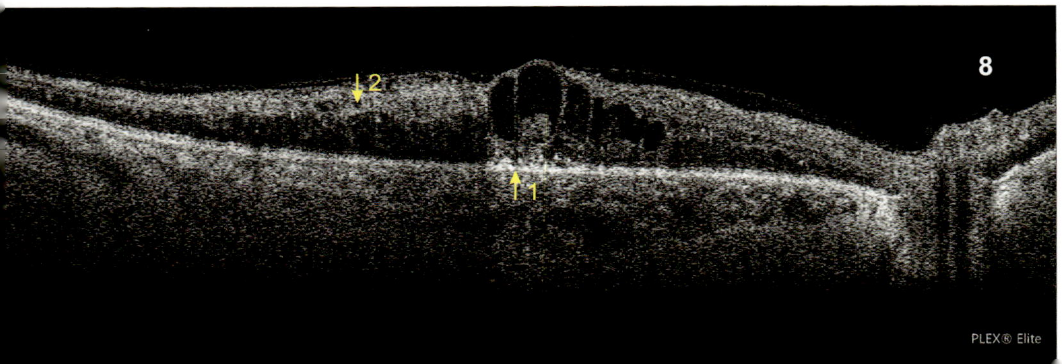


Figure 8 *Spectral domain OCT scan passing through the fovea shows gross intraretinal cystic fluid spaces with areas outer retinal disruptions (1) and disorganized inner retinal layers (2) due to ischemia.* □

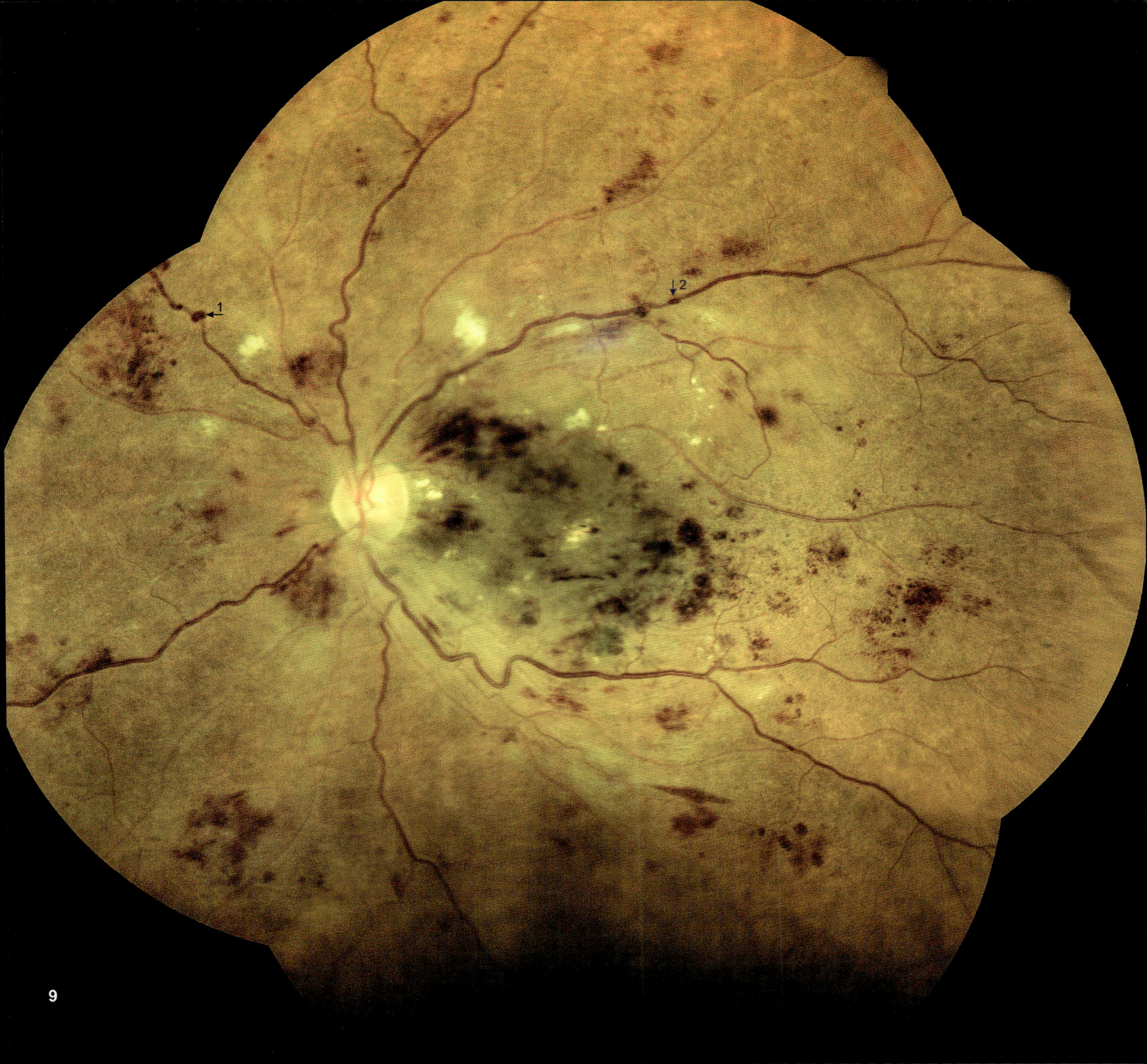


9

Figure 9 *Case of severe nonproliferative diabetic retinopathy demonstrating venous beading.*

As per the International Diabetic Retinopathy Severity Scale, presence of definite venous bleeding in two or more quadrants is suggestive of severe nonproliferative disease. Fundus image above shows venous bleeding along superonasal (1) and superotemporal (2) large vein, fulfilling the criteria of severe NPDR. Also note the presence of multiple superficial and deep retinal hemorrhages, cotton wool spots and macular edema.

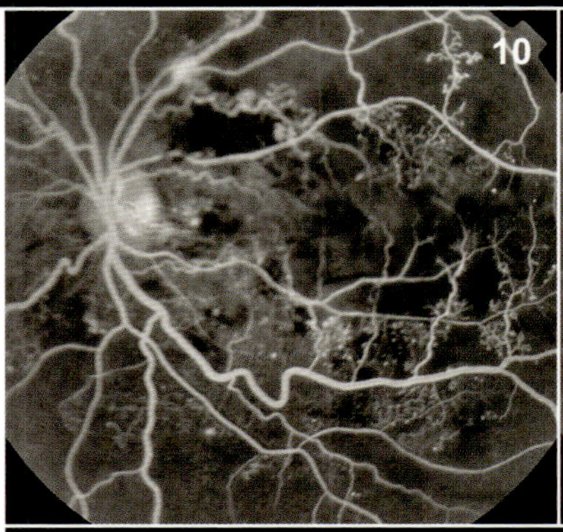

10

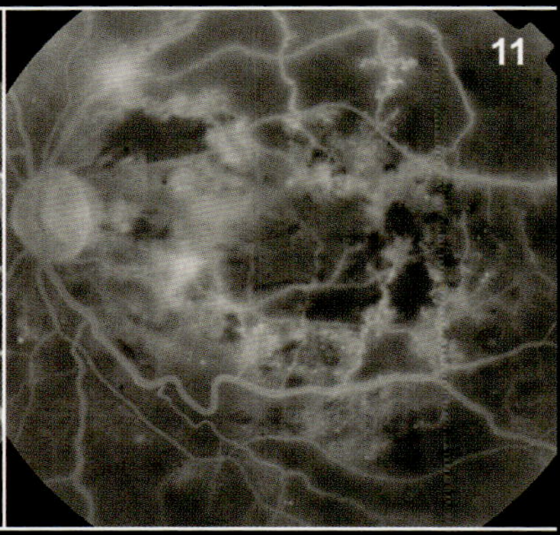

11

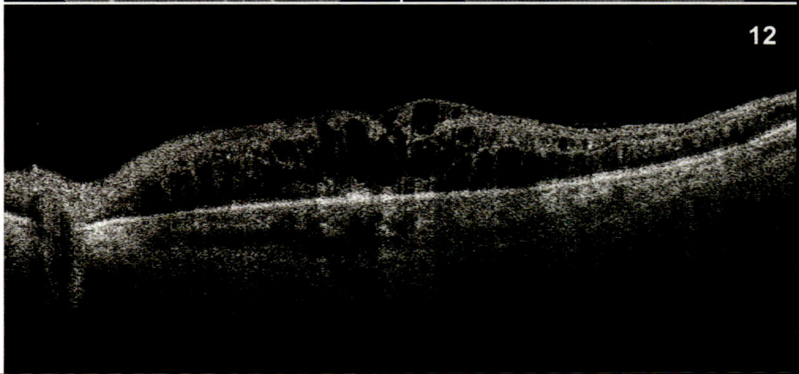

12

Figure 10 *Early frame of fundus fluorescein angiogram demonstrates complete capillary shut down with nonperfusion at the posterior pole, venous beading, blocked fluorescence from hemorrhages and IRMA. All these features are suggestive of severe NPDR.*

Figure 11 *Late frame of fundus fluorescein angiogram, shows diffuse leakage at the macula suggestive of macular edema. Note the absence of any neovascular leakage, confirming that this is a case of severe NPDR only.*

Figure 12 *OCT line scan passing through the fovea, demonstrates large intraretinal cystic fluid pockets and presence of an epiretinal membrane.* □

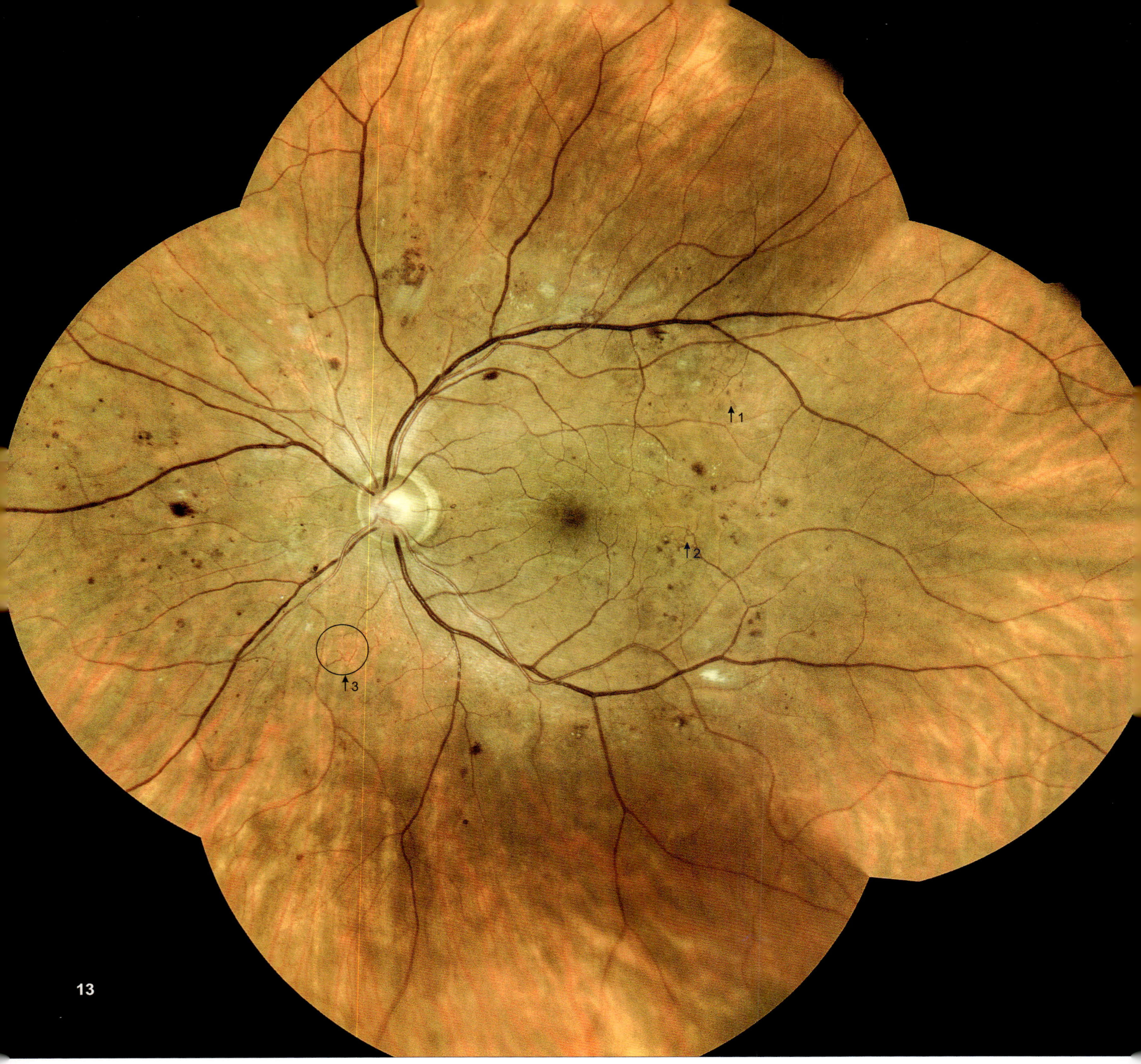


Figure 13 *Case of severe nonproliferative diabetic retinopathy demonstrating IRMAs (Intraretinal Microvascular Abnormality).*

Color fundus photograph of a case of severe NPDR. Besides microaneurysm, hemorrhages and cotton wool spots, note the presence of intraretinal microvascular abnormalities in all quadrants of retina (1, 2, 3).

IRMAs are either new vessel growth within the retinal tissue itself or shunt vessels through areas of poor vascular perfusion. It is common for intraretinal microvascular abnormalities to be located adjacent to cotton-wool spots. IRMA is one of the defining features of severe non-proliferative diabetic retinopathy, based on the "4-2-1" criteria from the Early Treatment Diabetic Retinopathy Study (ETDRS). When compared to neovascularization (NVE) in proliferative disease, IRMAs are slightly larger in caliber with a more broad arrangement and are always contained to the intraretinal space.

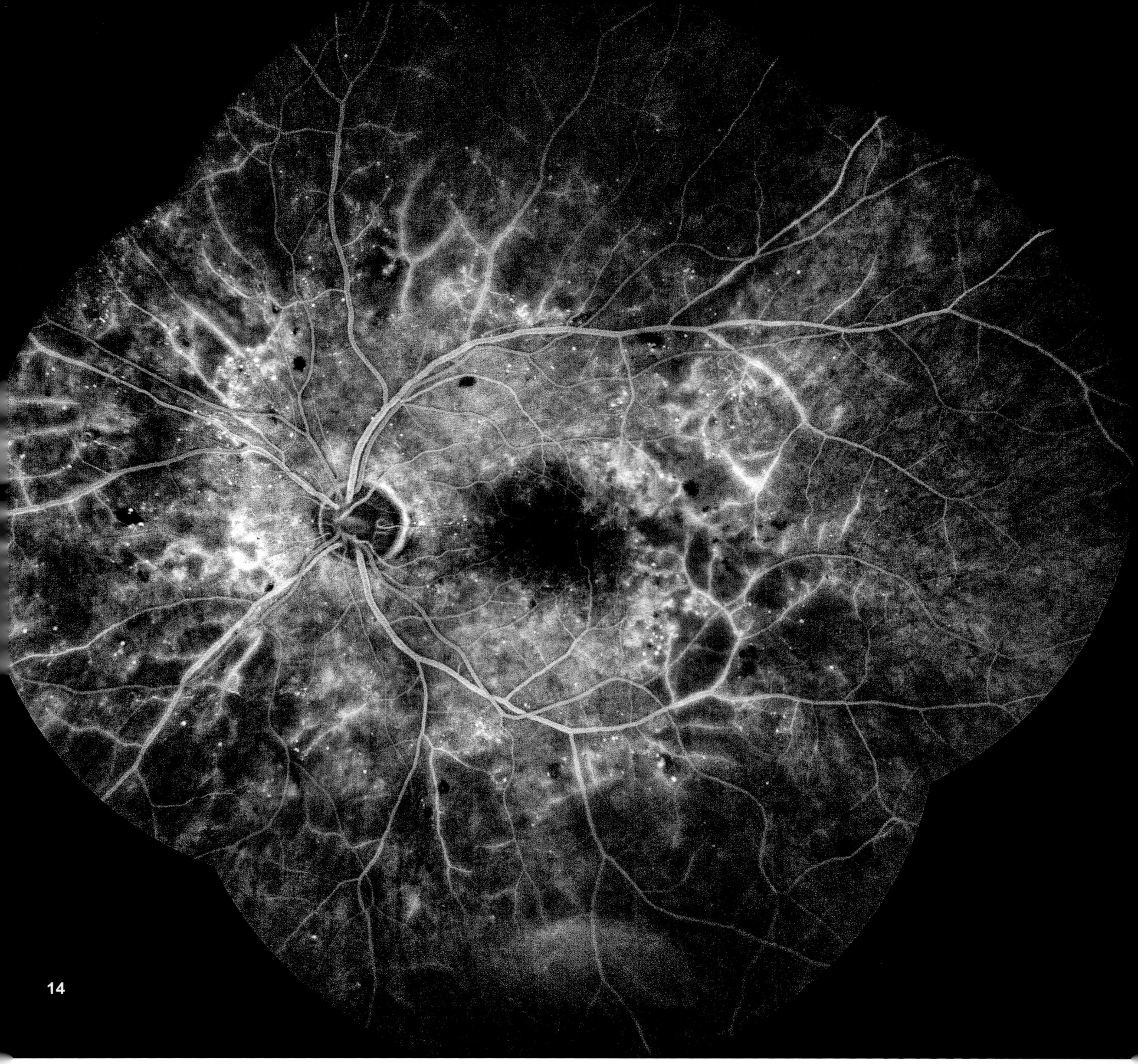


Figure 14 *Fundus fluorescein angiogram montage of a case of severe nonproliferative diabetic retinopathy.*

Note characteristic mid-peripheral areas of retinal ischemia, multiple pinpoint hyperfluorescent dots (microaneurysms), hypofluorescent dots (retinal hemorrhages) and intraretinal microvascular abnormalities that characteristically do not leak, thus differentiates it from retinal neovascularization.

Differentiation between IRMA and neovascularization is important as it helps to decide the need for treatment. If the patient has only developed IRMAs, he should be advised to optimize the diabetic control and careful 4–6 months observation is all that is needed. In case patient has developed neovascularization, panretinal photocoagulation is indicated. If NVE are small and diabetic control is good, some physicians may prefer to wait till it reaches a high risk PDR stage. □

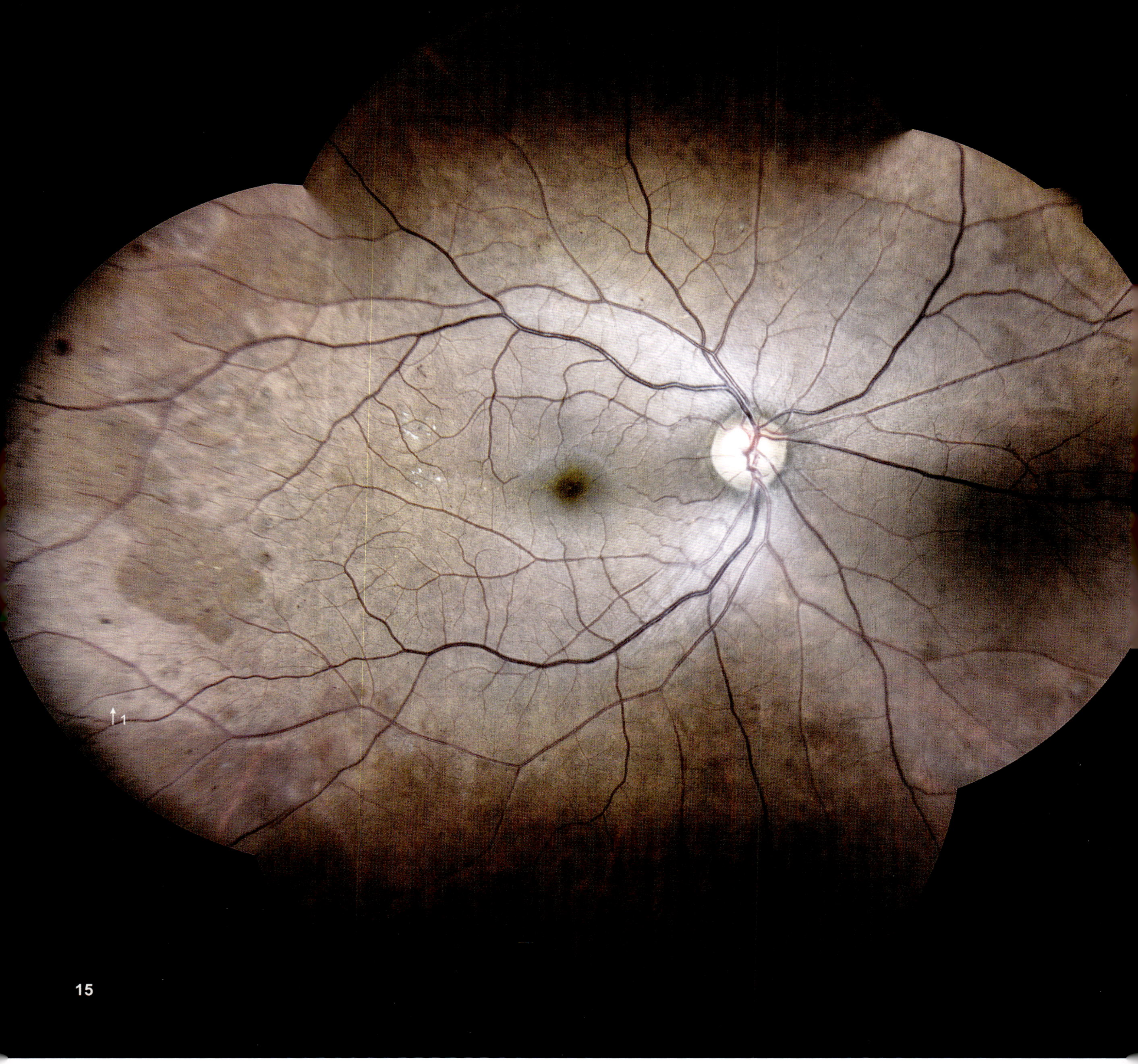


Figure 15 *Color fundus montage photograph demonstrating low-risk proliferative diabetic retinopathy, originating in the peripheral retina.*

Sixty four year old type 2 diabetic for the last 25 years was seen in the clinic for a routine check-up. The color fundus photograph shows that the posterior pole of the retina is remarkably normal without any diabetic changes, except few hard exudates. Note multiple pinpoint microaneurysms and dot hemorrhages in the temporal periphery and a frond of flat NVE (1) in the inferotemporal peripheral retina. Overall hypoxic state of the retina is driven by capillary occlusion and retinal nonperfusion which is found in the retinal periphery. About 11–17% of NVEs are found outside the standard seven-field imaging, thus, peripheral retinal examination is equally important in a diabetic patient.

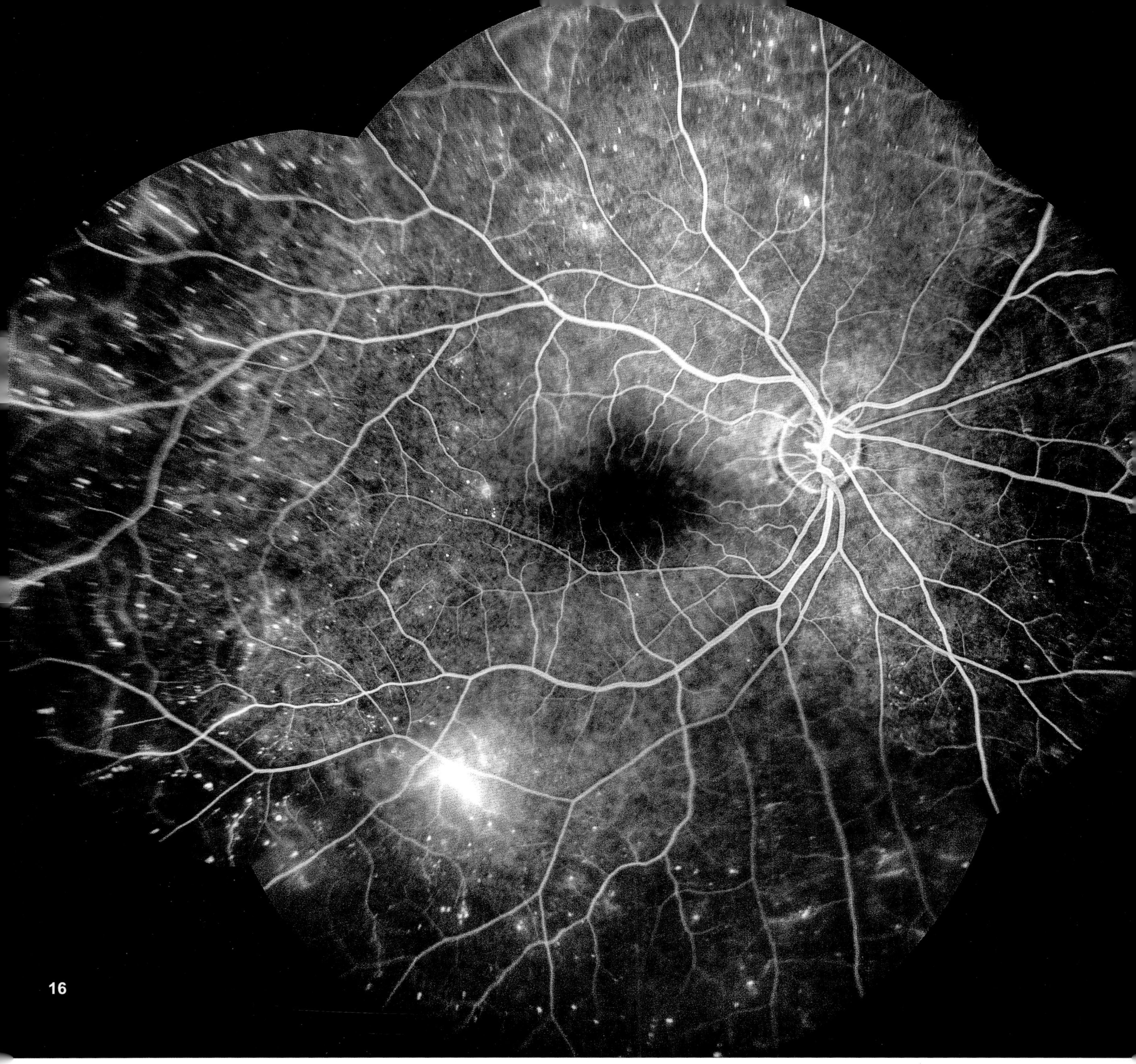

16

Figure 16 *FFA of the same patient illustrates much more detailed changes of diabetic retinopathy. It is to be noted that the posterior pole of the retina does not show any significant diabetic changes. Multiple pinpoint hyperfluorescent dots due to MA's are seen all along the retinal periphery. Peripheral ischemic areas of capillary nonperfusion are seen in the temporal periphery and leakage from the NVE.*

FFA is a useful tool to confirm the presence of neovascularization of retina. Any patient with long standing history of diabetes mellitus and any suspicious lesion in periphery should undergo fundus fluorescein angiogram to rule out the presence of proliferative disease. □

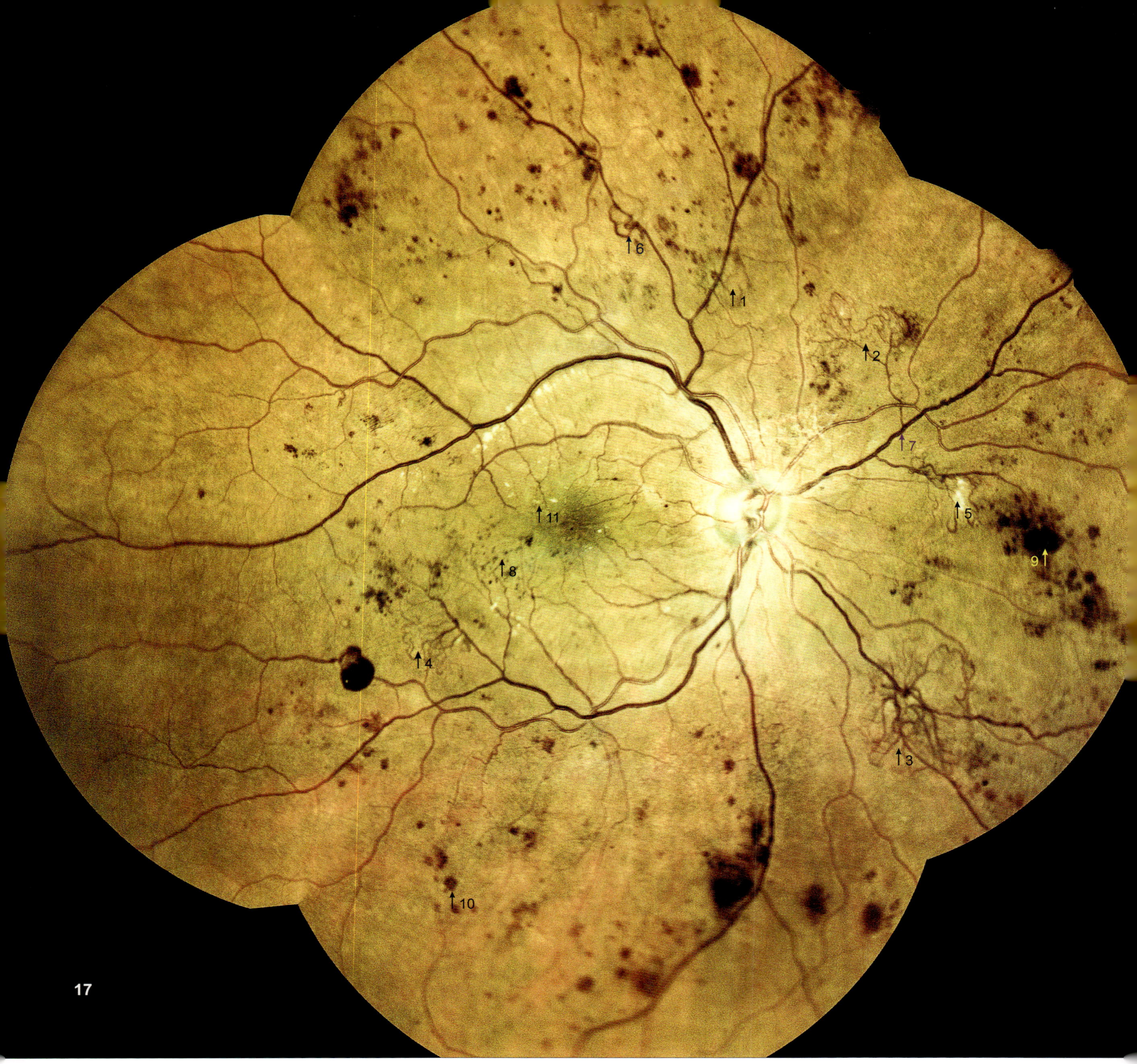


Figure 17 *Color fundus montage photograph of type II diabetic with early proliferative diabetic retinopathy.*

Multiple large fronds of flat NVE's are seen in all four quadrants (1 to 4).

Glistening preretinal fibrous tissue has started to develop at superior edge of optic disk adjacent to large NVE (5) suggestive of early fibrovascular proliferation. Small round preretinal bleed as an oil droplet is seen in inferotemporal arcade. Venous loops (6) and venous bleeding (7) is also visible along the superior and superonasal large retinal veins respectively. Venous beading is seen as intermittent dilated segment of retinal veins due to extensive capillary closure. To bypass these nonthrombotic occlusions, venous loops develop. Multiple microaneurysms (8), superficial hemorrhage (9) and deep hemorrhages (10) are also seen in all the four quadrants. Macula appears boggy secondary to diabetic macular edema with multiple leaking MA and hard exudates (11) visible in the color fundus image.

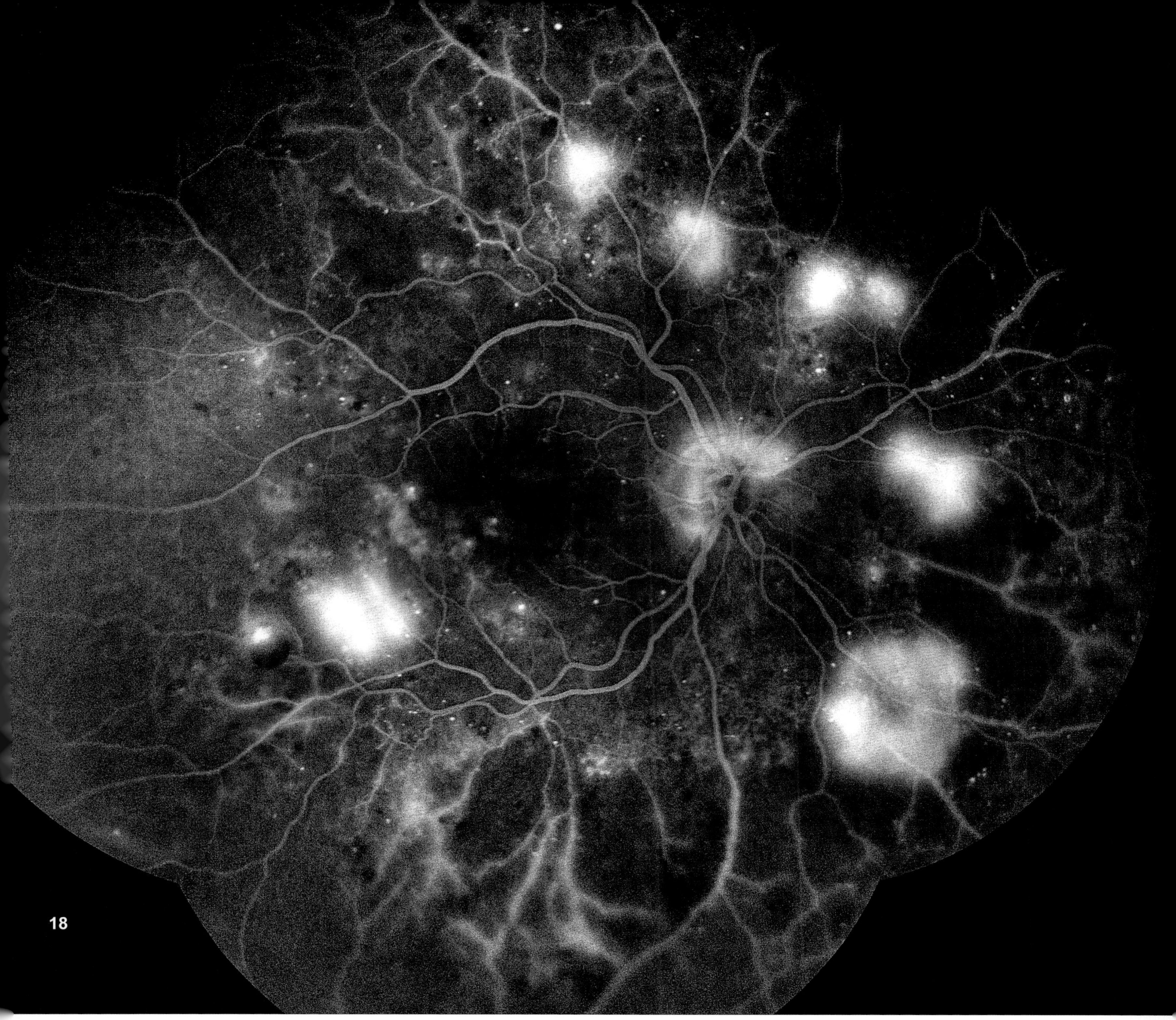


Figure 18 *Fundus fluorescein angiogram shows multiple hyperfluorescent dots corresponding to the microaneurysms, large scattered areas of capillary nonperfusion seen in the mid-periphery of the retina and leakages from the fronds of neovascularization at the optic disk and neovascularization elsewhere usually seen at the junction of perfused and nonperfused retina. All these findings were consistent with diagnosis of low-risk proliferative diabetic retinopathy.*

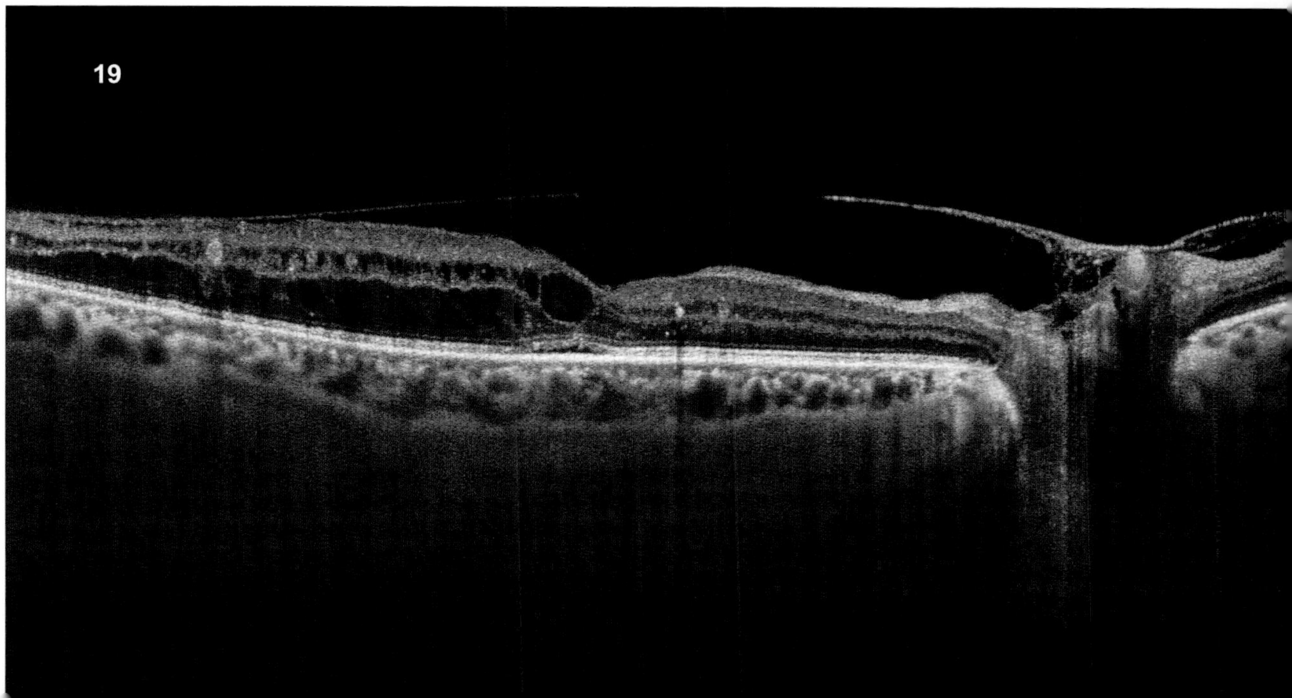


Figure 19

*Swept source optical coherence tomography scan passing through the fovea shows gross retinal thickening due to intraretinal cystic fluid and serous retinal fluid at the fovea. Also note preretinal hyperreflective band of vitreous at the optic disk causing vitreopapillary traction.* □

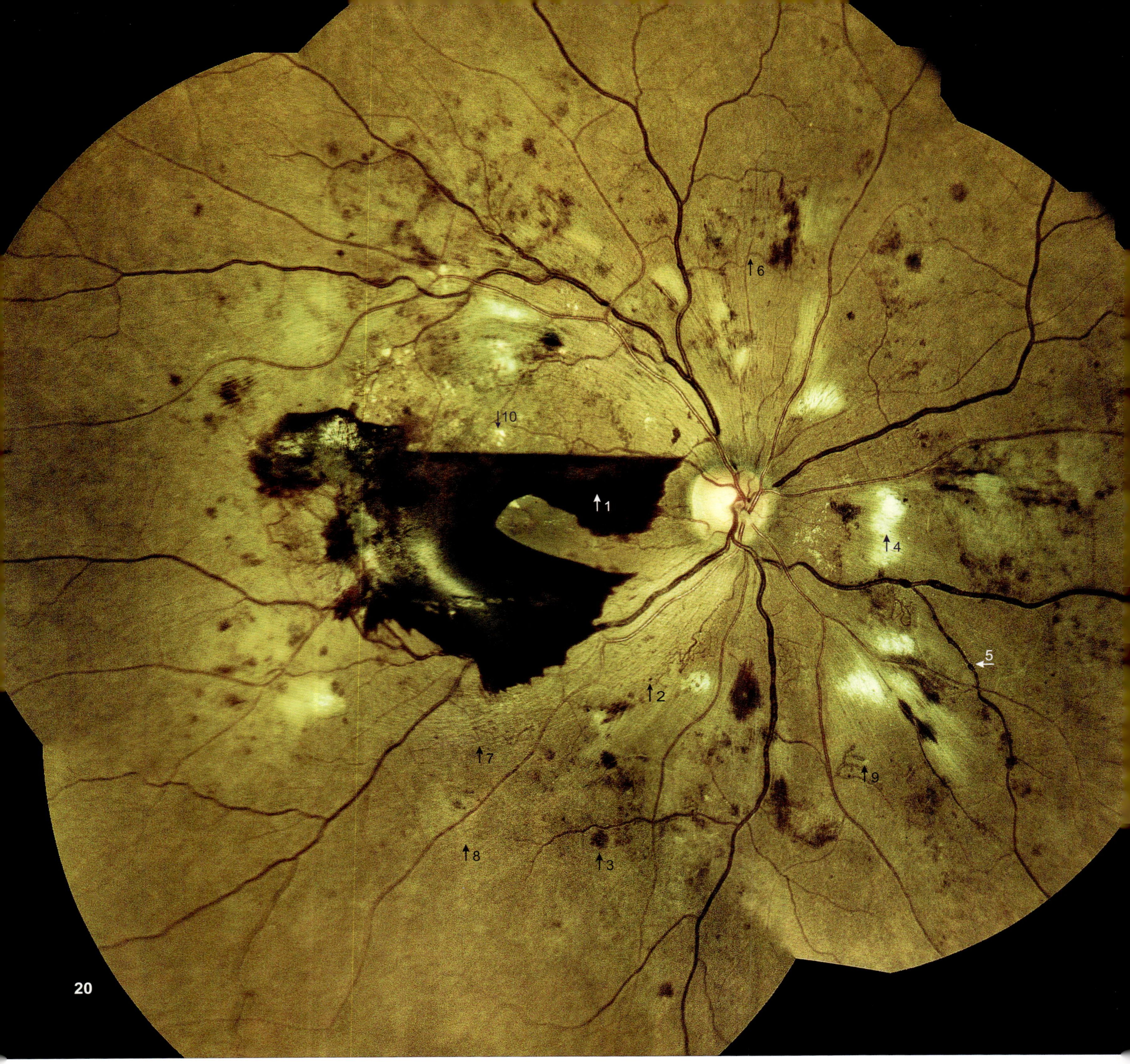


Figure 20 *Color fundus photograph demonstrates varying clinical signs in a case of proliferative diabetic retinopathy (PDR).*

Dense preretinal hemorrhage obscuring the retinal details is seen at the macula (1). It is located between the posterior limiting layer of vitreous and ILM of retina. Preretinal hemorrhage is darker at the bottom where the blood has settled with distinct horizontal line at the top known as 'D' or boat shaped. This occurs as a result of pooling of blood within the preretinal space due to gravity. Multiple round tiny microaneurysm (2) are seen in all the four quadrants of retina. They are focal dilations of the venous end of retinal capillaries and appear as small round red spots. Dot and blot hemorrhages (3) are again small round red spots slightly larger than the microaneurysms. They occur as a result of the rupture of an MA as in the deeper layers of the retina. Cotton wool spots are another hallmark of ischemic event in diabetic retinopathy. They appear as yellow white deposits (4) within nerve fiber layer that represent small patches of retinal infarction. Venous beading (5) is a pattern of nodular irregularity in retinal venous blood vessels as a result of ischemia. IRMAs are abnormal intraretinal shunt vessels with connection from arterioles to venules (6). They appear as flat tiny loops of retinal blood vessels (7) with adjacent featureless retina (8) suggesting nonperfusion/ischemia. They represent either new vessels growth within retina or remodeling of preexisting retina vessels stimulated by hypoxia. Multiple NVEs are seen in the retina. They form a small flat whorl like network (9). Hard exudates (10) appear as refractive yellow deposits at the macula as a result of protein or lipid fluid that leaks from blood vessels into surrounding retinal space.

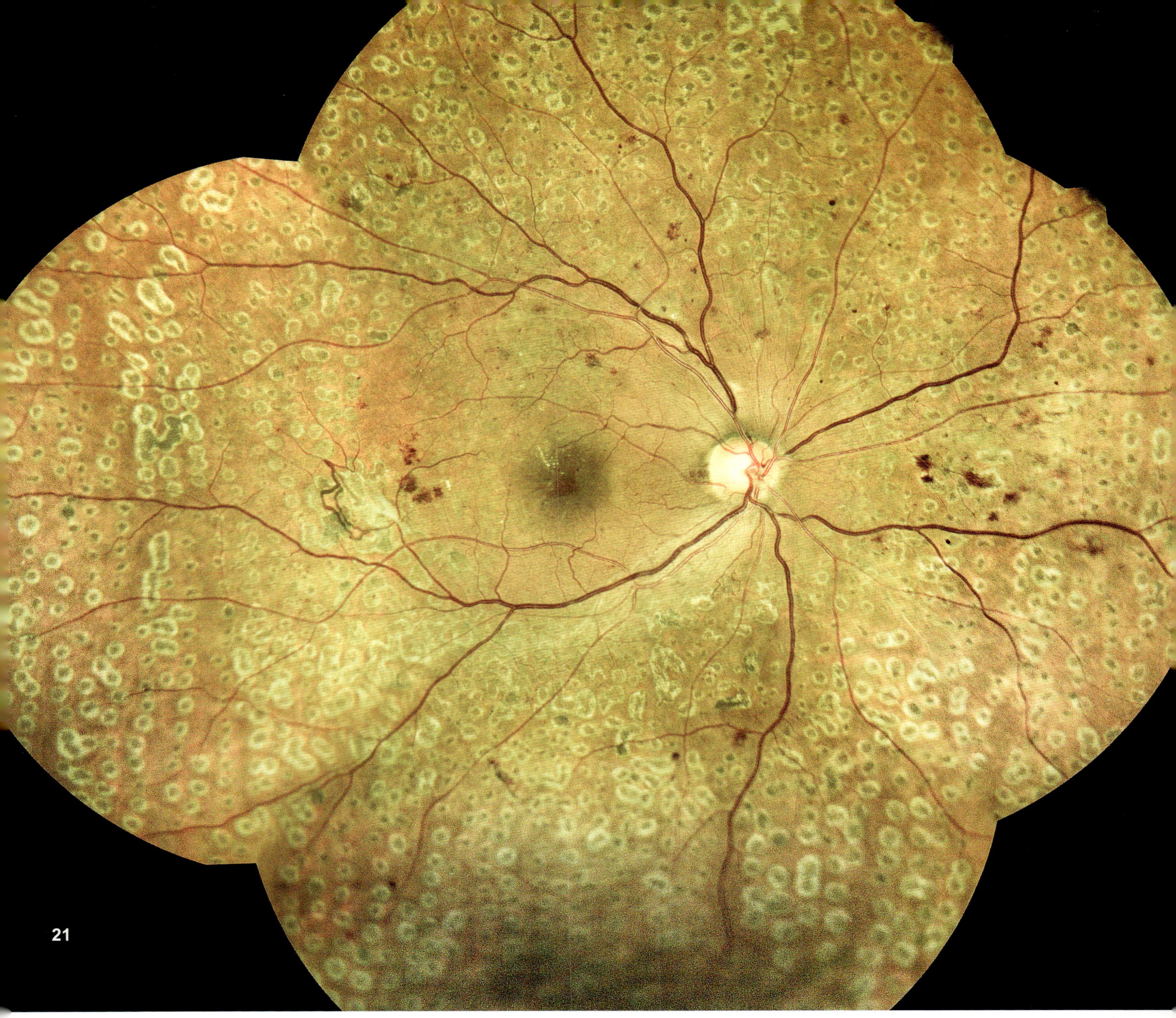

21

Figure 21 *Color fundus montage photograph of the same patient 6 months after treatment.*

Patient underwent a single intravitreal anti-VEGF injection and scatter panretinal photocoagulation sessions. Note the presence of panretinal laser photocoagulation scars in all the four quadrants of retina. Retinal bleed has resolved completely and disease is in its quiescent stage.

Figure 22 *Fundus fluorescein angiogram montage photograph shows inverted D-shaped patch of hypofluorescence due to blockage of fluorescein dye from preretinal bleed. Also note another patch of hypofluorescence in the nasal retina that is due to capillary nonperfusion. Hyperfluorescent patch with blurred margins is seen adjacent to the preretinal bleed in the temporal macula as a result of active neovascularization.*

Figure 23

*Swept source OCT scan depicts hyper-reflective preretinal bleed limited by a hyaloid anteriorly and extending into the superficial layers of the retina with underlying shadowing affect on the retinal layers. Also note presence of serous fluid and intraretinal fluid involving the fovea.* □

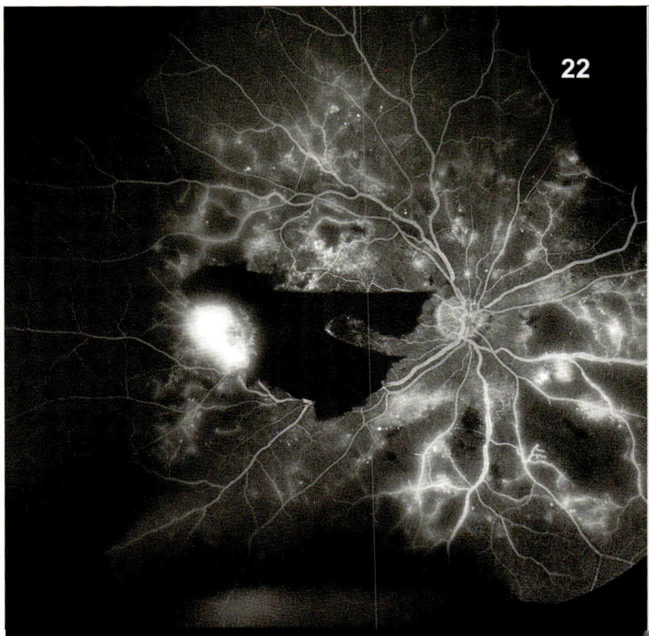

22

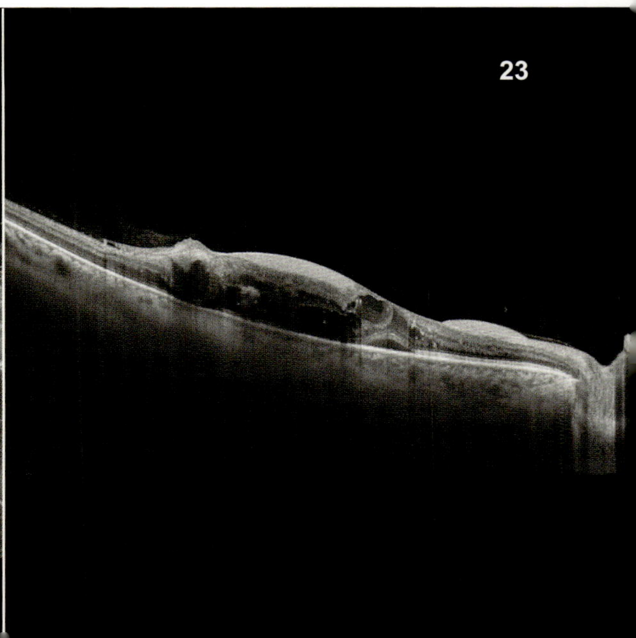

23

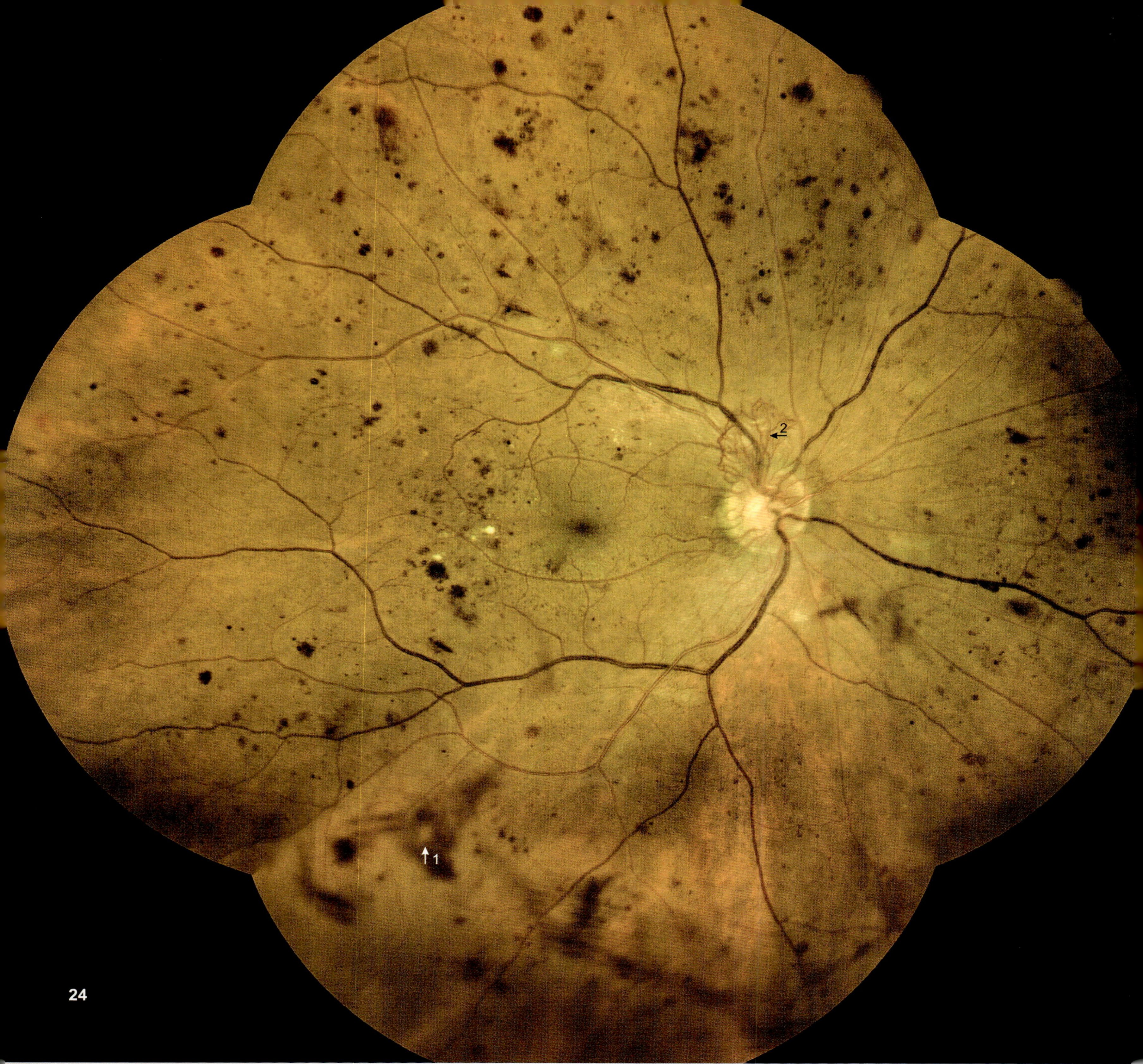


24

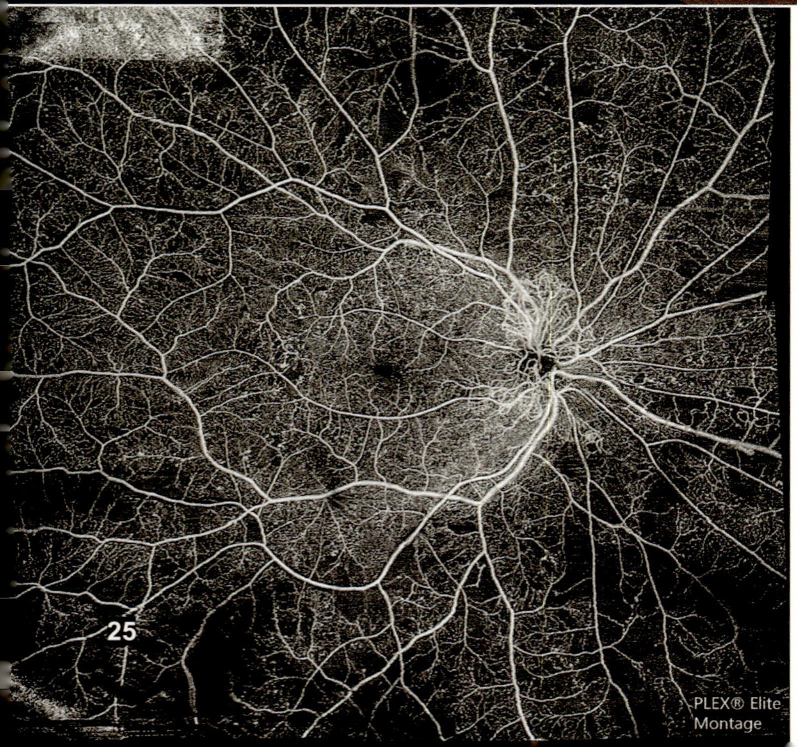


25

Figure 24 *Case of proliferative diabetic retinopathy demonstrating elevated neovascularization of the optic disk (NVD).*

A 64-year-old type 2 diabetic patient presented with recent onset floaters. The color fundus photograph shows multiple retinal hemorrhages in all four quadrants, mild vitreous hemorrhage (1) and large frond of elevated NVD (2) involving whole of optic nerve and extending beyond disk margin as well.

Urgent PRP laser was advised with adjuvant use of intravitreal anti-VEGF (Bevacizumab) injection as it is high-risk PDR. Full scatter photocoagulation was applied in 3 sessions 1 week apart with topical anesthesia. 2000 burns of 400 micron spot size (using super quad lens) 150 microsecond duration were applied ½-1 burn width apart. Also macular laser was done to leaking microaneurysms (0.1 second duration, 100 micron spot size using area centralis contact lens.

Figure 25 *12 × 12 mm wide field OCT angiography montage image at baseline.*

Retina slab demonstrated an elevated exuberant vascular proliferation arising from the optic disk suggestive of a neovascular frond. Also note the presence of peripheral capillary ischemia seen as hypofeatureless region.

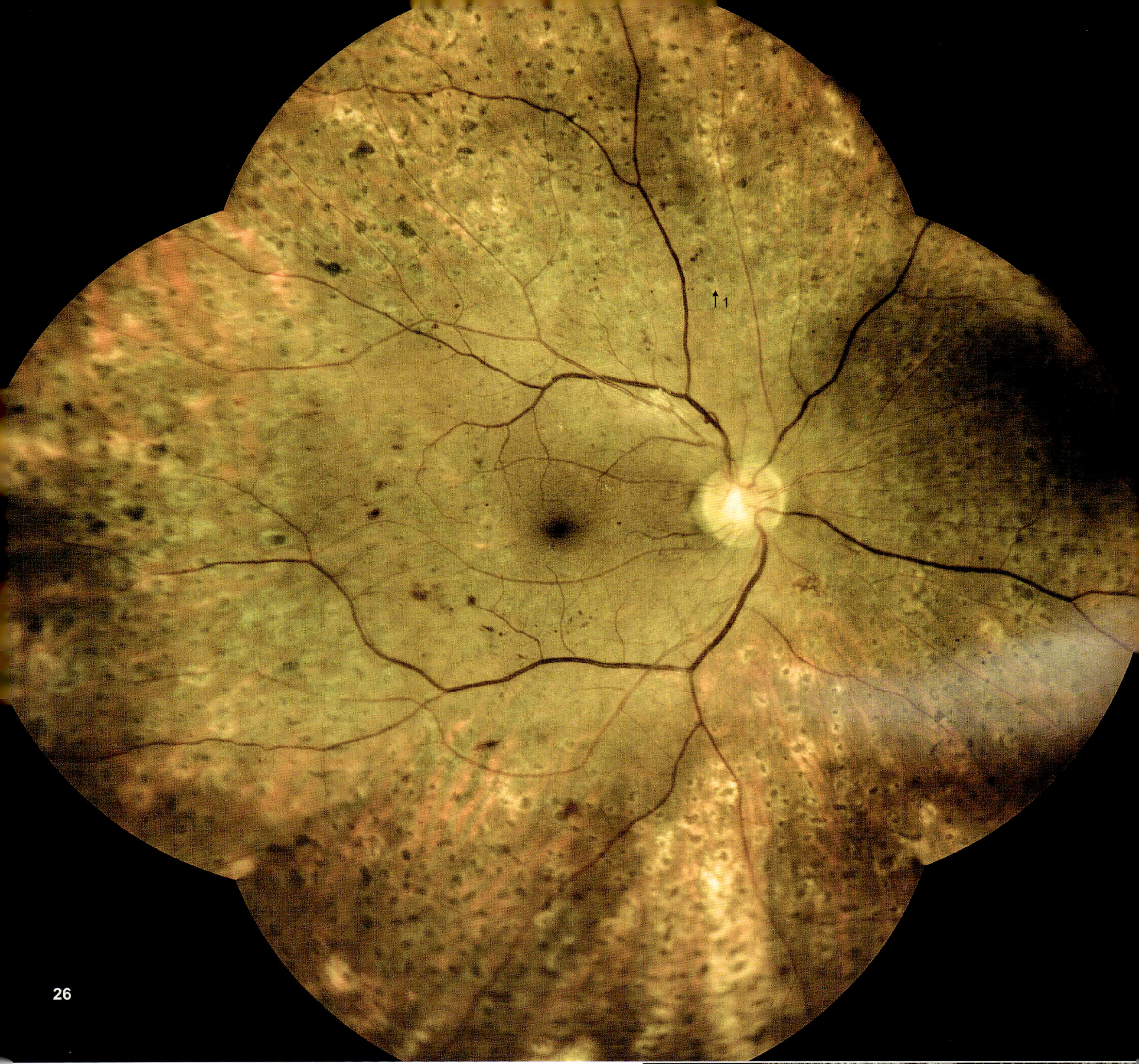


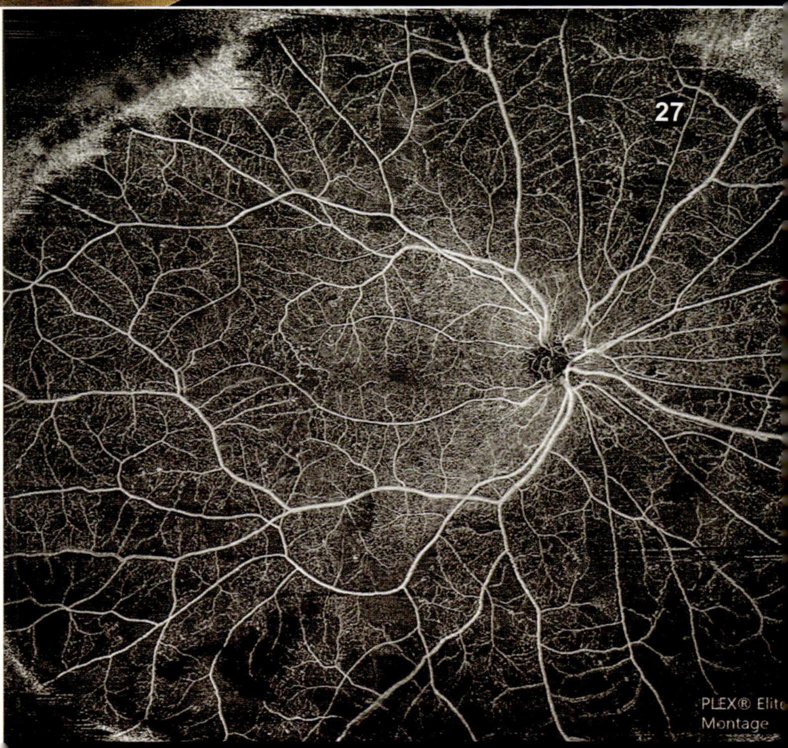


Figure 26 *Case of proliferative diabetic retinopathy 3 months post-treatment.*

After receiving one anti-VEGF injection and three sessions of panretinal photocoagulation, his disease has stabilized as seen on the color fundus montage image done 3 months later. Note the presence of PRP scars in all the four quadrants of retina (1), NVD has regressed completely and retinal hemorrhages have also reduced.

Figure 27 *Widefield OCT angiography montage image done 1 month later.*

Note drastic disappearance of NVD frond as compared to the baseline. Few small pruned vessels were still visible at the optic disk. Small multiple areas of capillary dropouts are scattered in the peripheral retina. □

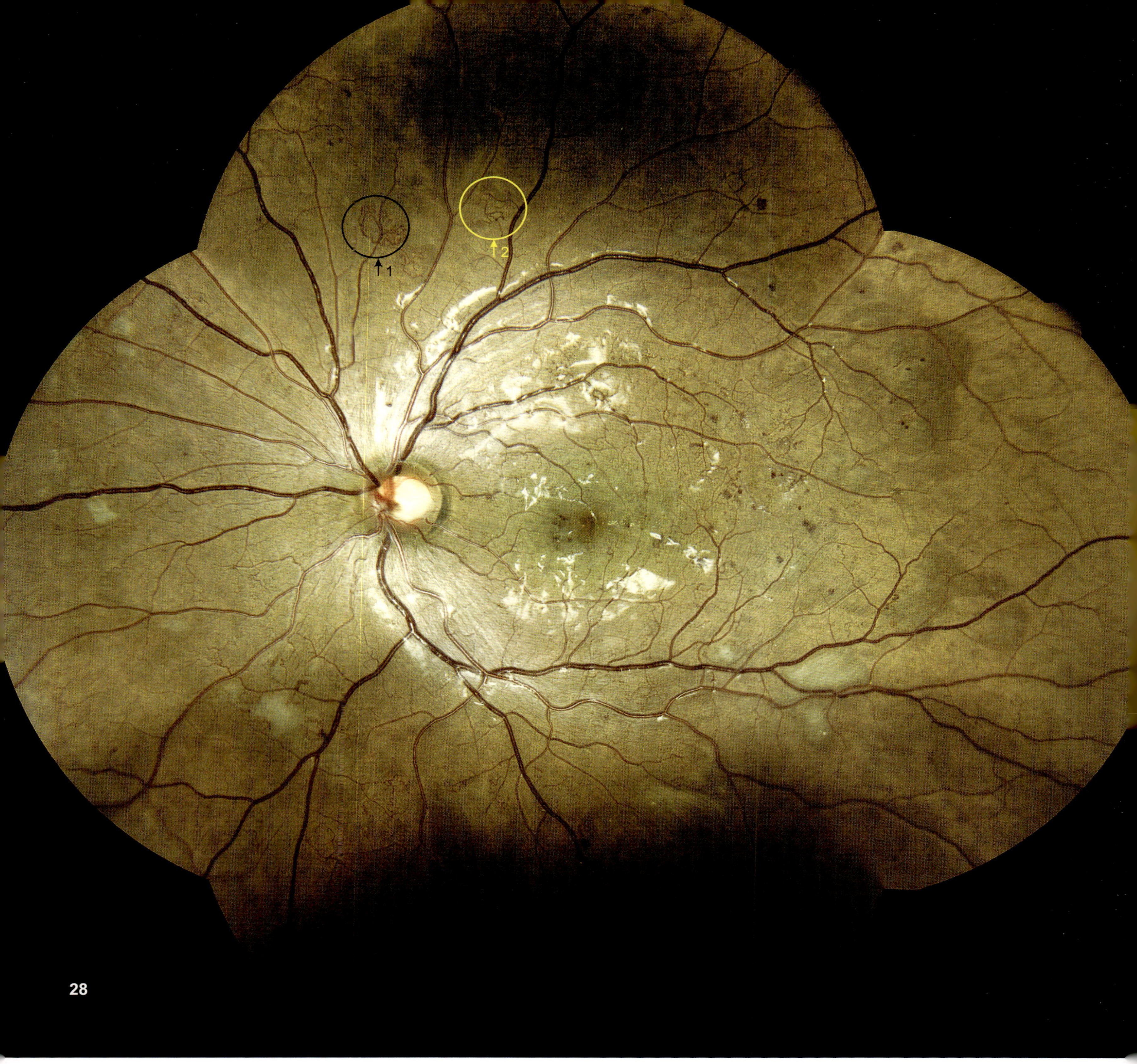


Figure 28 *Case of proliferative diabetic retinopathy demonstrating clinical difference in the appearance of neovascularization of retina and intraretinal microvascular abnormalities.*

Neovascularization is a consequence of retinal ischemia and new retinal vessels usually develop at the edge of perfused and nonperfused retina. Color photograph above shows that there is an abrupt termination of retinal vessels with surrounding silent capillary bed suggestive of peripheral ischemia and formation of new vessels on the surface of retina (1) adjacent to the area of nonperfusion.

Also note the presence of multiple flat intraretinal microvascular abnormalities (2). They are enlarged hypercellular capillaries appearing as dilated telangiectatic capillaries within the retina. As compared to IRMAs, NVE tend to be finer, delicate in caliber, and at much more superficial location. Multiple cotton wool spots and retinal hemorrhages are also seen. □

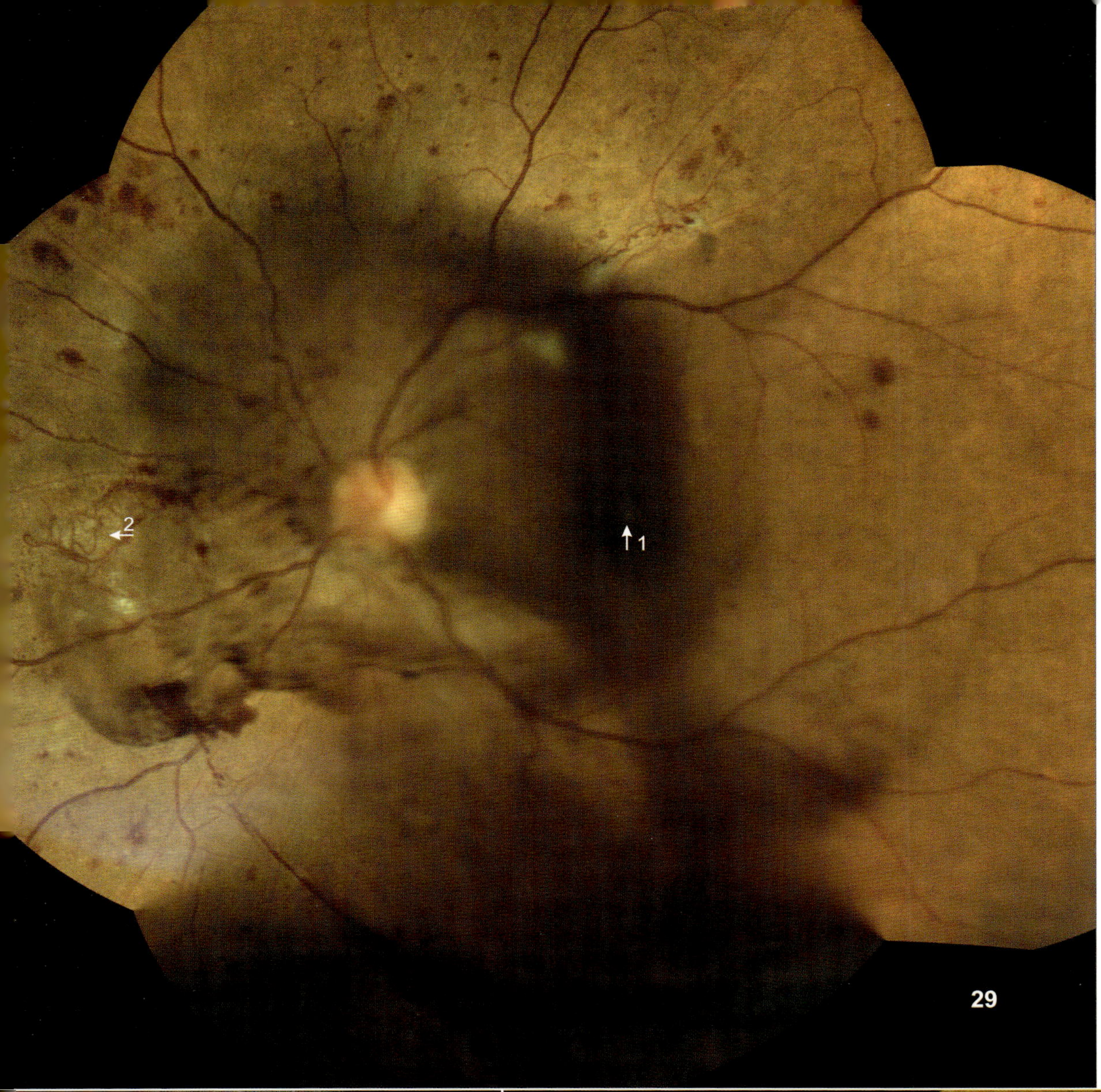


Figure 29

*Color fundus montage photograph of a case of high-risk proliferative diabetic retinopathy with vitreous hemorrhage.*

Sixty five year old with type 2 DM for 15 years presented with sudden onset floater and blurred vision for last 5 days. Color image demonstrates a blob of vitreous hemorrhage over the posterior pole (1) and large frond of NVE (2) in the nasal quadrant.

Figure 30

*Fundus fluorescein angiogram confirms disk leakage from NVD and NVE in the peripheral retina (Superotemporal and nasal). Also note that details of the macula are obscured due to media opacity (vitreous hemorrhage).*

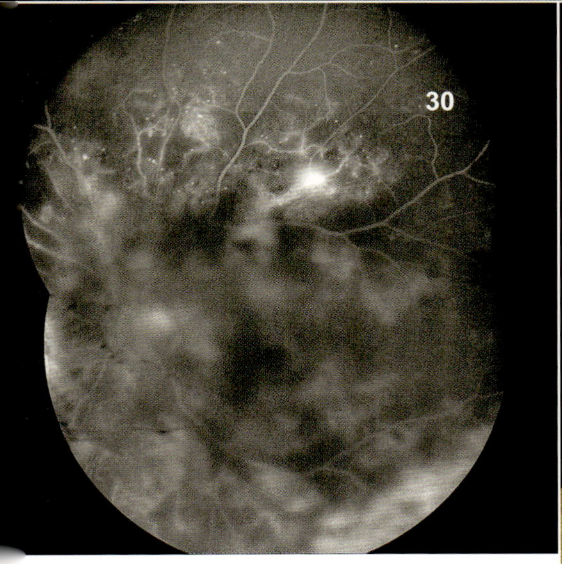


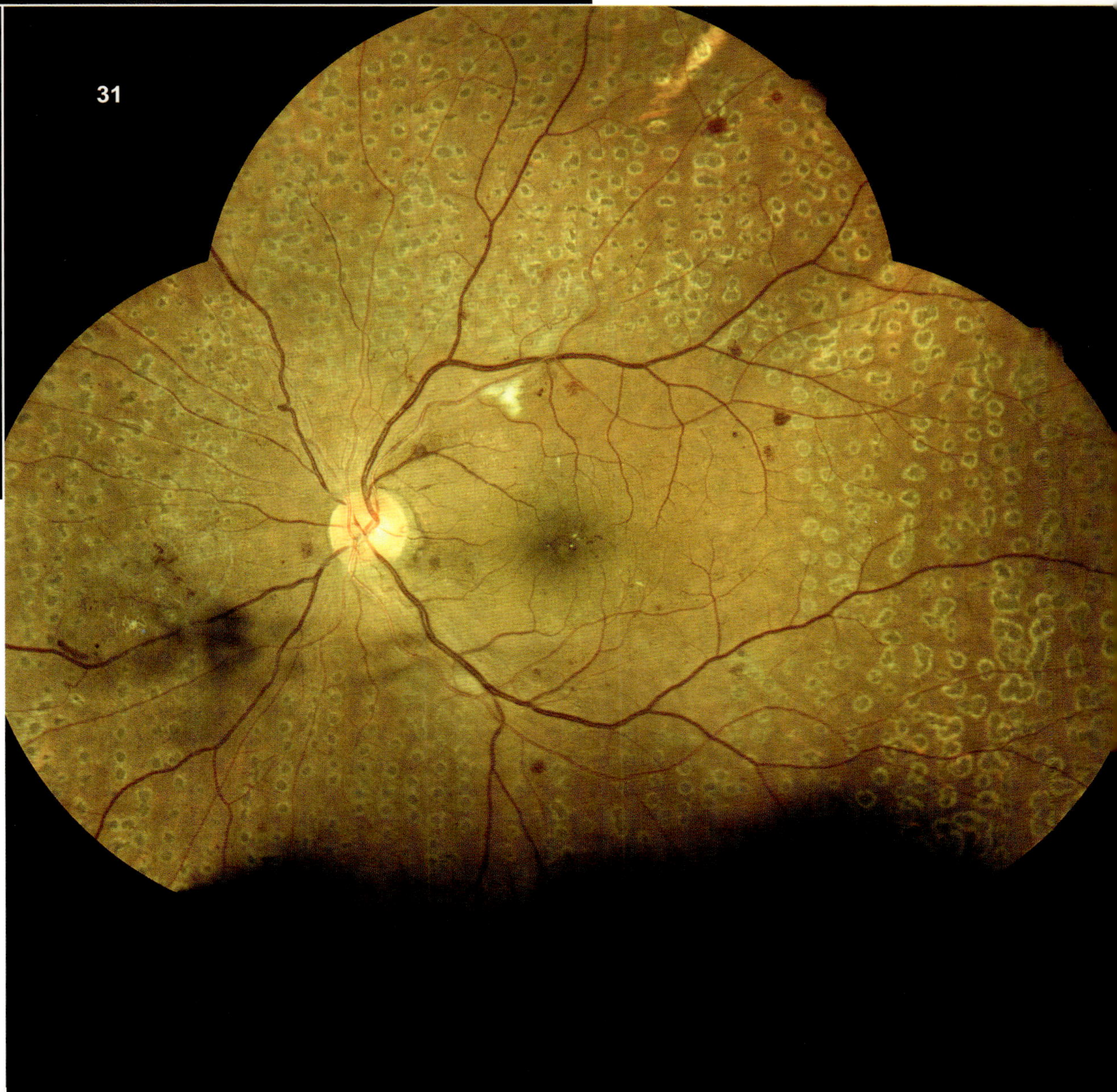


Figure 31

*Color fundus montage photograph after treatment.*

Patient underwent 3 sessions of laser photocoagulation 1 week apart with an adjuvant use of single intravitreal anti-VEGF injection. Vitreous hemorrhage has resolved drastically, NVE shows partial regression with minimal traction along the nasal retinal vessel. Laser photocoagulation scars are visible in all four quadrants. □

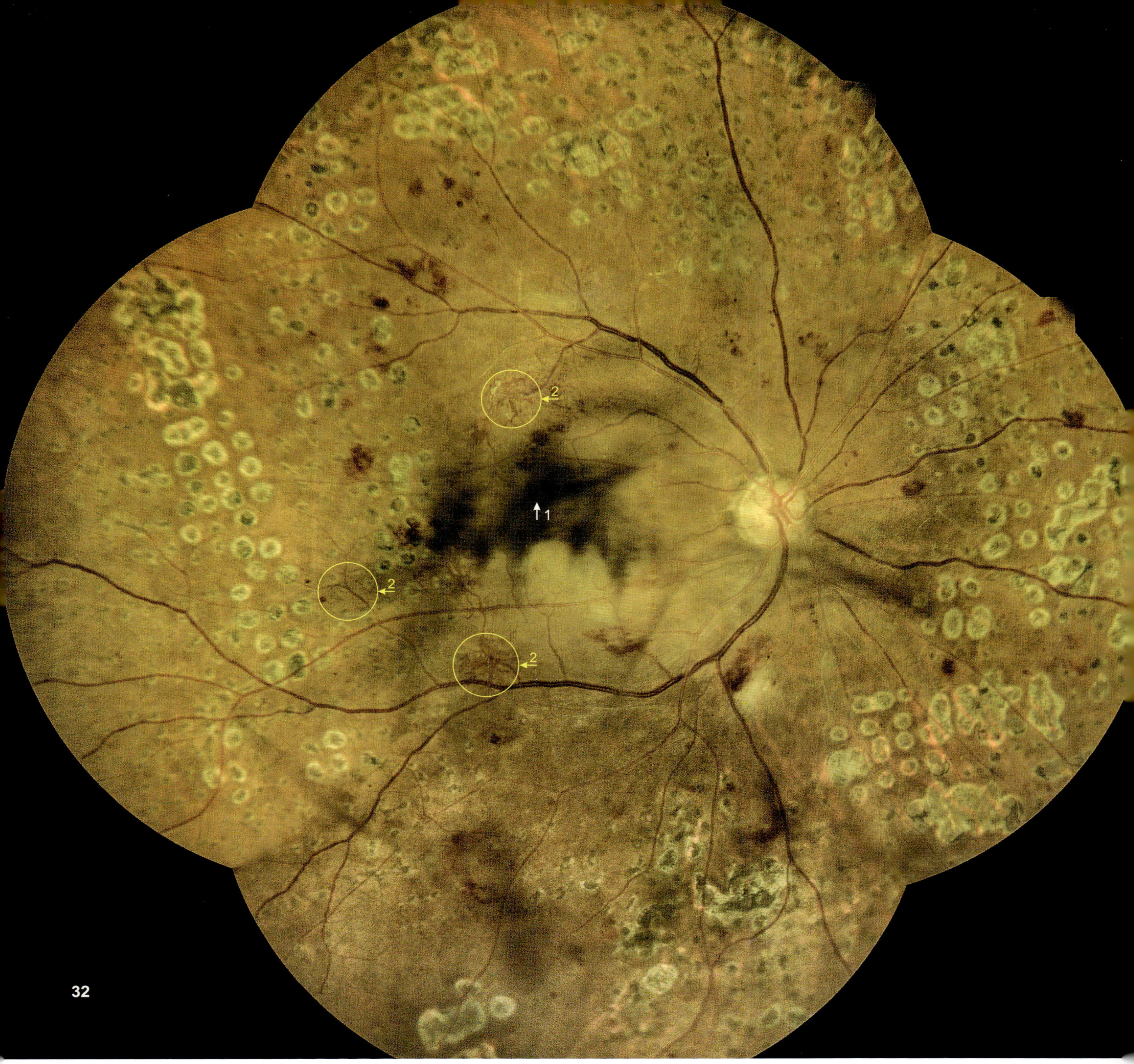


Figure 32 *Case of proliferative diabetic retinopathy with recurrent vitreous hemorrhage.*

Fifty four year old type 2 diabetic with history of previous treatment of diabetic retinopathy, presented with sudden onset floaters. Fundus photograph shows vitreous opacity obscuring the details of the macula (1). Scattered laser scars are visible. Also note the presence of multiple fronds of retinal neovascularization near the arcades (2).

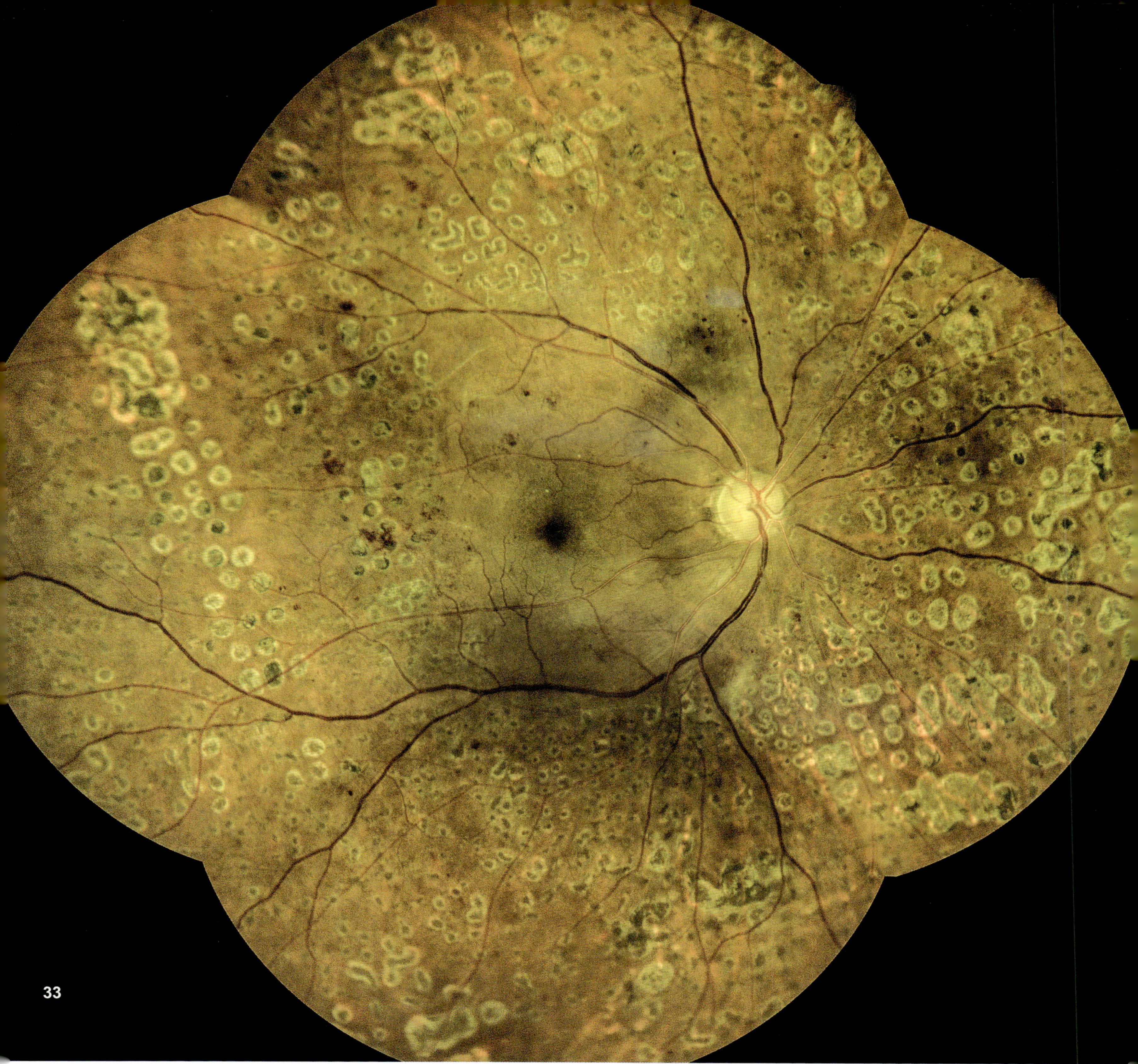


Figure 33 *Case of proliferative diabetic retinopathy 1 month after PRP laser augmentation.*

Color fundus montage image demonstrating regression of neovascularization and vitreous hemorrhage after treatment.

Patient underwent a single intravitreal anti-VEGF injection and augmentation of panretinal laser photocoagulation. Note the complete disappearance of neovascularization fronds and the resolution of vitreous hemorrhage.

Photocoagulation may improve oxygenation of the ischemic inner retinal layers by destroying some of the metabolically highly active photoreceptor cells and allowing the oxygen normally diffusing from the choriocapillaris to sustain remaining cells in the inner layers of the retina. It also relieves hypoxia and removes the stimulus for expression of angiogenic factors.

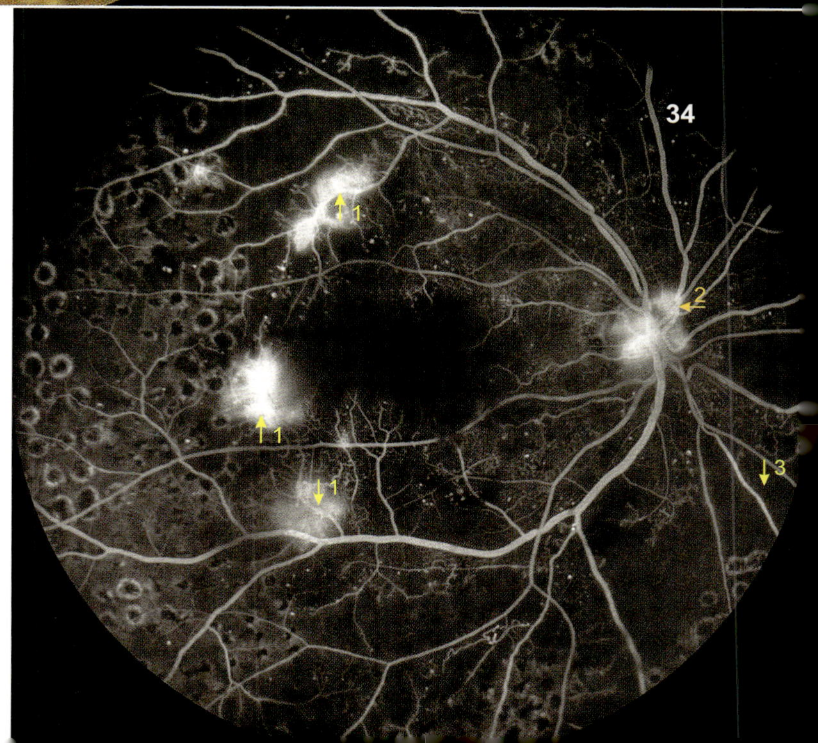


Figure 34 *Venous phase of fluorescein angiogram shows hyperfluorescent leaks from NVE (1) and NVD (2) and area of capillary nonperfusion in the nasal retina (3). Well-defined round laser scars are also visible at the temporal edge of the angiogram. They appear as hypofluorescence center with a hyperfluorescent ring.* □

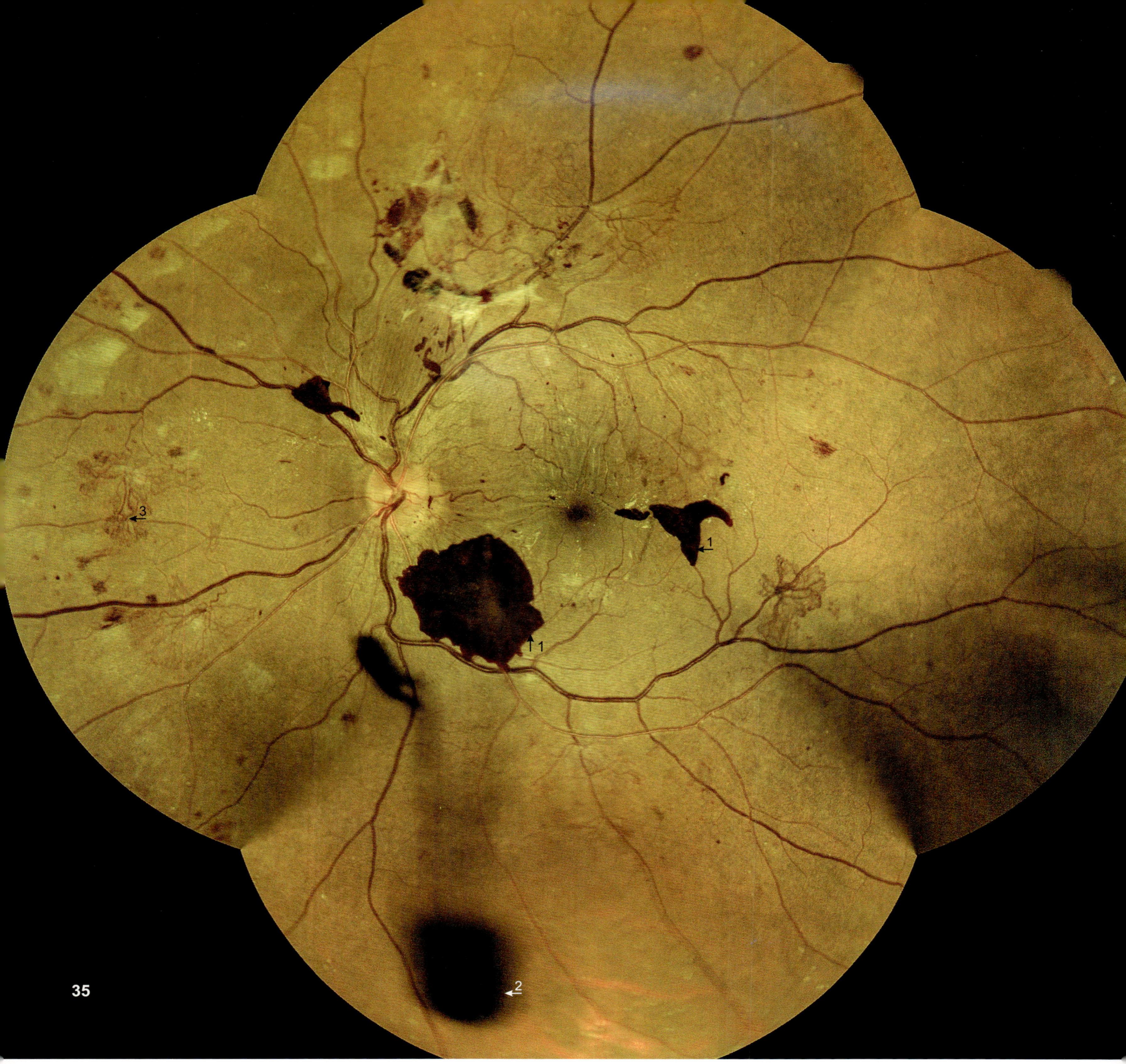


Figure 35 *Proliferative diabetic retinopathy in type 1 diabetic*.

Color fundus photograph of a 35-year-old poorly controlled type 1 diabetic female, with HbA1c of 12.0. She presented with sudden onset floaters in her left eye. Note presence of preretinal bleed (1), mild vitreous hemorrhage (2) and multiple NVEs (3) in the retina as a result of proliferative diabetic retinopathy.

Diabetic retinopathy is most frequent cause of blindness among adults aged 20–24 years. During 1st two decades of the disease, nearly all patients with type I diabetes have retinopathy. 3.6% of type I diabetics were legally blind as per Wisconsin Epidemiologic Study of Diabetic Retinopathy. Our case has high-risk proliferative diabetic retinopathy disease and was advised PRP laser as soon as possible. PRP is effective in stabilizing the PDR as it induces regression of existing neovascular tissue and present progressive neovascularization.

Patients with type I diabetes should have a dilated and comprehensive eye examination by an ophthalmologist within 3–5 years after the onset of diabetes. Subsequent examination should be repeated annually and more frequent examinations (3–4 months) are required if diabetic retinopathy has reached a preproliferative stage.

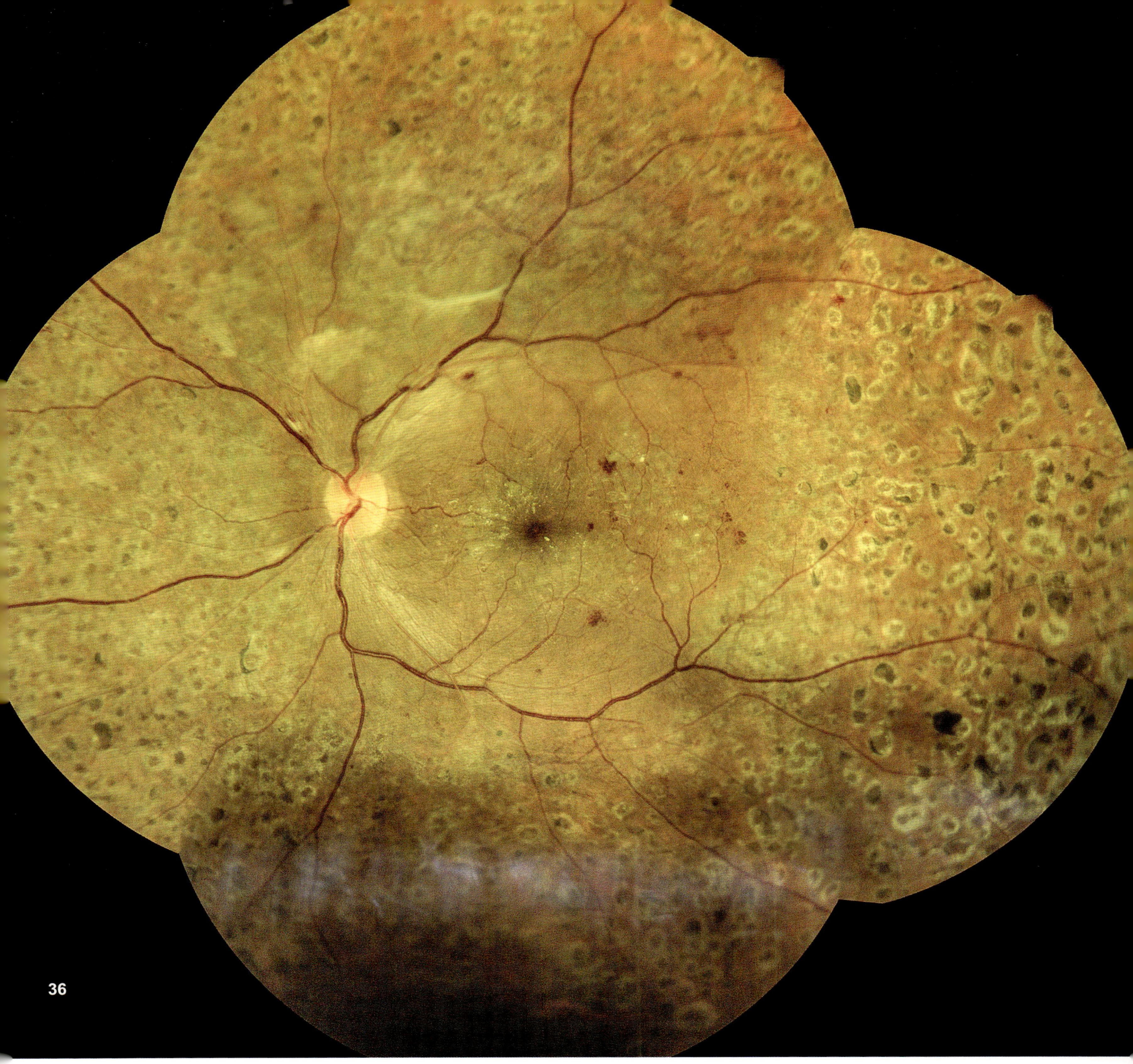


Figure 36 *Color fundus photograph 11 months after the treatment.*

Patient has received multiple laser treatment sessions over the last 11 months before regressed stage of PDR is achieved. Note presence of panretinal laser photocoagulation scars involving all the four quadrants.

PRP laser treatment was shown to significantly reduce the risk of severe vision loss (best acuity of 5/200 or worse) after only 2 years. This benefit persisted through the entire duration of follow-ups and greatest among patients who had high-risk characteristics. Treatment modalities exist to preserve vision, but timely detection of disease is of utmost importance. Regular and periodic diabetic retinopathy screening as per guidelines is of utmost importance.□

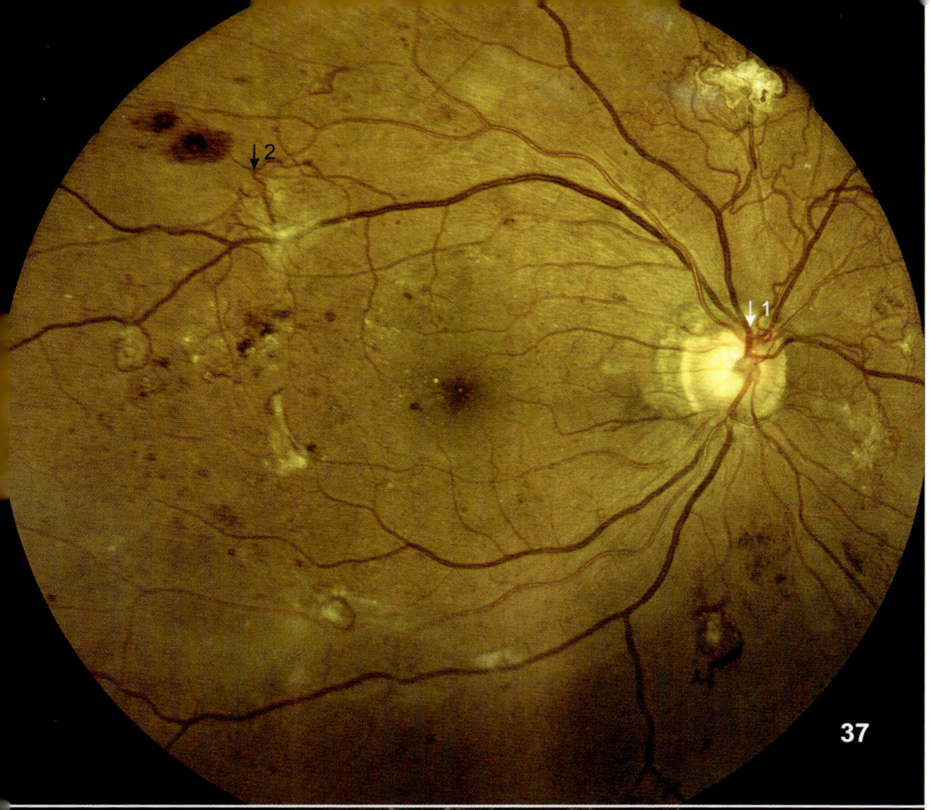


Figure 37 *Case of proliferative diabetic retinopathy at first presentation.*

Color fundus photograph shows the presence of a large frond of neovascularization of the disk involving the nasal vitreopapillary region (1). There early fibrotic changes and multiple NVEs at the posterior pole (2).

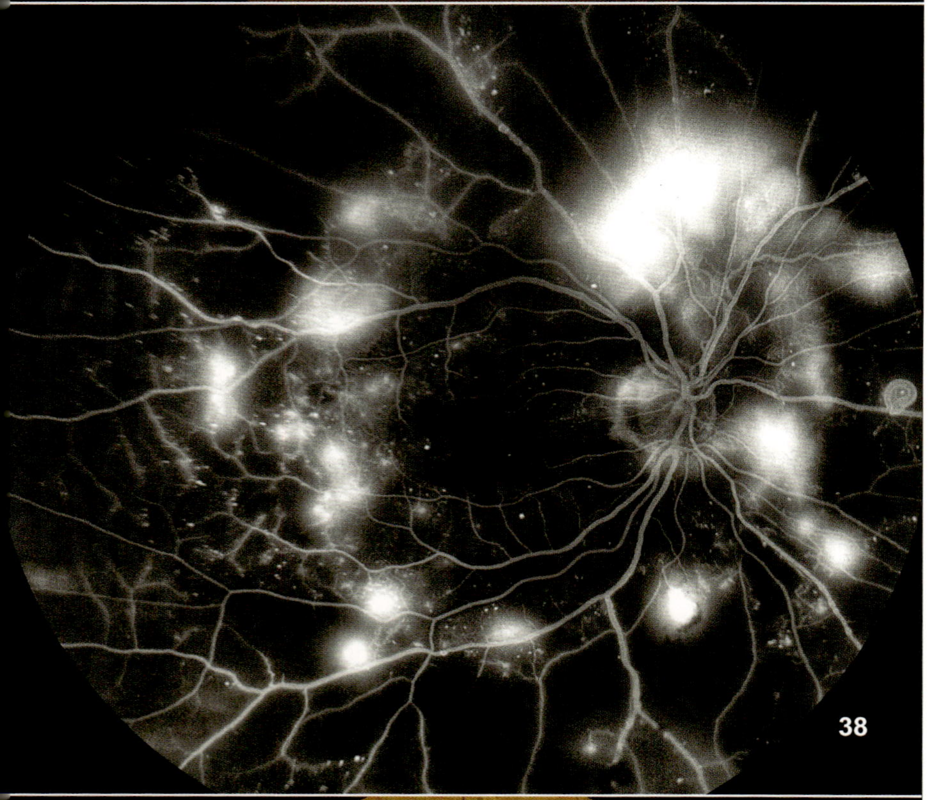


Figure 38 *FFA confirms the presence of PDR as it shows multiple leaky NVE, NVD and capillary nonperfusion areas in the mid-periphery.*

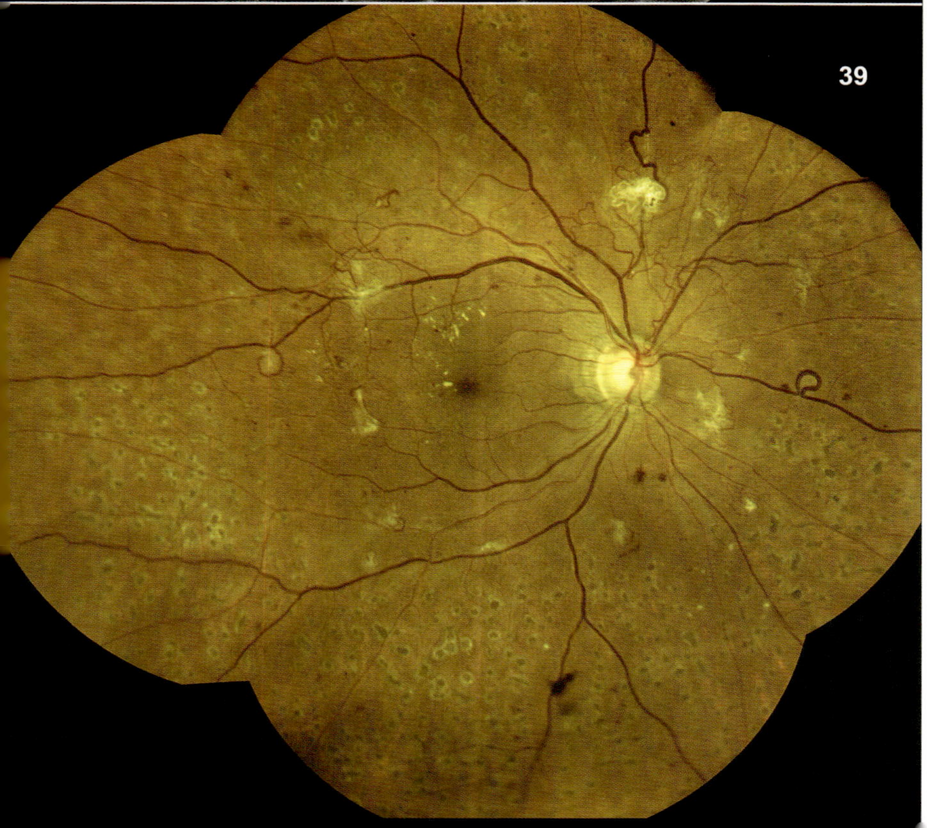


Figure 39 *Case of proliferative diabetic retinopathy 3 months after initiation of treatment.*

She received 3 sessions of scatter laser photocoagulation. Color fundus photograph 3 months later showed partial regression of NVE with laser photocoagulation scars in all the four quadrants.

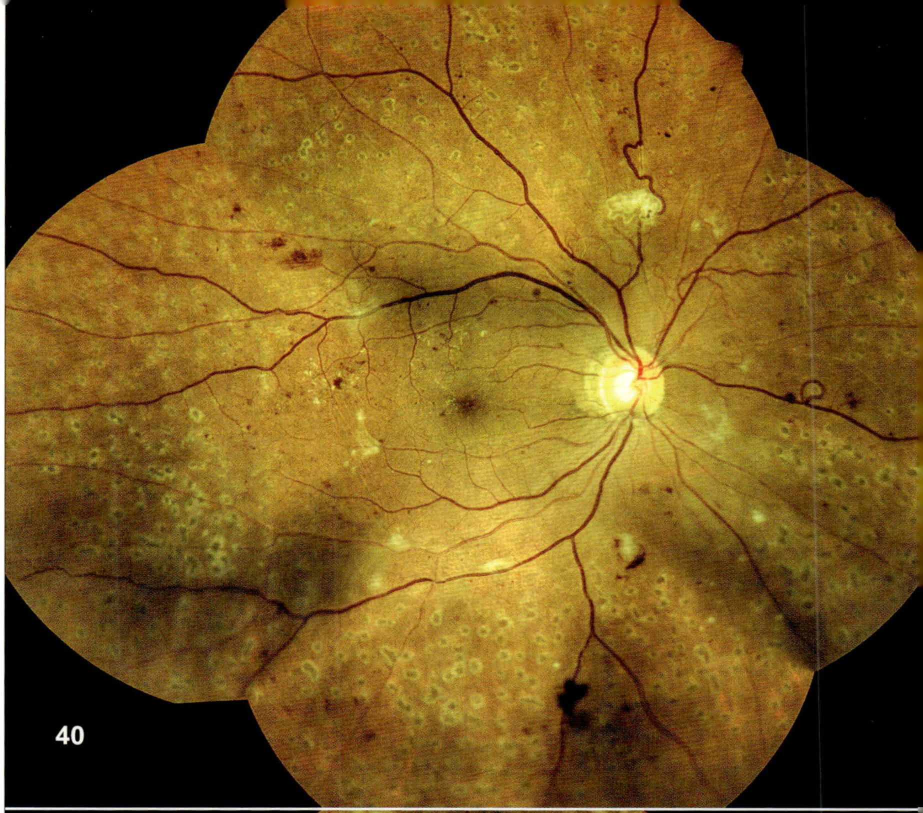


Figure 40 *Case of proliferative diabetic retinopathy 4 months after initiation of treatment.*

Four months later, NVE patches have enlarged and a new inferotemporal NVE patch has developed. At this stage patient was advised PRP augmentation.

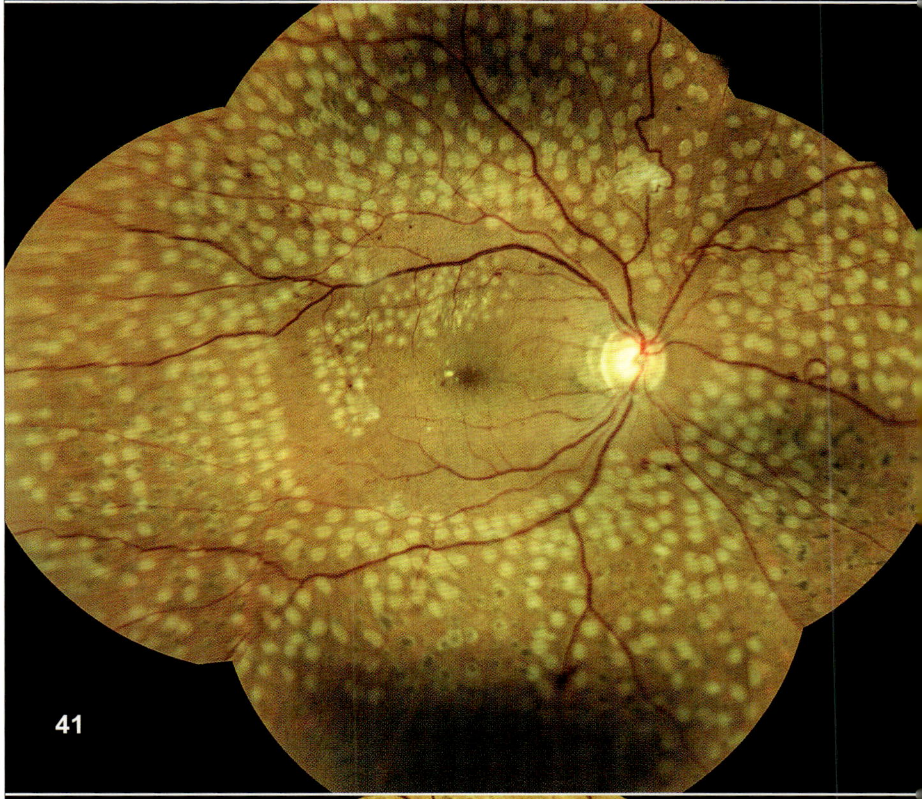


Figure 41 *Case of proliferative diabetic retinopathy immediately after retinal laser augmentation.*

As per ETDRS guidelines additional treatment was indicated as there is enlargement of NVE. Studies have documented that only two-thirds of treated eyes will show complete regression after three initial scatter laser session and rest one-third need more laser augmentation to achieve regression. Color fundus image is done immediately after laser augmentation. Retinal photocoagulation was done to previously untreated areas and extended up to the vascular arcade anteriorly. Modified grid laser was done to area of retinal thickening.

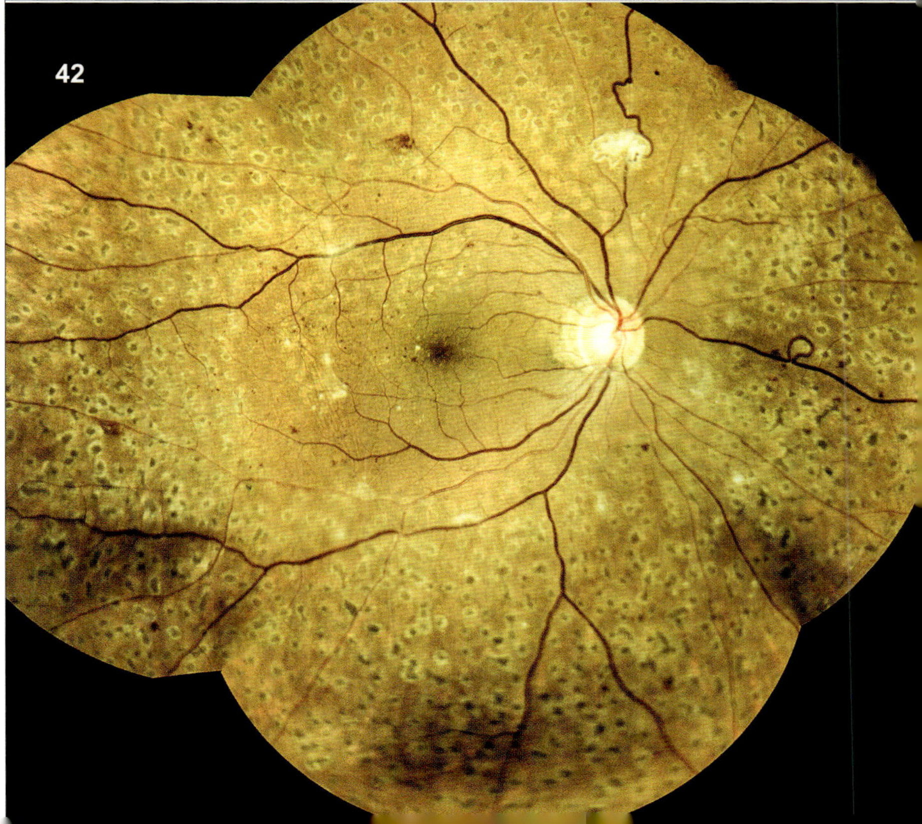


Figure 42 *Case of proliferative diabetic retinopathy 6 months after initiation of treatment.*

Color fundus image 1 month after laser augmentation. Note that there is a complete regression of NVE. No new lesion has developed. Laser scars were visible covering all the four quadrants of the retina periphery and posterior pole looks stable. □

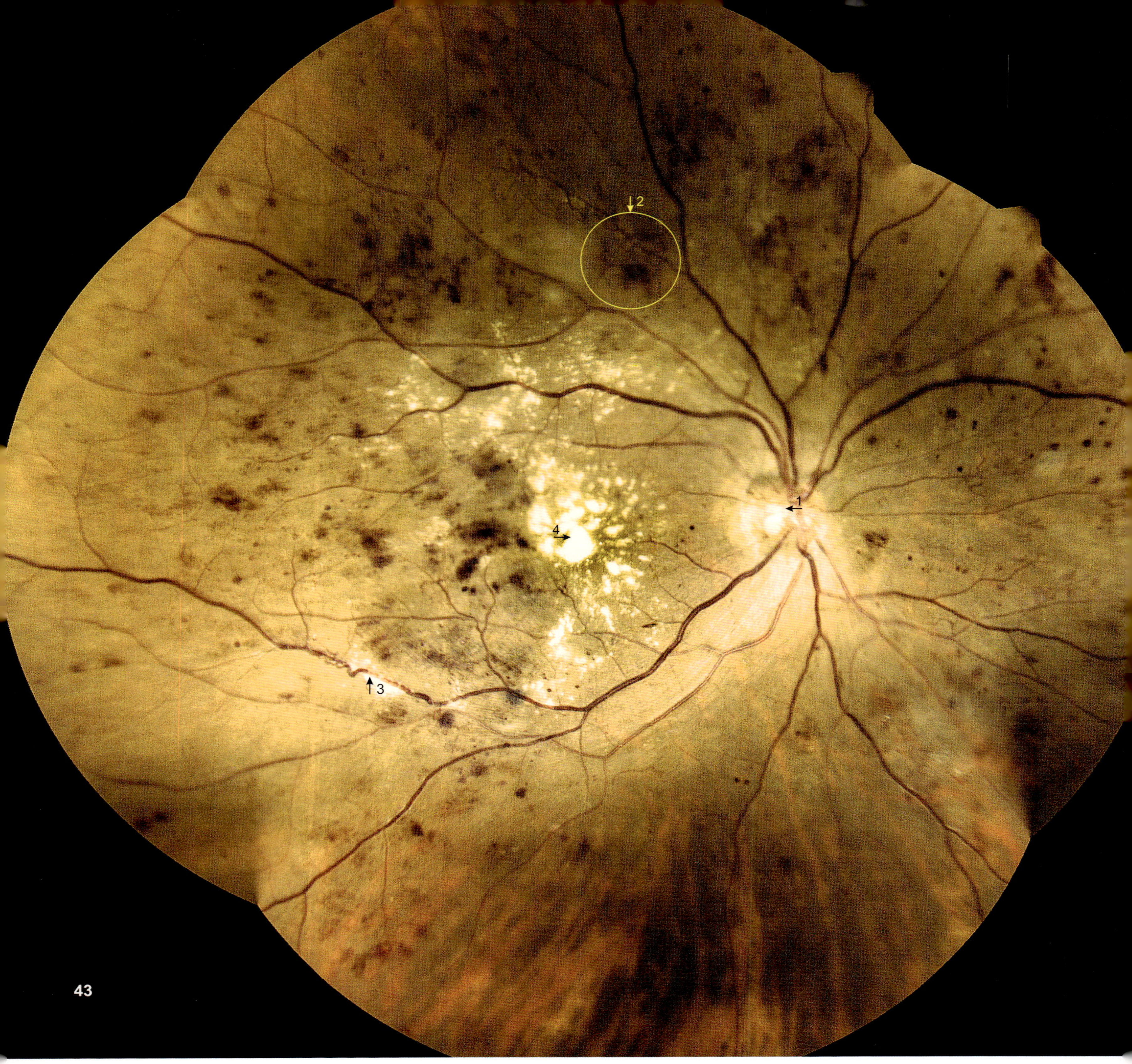


Figure 43 *Color fundus image demonstrating a case of high-risk proliferative diabetic retinopathy without treatment.*

Note the presence of flat neovascularization at the disk that involves more than half of the disk area (1).

Multiple NVEs (2), venous beading (3), and a plaque of hard exudates at the macula (4).

This patient is a 55-year-old female, type 2 diabetic who presented with high-risk proliferative diabetic retinopathy and severe diabetic macular edema. Such cases are at a risk of severe visual loss and if the disease continues to progress can result in complete blindness. Panretinal photocoagulation along with anti-VEGF injections can reduce the risk of blindness and has to be administered as soon as possible.

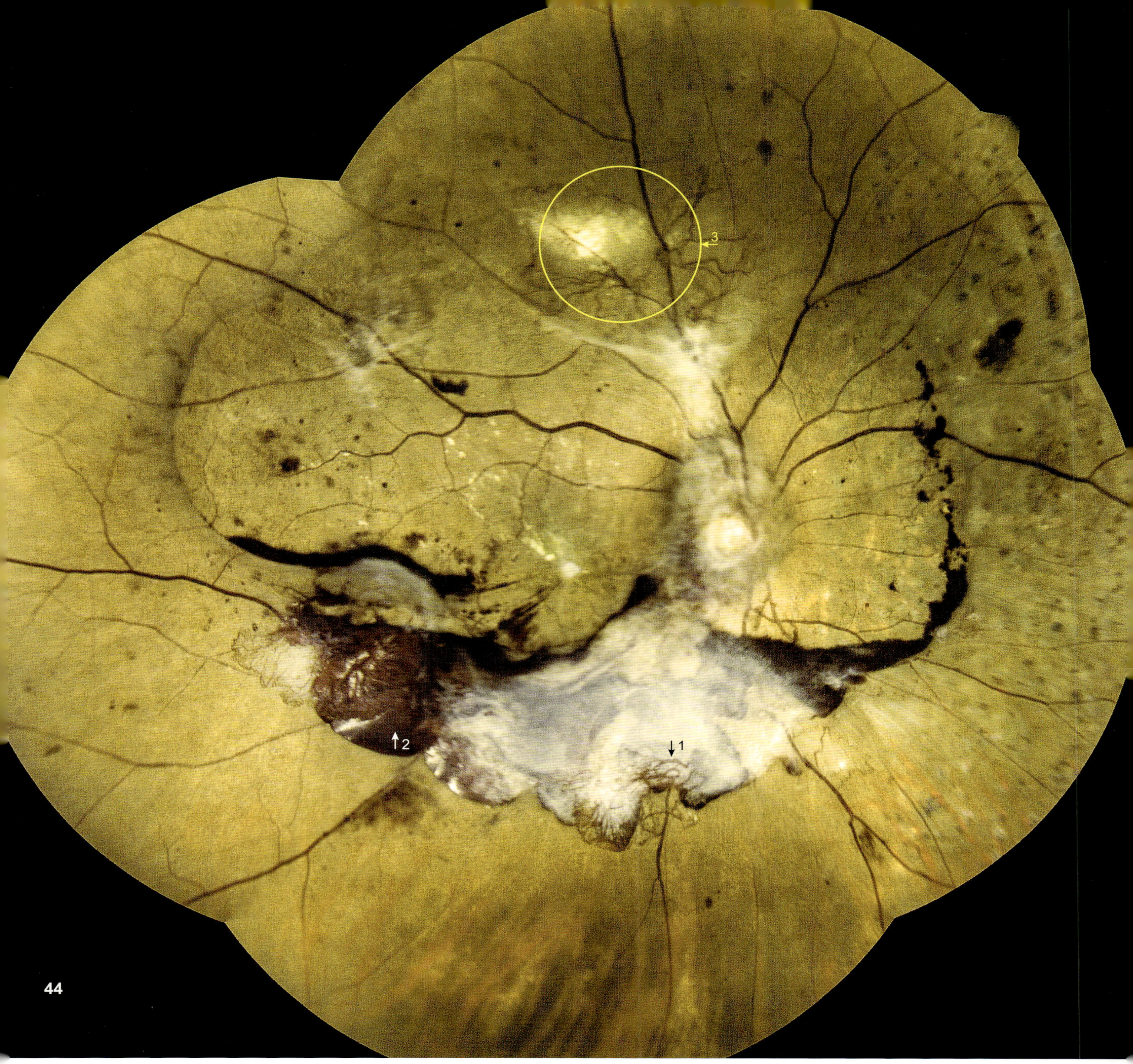


Figure 44 *Color fundus image 9 months later demonstrating progression to tractional retinal detachment.*

Patient failed to complete the treatment and presented 9 months later with tractional retinal detachment (1) and sub hyaloid bleed (2). Note the NVEs have increased in size (3). Broad fibrovascular adhesions have formed between the neovascularization at the optic disk and the inferotemporal arcade resulting in contraction and pulling of the retina and associated retinal bleed.

Few scattered laser photocoagulation scars are seen in the nasal quadrant. This case highlights the importance of panretinal photocoagulation in cases with high-risk PDR. Landmark DRS study has demonstrated 50% reduction in the risk of severe vision loss following treatment with PRP laser. □

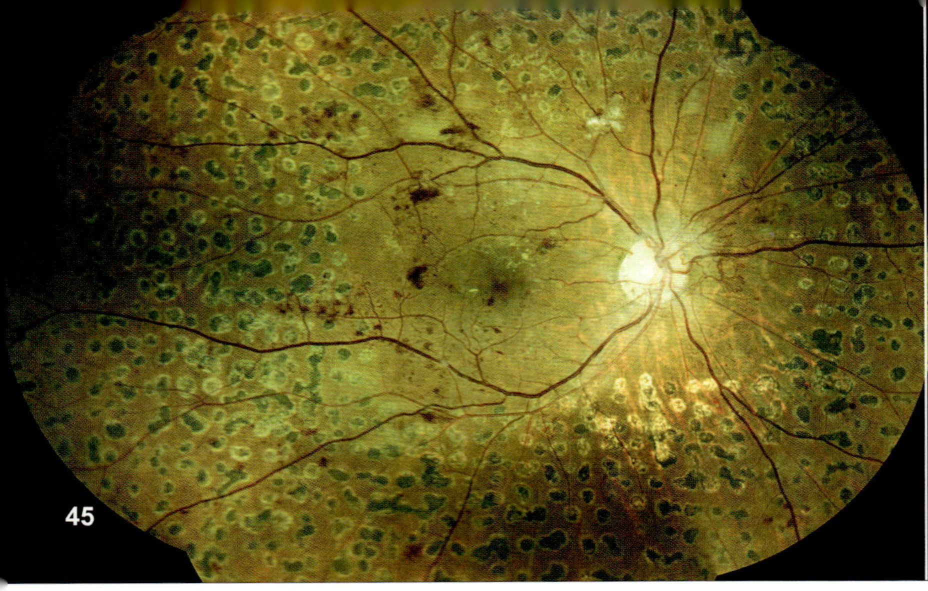

45

Figure 45 *Case of proliferative diabetic retinopathy treated with laser photocoagulation. (Right Eye)*

Color fundus photograph of a poorly controlled type 1 diabetic shows adequately spaced laser scars in the retina. Despite the laser, patient has developed NVEs and NVD.

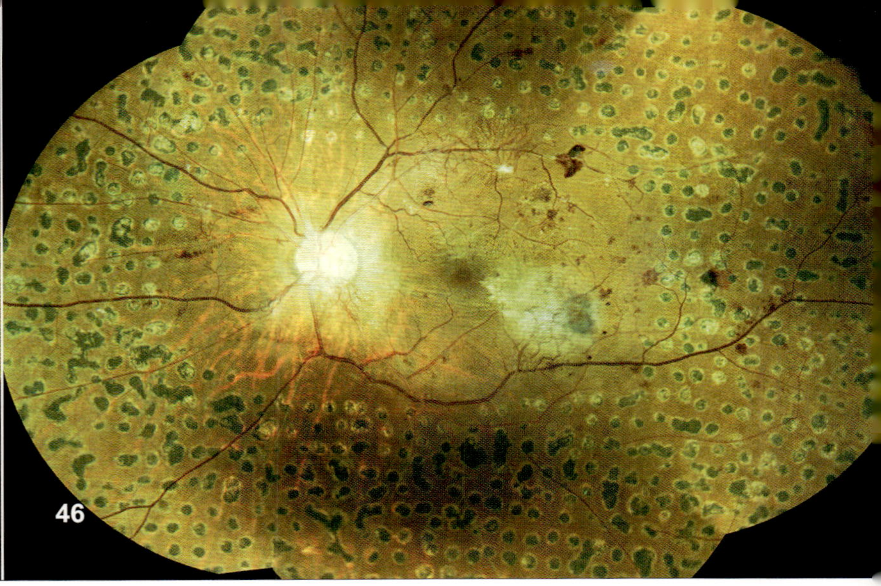

46

Figure 46 *Case of proliferative diabetic retinopathy treated with laser photocoagulation.(Left Eye)*

Note the presence of NVEs and localized area of fibrovascular traction at the temporal macula.

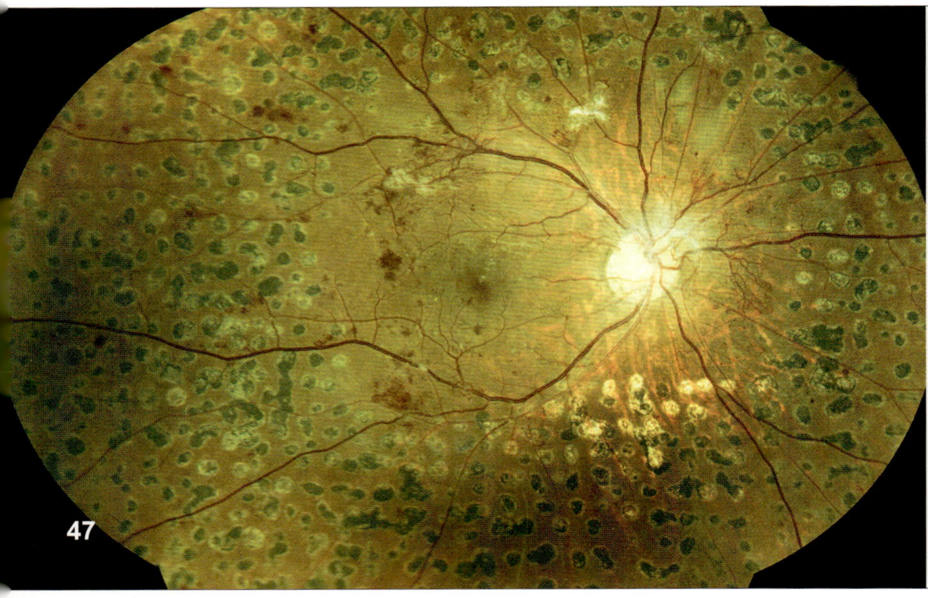

47

Figure 47 *Patient did not seek any treatment. Color fundus photograph at 6 months shows further progression of NVE.*

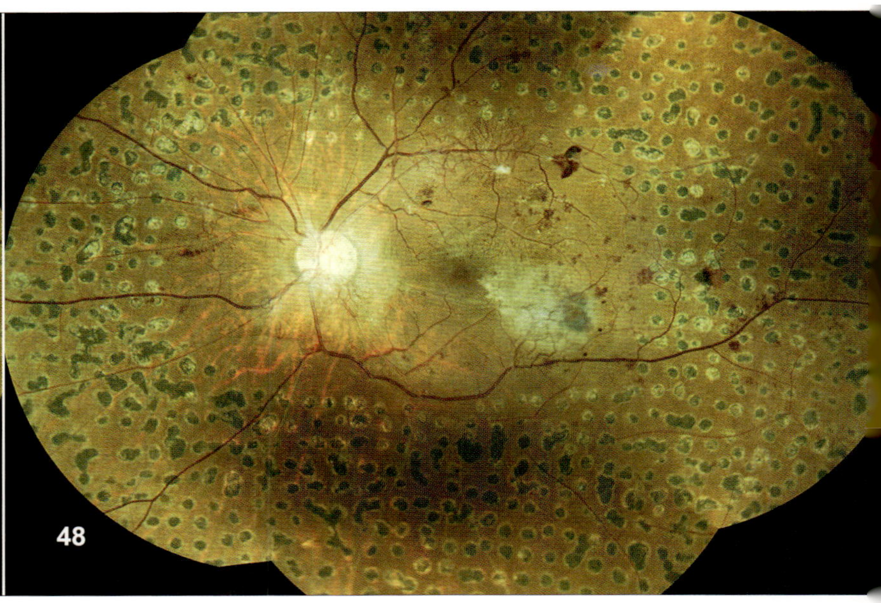

48

Figure 48 *At 6 months, fibrovascular traction at the temporal macula has further increased and is threatening the fovea.*

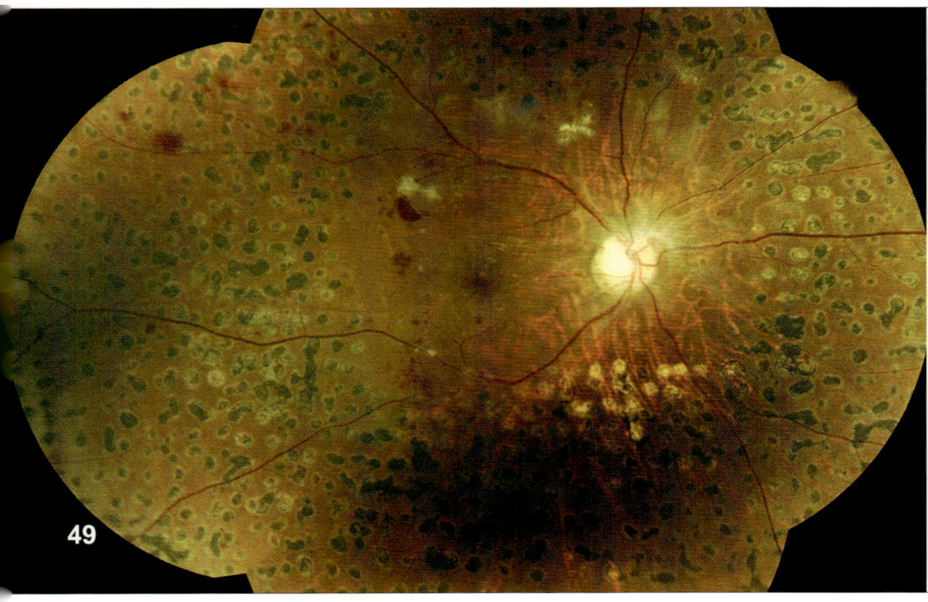

49

Figure 49 *Case of proliferative diabetic retinopathy, 1 month after treatment.*

Patient was advised intravitreal anti-VEGF injection. It induced rapid regression of NVE.

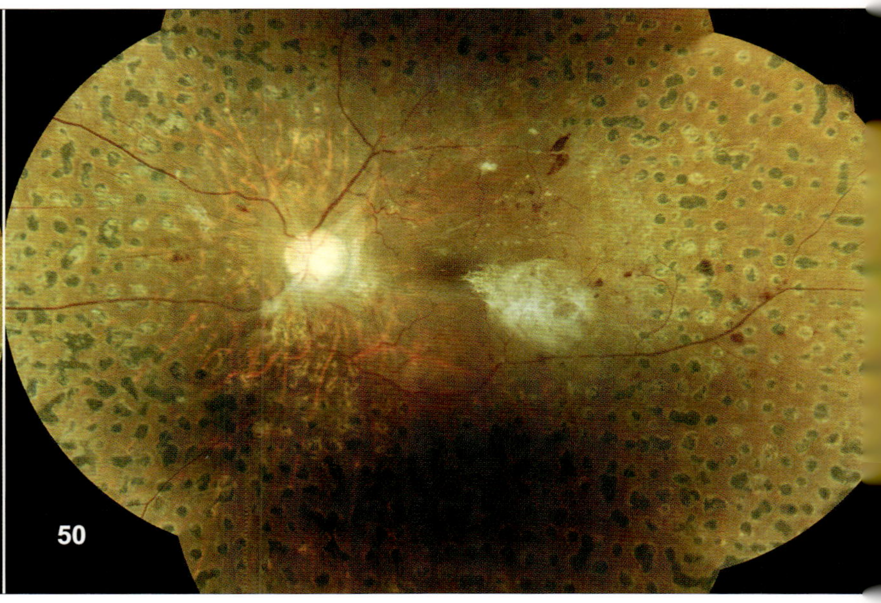

50

Figure 50 *Case of proliferative diabetic retinopathy 1 month after treatment.*

Note regression of NVE, and stabilization of retinal traction following laser augmentation. □

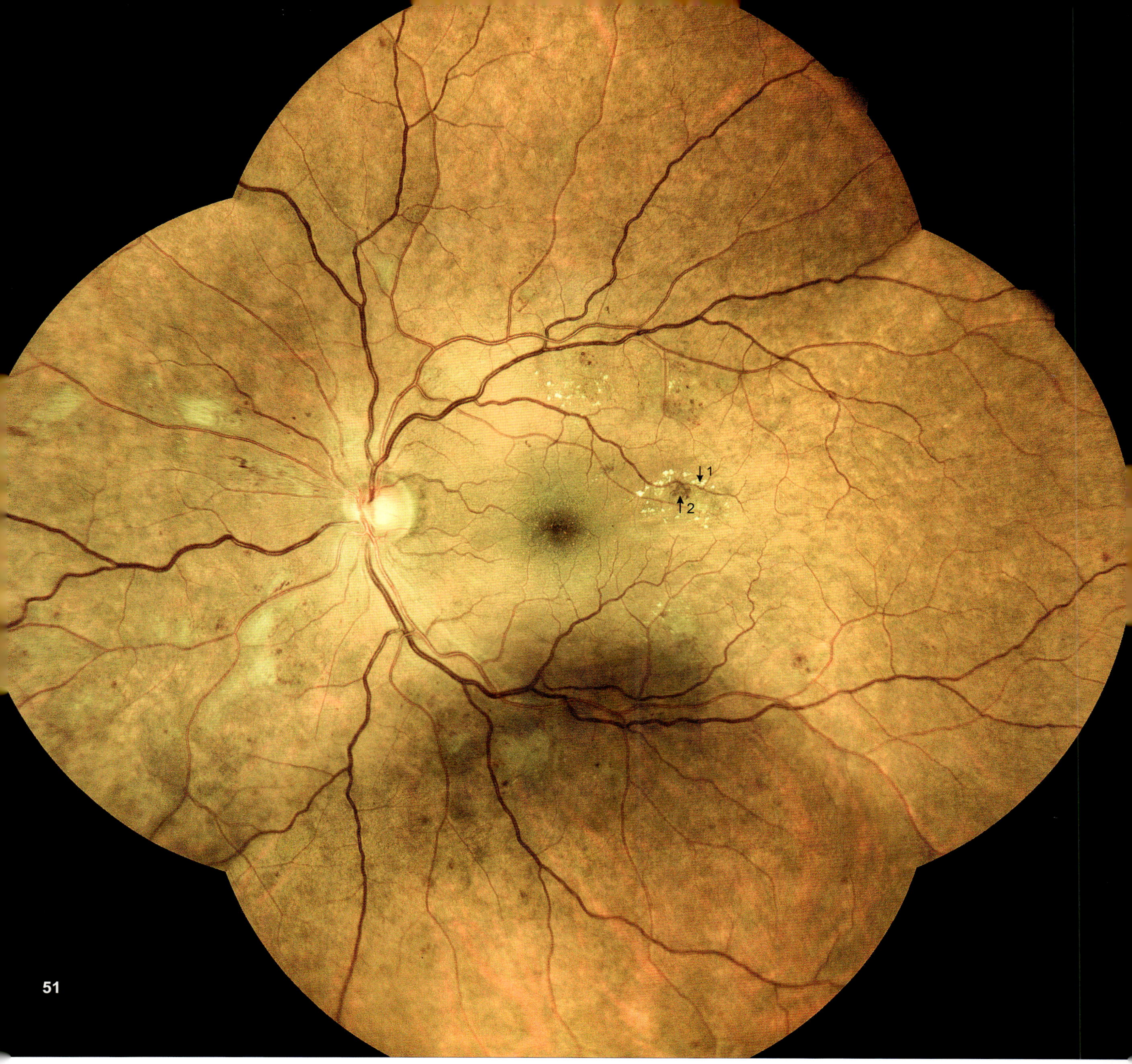


Figure 51 *Moderate nonproliferative diabetic retinopathy with mild diabetic macular edema: Color fundus photograph shows hard exudates (1) arranged in circinate pattern around the leaking microaneurysms (2) at the posterior pole but far from macula center. Also note the presence of whitish fluffy cotton wool spots in the nasal mid-periphery.*

Diabetic macular edema (DME) is an accumulation of fluid in the macula due to leaking blood vessels resulting in visual impairment. As per the International Clinical Diabetic Macular Edema Disease Severity Scale, Mild DME is defined as the presence of some retinal thickening or hard exudates in the posterior pole but distant from the center of the macula. Management at this stage involves optimizing diabetic control and optimize the lipid control if deranged. 4–6 monthly routine observation by a retina specialist is recommended and treatment should be indicated if it progresses further and become fovea threatening. □

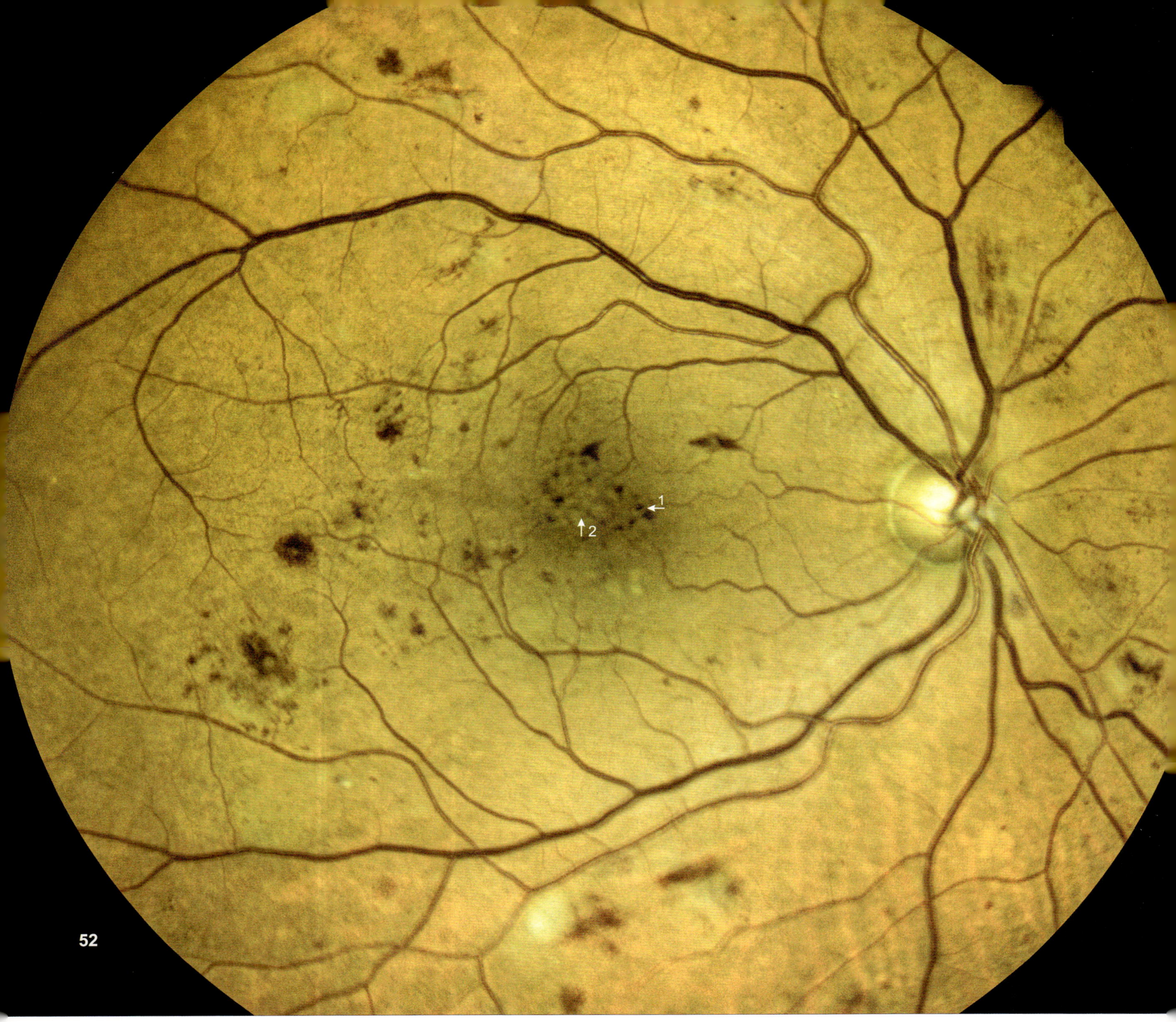


Figure 52 *Fundus photograph of another variant of severe diabetic macular edema.*

Note there are no hard exudates seen in the macula, but foveal region appears thickened with loss of foveal reflex, multiple microaneurysms (1) and cystic pattern of thickening (2). Retinal thickening greater than 300 microns can be seen on clinical biomicroscopic examination. Retinal thickening less than 300 microns is subclinical diabetic macular edema and is usually picked up by the Optical Coherence Tomography only.

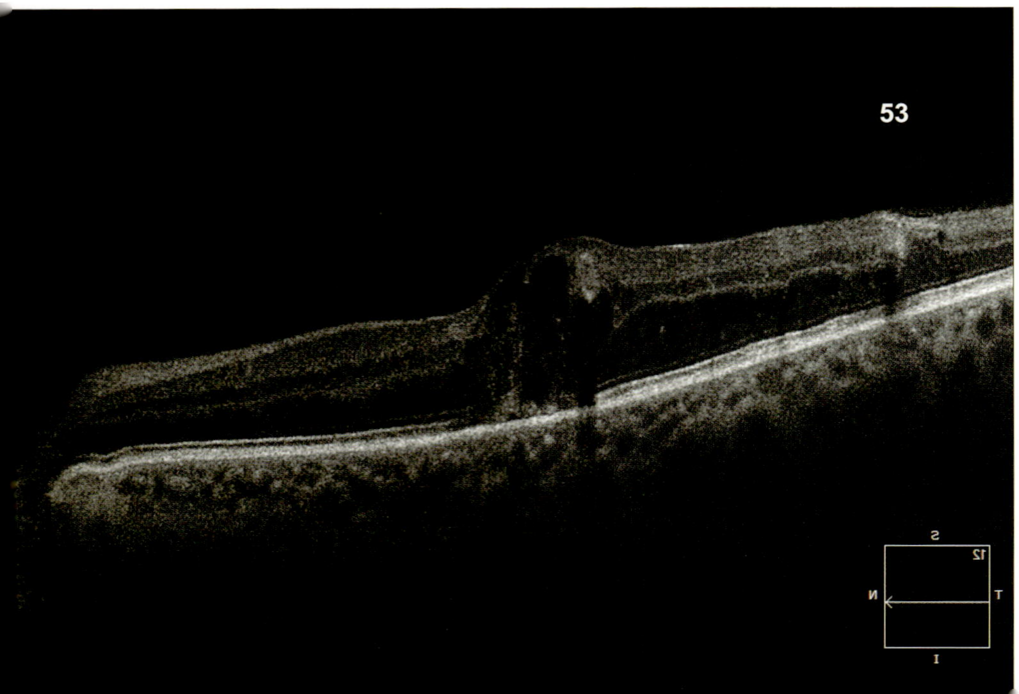


Figure 53 *Spectral domain OCT confirms the presence of diabetic macular edema.* □

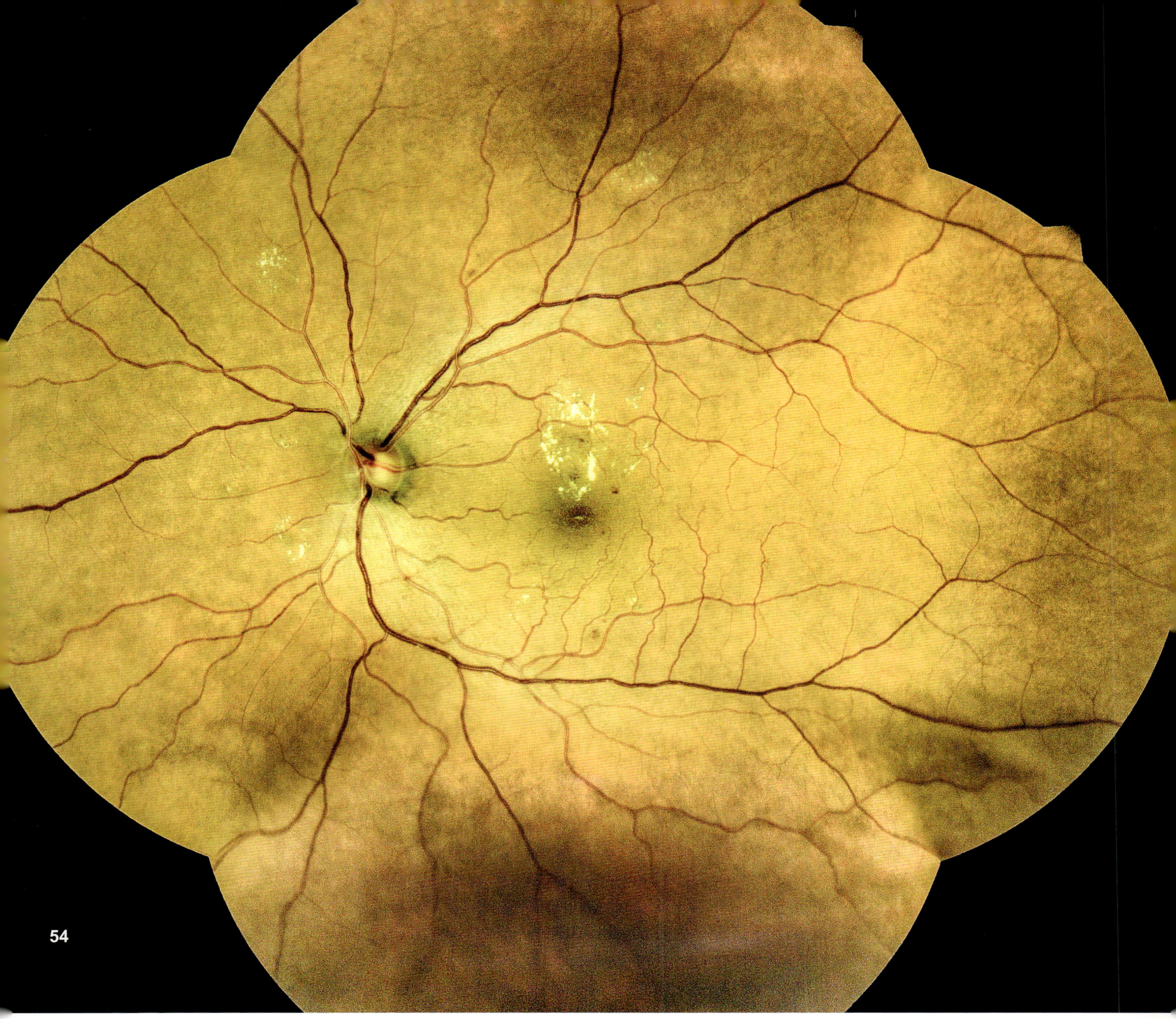

54

Figure 54 *Case of moderate diabetic macular edema.*

Color fundus photograph shows multiple hard exudates approaching the macula center but is not involving it. This classifies as moderate DME. Since DME is still nonfoveal center involving, patients visual acuity is maintained at 6/6. Strict diabetic control, optimization of lipid profile and focal laser photocoagulation is indicated to stop the further progression.

Figure 56 *Color fundus photograph 9 months postlaser treatment.*

Note the resolution of hard exudates with normal fovea. Laser photo-coagulation is still a treatment of choice especially in noncenter diabetic macular edema and provide long-term stability unlike anti-VEGF injections where treatment has to offered repeatedly. □

Figure 55

*Color fundus photograph immediately after laser photo-coagulation.*

Patient underwent focal laser to microaneurysms, modified light grid laser to adjacent areas of retinal thickening using mild intensity yellow laser.

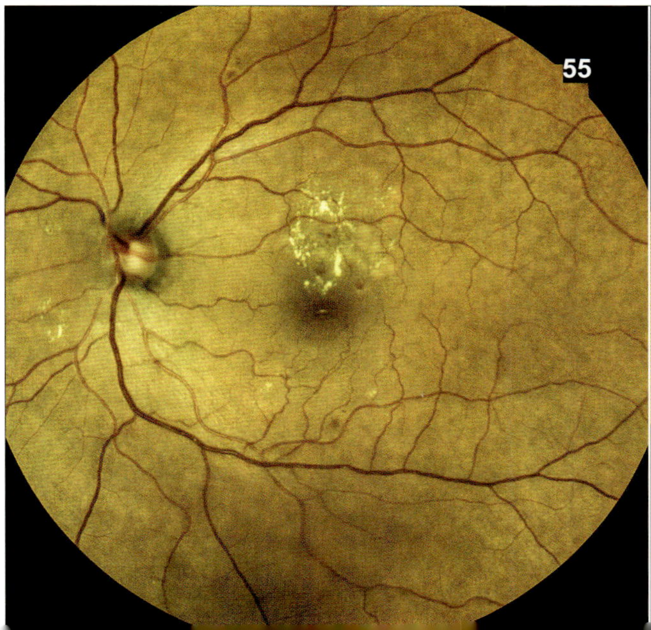

55

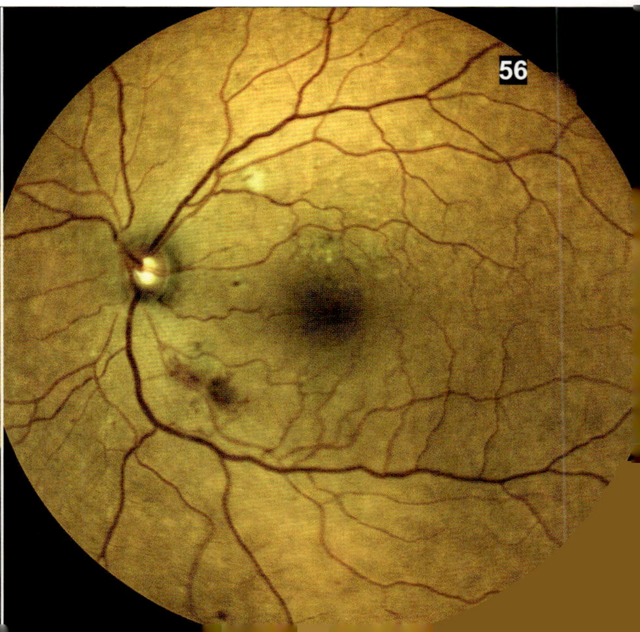

56

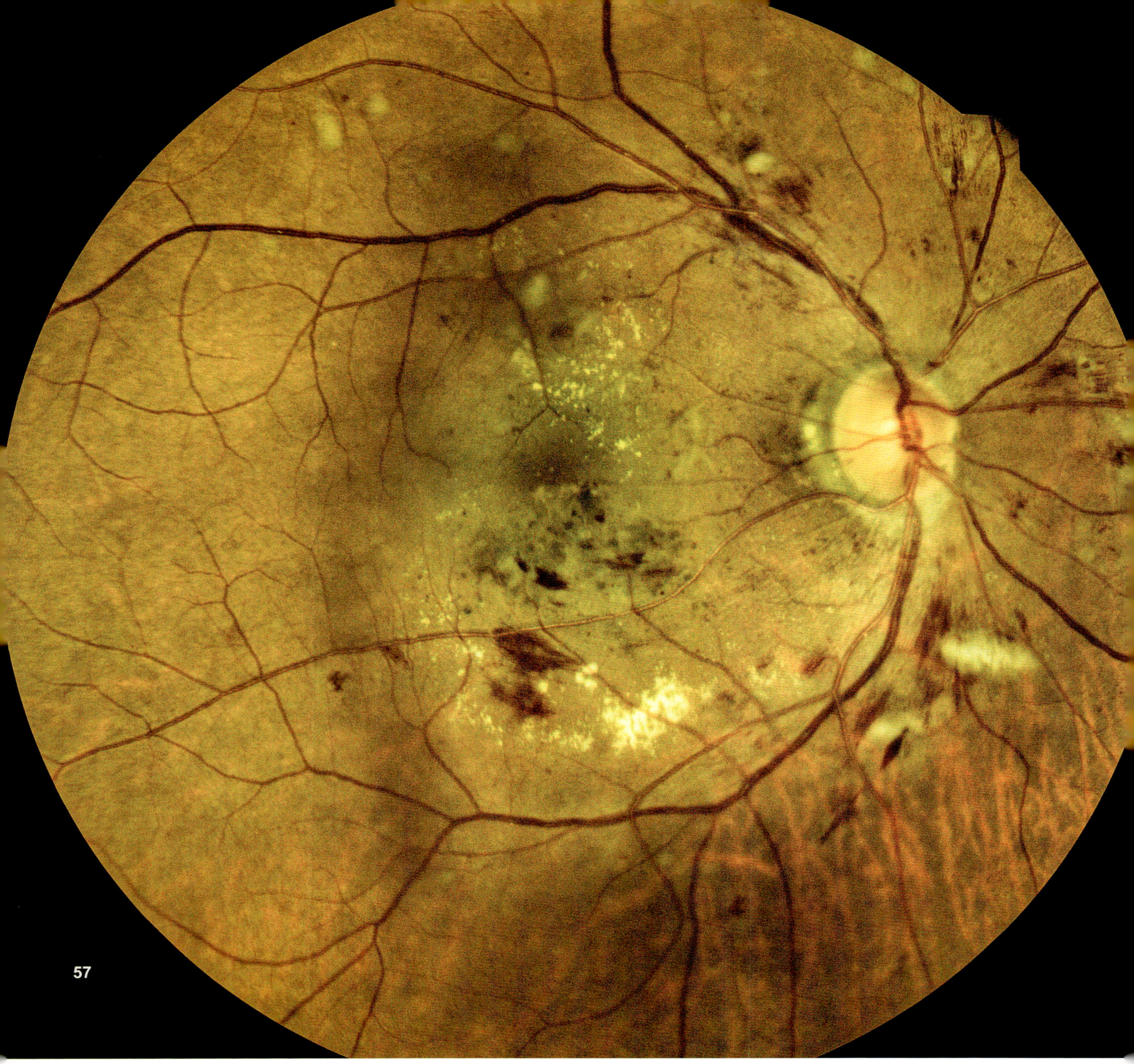


Figure 57 *Case of severe diabetic macular edema with moderate nonproliferative diabetic macular edema.*

Color fundus photograph shows retinal thickening and hard exudates involving the macula center, classifying it as severe DME as per the International Clinical Diabetic Macular Edema Disease Severity Scale. He is a 65-year-old type 2 diabetic hypertensive patient who presented with complaints of blurred vision for the last 2 months. He underwent FFA/OCT that confirmed the diagnosis of severe diabetic macular edema. Complete metabolic profile was advised with anti-VEGF injections. Anti-VEGF injection can improve the central vision but is usually required to give multiple treatment sessions. Optimizing diabetes mellitus and lipid levels is equally important in management. Visual acuity is recorded as 6/36 due to diffuse retinal edema involving the foveal center such cases need treatment in the form of multiple intravitreal anti-VEGF injections.

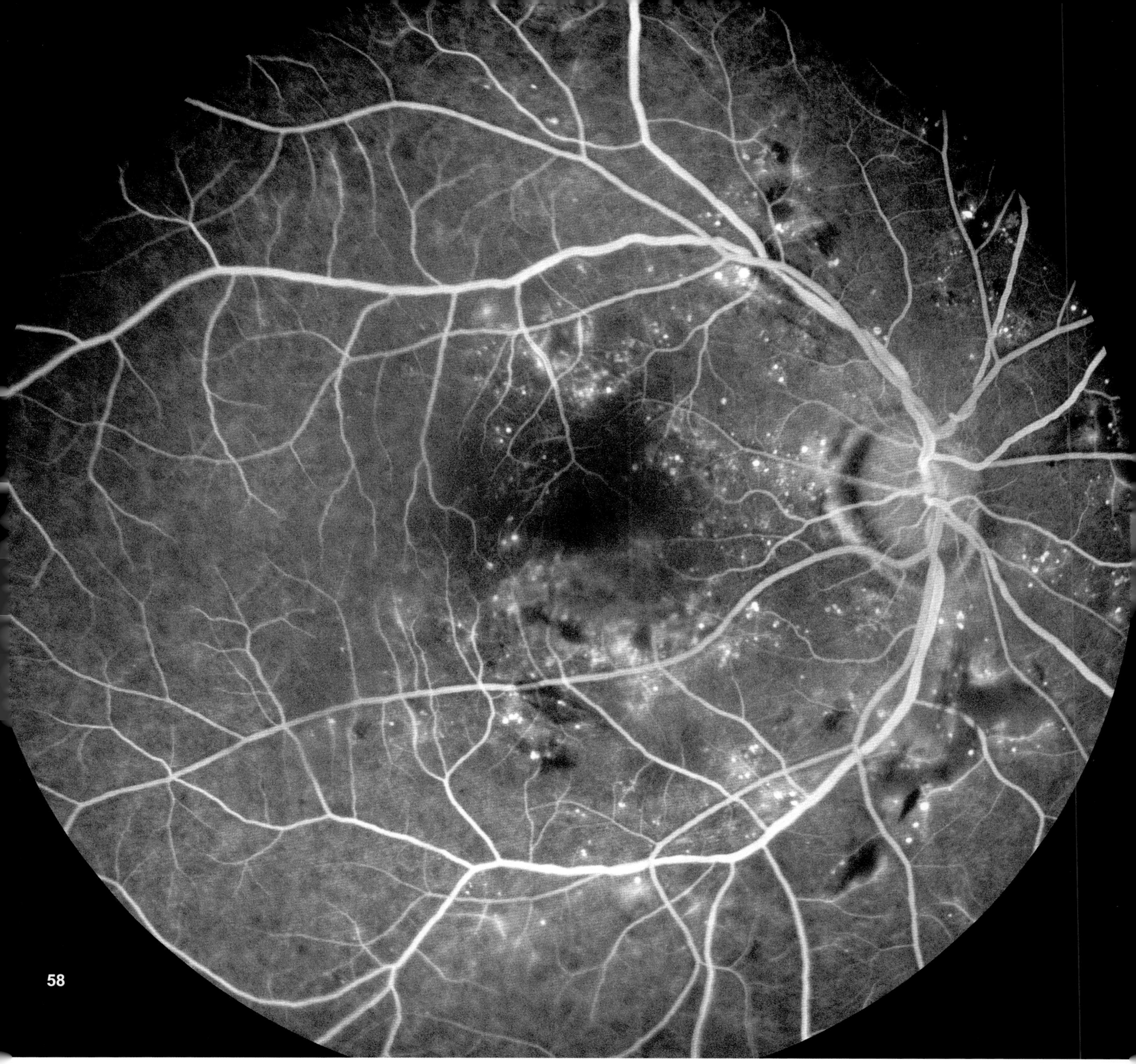


Figure 58 *Early frame of fluorescein angiogram demonstrating multiple pinpoint hyperfluorescent microaneurysms around the fovea and blocked hypofluorescence from retinal hemorrhages.*

Figure 59 *Late phase of fluorescein angiogram shows diffuse leakage involving whole of the macula.*

Figure 60 *Swept source OCT scan demonstrating gross retinal thickening from presence of subretinal and intraretinal fluid in this case of diabetic macular edema. Also note the presence of hard exudates that are seen as hyper-reflective intraretinal dot lesions.*□

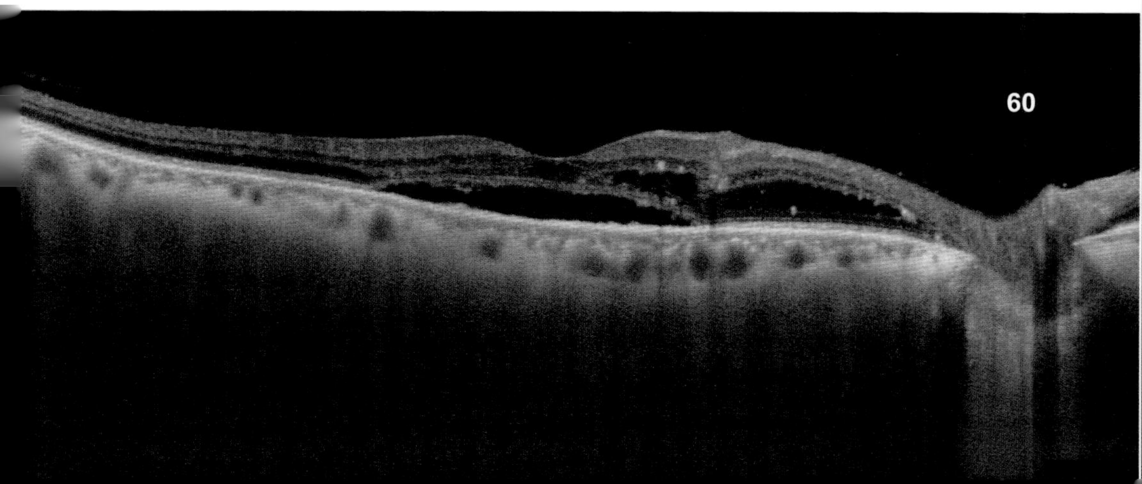


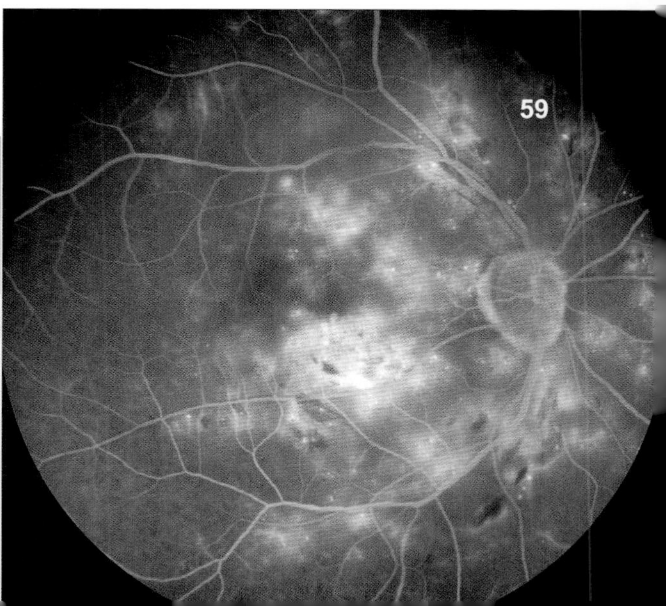

Figure 61

*Moderate nonproliferative diabetic retinopathy with diabetic macular edema. Multiple dot (1), superficial hemorrhages (2) cotton wool spots (3) can be seen at posterior pole and mid-peripheral retina. Circinate pattern of hard exudates (4) are seen at posterior pole as well.*

Figure 62

*Spectral domain OCT scan in a case of moderate nonproliferative diabetic retinopathy with diabetic macular edema.*

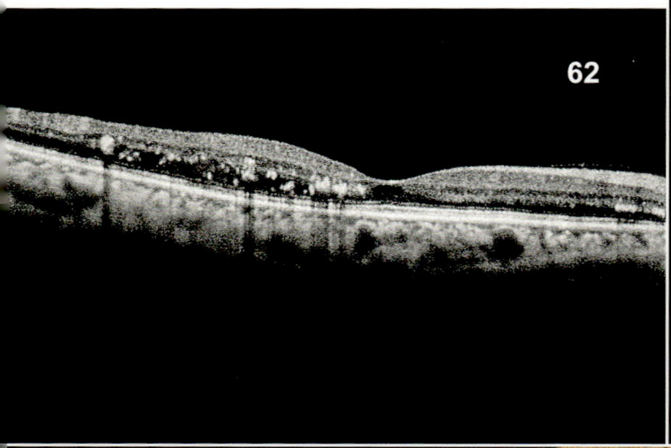

62

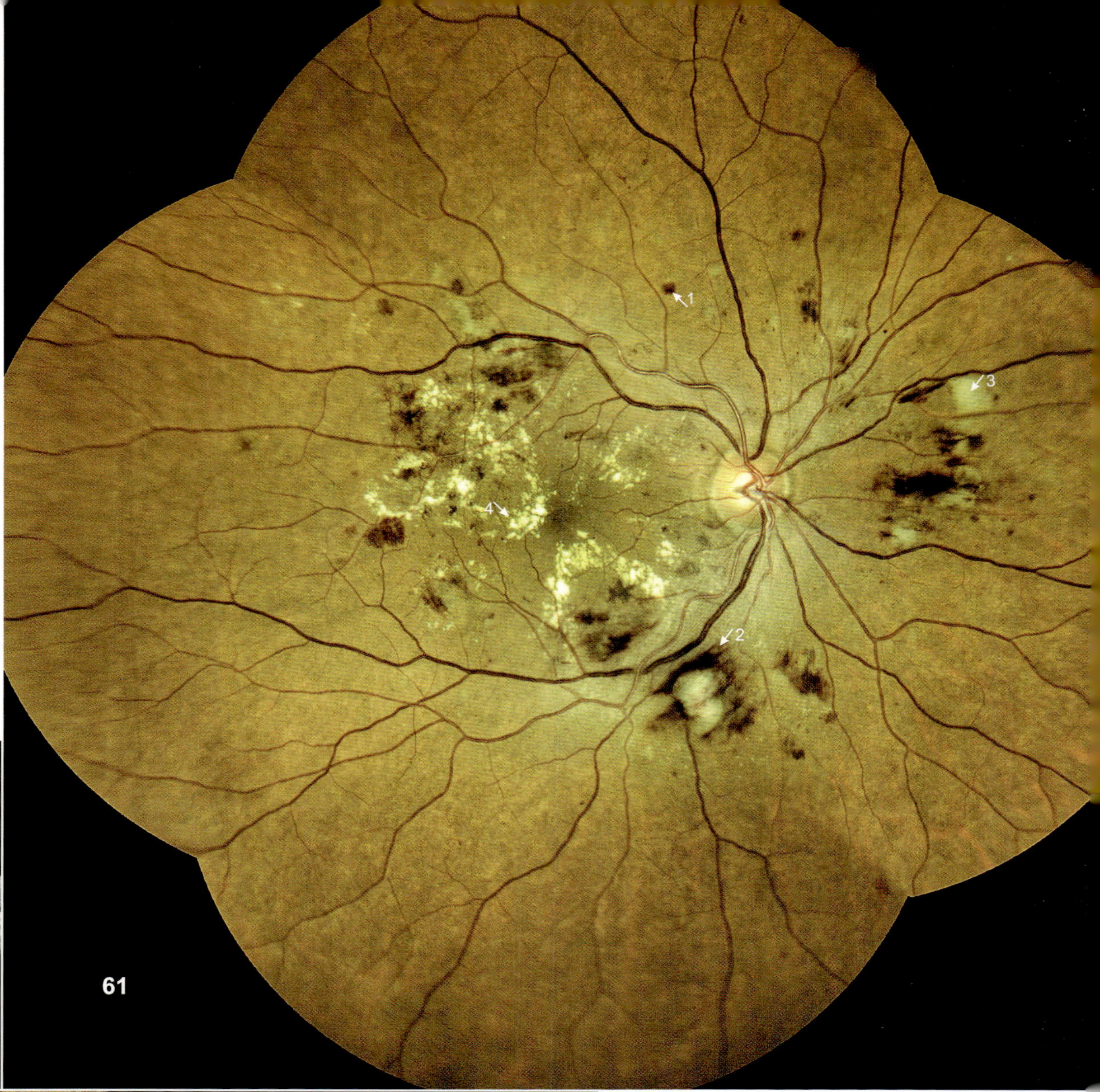


61

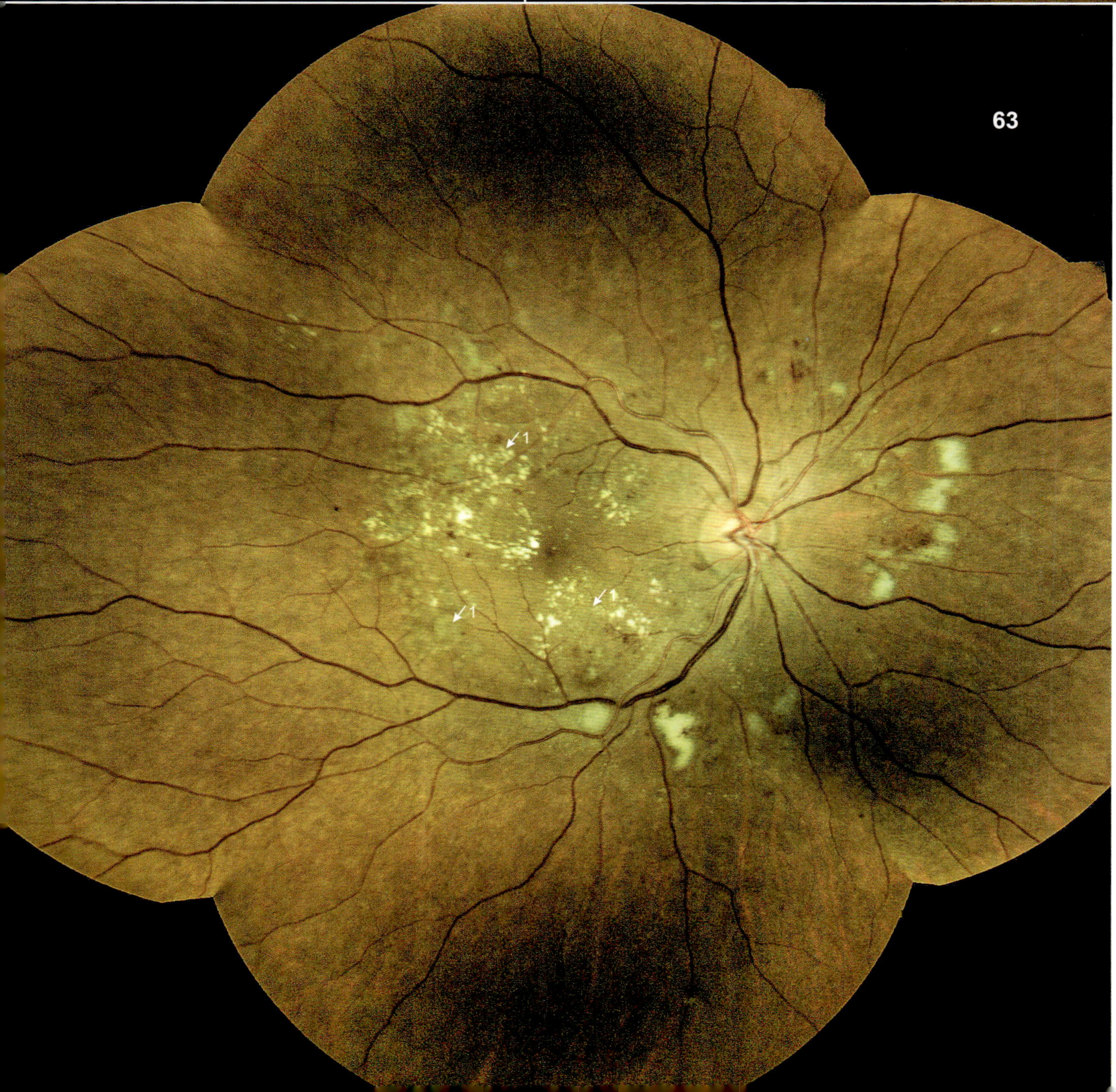


63

Figure 63

*Color fundus montage of the same patient 6 months after macular laser treatment and anti-VEGF injection. Note significant reduction in retinal hemorrhages and hard exudates as compared to Figure 61. Tiny gray colored round macular laser spots (1) can be seen in a modified grid pattern.*

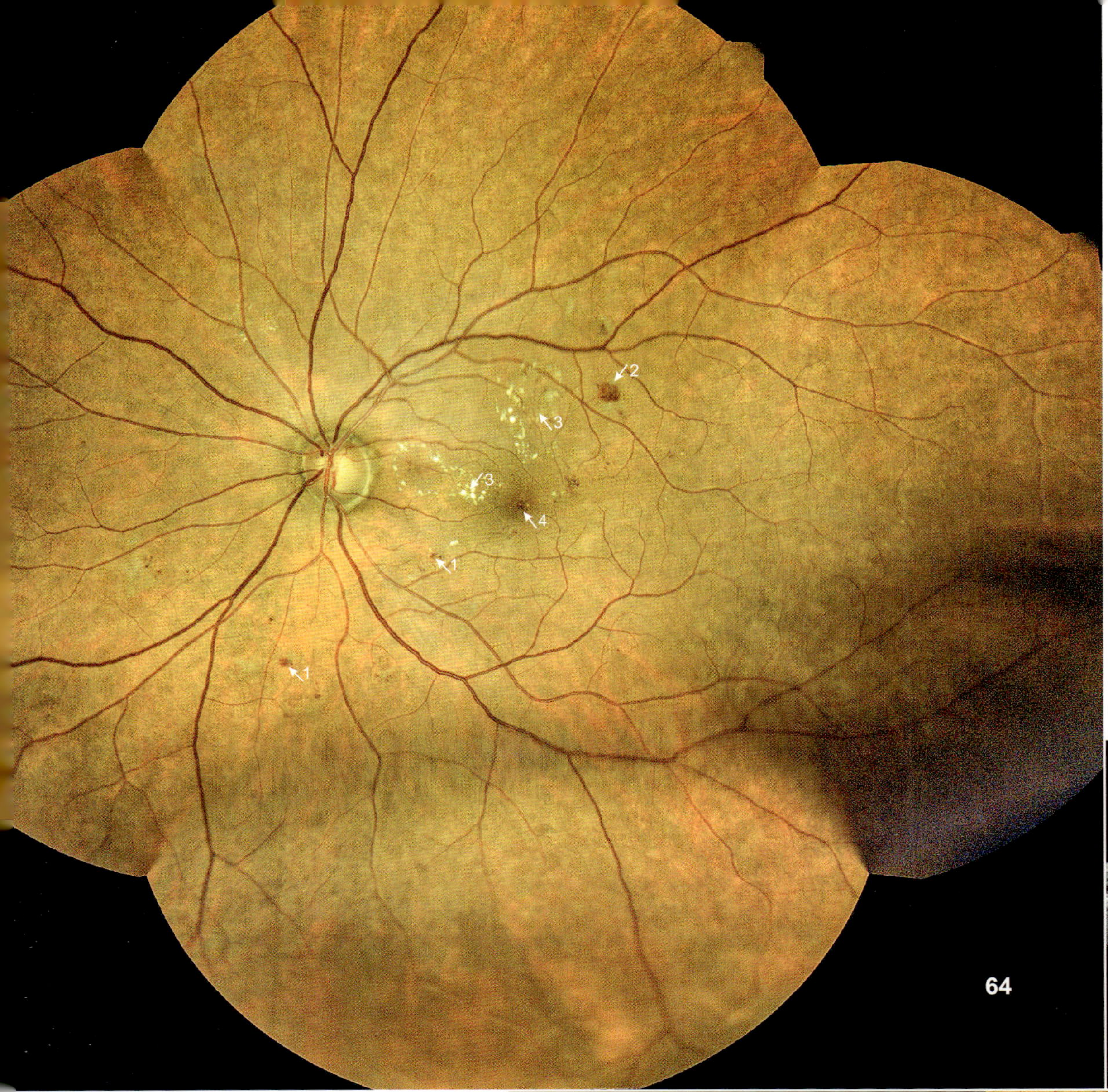


Figure 64

*Moderate nonproliferative diabetic retinopathy with diabetic maculopathy. Note the presence of microaneurysm (1), dot hemorrhage (2) and hard exudates superonasal and superotemporal to the fovea (3). Foveal reflex is normal (4).*

Figure 65

*Spectral domain OCT scan in a case of moderate nonproliferative diabetic retinopathy. Microaneurysm (oval hyporeflective pattern) (1) and few hard exudates can be seen (hyper-reflective dots)(2). Foveal profile is normal and there is no retinal thickening.*

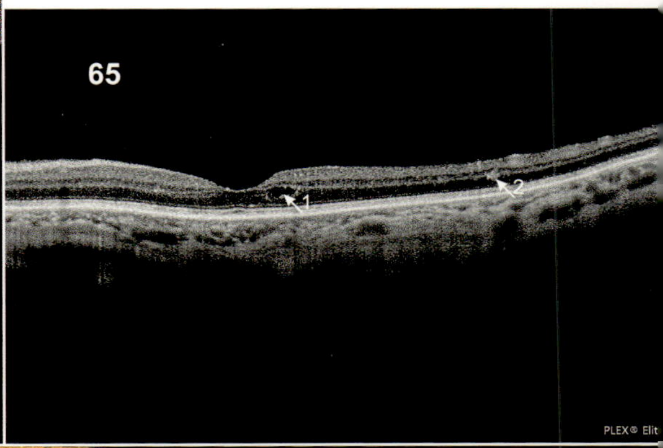


Figure 66

*Color fundus montage image of same patient with moderate nonproliferative diabetic retinopathy and diabetic maculopathy 6 months after treatment with Tab. Fenofibrate (lipid lowering medication). Significant reduction in hard exudates could be seen as compared to figure 64 (1).*

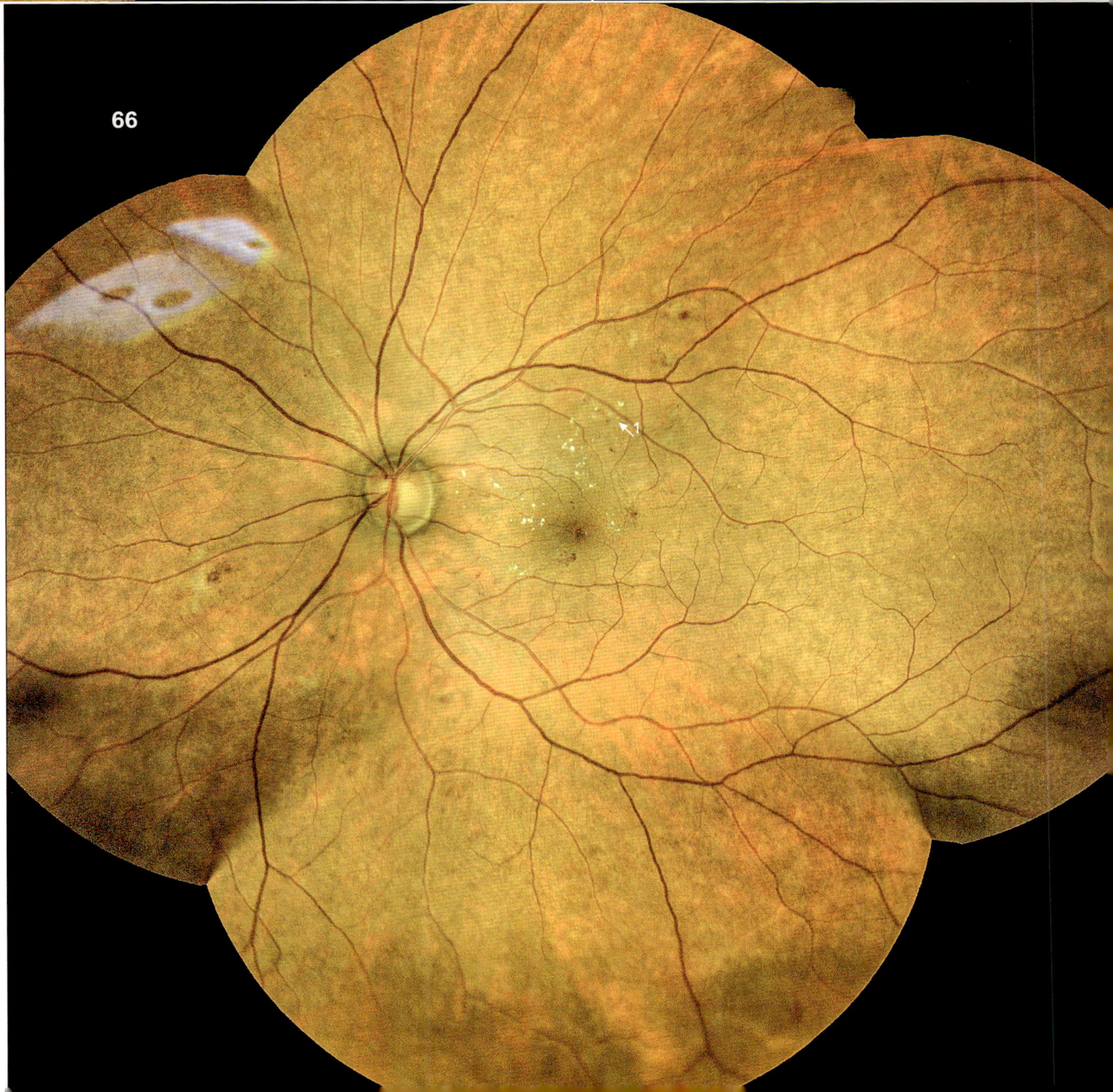

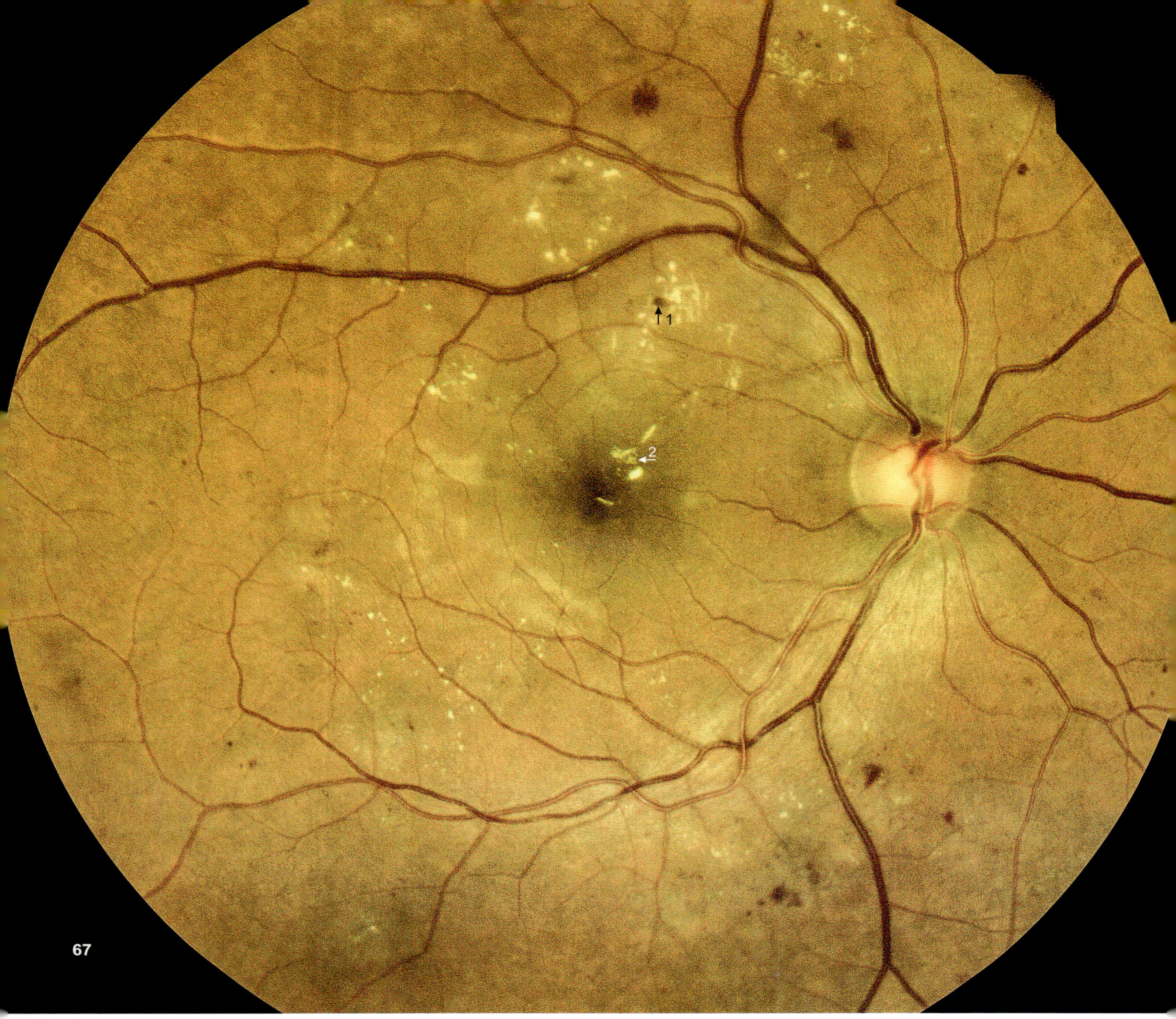


Figure 67 *Color fundus photograph of a case of moderate diabetic macular edema with hard exudates at the posterior pole scattered around the leaking microaneurysms (1), with retinal thickening and hard exudates encroaching the fovea superonasally (2). Its a non-center DME, threatening the fovea center.*

Figure 68 *Early frame of fundus fluorescein angiogram shows multiple hyperfluorescent dots due to presence of microaneurysms at the posterior pole. Foveal avascular zone is well preserved.*

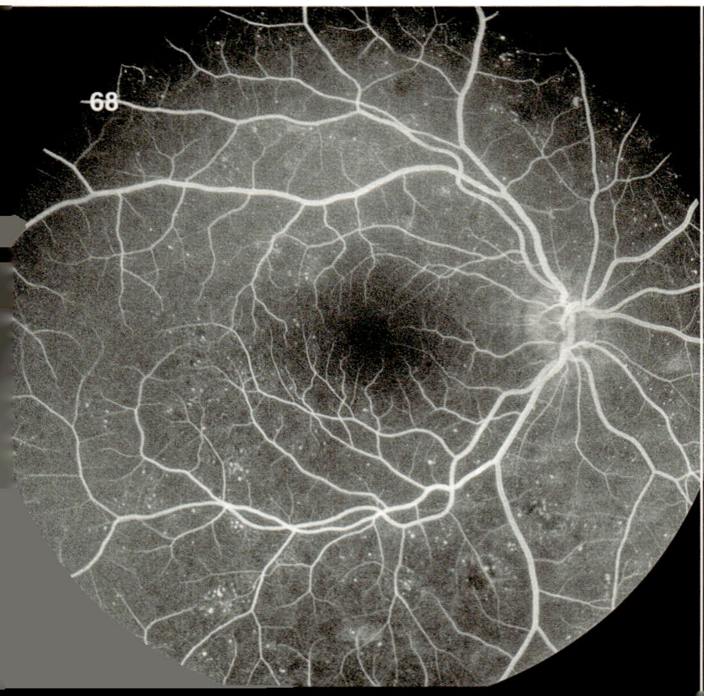

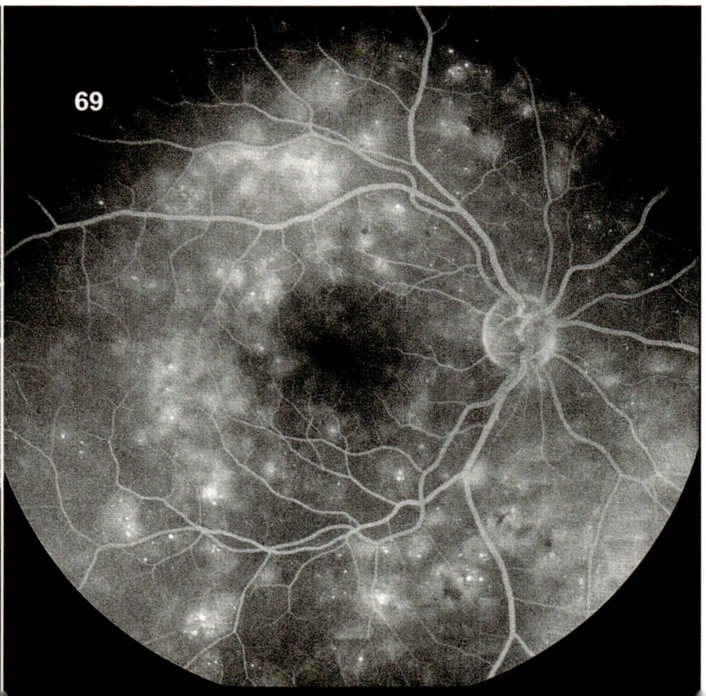

Figure 69

*Late phase of fluorescein angiogram demonstrates focal and diffuse late leakage at the posterior pole with sparing of the fovea in a case of non-center fovea threatening DME.*

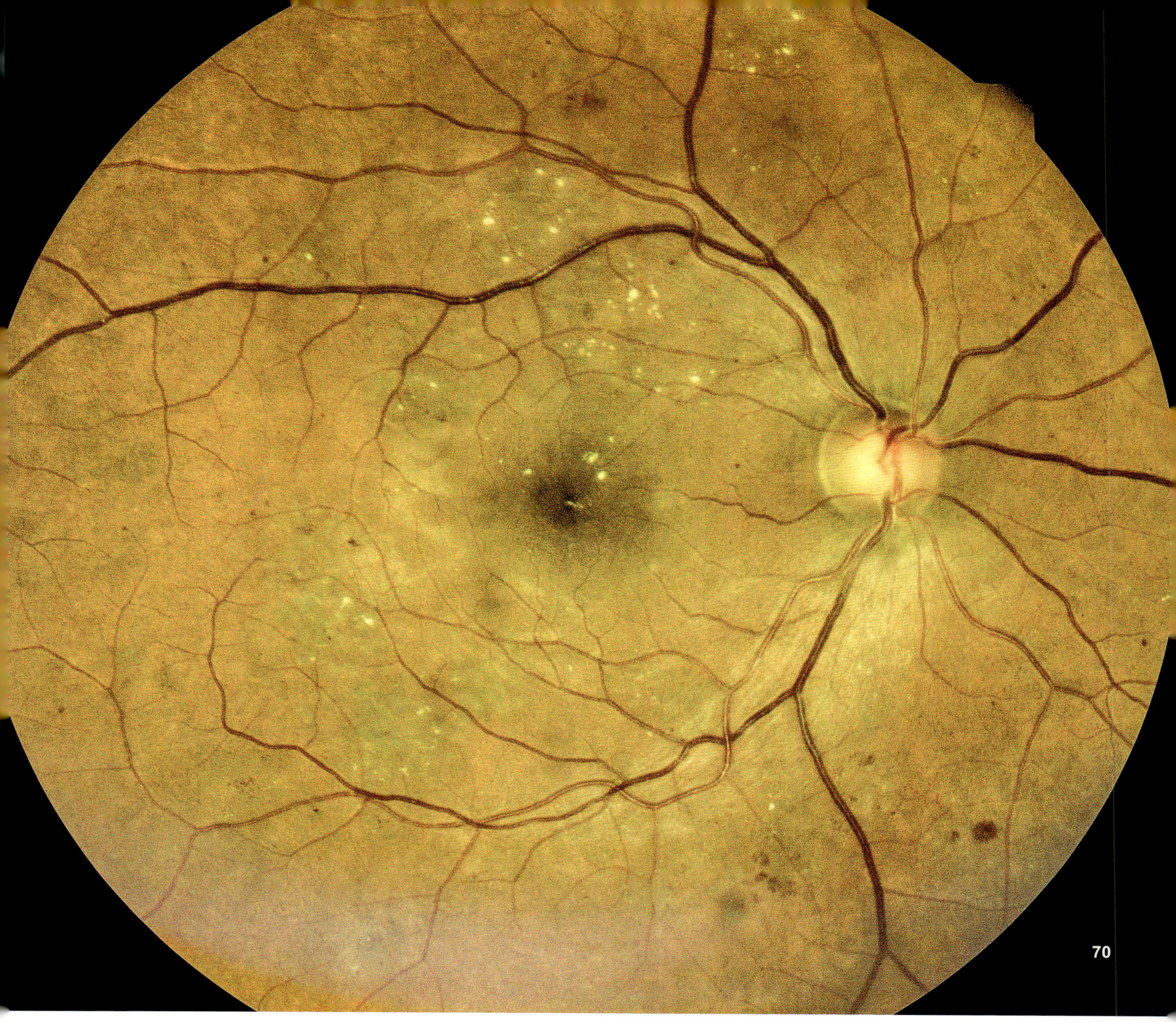

Figure 70 *Color fundus photograph of the same patient done at 3 months: Macular laser photocoagulation is still treatment of choice for noncenter involving DME. She was treated with macular laser burns of mild-moderate intensity, 50 micron spot size and 100 millisecond duration. Color photograph demonstrates reduction in the amount of hard exudates. Laser scars are visible where the treatment was offered and foveal exudates have also reduced.*

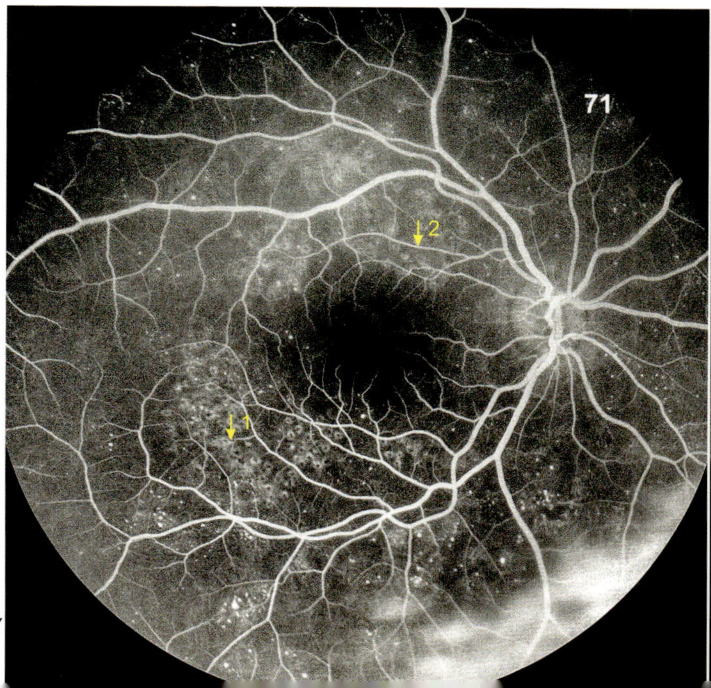

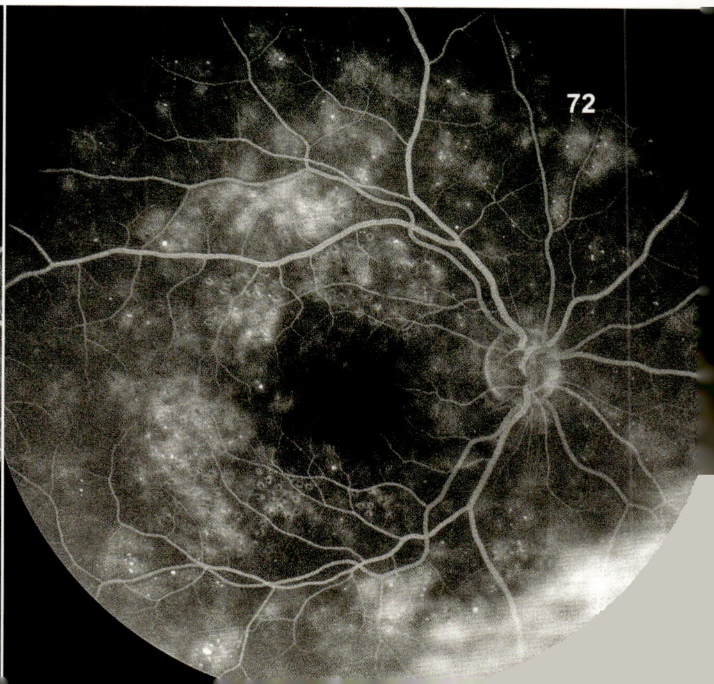

Figure 71

*Early frame of fundus fluorescein angiogram done at 3 months shows well-defined round laser scars in the infero-temporal area (1) and superior to macula (2).*

Figure 72

*Late phase of fluorescein angiogram shows drastic reduction in the amount of leakage as compared to the baseline FFA.* □

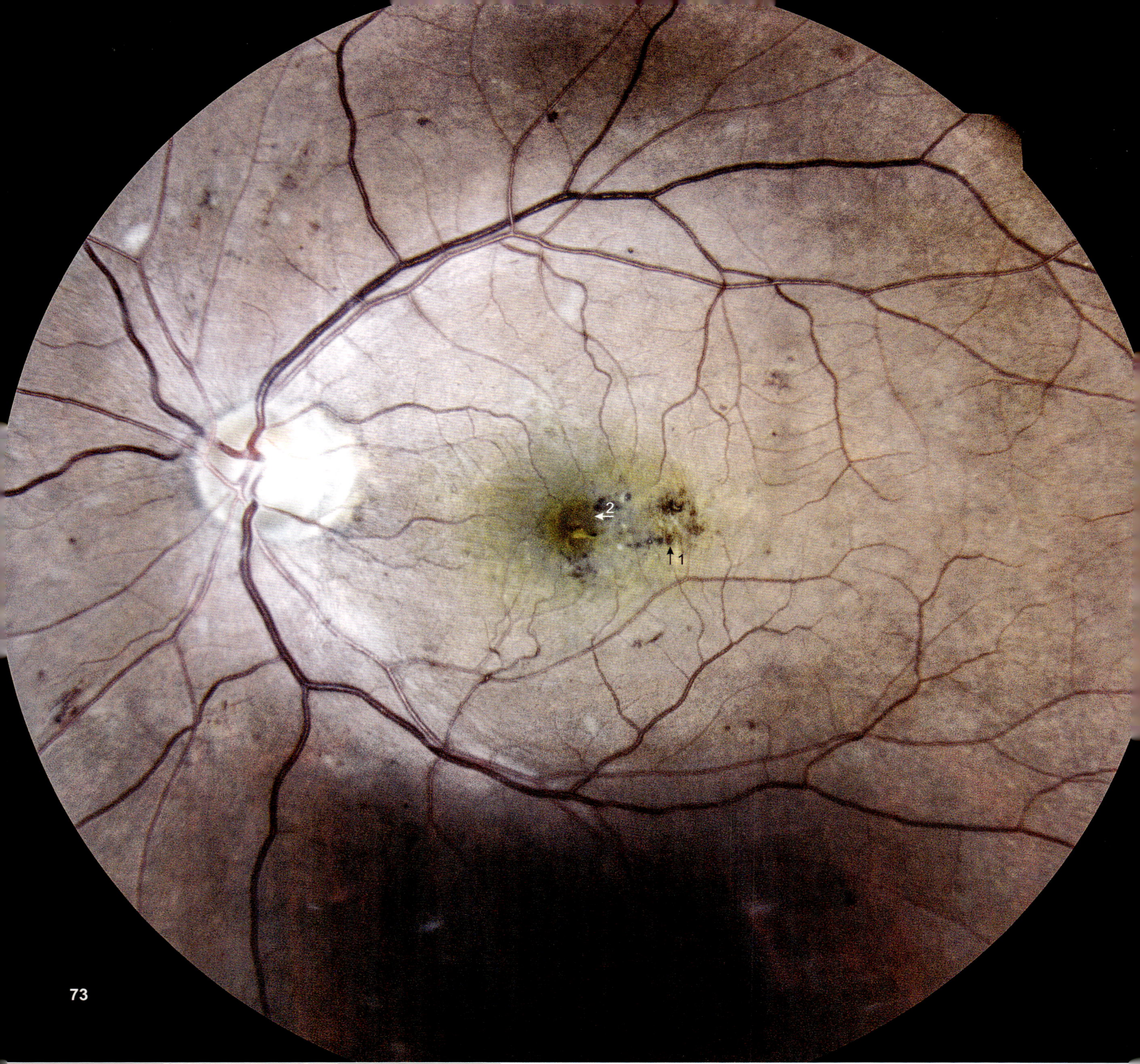


73

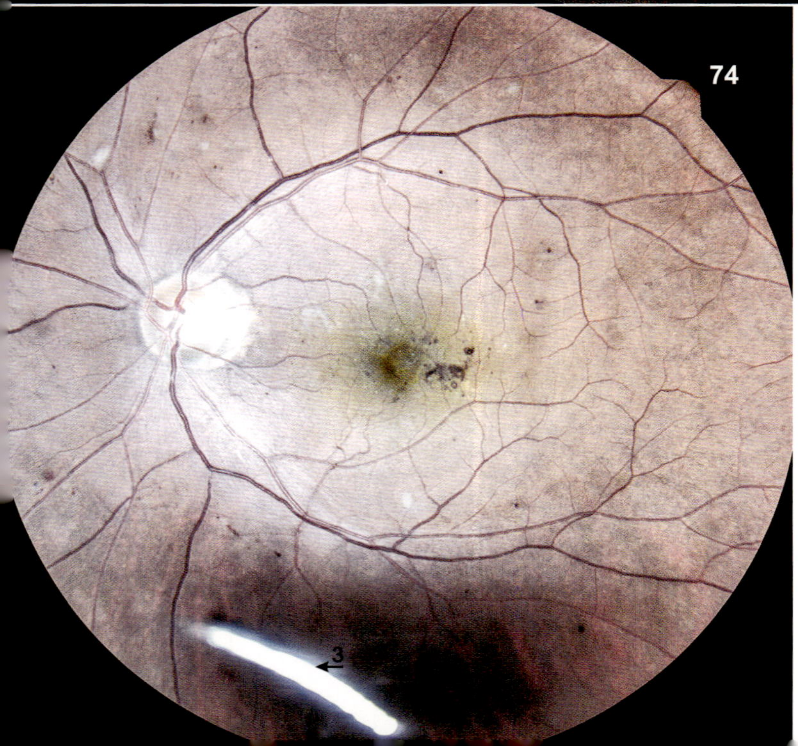


74

Figure 73 *Color fundus photograph of a patient with moderate NPDR and center involved DME. Note presence of multiple microaneurysms (1) at the fovea with associated retinal thickening and foveal cyst (2).*

Patient is pseudophakic and had gross DME as seen on the OCT scan. He underwent an intravitreal Ozurdex implant to reduce the macular edema. Note presence of Ozurdex implant (3) in the inferior mid-periphery.

Figure 74 *Color fundus photograph post-treatment: Note the reduction in retinal hemorrhages and presence of whitish vitreous opacity at the inferotemporal macula due to presence of the intravitreal Ozurdex implant that has migrated at the posterior pole.*

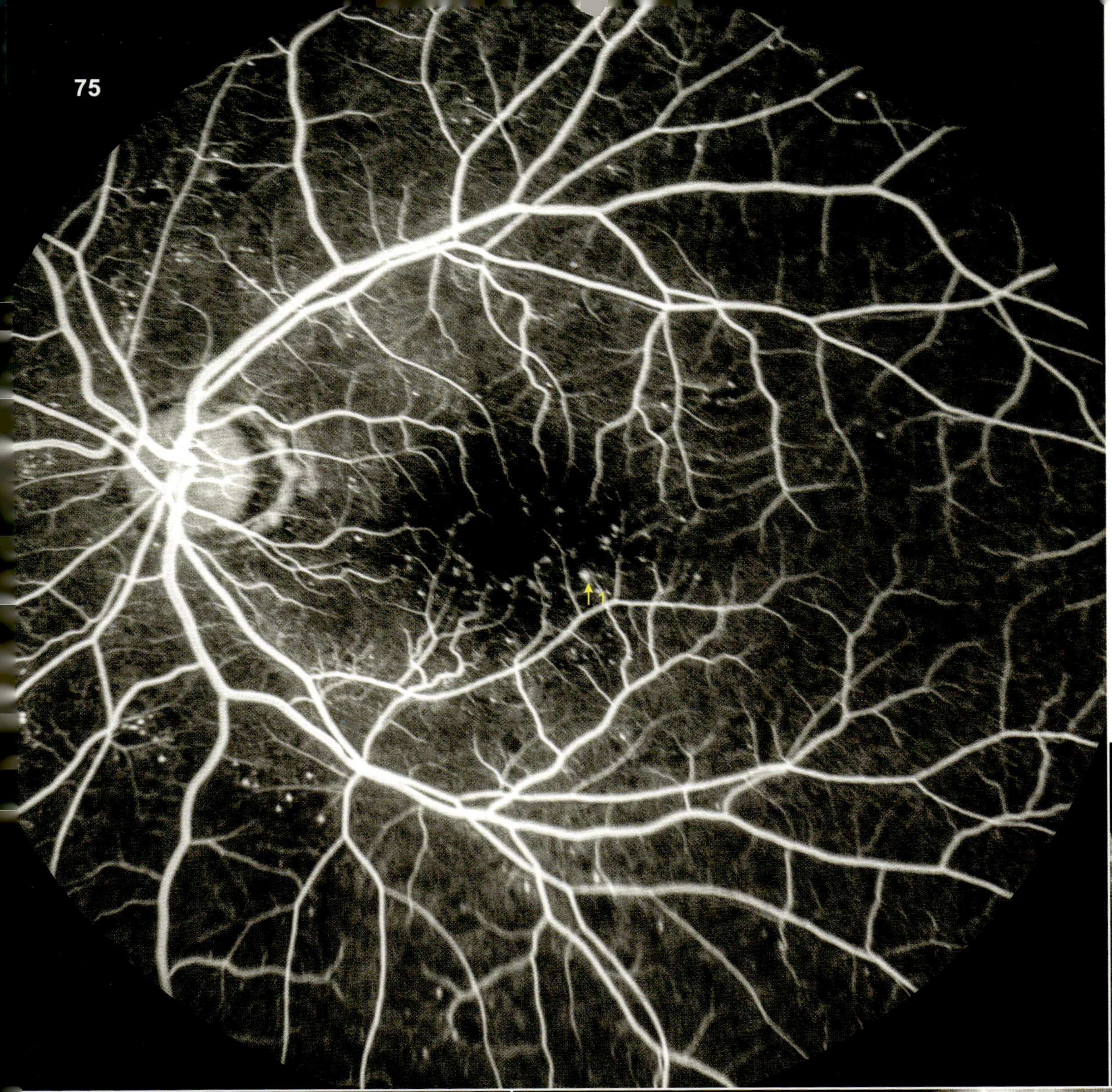


Figure 75

*Early frame of fundus fluorescein angiogram shows multiple hyper-fluorescent dot-like microaneurysm characteristically distribute around the foveal edge (1).*

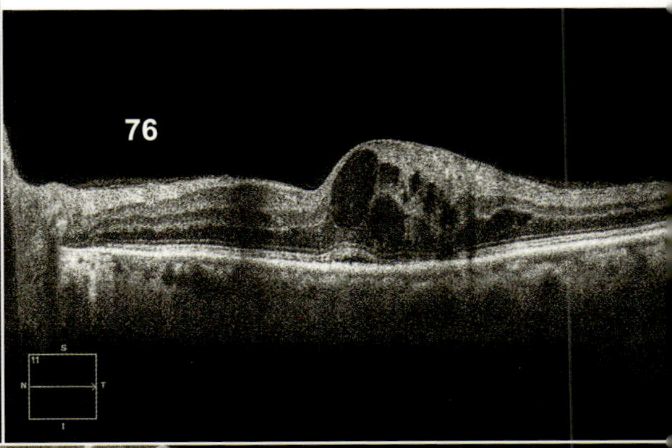


Figure 76

*Spectral domain OCT scan through the fovea demonstrates large cystic fluid spaces and a small subretinal fluid pocket at the fovea.*

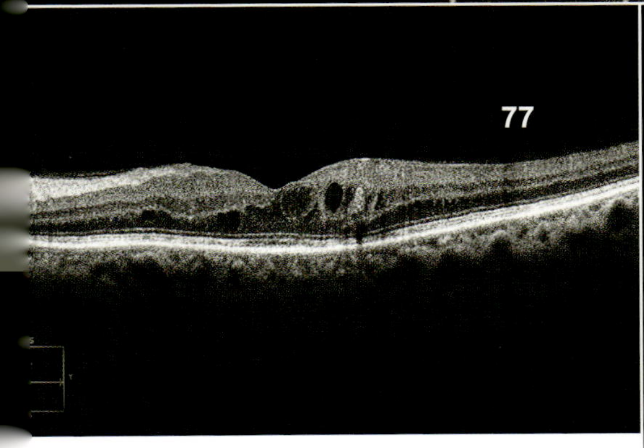


Figure 77

*Spectral domain OCT scan done 1 month after treatment with Ozurdex implant shows massive reduction in the retinal fluid with normal foveal contour. Although few cystic fluid pockets are still persisting.*

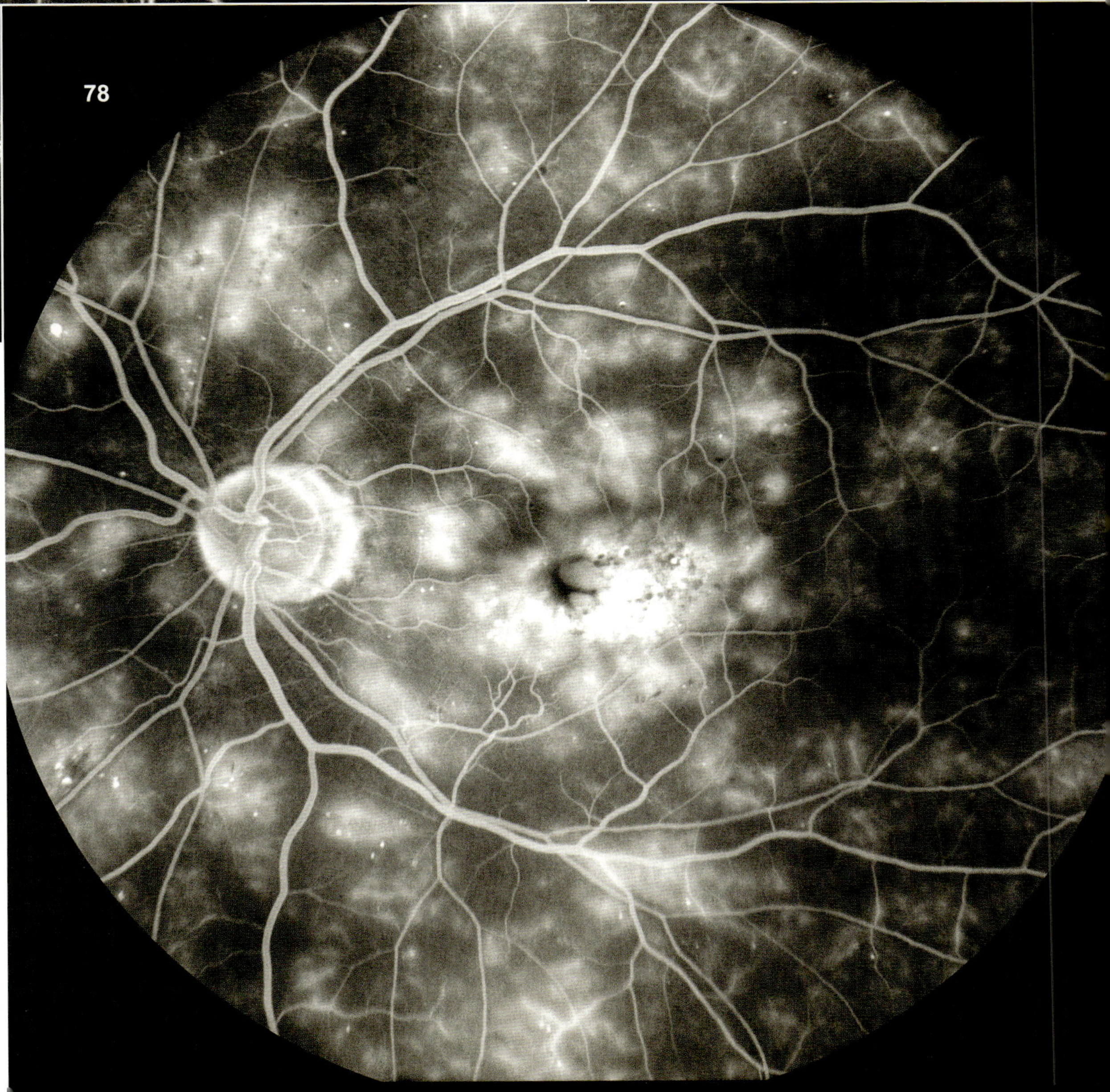


Figure 78

*Late phase of the fluorescein angiogram shows petalloid pattern of leakage due the leakage of retinal fluid and its accumulation in the outer Henle layer.* □

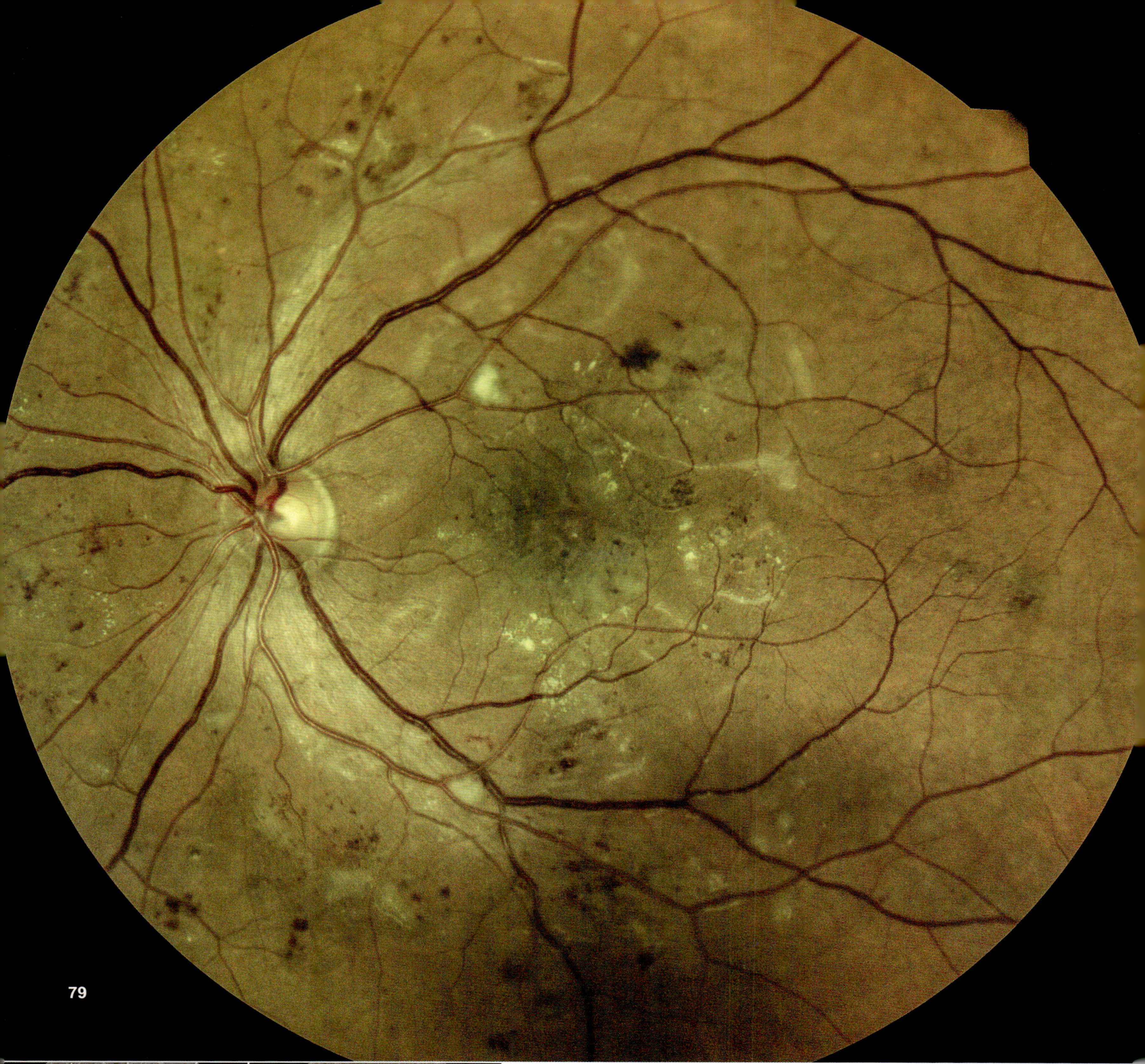

79

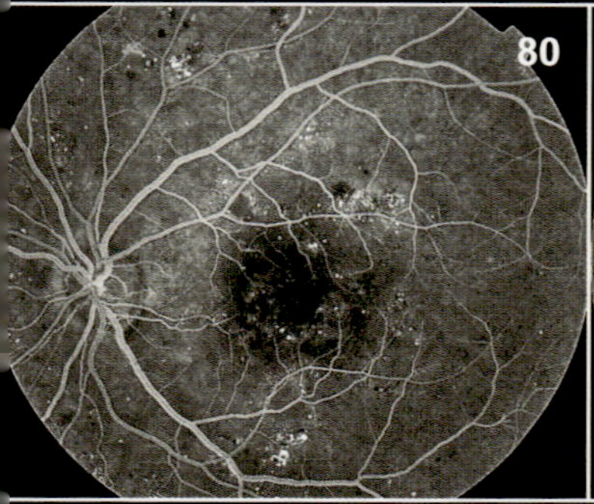

80

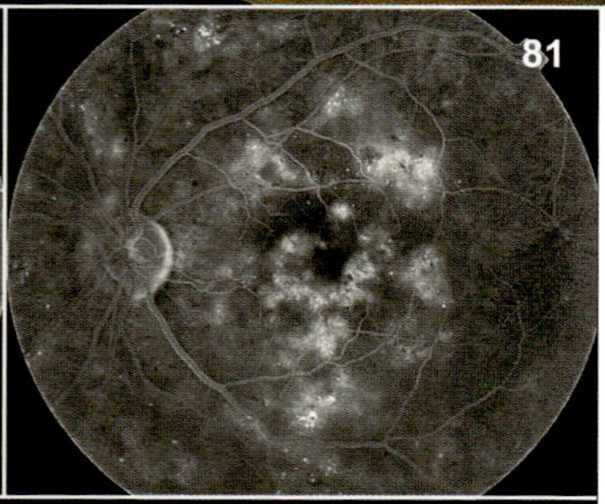

81

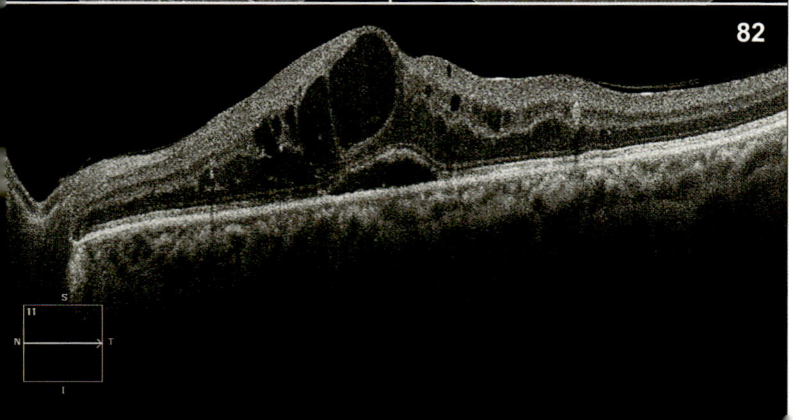

82

Figure 79 *Case of moderate NPDR with macular edema: color fundus shows retinal hemorrhages, cotton wool spots, microaneurysms, dot hemorrhages consistent with diagnosis of moderate NPDR. Foveal reflex is dull and there is retinal thickening at the macula.*

Figure 80 *Early frame of fundus fluorescein angiogram demonstrates hyper-fluorescent dots due to microaneurysms at the fovea and scattered all around the posterior pole.*

Figure 81 *Late phase of FFA shows leakage at the macula arising from the leaky microaneurysms suggestive of diabetic macular edema with foveal involvement.*

Figure 82 *Spectral domain OCT scan passing through the foveal center shows massive intraretinal cystic fluid and subretinal fluid confirming macular edema.* □

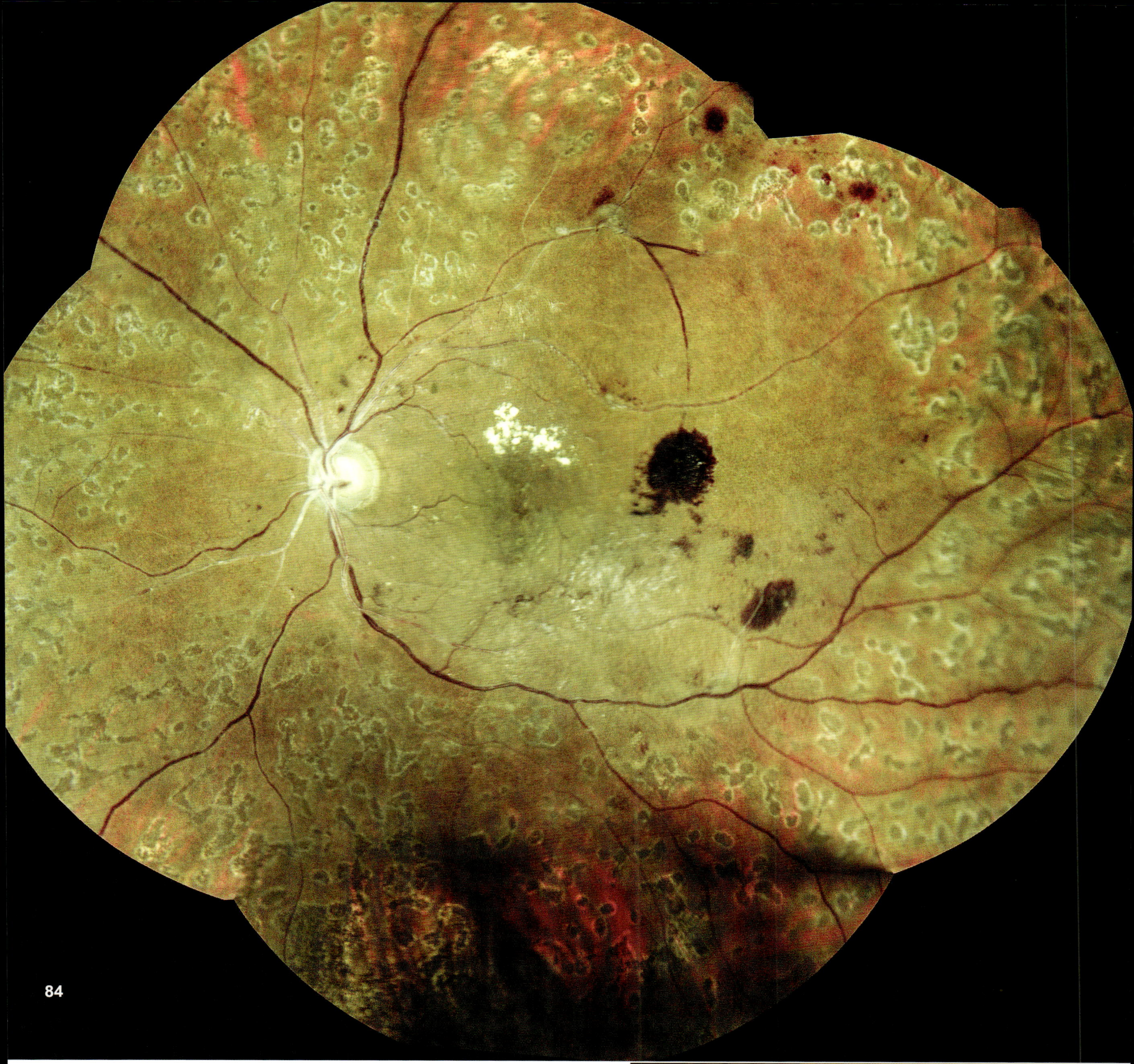

84

Figure 83 *A case of proliferative diabetic retinopathy with dense vitreous hemorrhage and fibrovascular proliferation managed with microincision pars vitrectomy.*

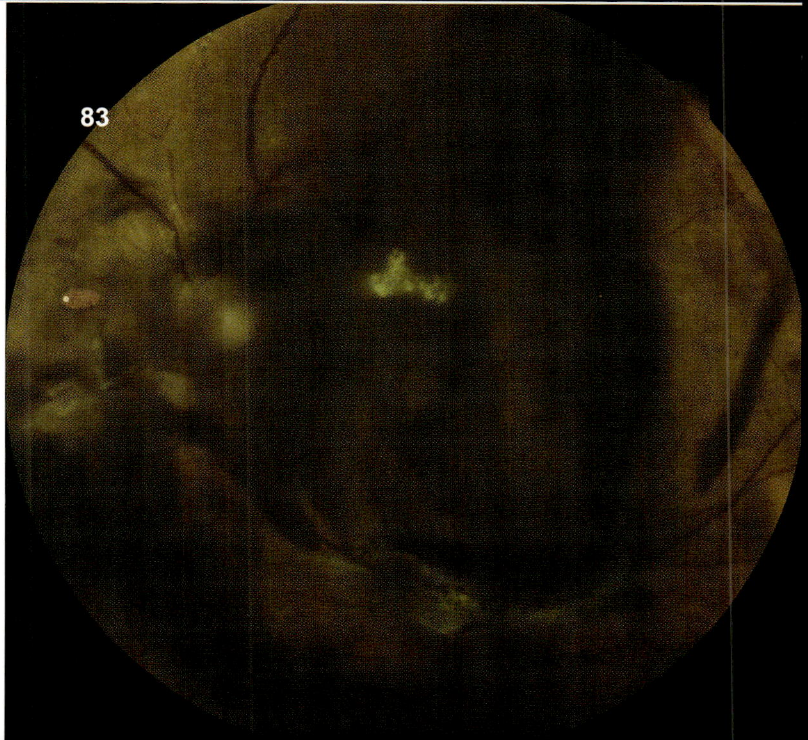

83

A 58-year-old female, known case of diabetes mellitus type 2, complained of sudden appearance of floaters in her left eye along with diminution of vision since 15 days.

Fundus photo of left eye shows vitreous hemorrhage obscuring most of view of macula. Hard exudates at the macula can be seen faintly through the bleed. Grayish white fibrous proliferation can be seen along the inferotemporal arcade. She gave no history of prior laser photocoagulation.

Figure 84 *Treatment naïve eyes with vitreous hemorrhage blocking most of the view of fundus require vitrectomy on emergent basis. One month post-vitrectomy media clarity is grade 1, 360 degree endolaser PRP marks are seen, hard exudates and retinal hemorrhage at the macula are seen. Arteriosclerosis can be seen along most of the blood vessels resulting from ischemic diabetic damage.*□

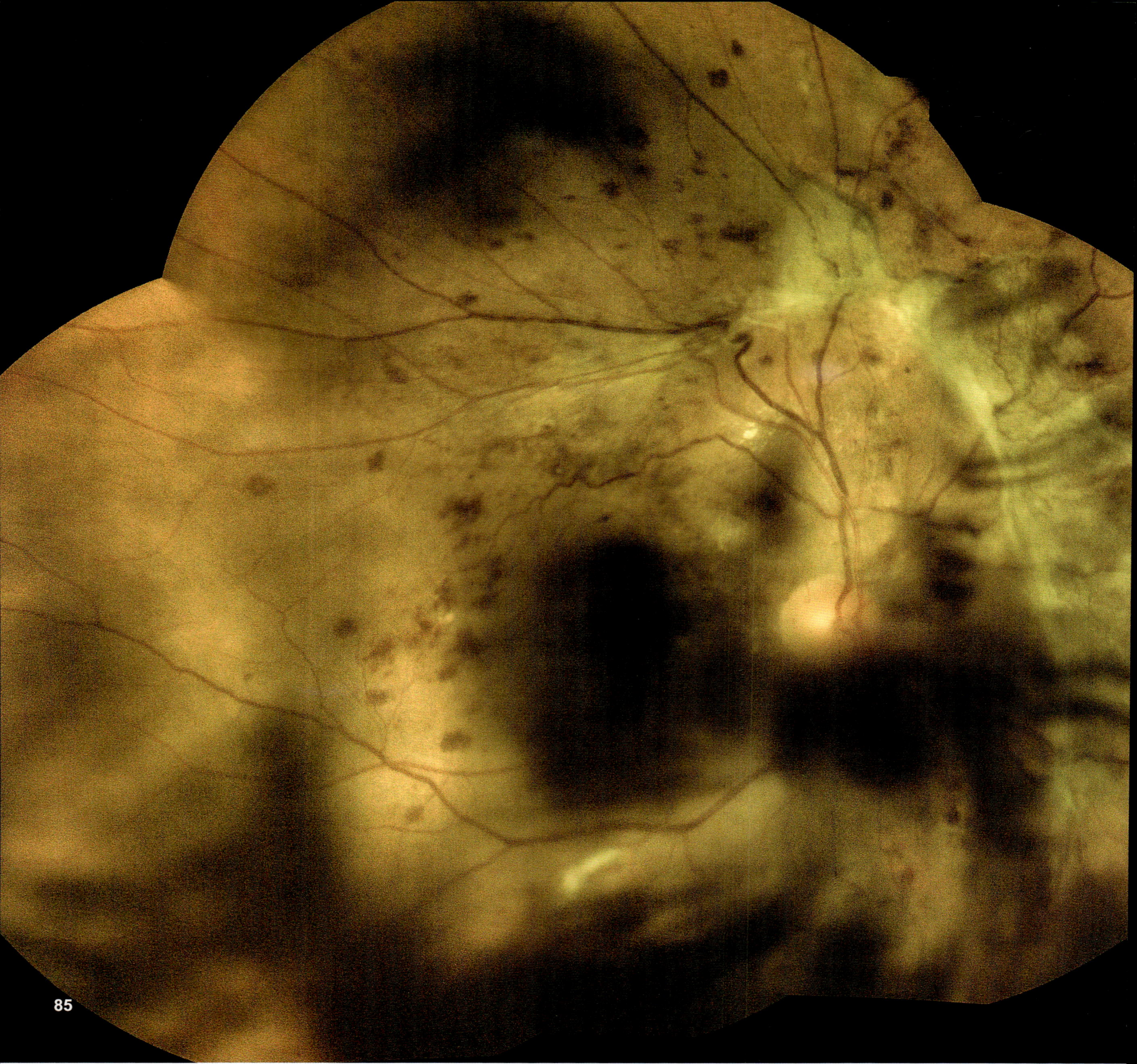

Figure 85 *A 58-year-old male, best corrected visual acuity of counting finger two meters, fundus photo of OD shows advanced proliferative diabetic retinopathy with fibrovascular proliferation along the nasal and superonasal aspect of retina. It is dragging retina along superotemporal arcade. Cotton wool spots and dot blot hemorrhages can be seen throughout the fundus. Vitreous hemorrhage is present obscuring most of the view of macula and inferior retina.*

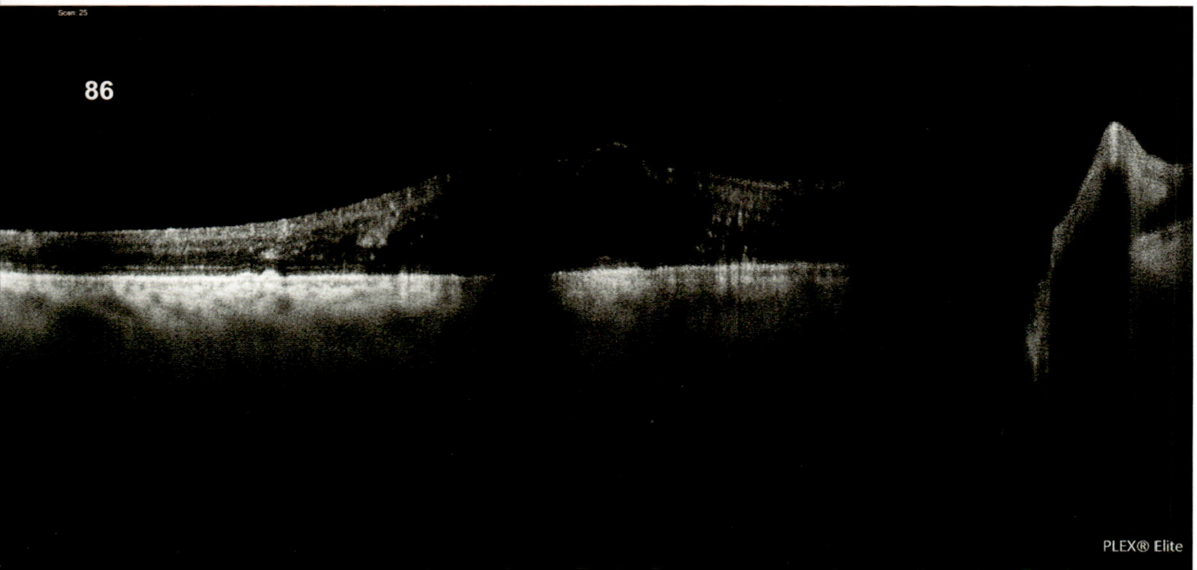


Figure 86 *OCT scan preoperatively demonstrates areas of vitreous hemorrhage obscuring underlying retina with significant large hyporeflective cystoid spaces suggestive of macular edema.*□

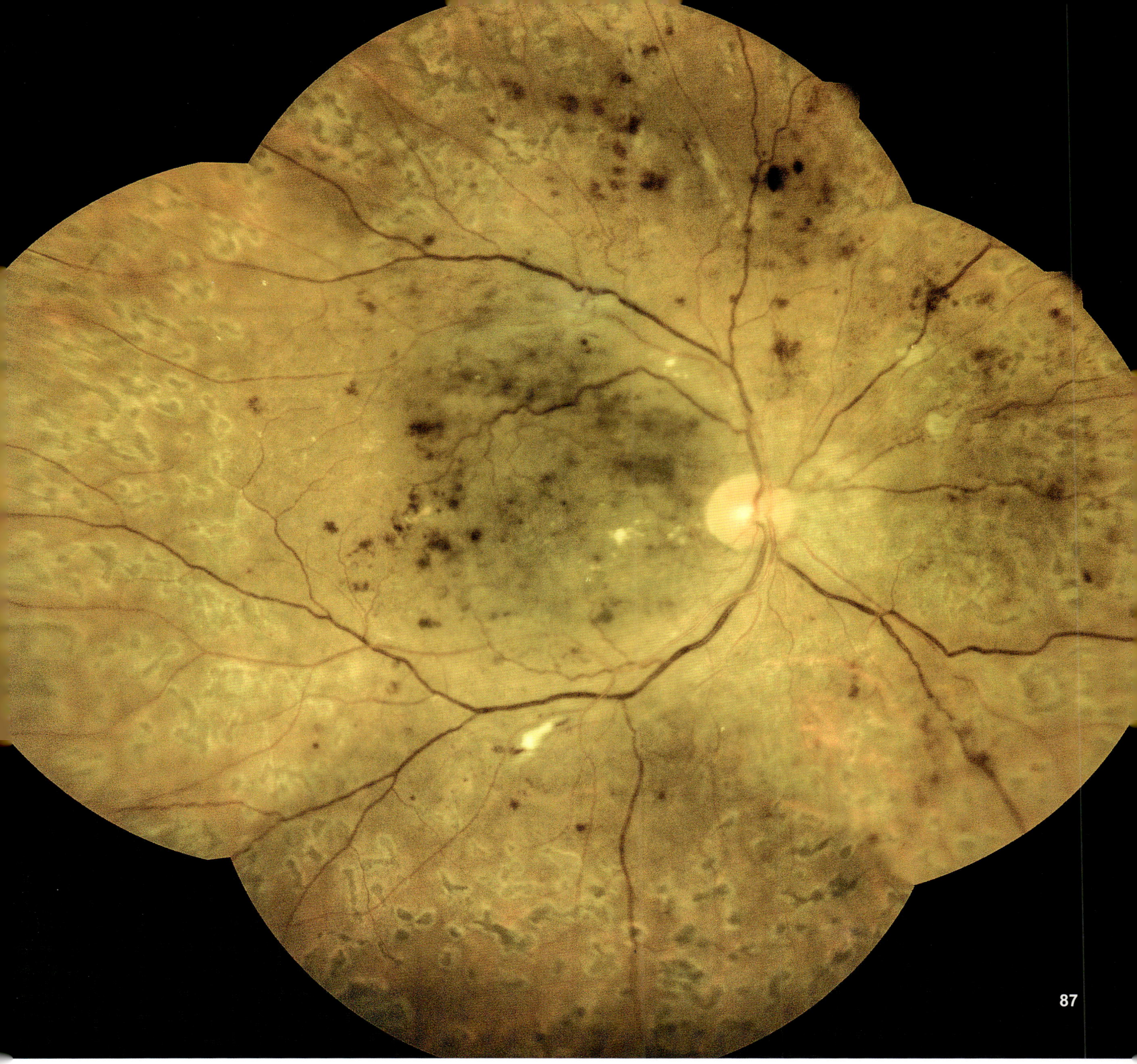


Figure 87 *Six weeks post-25 gauge pars plana vitrectomy media clarity improve to grade, PRP marks can be seen all around. Some residual dot and blot hemorrhages persist which may resolve with metabolic control.*

Figure 88 *OCT postoperatively demonstrates macular edema which requires management with intravitreal injections.*□

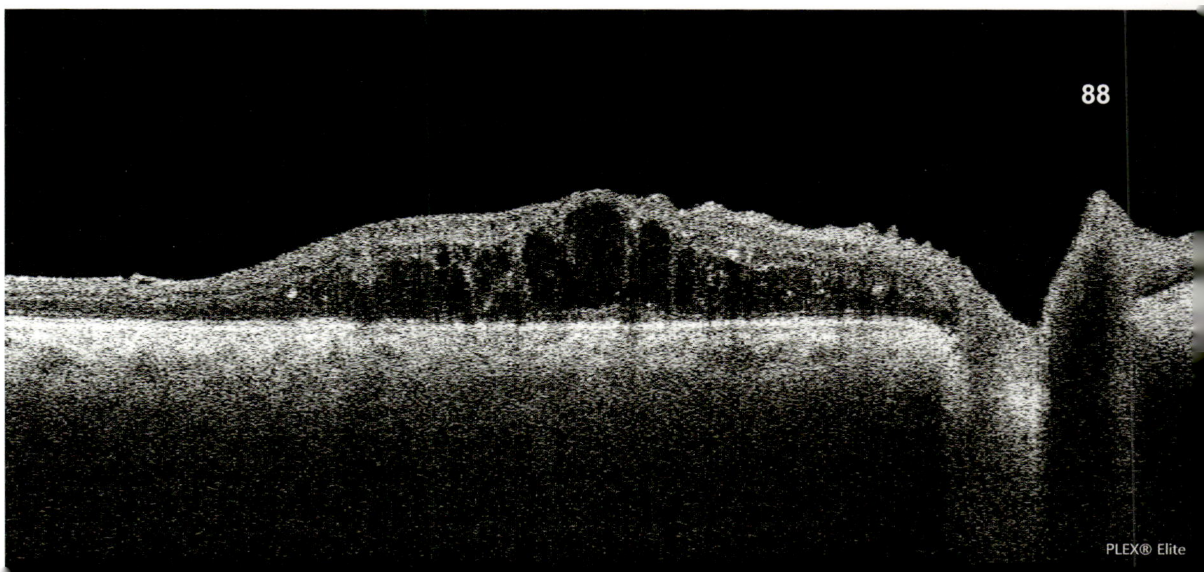

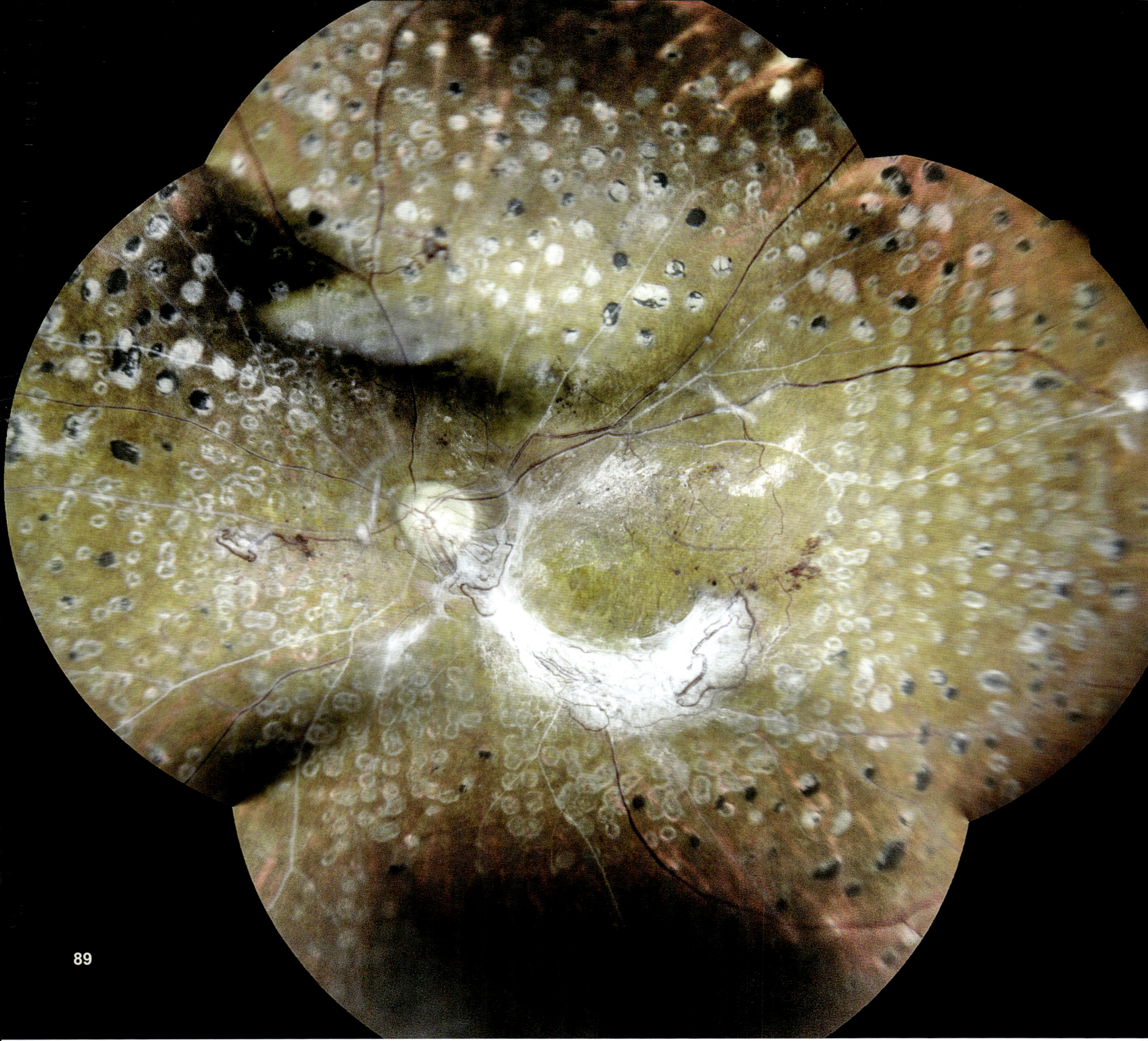

89

Figure 89 *A case of proliferative diabetic retinopathy with recalcitrant macular edema secondary to fibrovascular proliferation managed with micro-incision pars plana vitrectomy.*

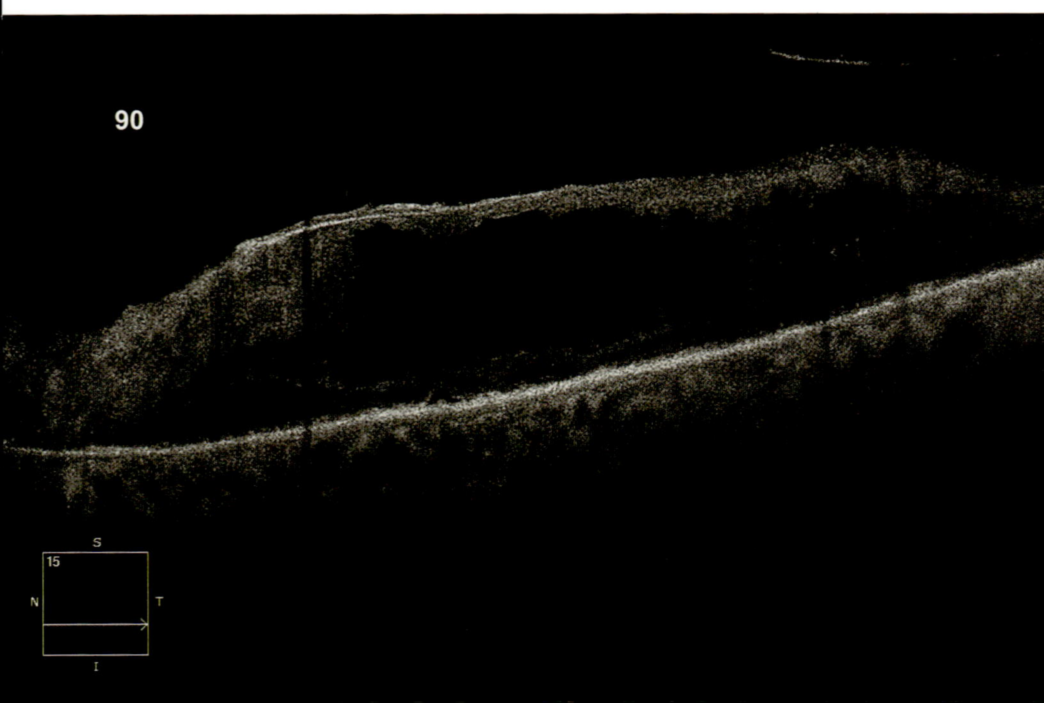


A 68-year-old male with uncontrolled diabetes complained of gradual diminution of vision in both eyes for 1 month. Advanced proliferative diabetic retinopathy changes are seen in left eye. Grayish white fibrovascular proliferation can be seen inferotemporal to the disk involving the fovea, small cystic spaces on the fovea can be seen clinically. Endolaser marks can be seen 360 degree. Neovascular fronds can still be seen in nasal and superonasal retina.

Sclerosed retinal vessels are seen 360 degree and optic nerve head also appears pale due to advance diabetic ischemic damage.

Figure 90 *OCT demonstrates retinal schisis, distortion of architecture of all layers of retina, and a thick hyper-reflective layer on retinal surface indicative of epiretinal fibrovascular proliferation.*

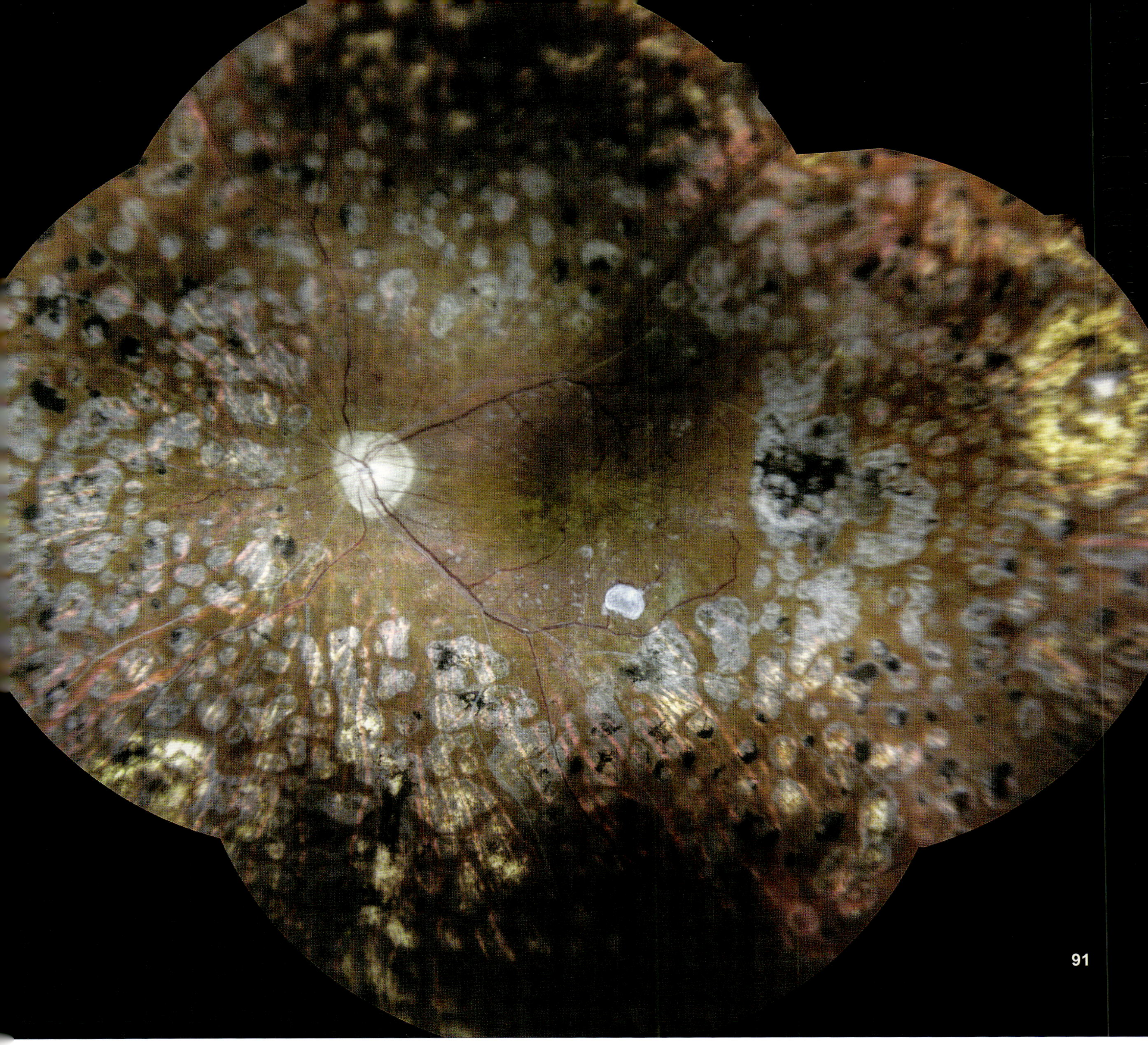


Figure 91 *Six months postoperatively silicone oil removal was done, media clarity was grade 1, 360 endolaser marks and residual stump could be seen.*

Figure 92 *OCT reduction in retinal schisis, few hypo-reflective spaces temporally and disruption of IS-OS junction and retinal pigment epithelium layer which was present preoperatively.*□

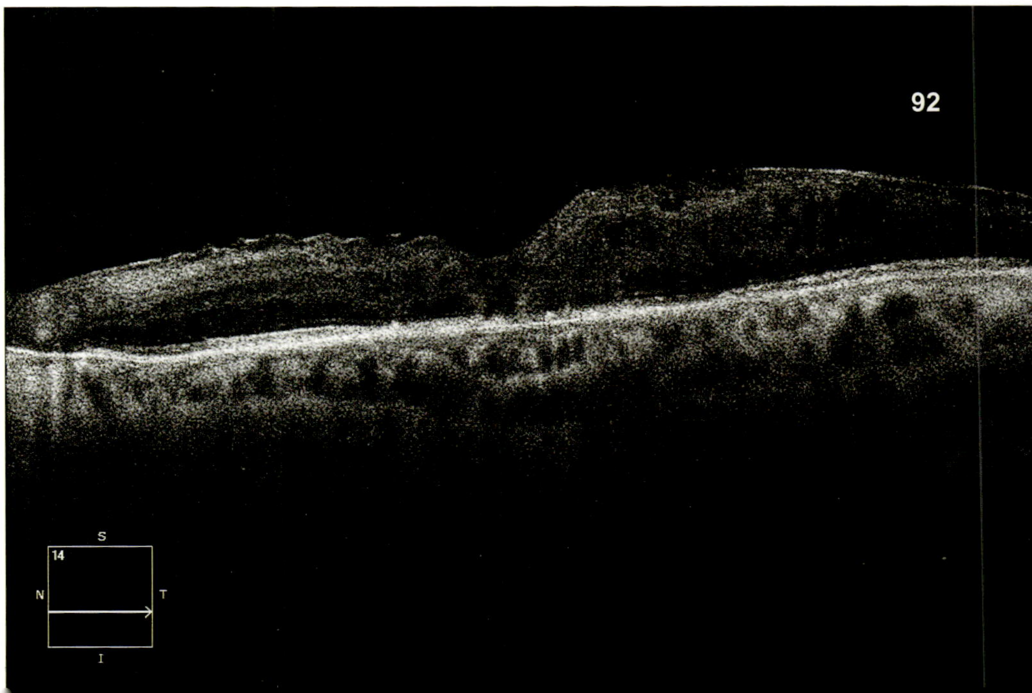

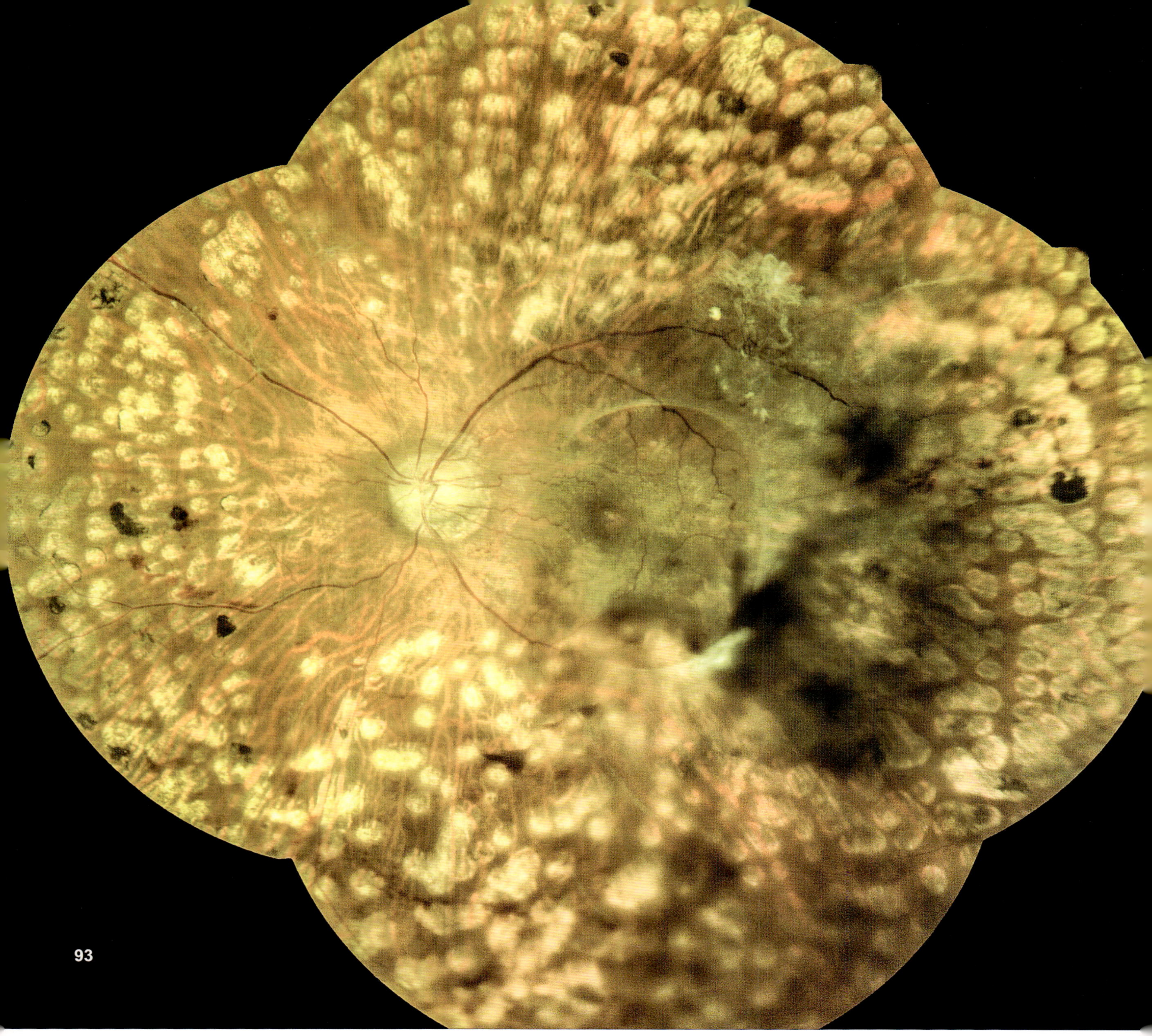

93

Figure 93 *A case of proliferative diabetic retinopathy with tractional maculopathy managed with pars plana vitrectomy. Faint amount of vitreous hemorrhage can also be seen temporal to the macula.*

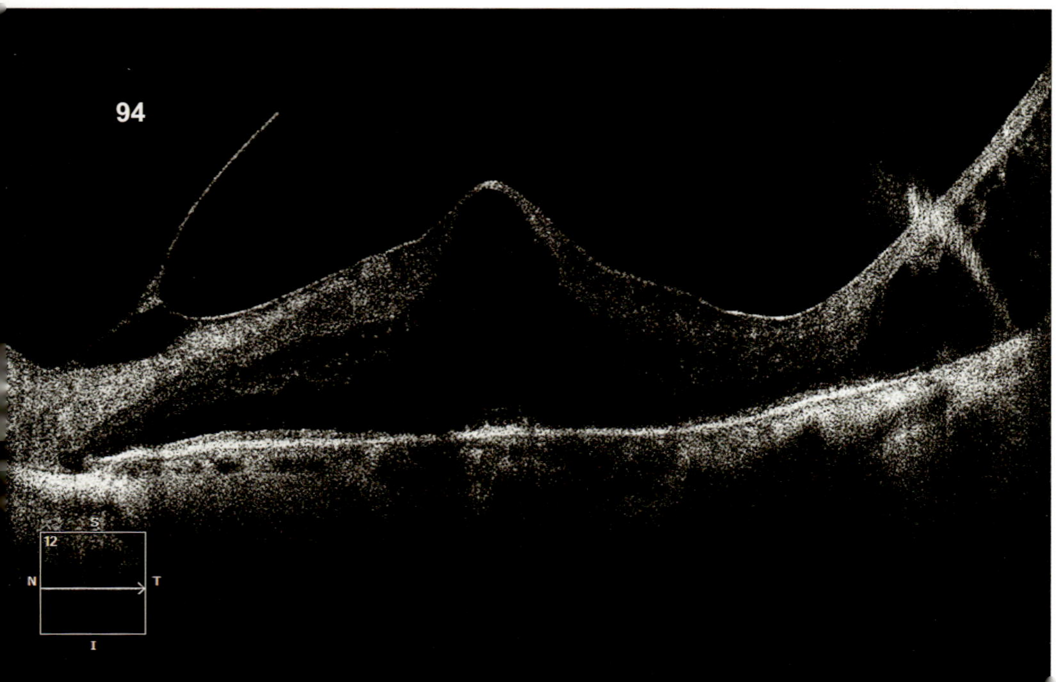



A 62-year-old male presented with complaints of blurring of vision from his left eye for 4 months. He was known case of diabetes mellitus type 2. Fundus photo shows taut grayish thick fibrous membrane temporal fovea and extending towards it. 360 degree endolaser marks can be seen.

Figure 94 *OCT scan preoperatively shows large vertically elongated cystoid space at fovea and thick hyper-reflective membrane on surface of retina suggestive of epiretinal membrane. Retinal schisis can be appreciated temporal to the fovea.*

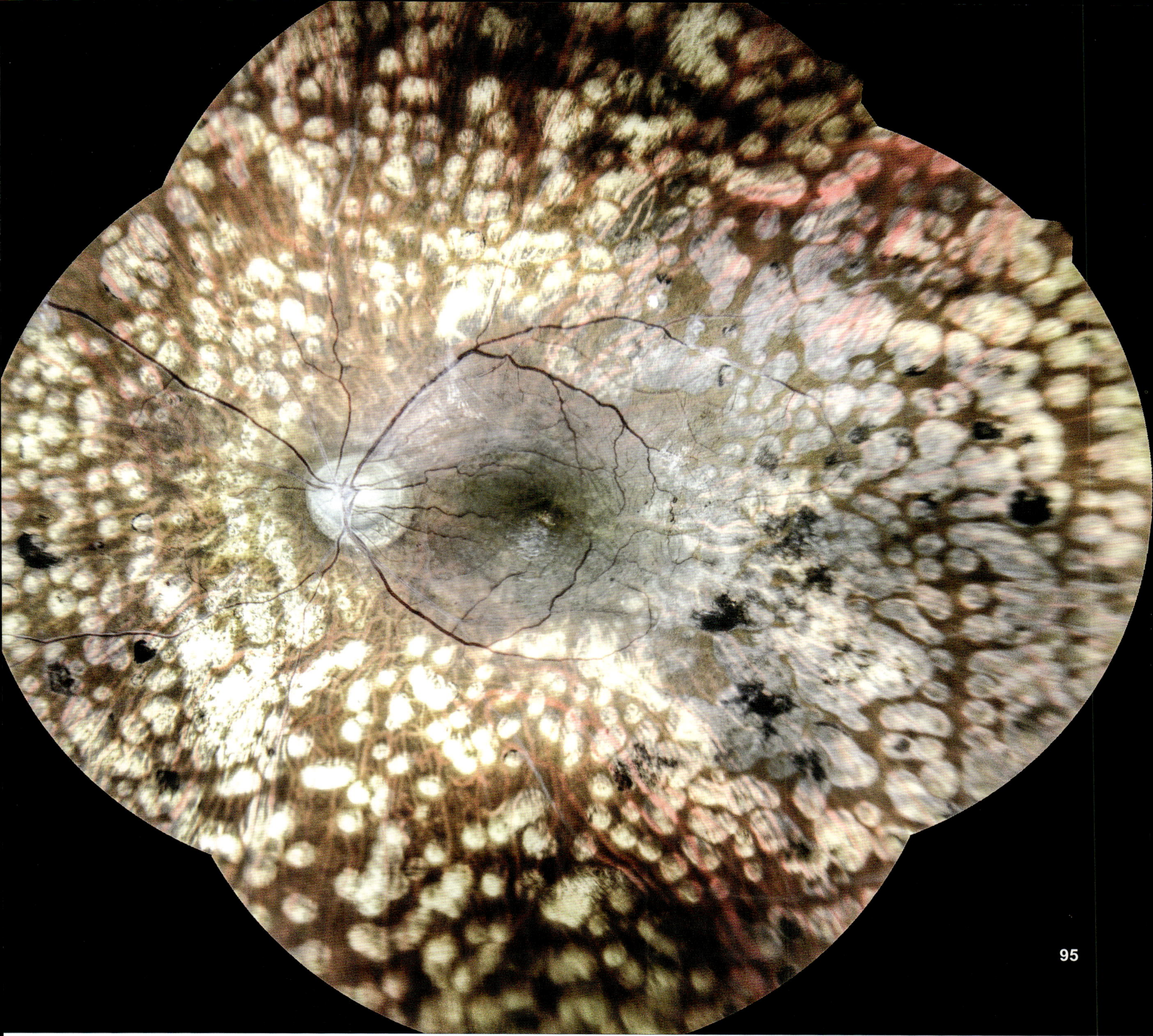

Figure 95 *25-gauge pars plana vitrectomy was done and fibrous proliferation was very gently peeled using transvitreal forceps and proportional reflux hydrodissection mode in Alcon constellation vitrectomy module. Fundus photo shows media clarity grade 1 with complete removal of epiretinal membrane with restoration of normal anatomy.*

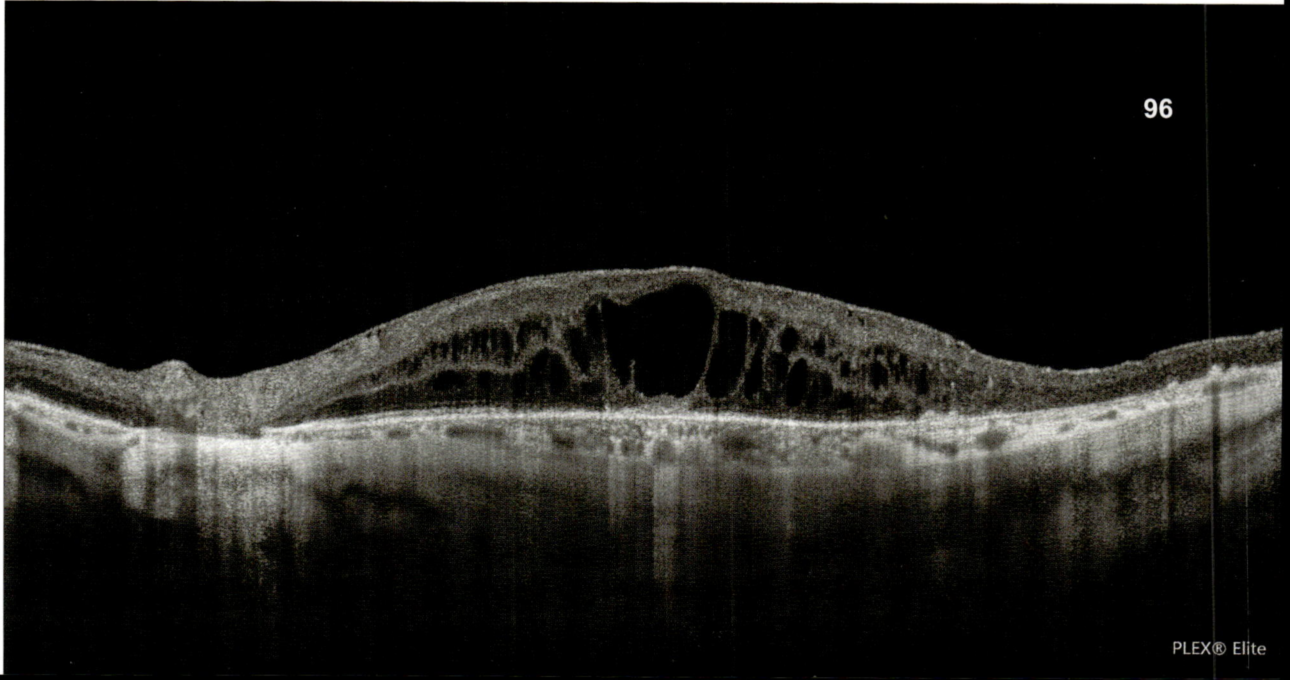


Figure 96 *OCT scan postoperatively shows reduction in cystoid spaces and complete removal of epiretinal membrane.* □

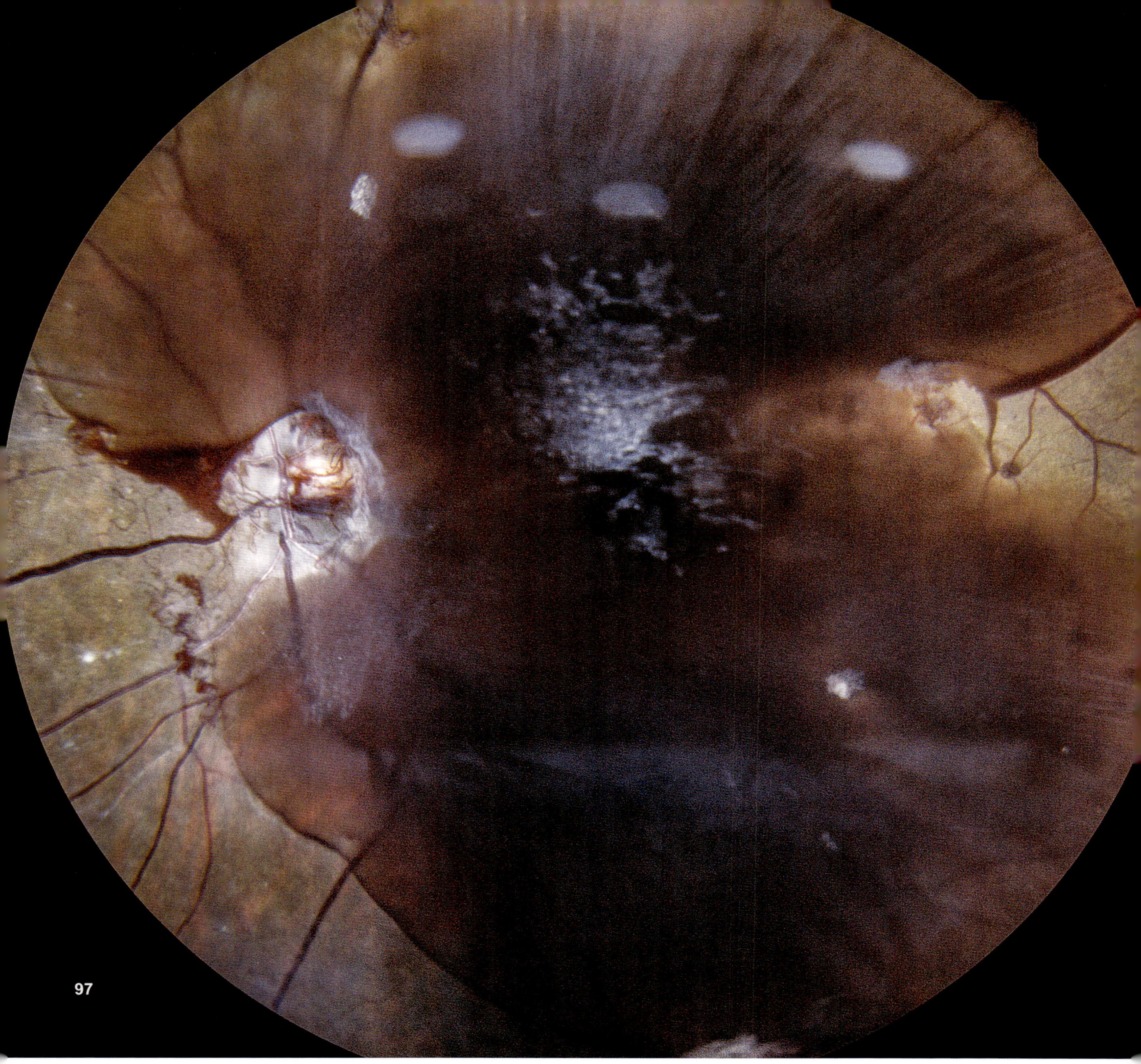



Figure 97 *A case of treatment naive advance proliferative diabetic retinopathy with preretinal hemorrhage managed with 25-gauge pars plana vitrectomy.*

A 62-year-old male presented with complaints of sudden drop in vision in his right eye for the last 2 days. Fundus photo shows advance proliferative diabetic retinopathy changes. Fresh preretinal dense hemorrhage can be seen in the right eye. neovascularization can be seen at the disk, nasal to disk and superiorly. Adherent fibrovascular tissue proliferation can be seen on the disk margin in the right eye.

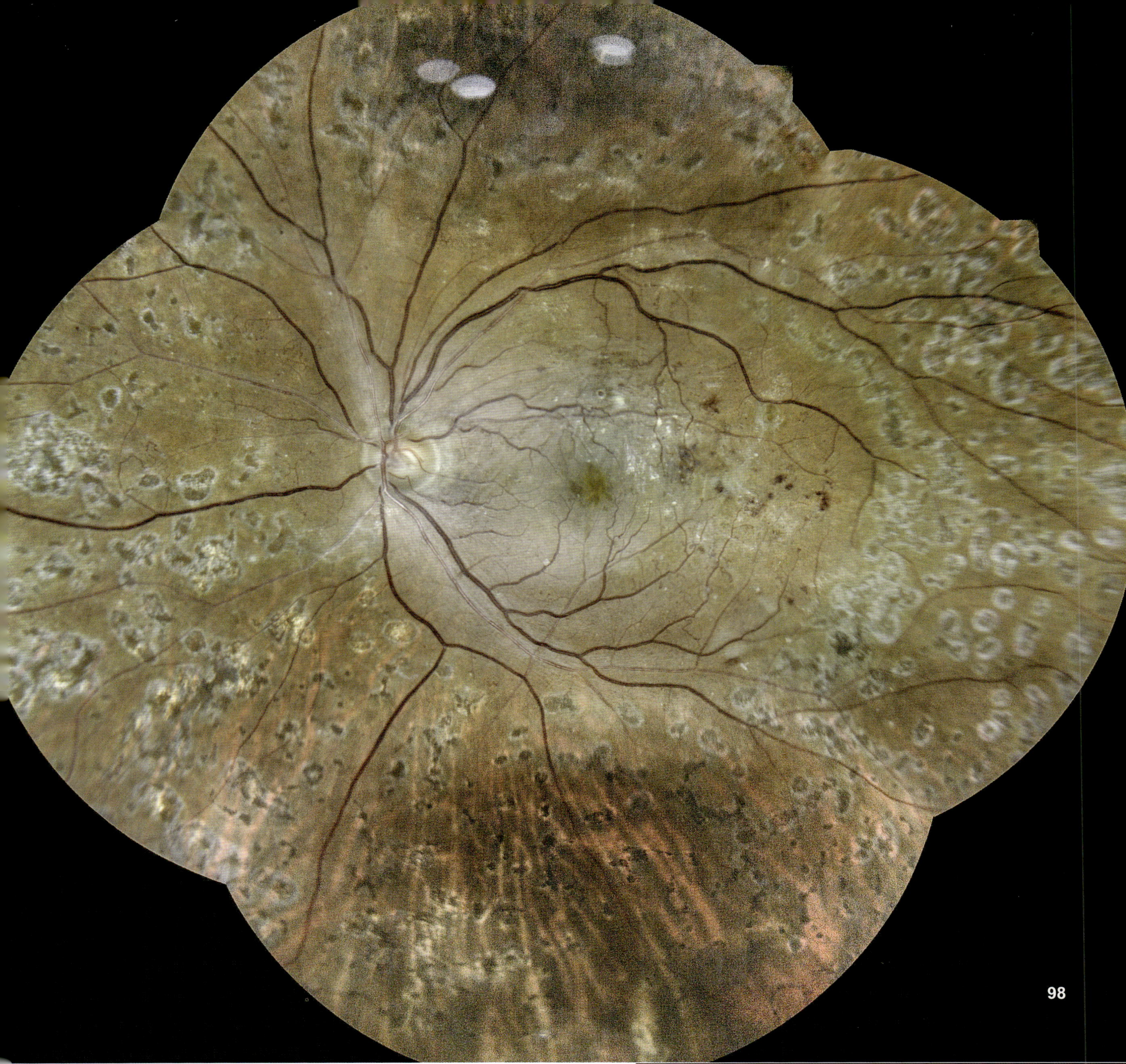

98

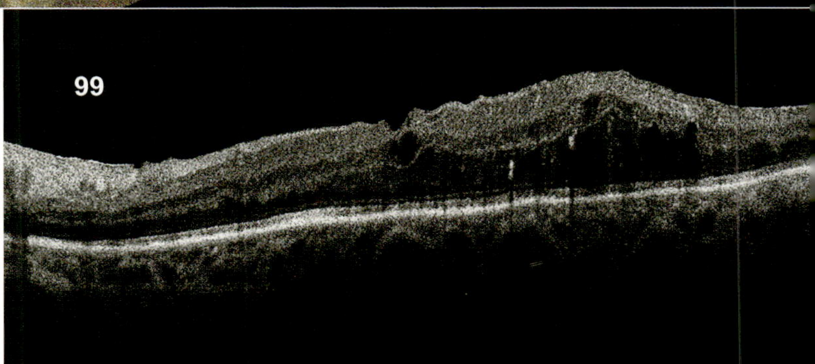

99

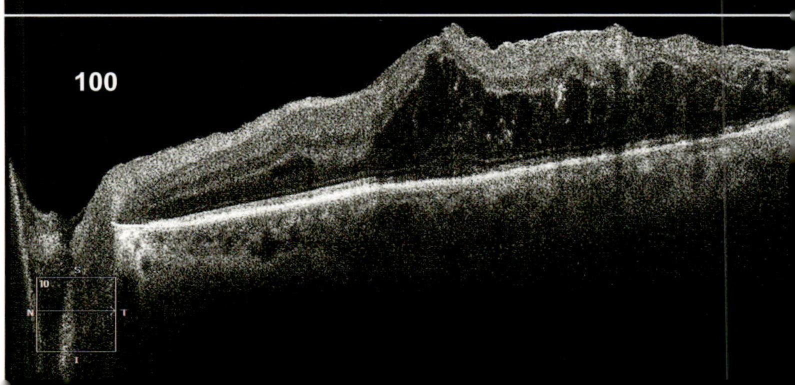

100

Figure 98 *Following 25-gauge pars plana vitrectomy the vitreous hemorrhage has been completely cleared with media clarity grade 1 and 360 endolaser marks of intraoperative panretinal photocoagulation are visible.*

Figure 99 *OCT could be acquired postoperatively after media clarity improved and showed few cystoid spaces and mild retinal thickening temporally.*

Figure 100 *Two months postoperative OCT showed increase in cystoid spaces and macular thickening. Diabetic macular edema postoperatively will require treatment with intravitreal injection of anti-VEGF or steroids.* □

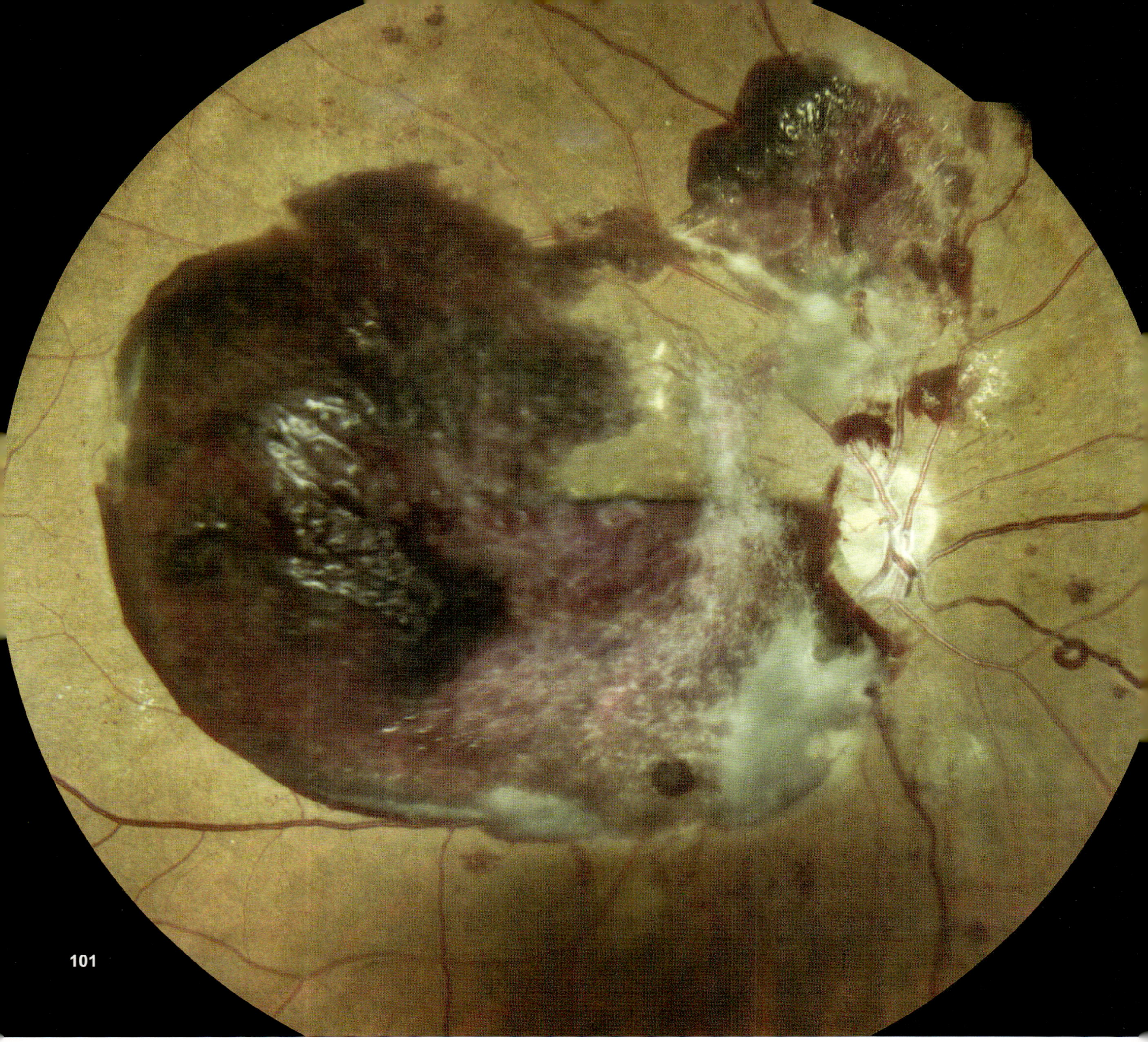


Figure 101 *Case of proliferative diabetic retinopathy with preretinal bleed with fibrovascular proliferation managed with microincision pars plana vitrectomy.*

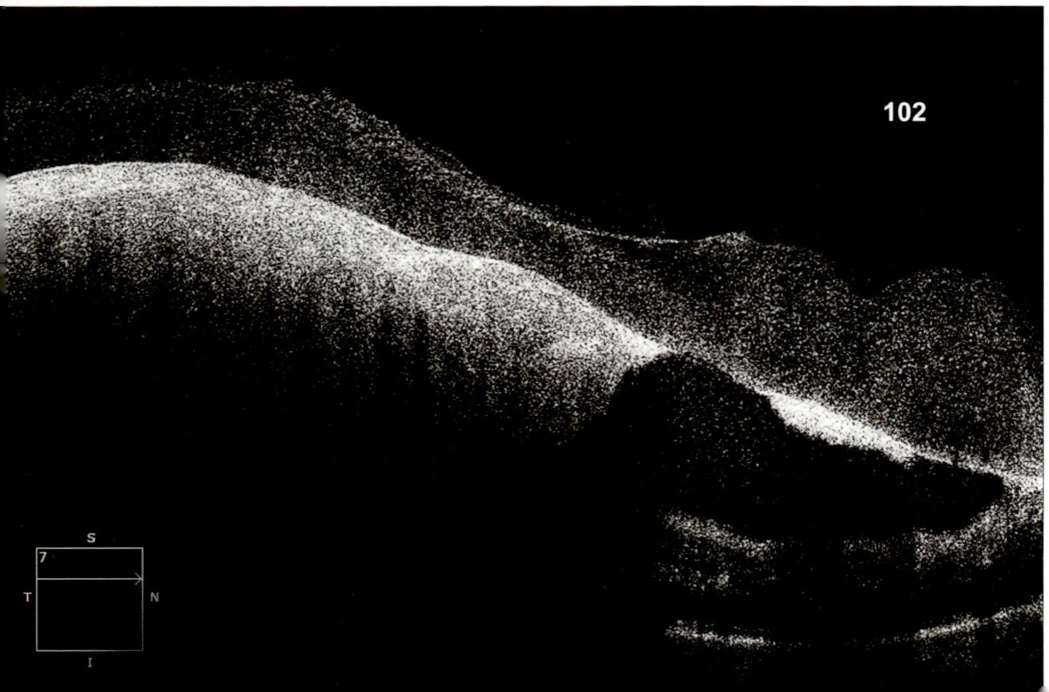


A 56-year-old female presented with complaints of sudden diminution of vision from her right eye for 5 days. Fundus photo of right eye shows dense preretinal subhyaloid bleed which tend to confirm to contours of hyaloid attachment. Grayish fibrovascular tissue proliferation can be seen along the inferotemporal arcade as well superior to the optic nerve head. Arteriosclerosis can be seen along the vessel wall. Venous beading is also apparent suggestive of ischemic insult.

Figure 102 *SS-OCT preoperatively shows hyper-reflective dense preretinal hemorrhage contained in subhyaloid space, faint view of retina on nasal aspect is seen owing to good penetration of SS-OCT.*

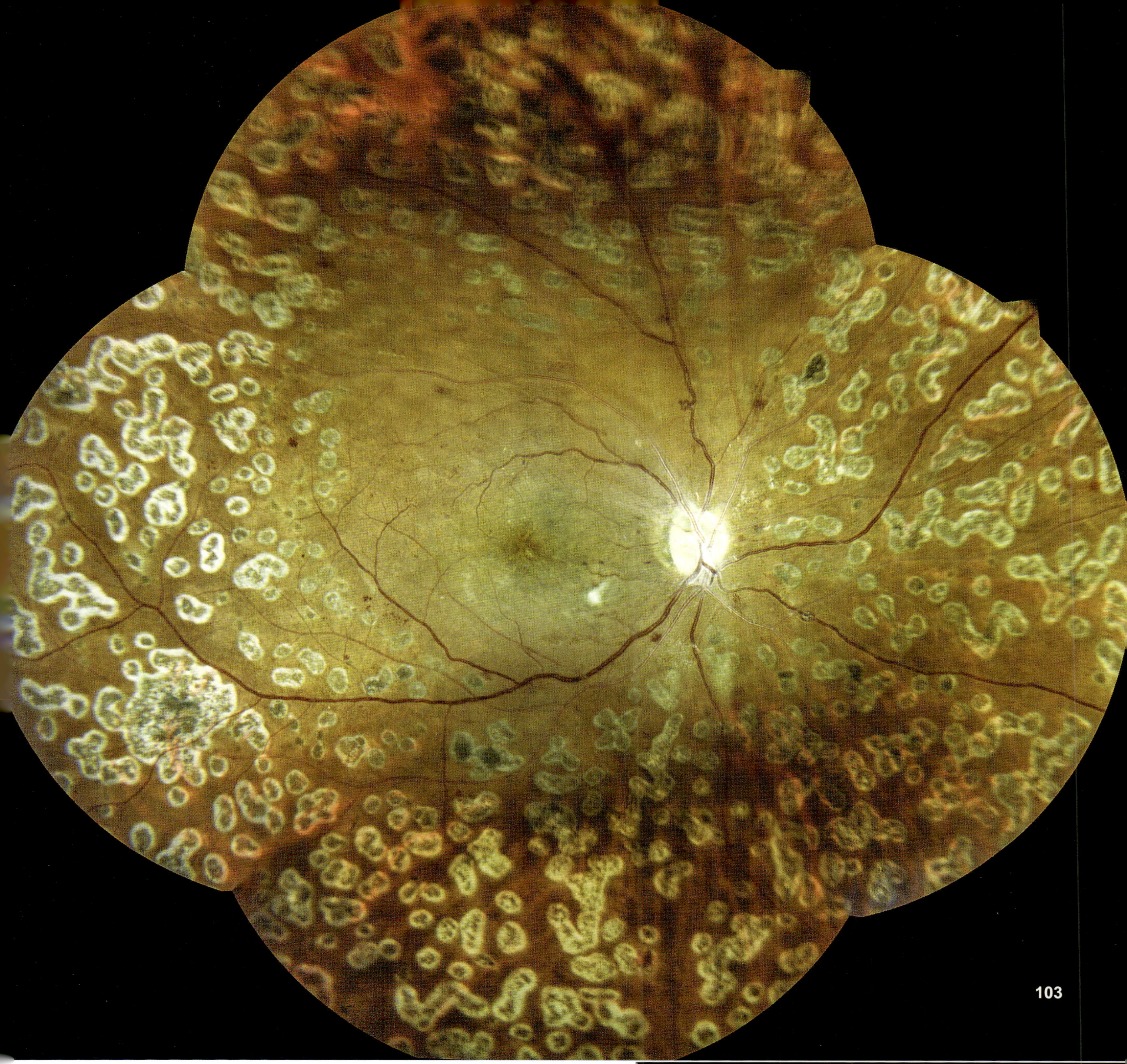

103

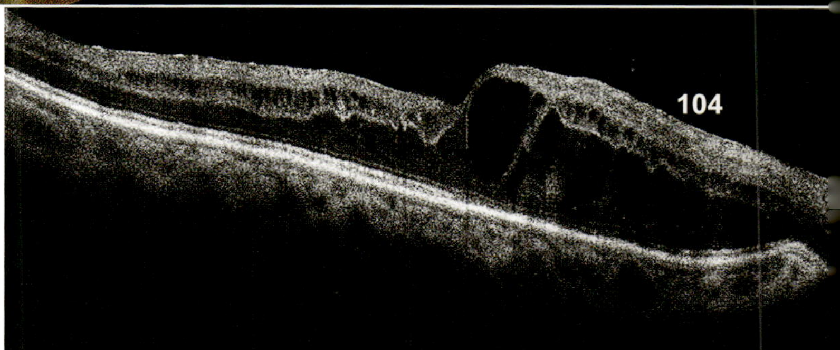

104

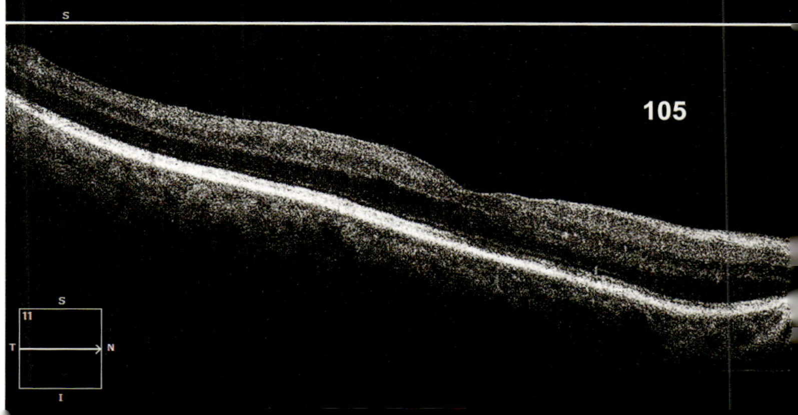


105

Figure 103 *Post-Ozurdex, resolution of hard exudates can also be seen at the macula and also reduction in dot and blot hemorrhages which good metabolic control.*

Figure 104 *OCT postoperative showed large cystic spaces involving the fovea and nasal aspect of macula along with diffuse thickening suggestive of macular edema.*

Figure 105 *Following intravitreal Ozurdex implant over a period of 2 months the cystoid macular edema subsided significantly. There was corresponding improvement in visual acuity.* □

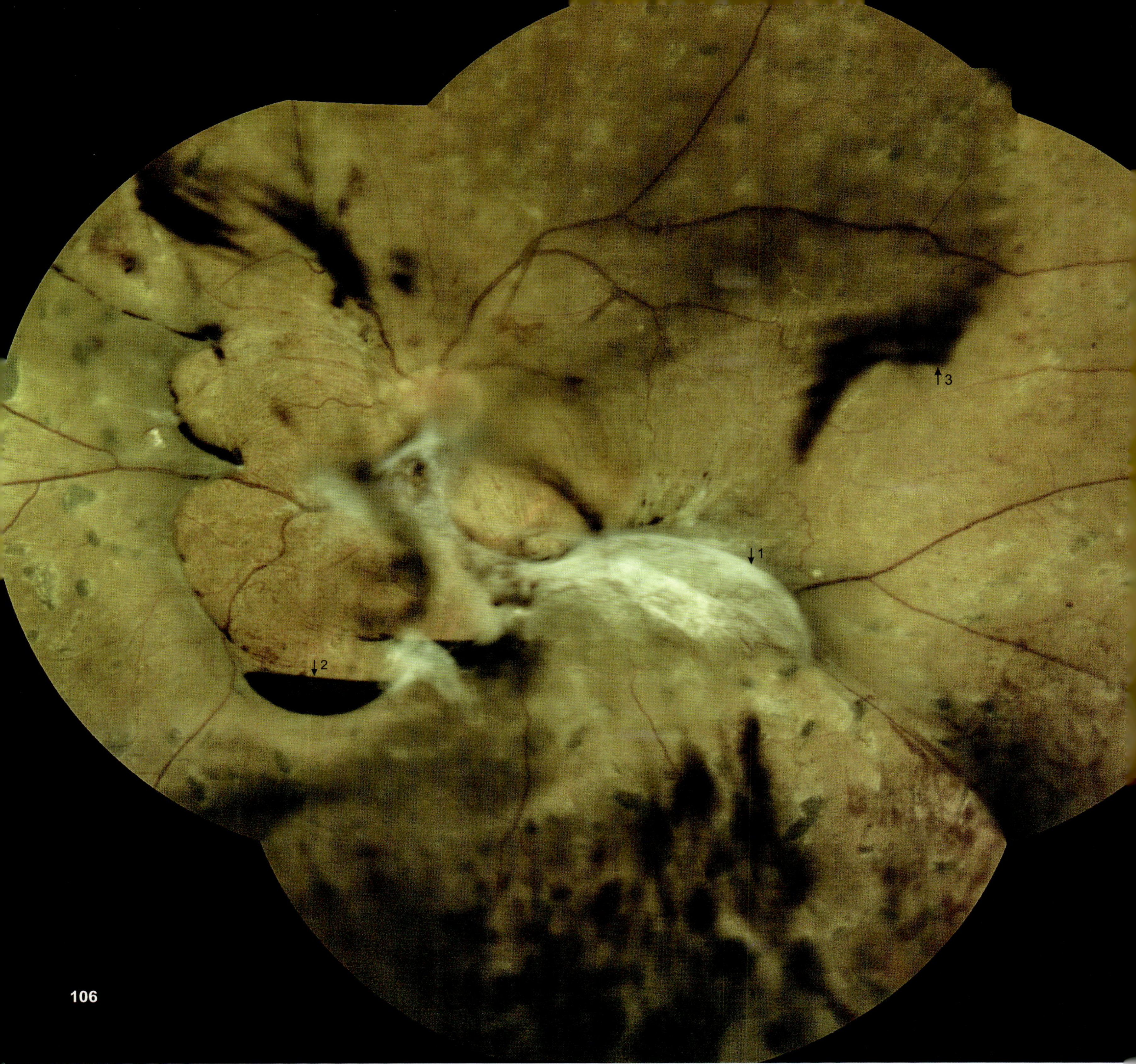


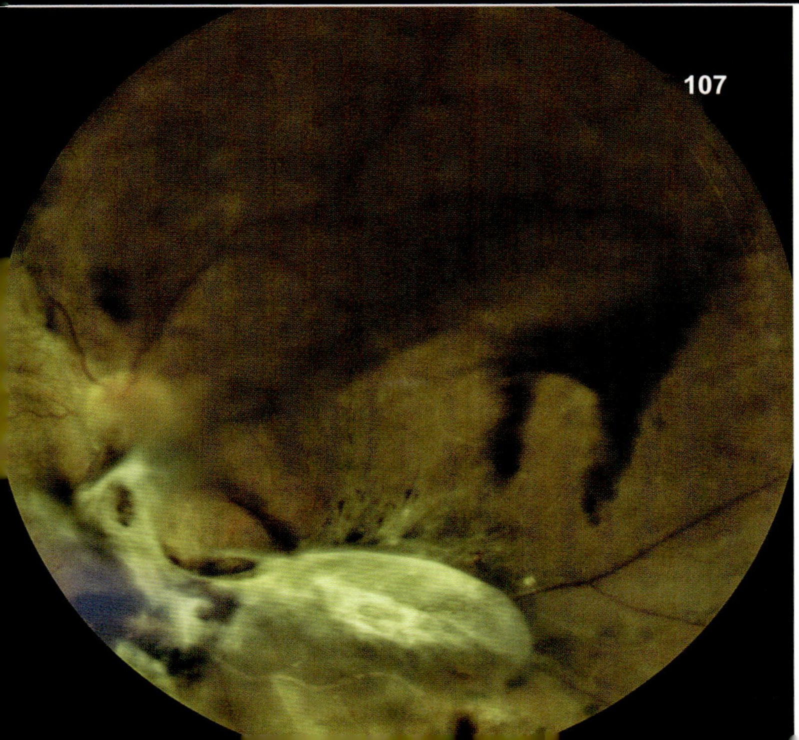


Figure 106 *Color fundus montage image in a case of diabetes mellitus type 2 with advanced proliferative diabetic retinopathy with tractional retinal detachment involving the macula. The case was managed with pars plana vitrectomy "proportional reflux hydrodissection" technique.*

A 42-year-old male presented with complaints of diminution of vision from his left eye for the last 3 weeks. Best corrected visual acuity was hand motion close to face. Color fundus photo demonstrates grayish white fibrovascular proliferation in the nasal quadrant, also, extending from the disk involving the macula and causing a drag on the fovea (1). Preretinal boat-shaped subhyaloid hemorrhage can be seen inferonasal to the disk (2). Dense reddish colored vitreous hemorrhage can also be seen (3).

Scant panretinal photocoagulation marks are visible in the periphery.

Figure 107 *Color fundus image of the same patient with PDR-related vitreous hemorrhage and fibrovascular traction. Note the central fundus image is not enough to define the extent of fibrovascular membranes.*

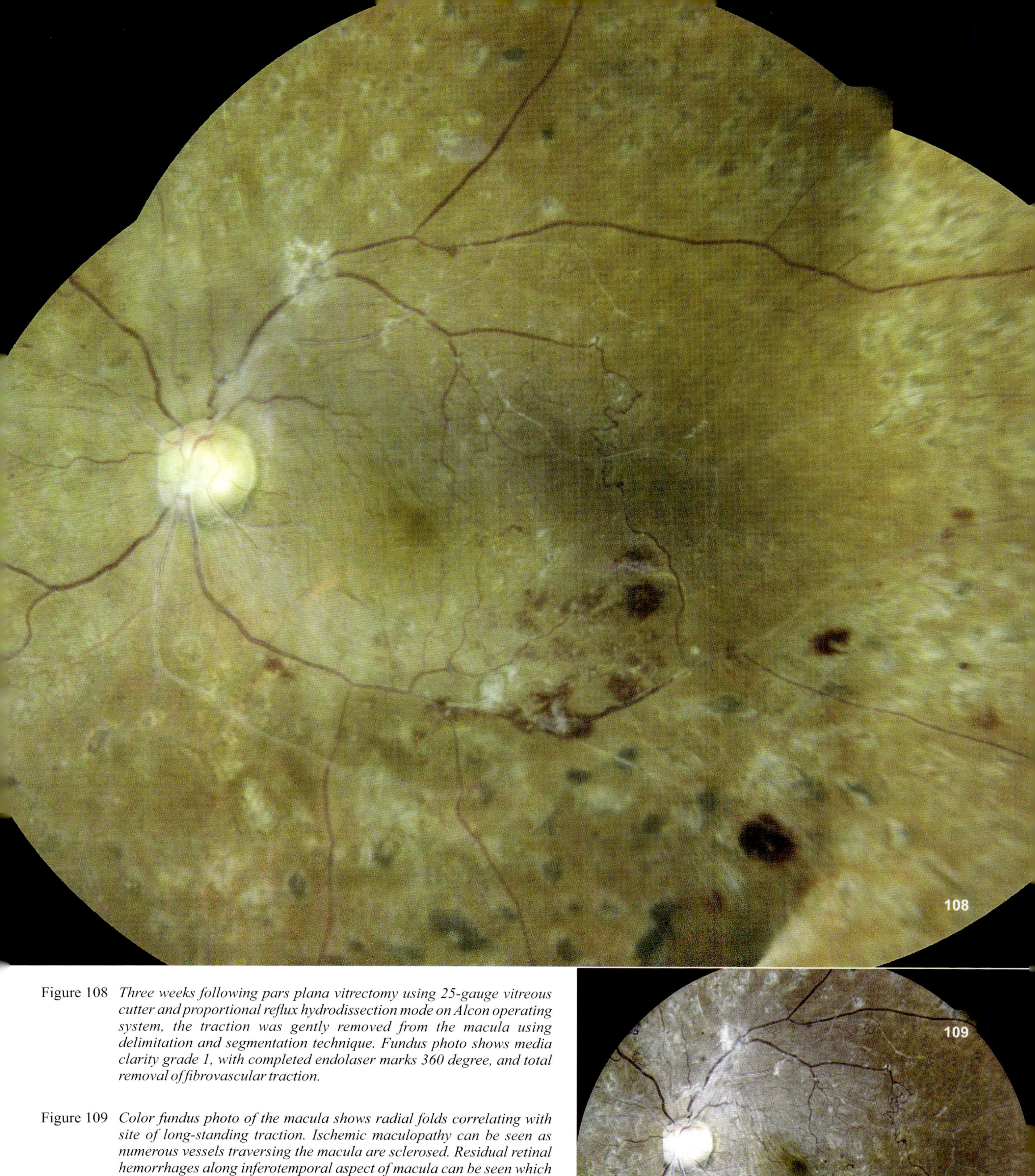


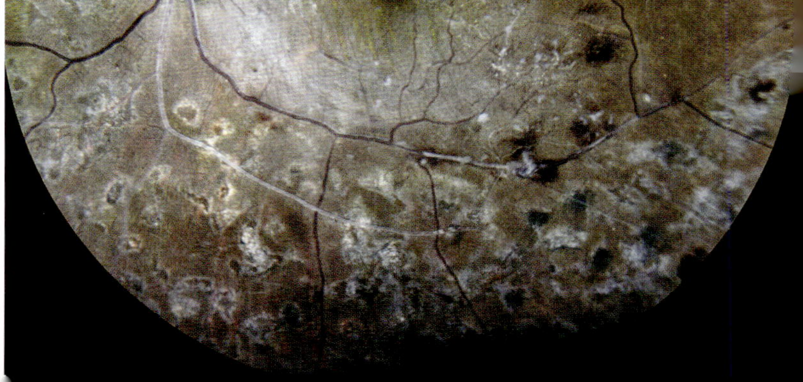


Figure 108 *Three weeks following pars plana vitrectomy using 25-gauge vitreous cutter and proportional reflux hydrodissection mode on Alcon operating system, the traction was gently removed from the macula using delimitation and segmentation technique. Fundus photo shows media clarity grade 1, with completed endolaser marks 360 degree, and total removal of fibrovascular traction.*

Figure 109 *Color fundus photo of the macula shows radial folds correlating with site of long-standing traction. Ischemic maculopathy can be seen as numerous vessels traversing the macula are sclerosed. Residual retinal hemorrhages along inferotemporal aspect of macula can be seen which may resolve with time.* □

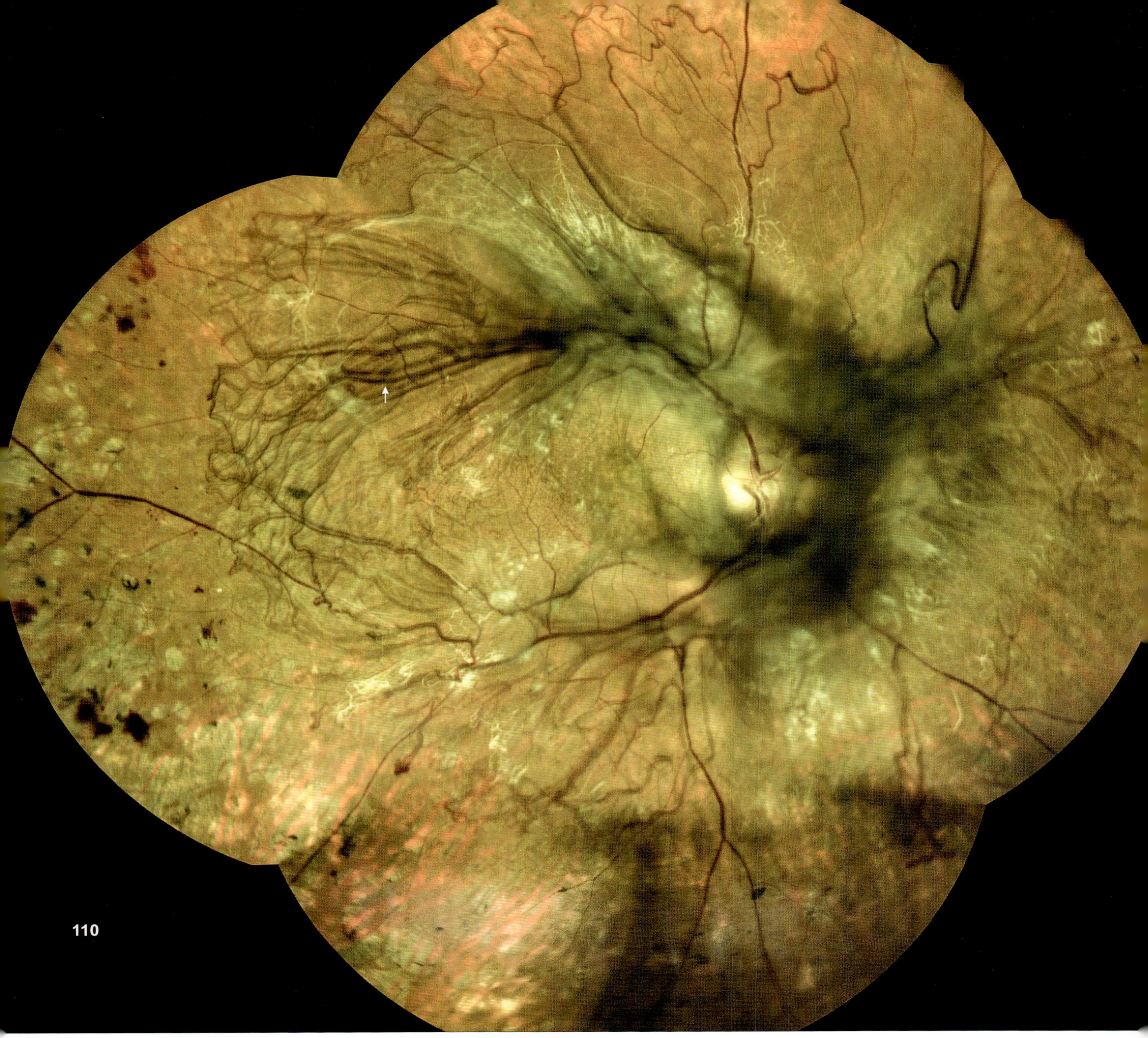


Figure 110 *A case of severe proliferative diabetic tractional retinal detachment with extensive neovascularization managed with preoperative anti-vascular endothelial growth factor (VEGF) injection and microincision pars plana vitrectomy with silicone oil tamponade.*

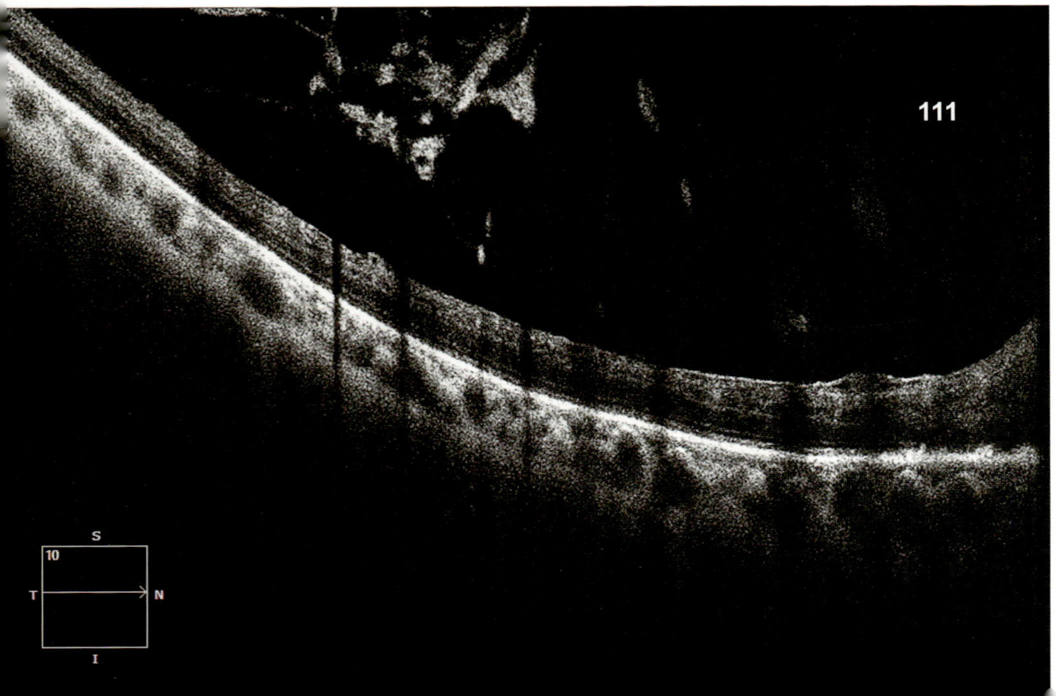


A 48-year-old male known case of diabetes mellitus type 2 for the last 20 years, complained of diminution of vision from his right eye for 6 months. Best corrected visual acuity was counting finger close to face.

Color fundus photo shows dense fibrovascular network extending from the disk involving the macula and extending up to the mid-periphery. The extensive abnormal vascular proliferation is forming an interlacing web-like network (arrow). Few laser photocoagulation marks can be seen in the periphery. Risk of preoperative and perioperative hemorrhage is very high in such cases. Judiciously timed preoperative anti-VEGF is very useful to reduce risk of same.

Figure 111 *OCT shows dense fibrovascular network in the vitreous cavity extending anterior to the retinal surface. Thick hyper-reflective membrane on retinal surface can be seen suggestive of epiretinal fibrous proliferation.*

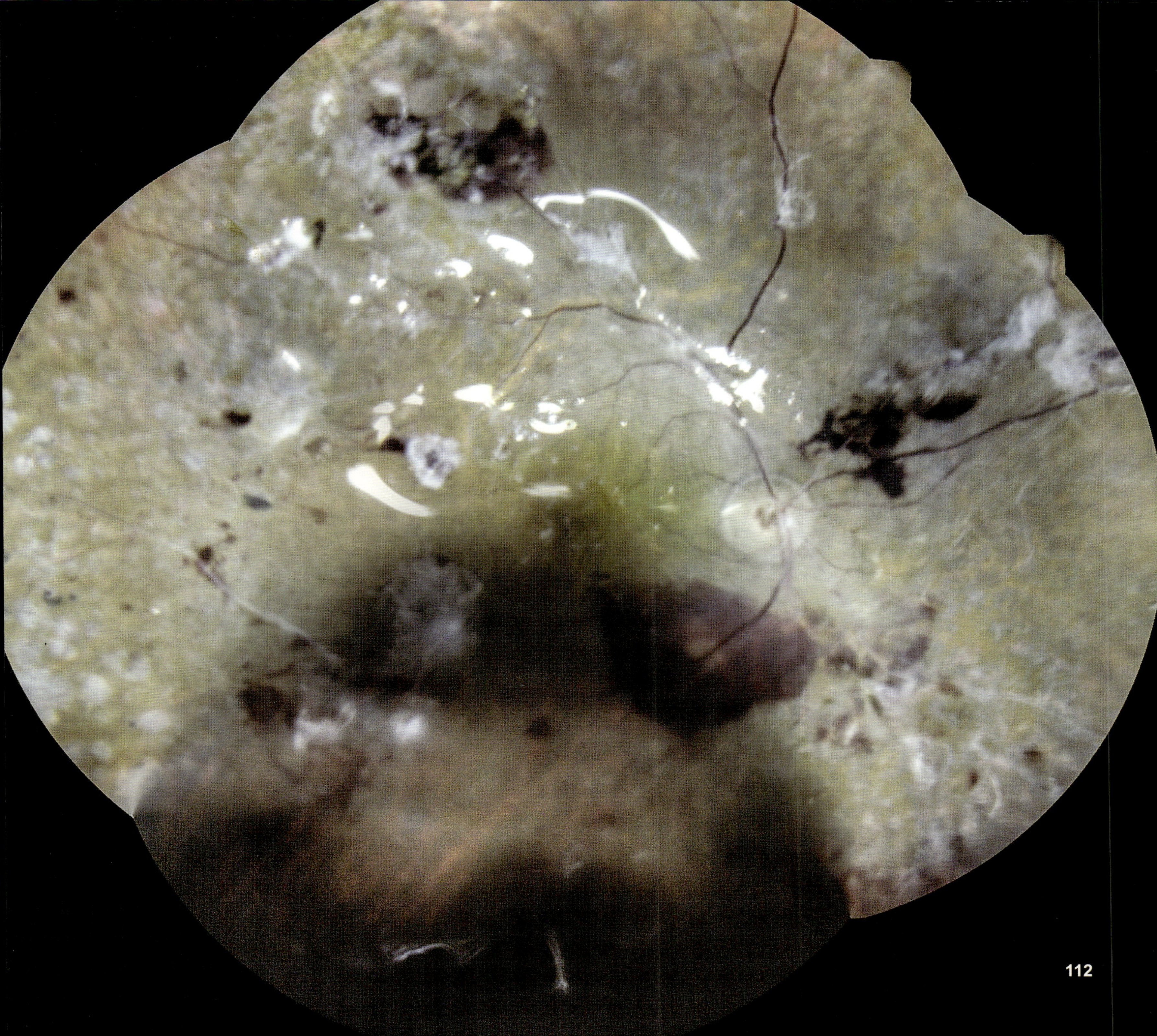



Figure 112 *25-gauge pars plana vitrectomy was performed with dissection of fibrovascular proliferation using vitreous cutter and delicate transvitreal forceps. Very adherent residual fibrovascular stump can be seen temporal to the macula. Endolaser was completed 360 degree in all quadrants and silicone oil tamponade was put in-situ. Best corrected visual acuity postoperatively was 6/60.*

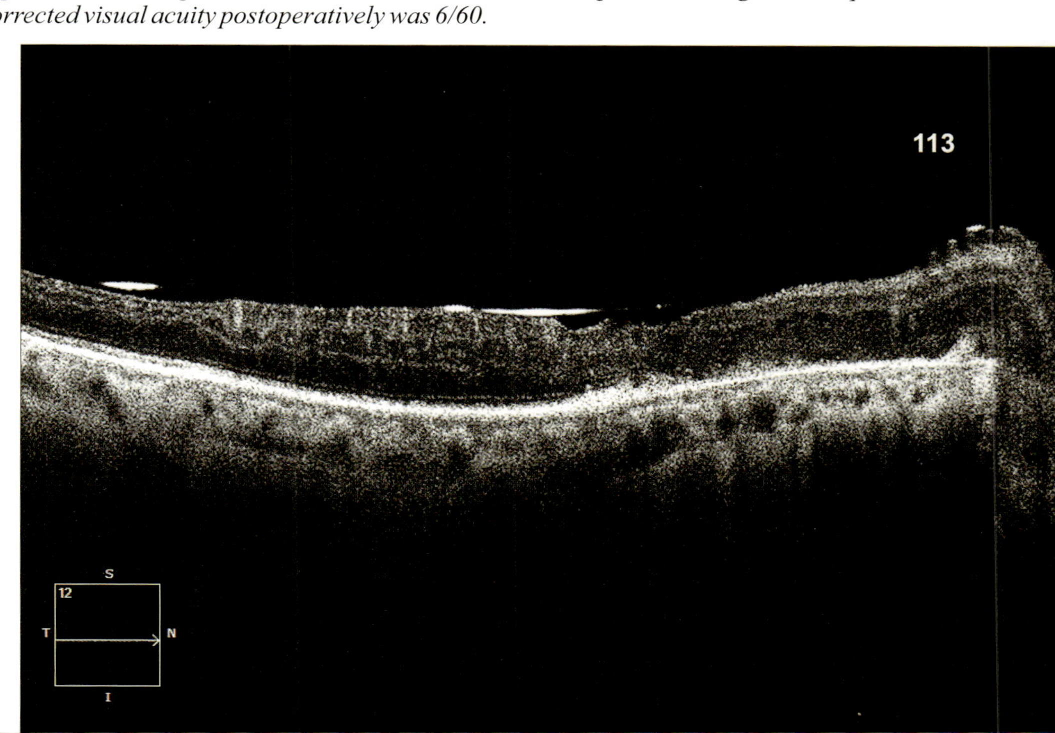



Figure 113 *OCT postoperatively shows well-attached retina with silicone oil meniscus over the retinal surface.*□

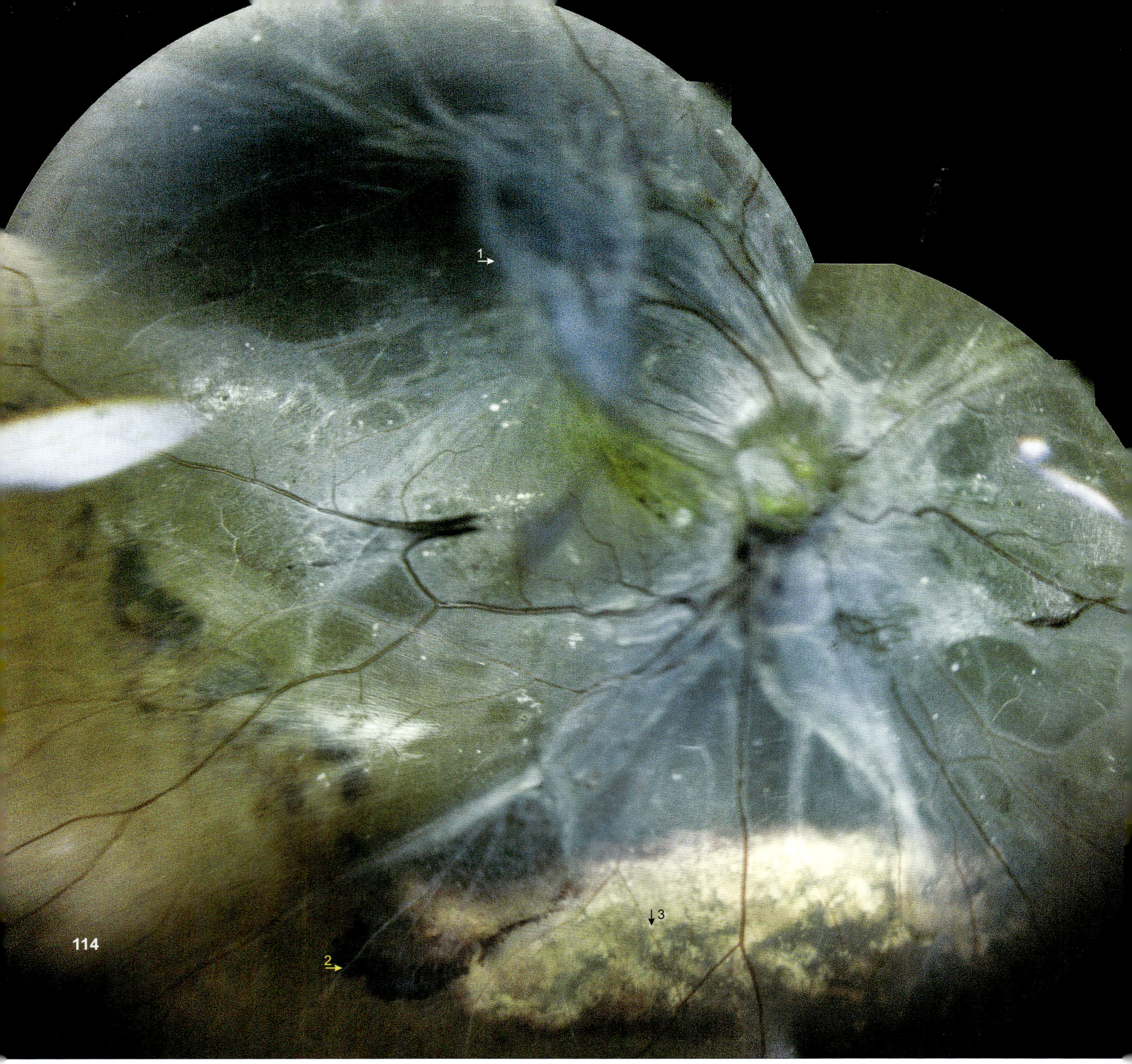


Figure 114 *Combined tractional—rhegmatogenous retinal detachment in diabetics can be extremely challenging to tackle intraoperatively. It usually requires long-acting tamponade with modest improvement in visual acuity despite good anatomical outcomes.*

A 60-year-old male, known case of type 2 diabetes mellitus presented with loss of vision in right for past 6 months. Fundus photo demonstrates combined tractional and rhegmatogenous retinal detachment involving the macula. Extreme temporal and inferior retina was on. A stretch break was identified at 12 o'clock using indirect ophthalmoscopy. A thick grayish membrane can be seen at the macula dragging it upwards and temporally and disrupting its normal architecture indicative of proliferative vitreoretinopathy (1). Dark red colored bleed can be visualized which is subretinal and inferior to the disk (2). There is old de-hemoglobinized blood which can be identified inferior to it indicative of long-standing nature of the pathology (3). Sclerosed vessels could be seen 360 degree indicative of severe retinal ischemia.

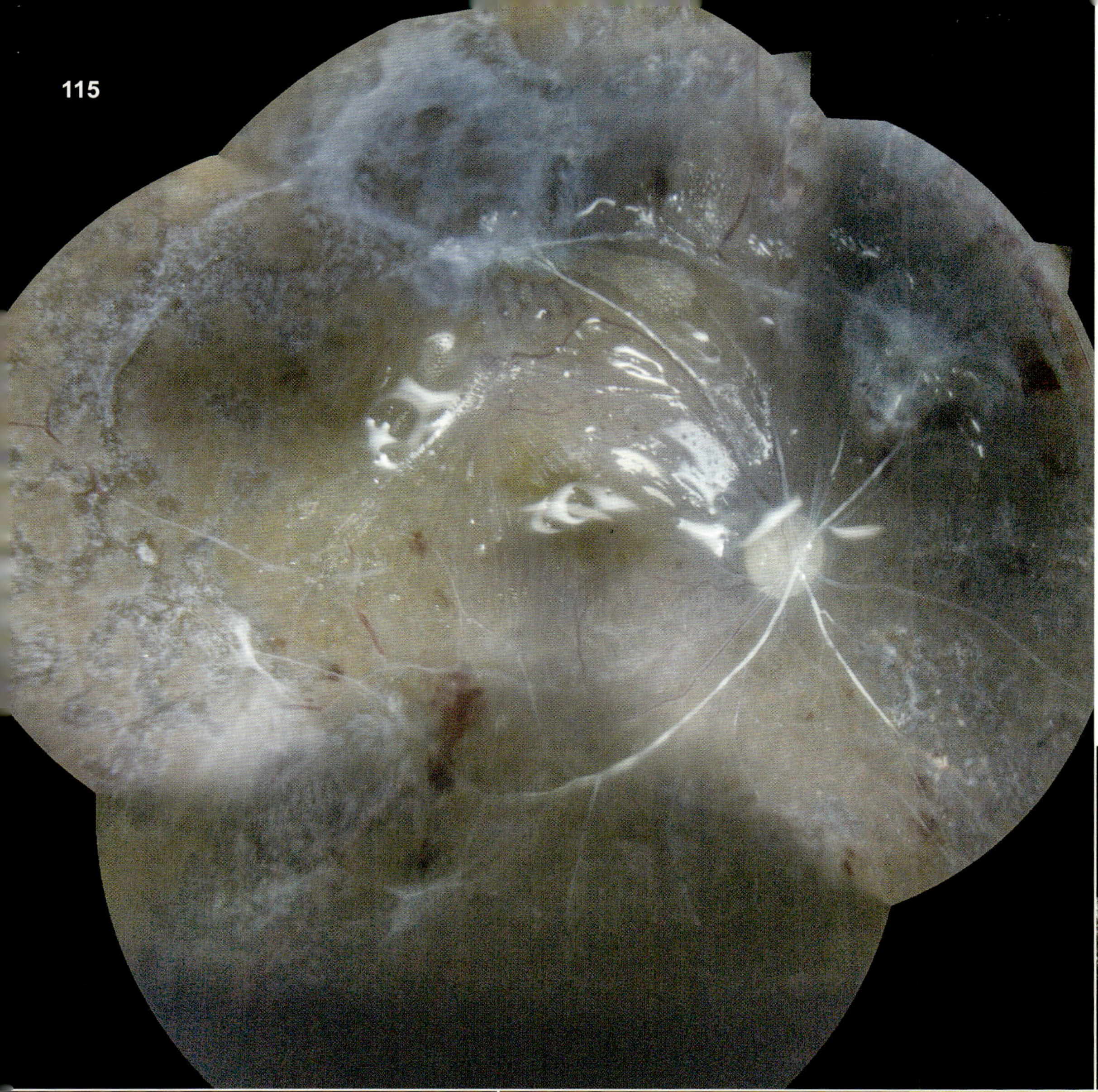

Figure 115

*25-gauge pars plana vitrectomy was performed in right eye with silicone oil tamponade. Bimanual dissection using chandelier illumination provides an indispensable tool to tackle such cases allowing the surgeon to use both hands to proceed with surgical removal of fibrovascular proliferation. Postoperative fundus photo shows successful reattachment of detached retina with silicone oil in situ. Sclerosed vessels can be seen in all quadrants of retina indicative of severe ischemia. Endolaser marks can be seen 360 degree.*

Figure 116

*OCT scan preoperatively demonstrates detached neurosensory layer of retina with a thick hyper-reflective layer of epiretinal membrane causing traction.*

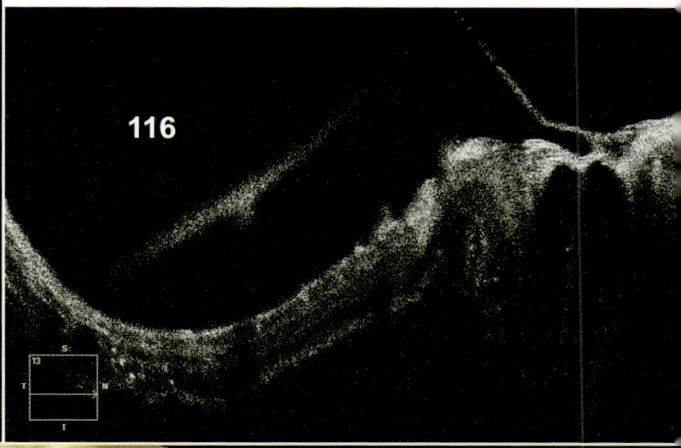

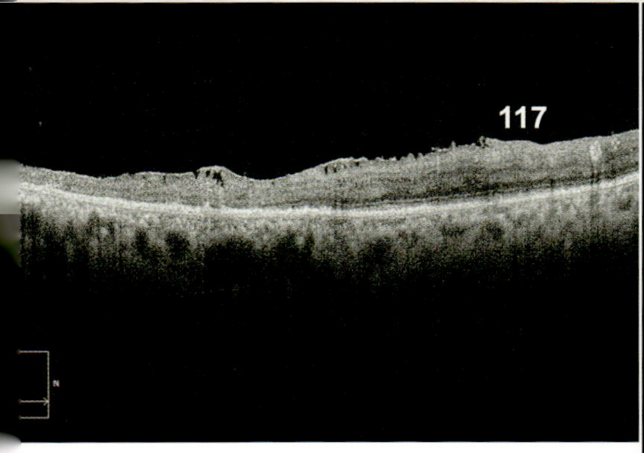

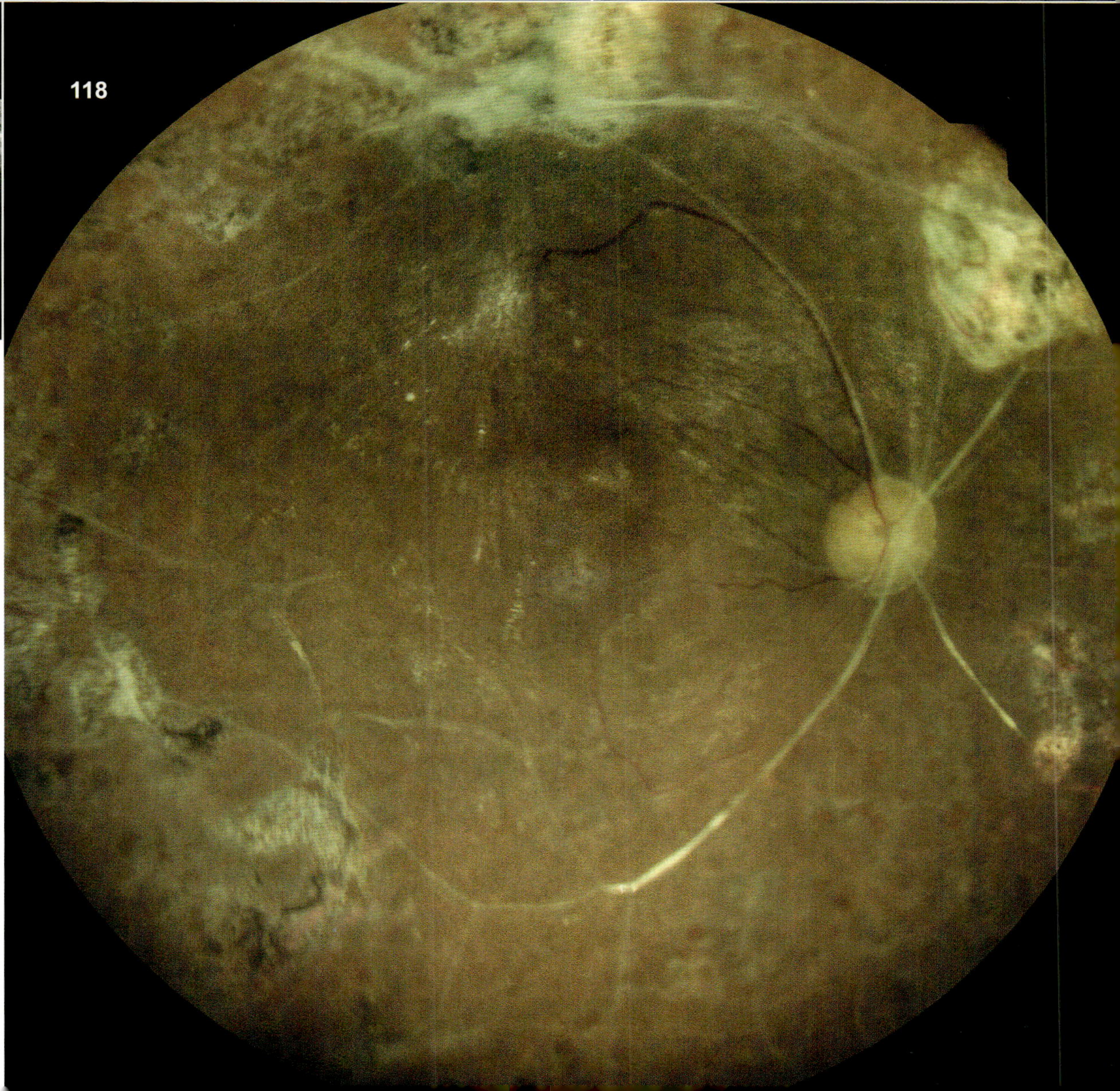

Figure 117

*OCT scan postoperatively after silicone oil removal demonstrated re–attachment of neurosensory retina to underlying retinal pigment epithelium with some residual epiretinal membrane. Disruption of inner layers of neurosensory retina and retinal pigment epithelium can be seen clearly with thinning of temporal half of retina owing to severe ischemia.*

Figure 118

*Six months postoperatively retina remained well attached and post-silicone oil removal visual acuity improved to 6/60.* □

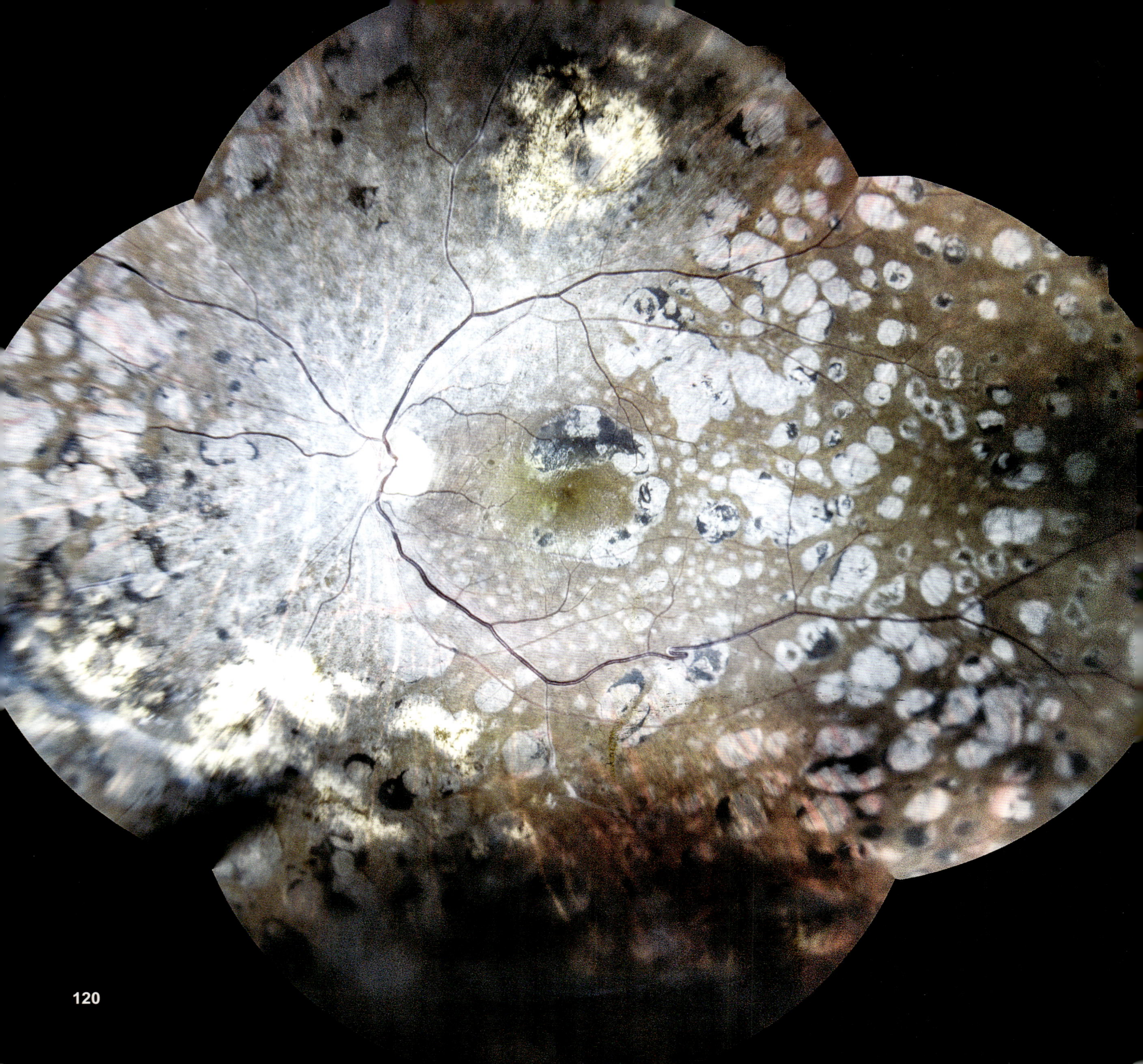

120

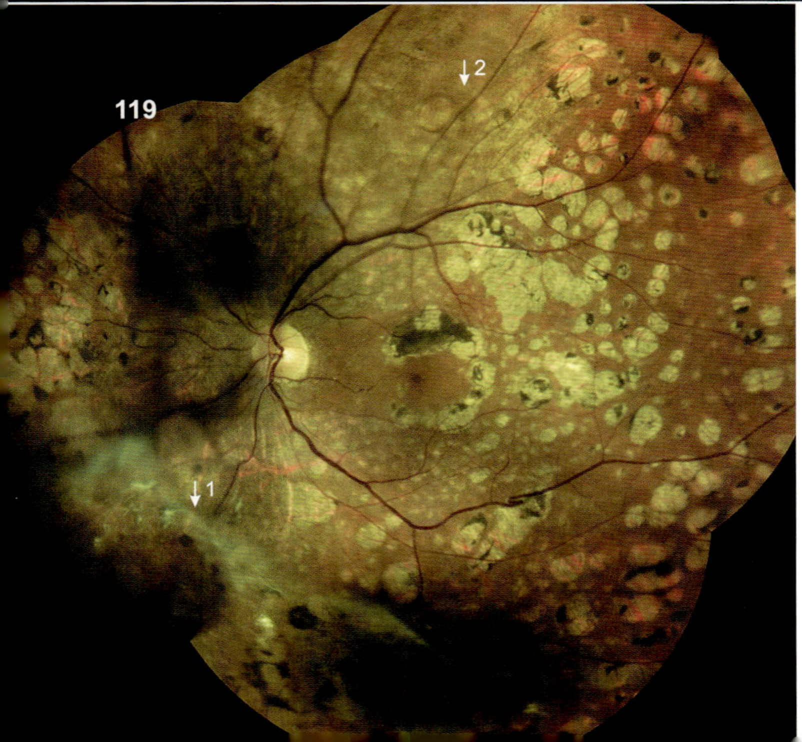



119

Color fundus montage image in a case of combined tractional and rhegmatogenous retinal detachment.

Figure 119 *Color fundus photo shows media clarity grade 1 with 360 degree endolaser marks of previous panretinal photocoagulation. Heavy macular laser scars are also visible. Inferonasal grayish vascular proliferation can also be seen (1). One can identify a small atrophic hole superior to the superior arcade (2) leading to small amount of retinal fluid percolating superonasally and leading to shallow subtotal retinal detachment. Superior detachment tends to progress at a rapid pace, hence he underwent an early 25 gauge pars plana vitrectomy with dissection of fibrovascular adherent tissue with transvitreal forceps and vitreous cutter. Complete removal of hyaloid and base excision 360 degree was done. Meticulous removal of hyaloid in diabetic is required to prevent proliferative vitreoretinopathy and re-detachment.*

Figure 120 *At 6 months after silicone oil removal, color fundus photo shows attached retina with endolaser marks visible 360 degrees. There is complete removal of inciting traction and no residual subretinal fluid is left.*□

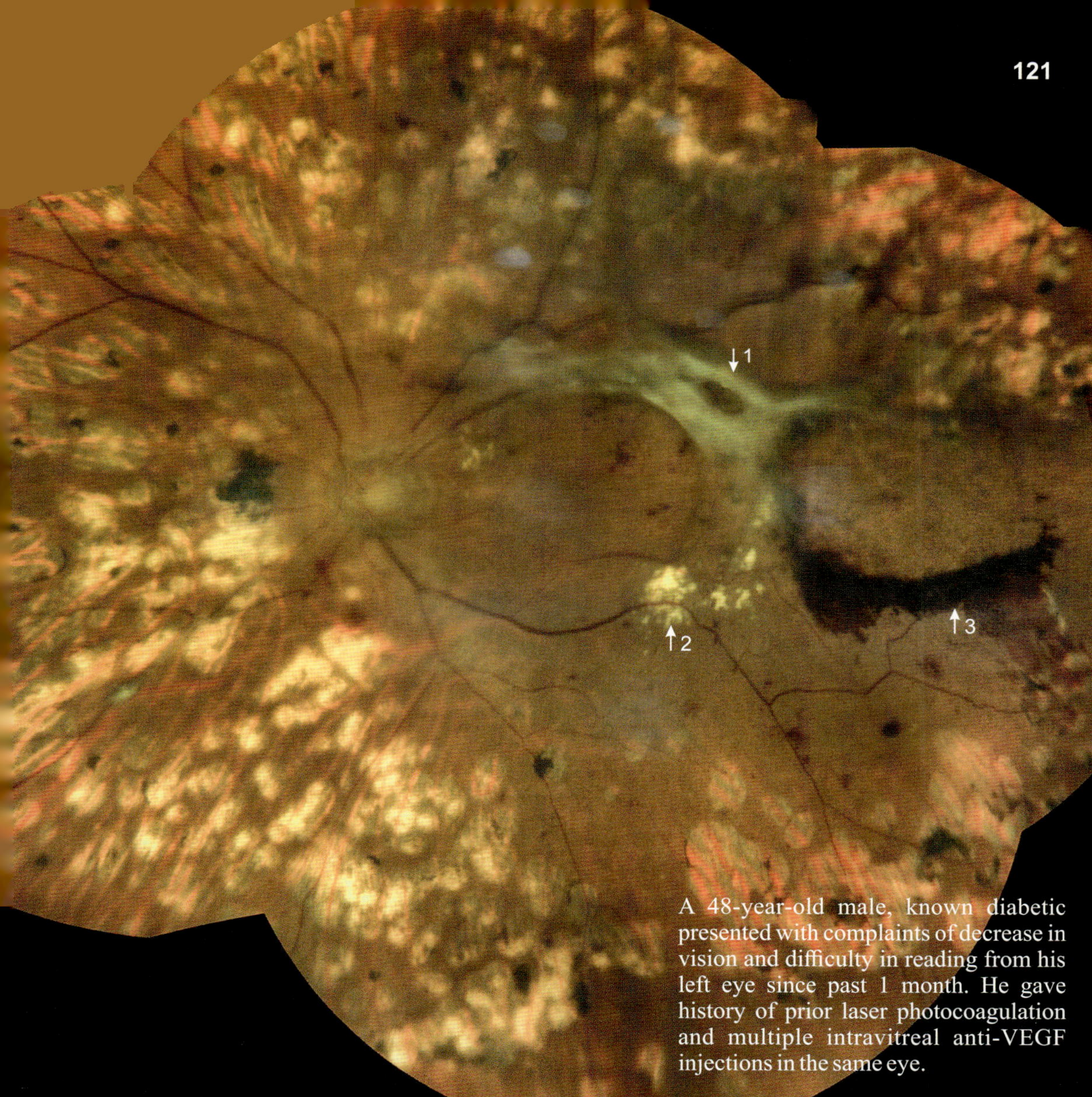


A 48-year-old male, known diabetic presented with complaints of decrease in vision and difficulty in reading from his left eye since past 1 month. He gave history of prior laser photocoagulation and multiple intravitreal anti-VEGF injections in the same eye.

Figure 121

*Color fundus photo demonstrates a thick grayish epiretinal fibrotic membrane superior and temporal to the macular (1), few yellow colored diskrete hard exudates can also be seen temporal to the macula (2). Fresh red colored preretinal hemorrhage (3) is also seen temporal to the macula. 360 degree scatter laser marks can be seen in the periphery.*

Figure 122

*OCT through the retina shows thick epiretinal membrane causing traction on temporal aspect of macula threatening the fovea and leading to large cystoid spaces in temporal aspect of retina "Recalcitrant macular edema", there is also significant thinning of neurosensory retina at the fovea along with disruption of architecture of retinal inner and outer layers at fovea.*

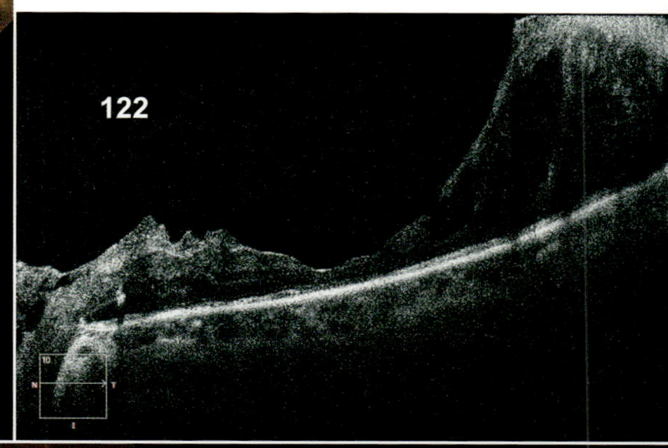


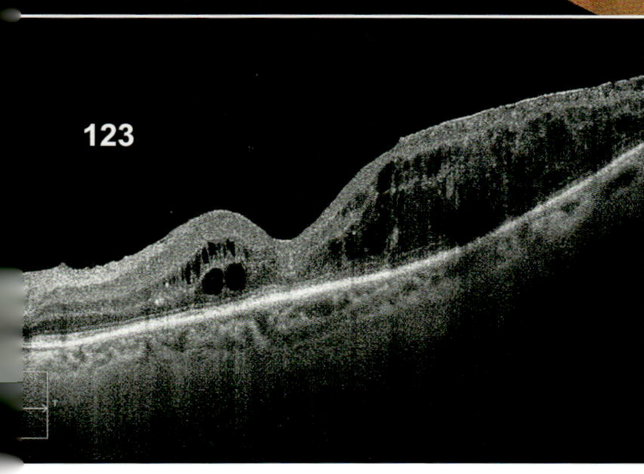


Figure 123

*Postoperative OCT shows significant reduction in macular thickness, resolution of cystoid spaces and complete removal of epiretinal fibrotic membrane. Few cystoid spaces persisted nasally which were managed conservatively.*

Figure 124

*In view of significant epiretinal fibrous traction causing macular edema threatening the fovea he was advised 25-gauge pars plana vitrectomy with removal of epiretinal fibrous proliferation using delicate ILM forceps and proportional reflux hydrodissection mode. Complete removal of epiretinal fibrosis with media clarity grade 1 can be seen postoperatively. Streak amount of preretinal hemorrhage persists temporally which usually resolves over course of time.* □

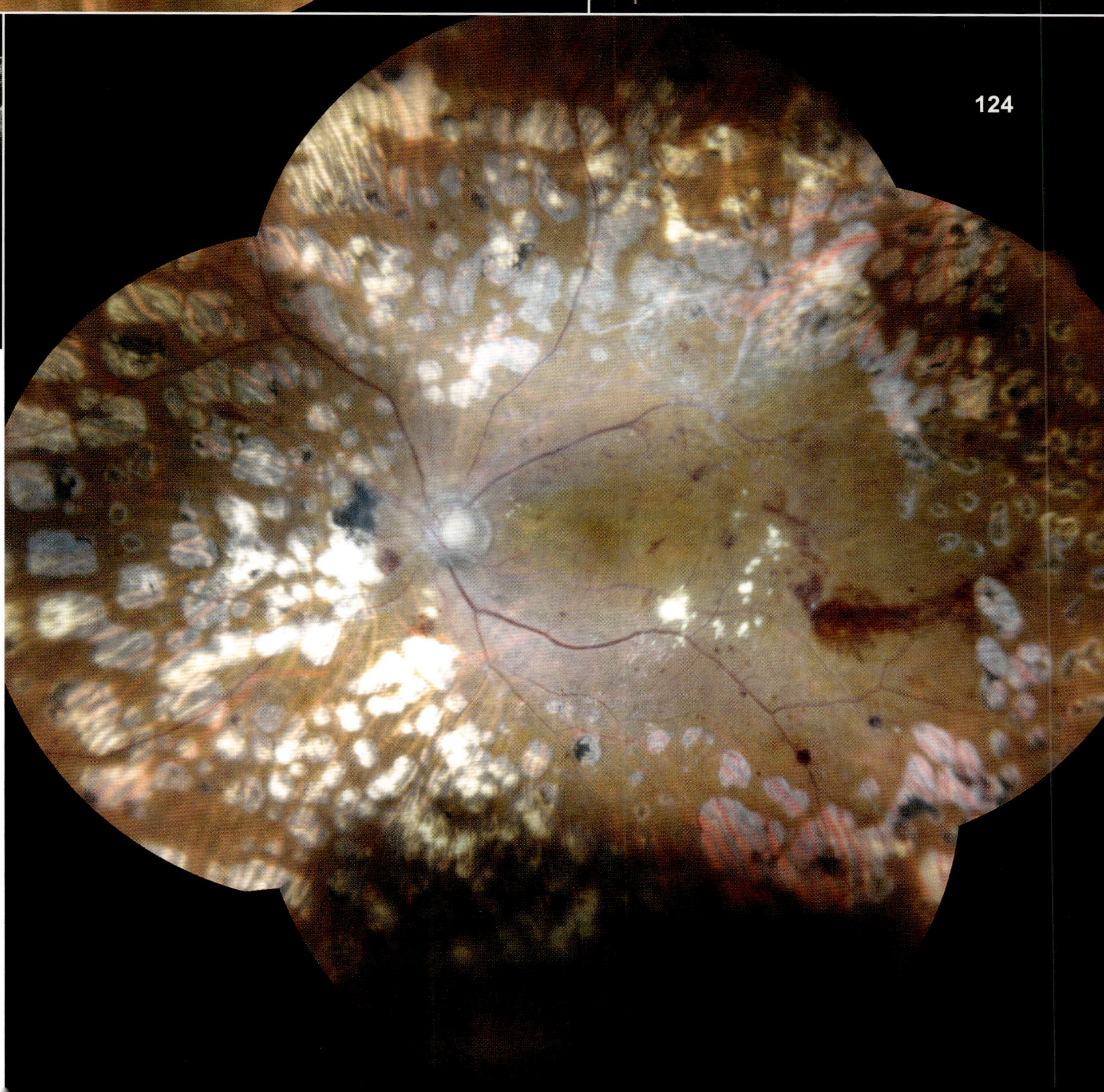

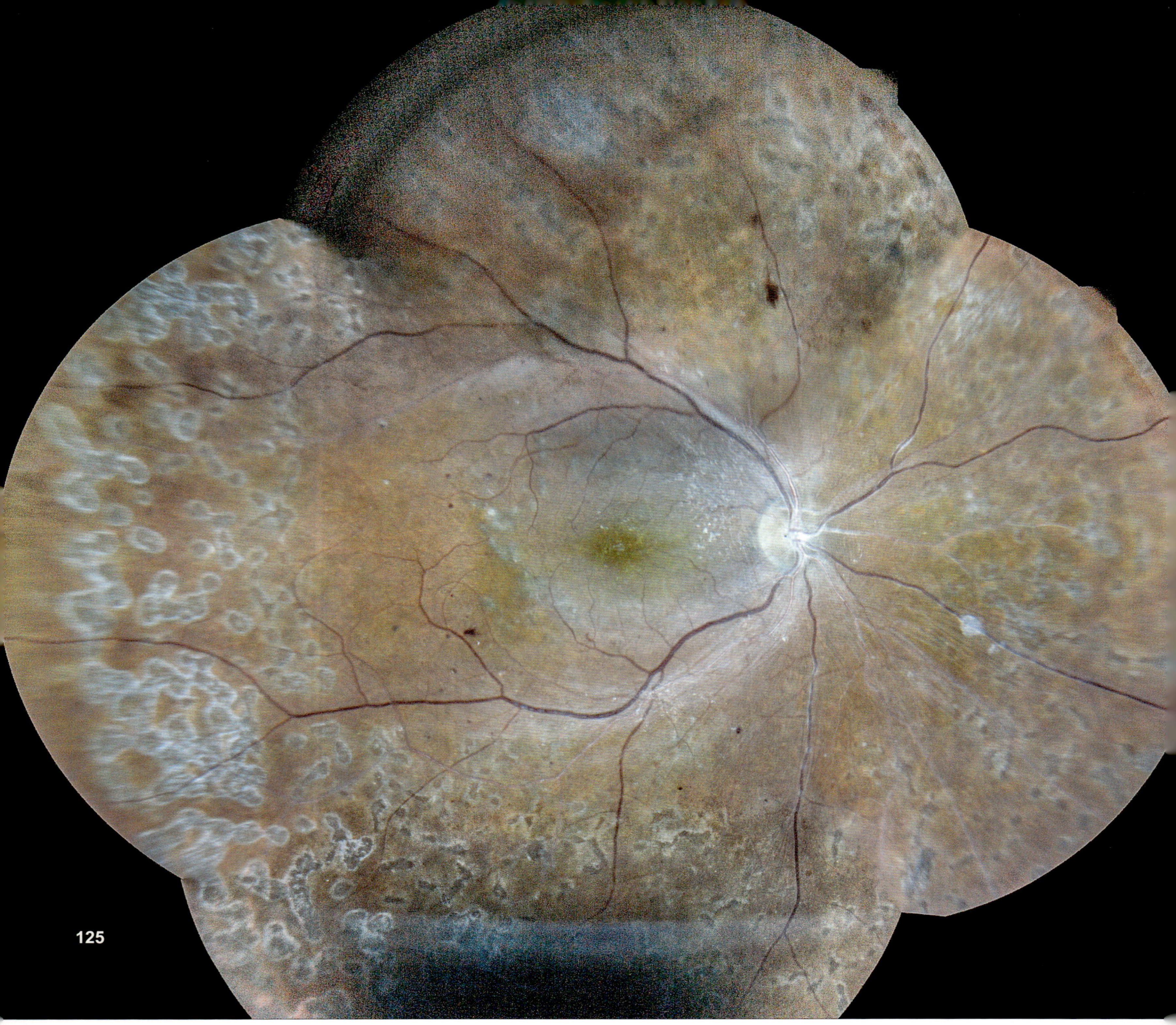


Figure 125 *25-gauge pars plana vitrectomy was performed. Two months postoperatively visual acuity improved to 6/24. Media clarity was grade 1 and 360 degree laser marks are visible which were applied intraoperatively.*

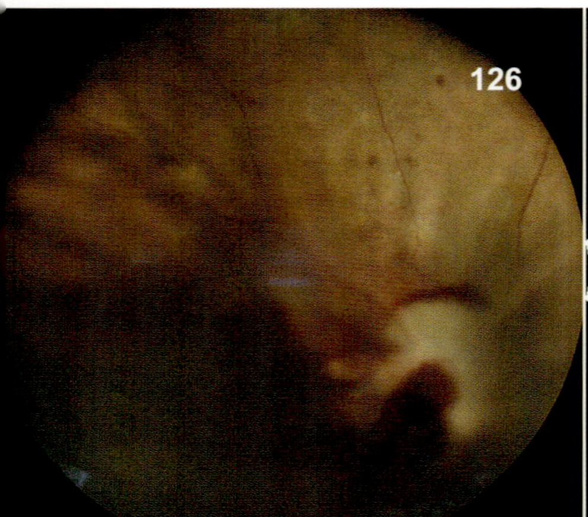


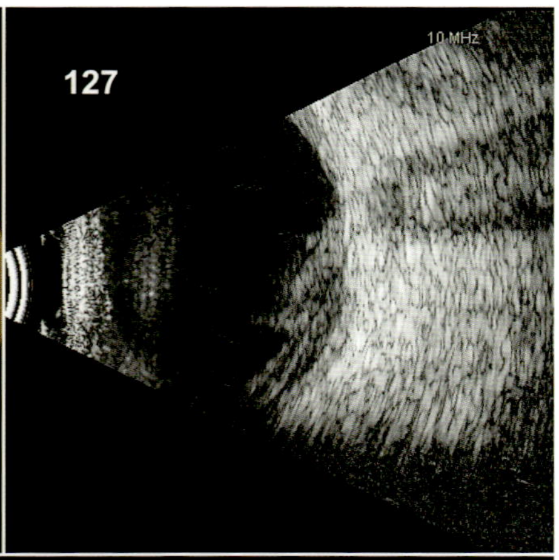


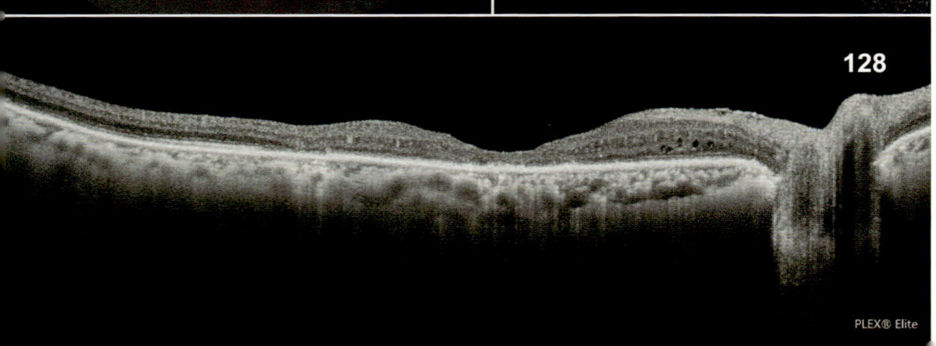


Figure 126 *A 60-year-old female with history of DM, presented with complaint of sudden decrease in vision in both eyes since 1 month. Fundus photo of the right eye shows vitreous hemorrhage obscuring most details of retina in central and inferior half, superior retinal details were visible hazily.*

Figure 127 *Ultrasound demonstrates vitreous hemorrhage with moderate amplitude echoes which are prominent near retinal surface, with no evidence of retinal detachment.*

Figure 128 *Optical coherence tomography image, postoperative showed disruption of retinal pigment epithelium, IS-OS receptors, at the macular area, with few hyporeflective spaces nasally, accounting for limited postoperative visual recovery.*

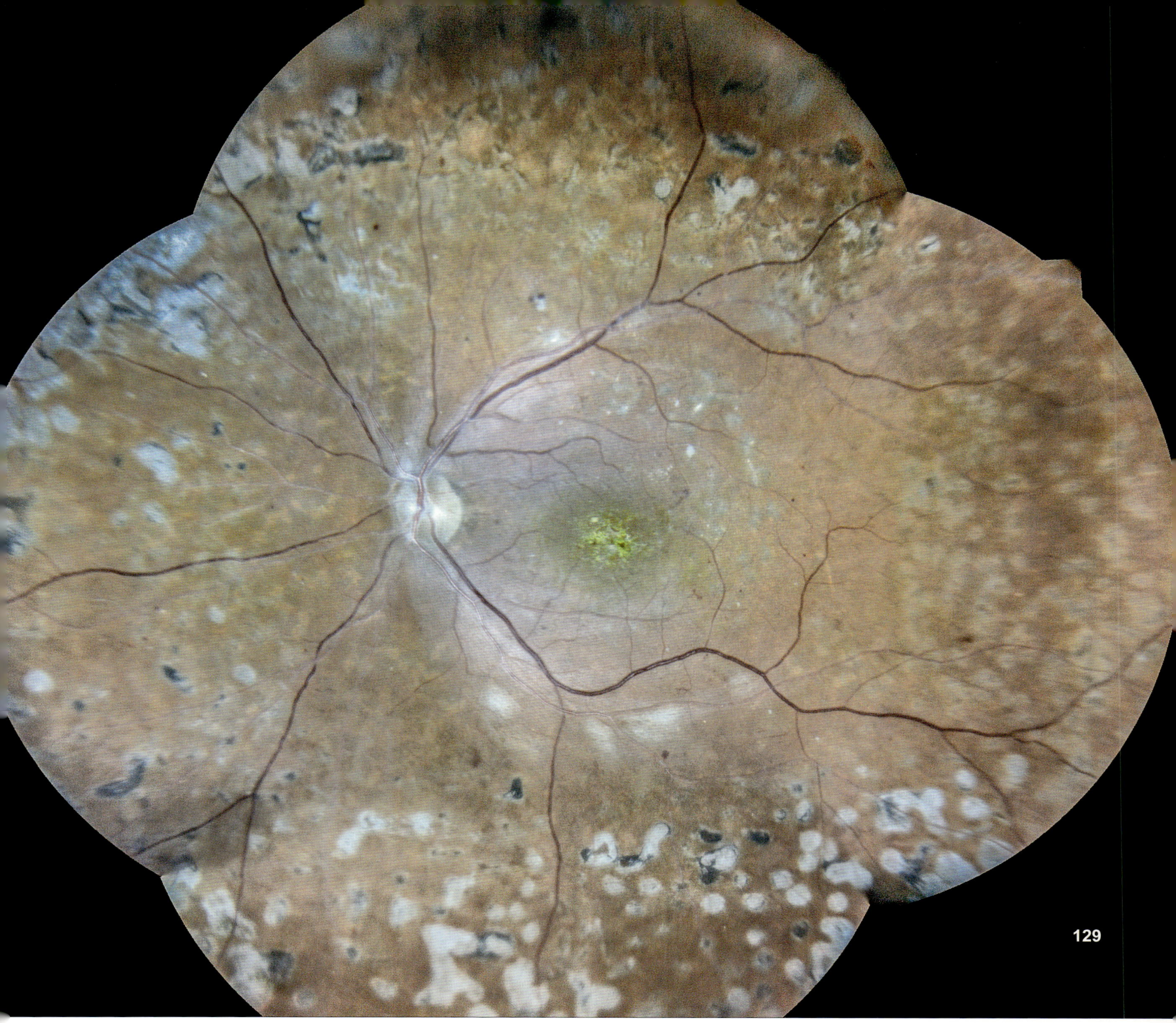

Figure 129 *Left eye 25-gauge PPV, one month postoperatively visual acuity improved to 6/36. Media clarity was grade 1 and 360 degree laser marks are visible. At the macular area, area of retinal pigment atrophy is seen contributing to limited amount of visual improvement despite good anatomical outcome.*

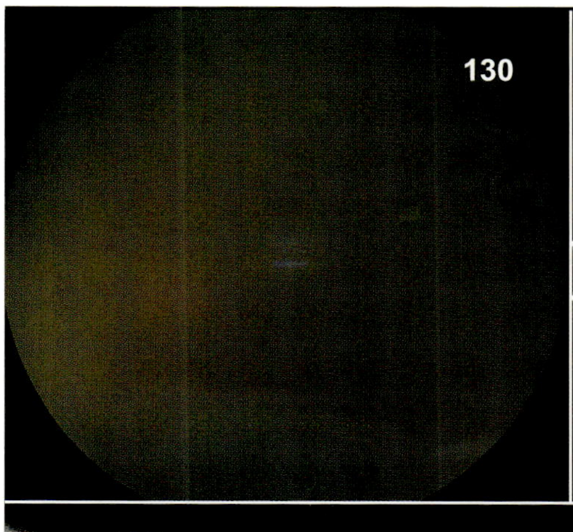

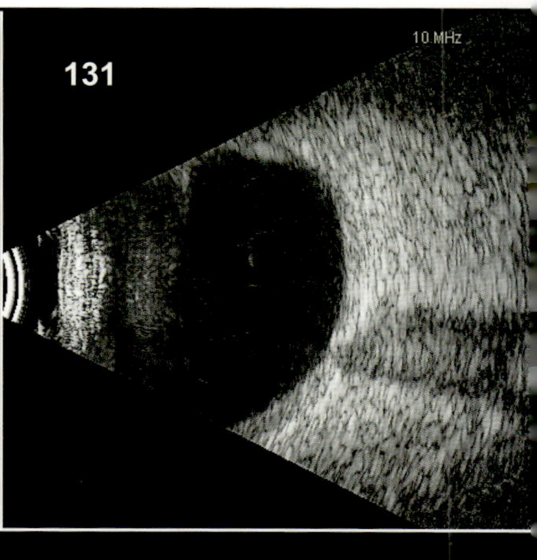


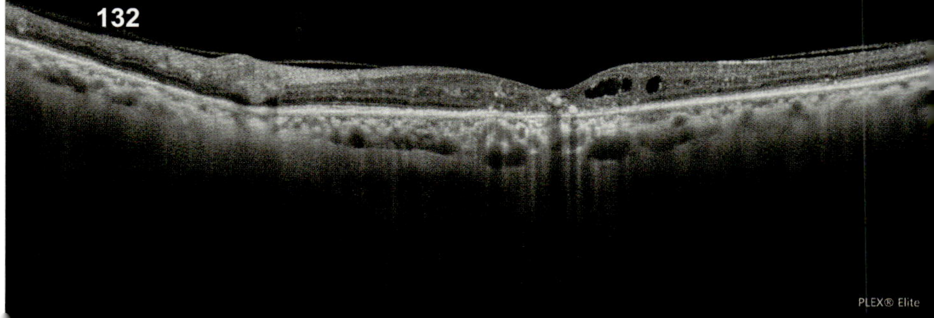


Figure 130 *No details of retina were visible in the left eye fundus, due to dense vitreous hemorrhage. Ultrasonography in left eye demonstrated moderate echoes in vitreous cavity suggestive of vitreous hemorrhage with no element of retinal detachment.*

Figure 131 *Ultrasound of the left shows moderate echoes primarily in anterior vitreous cavity suggestive of vitreous hemorrhage, no element of traction was seen on retina.*

Figure 132 *Postoperatively as media clarity improved OCT scan could be performed, shows loss of integrity of inner retinal layers and diffuse retinal pigment epithelium atrophy account for limited visual improvement despite complete removal of vitreous hemorrhage in both eyes. Few hyporeflective spaces can be seen temporal to disk.*□

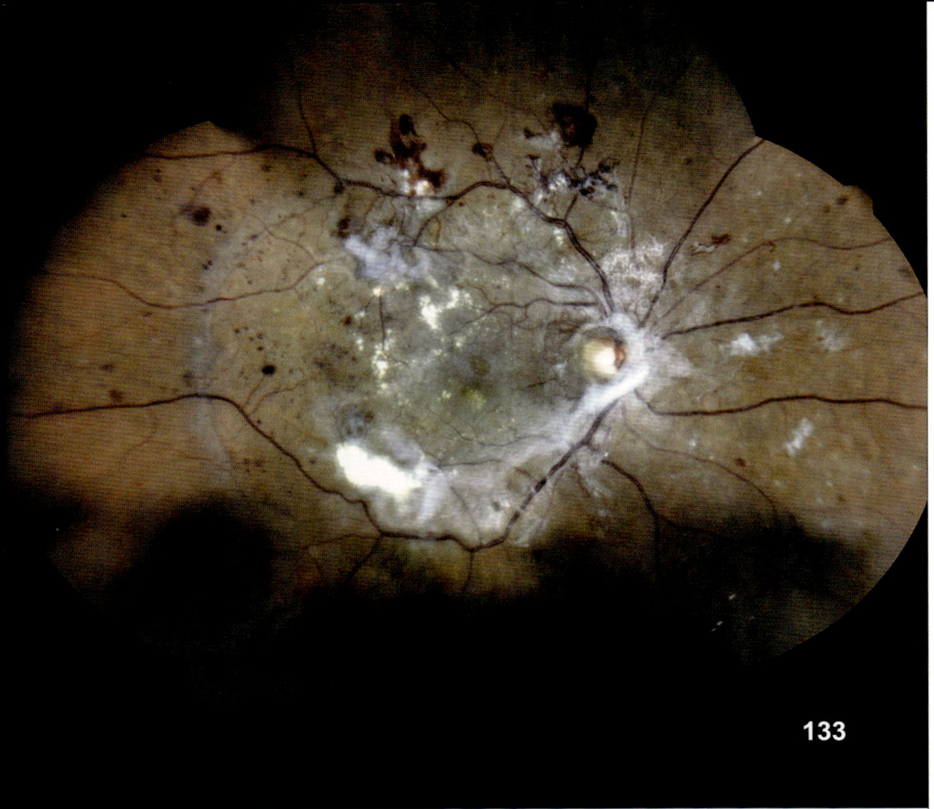


Figure 133 *A case of bilateral advanced proliferative diabetic retinopathy with fibrovascular proliferation managed with sequential pars plana vitrectomy.*

A 54-year-old male with uncontrolled diabetes mellitus type 2 presented with complaints of decrease in vision from both eyes gradually over a period of 4 months.

Best corrected visual acuity of right eye was 6/60. Color fundus photo of his right eye shows thick grayish white fibrovascular proliferation over the macula extending from the disk nasally to encompass the whole retina.

Extensive neovascularization of the disk and also elsewhere superior to the superior arcade along with preretinal bleed are also visible.

There is a pseudomacular hole-like appearance at the fovea due to the epiretinal membrane which can be confirmed on OCT.

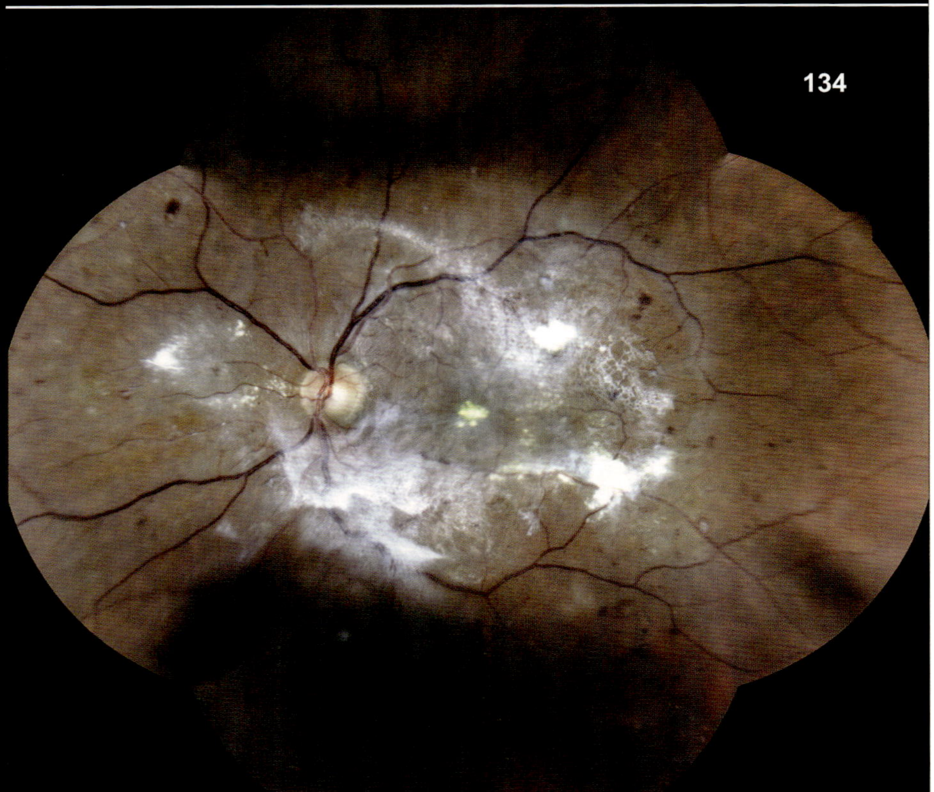


Figure 134 *Left eye best corrected visual acuity was counting finger 3 meters. Color fundus photo similar to the right eye shows thick grayish white fibrovascular proliferation over the macula extending from the disk nasally to encompass the whole retina. Traction can also be seen extending nasal to the disk. Numerous yellowish colored hard exudates can be seen deposited on the retinal surface. Dot and blot hemorrhages are seen in the periphery. The subfoveal fibrosis in this eye has a significant correlation with poor visual acuity gain even after intervention owing to damage to the photoreceptors at fovea.*

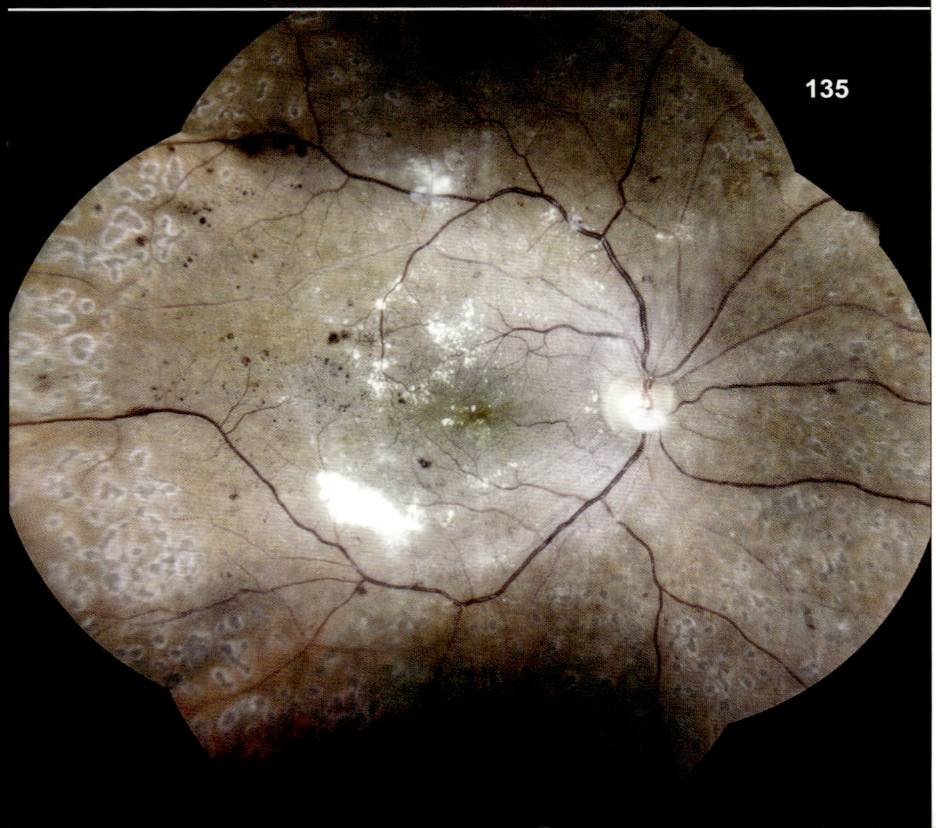


25-gauge pars plana vitrectomy with preoperative intravitreal anti-VEGF was done sequentially in both eyes with removal of epiretinal fibrosis using ILM forceps and 25-gauge vitreous cutter and proportional reflux hydrodissection technique.
It is imperative to apply endolaser 360 degree to prevent recurrent bleeding and regress neovascularization completely.

Figure 135 *Color fundus photo right eye shows media clarity grade 1 with 360 degree endolaser marks, significant amount of hard exudates are present at the macula. Residual stump of fibrous tissue can be seen at the disk.*

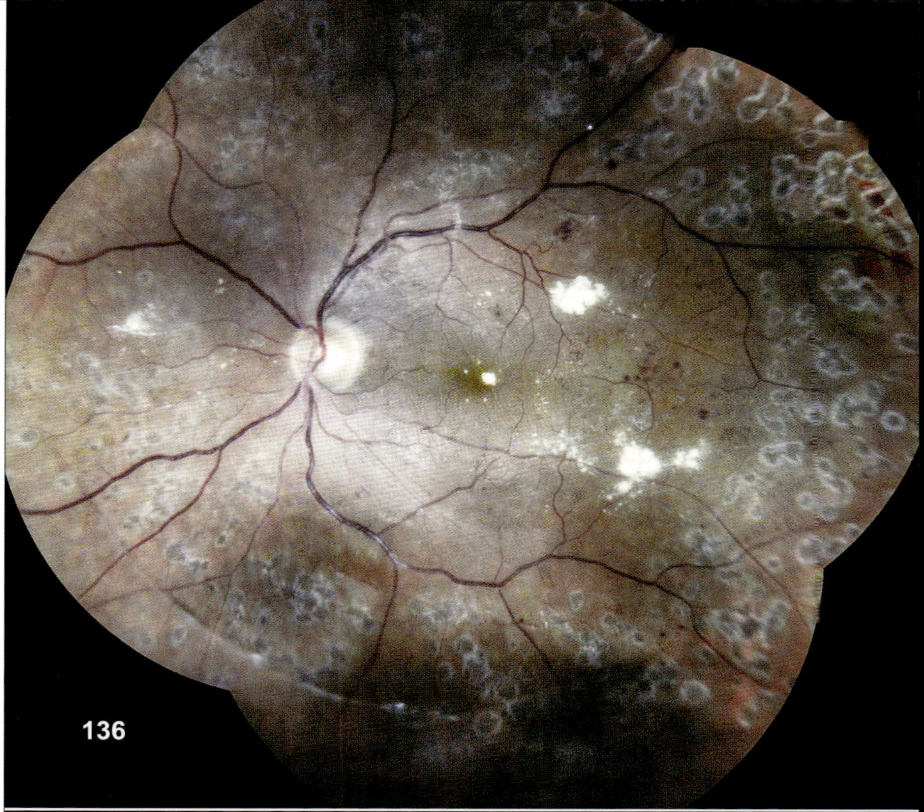


Figure 136 *Fundus photo of the left eye shows media clarity grade 1 with 360 degree endolaser marks with complete removal of fibrovascular proliferation, residual hard exudates and subfoveal fibrosis can be seen at the macula.*

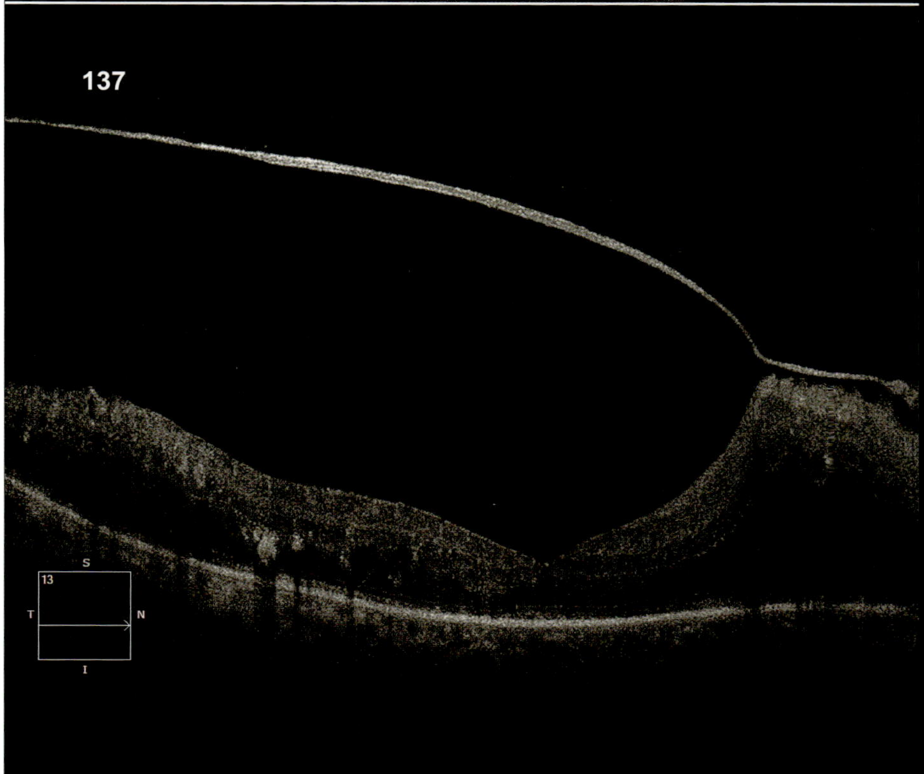


Figure 137 *OCT of the left demonstrates a thick hyper-reflective epiretinal membrane causing traction at the macula sparing the fovea more so in the nasal aspect. There is significant increase in central retinal thickness due to tractional pull of epiretinal membrane.*

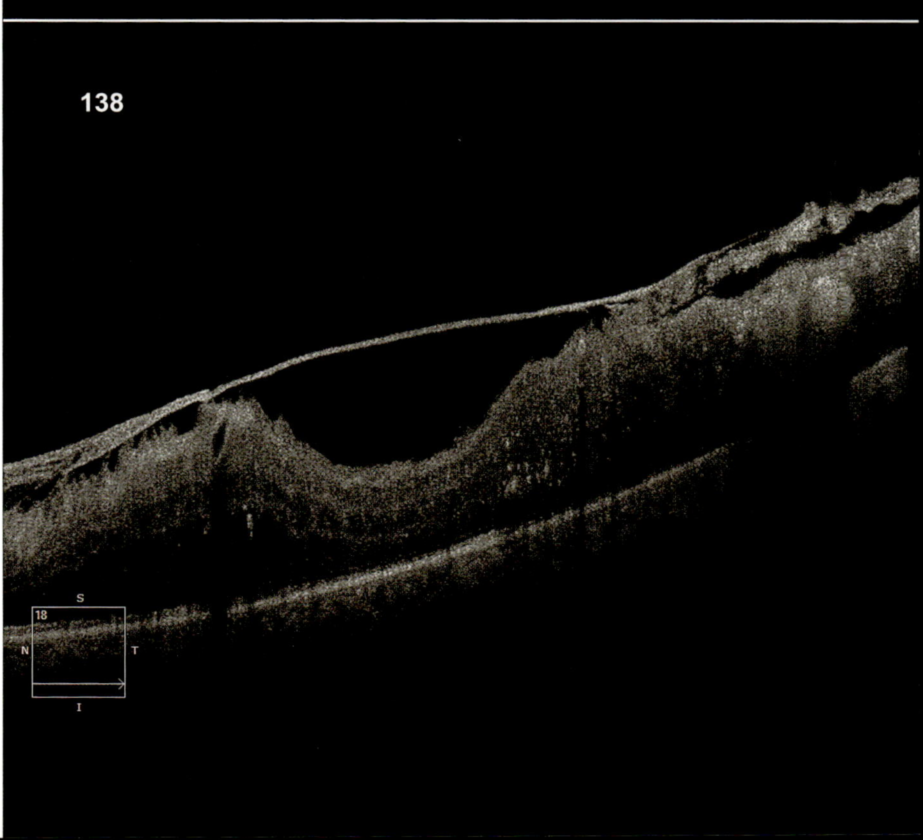


Figure 138 *OCT of the right eye demonstrates a thick hyper-reflective epiretinal membrane causing traction at the macula sparing the fovea. There is significant increase in central retinal thickness due to tractional pull of epiretinal membrane.* □

# CHAPTER 3

## RETINAL VASCULAR DISORDERS

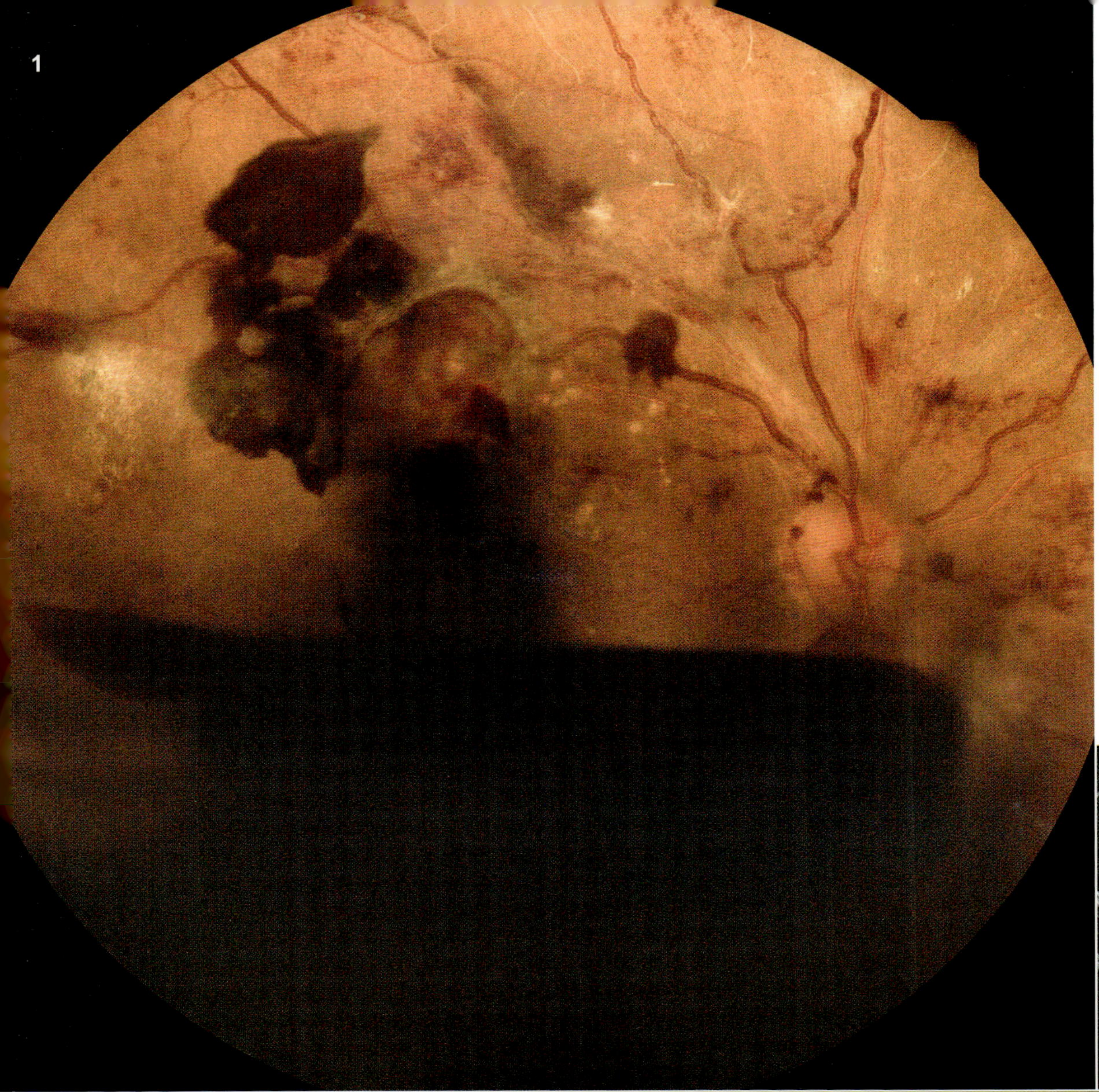


Figure 1

*A 47-year-old male presented with history of decrease in vision in right eye for the last 4 months. Fundus photo shows advanced proliferative diabetic retinopathy, a preretinal dense dark red boat-shaped sub-hyaloid hemorrhage obscuring most of the view of macula. Superficial flame-shaped hemorrhages are seen in superior and superonasal quadrant of retina. Venous beading and diffuse arterial sclerosis are seen in visible areas of retina suggestive of severe retinal ischemia.*

Figure 2

*Preretinal hyper-reflective sub-hyaloid bleeding contained in the vitreous cavity is visible with thickening of underlying neurosensory retina suggestive of macular edema.*

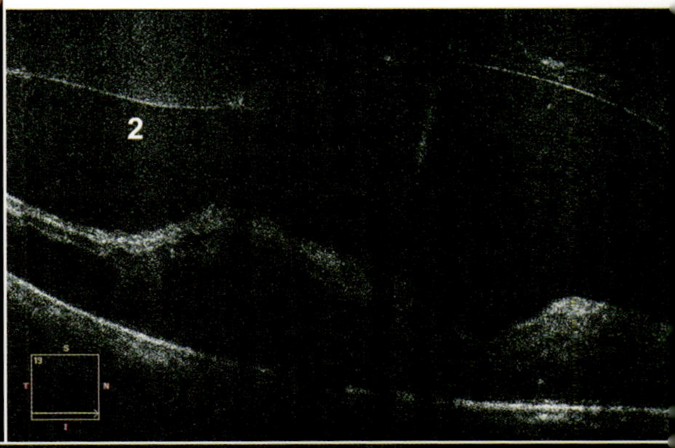


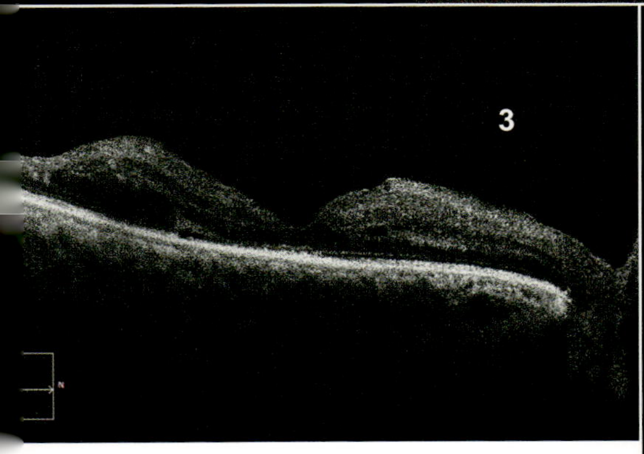


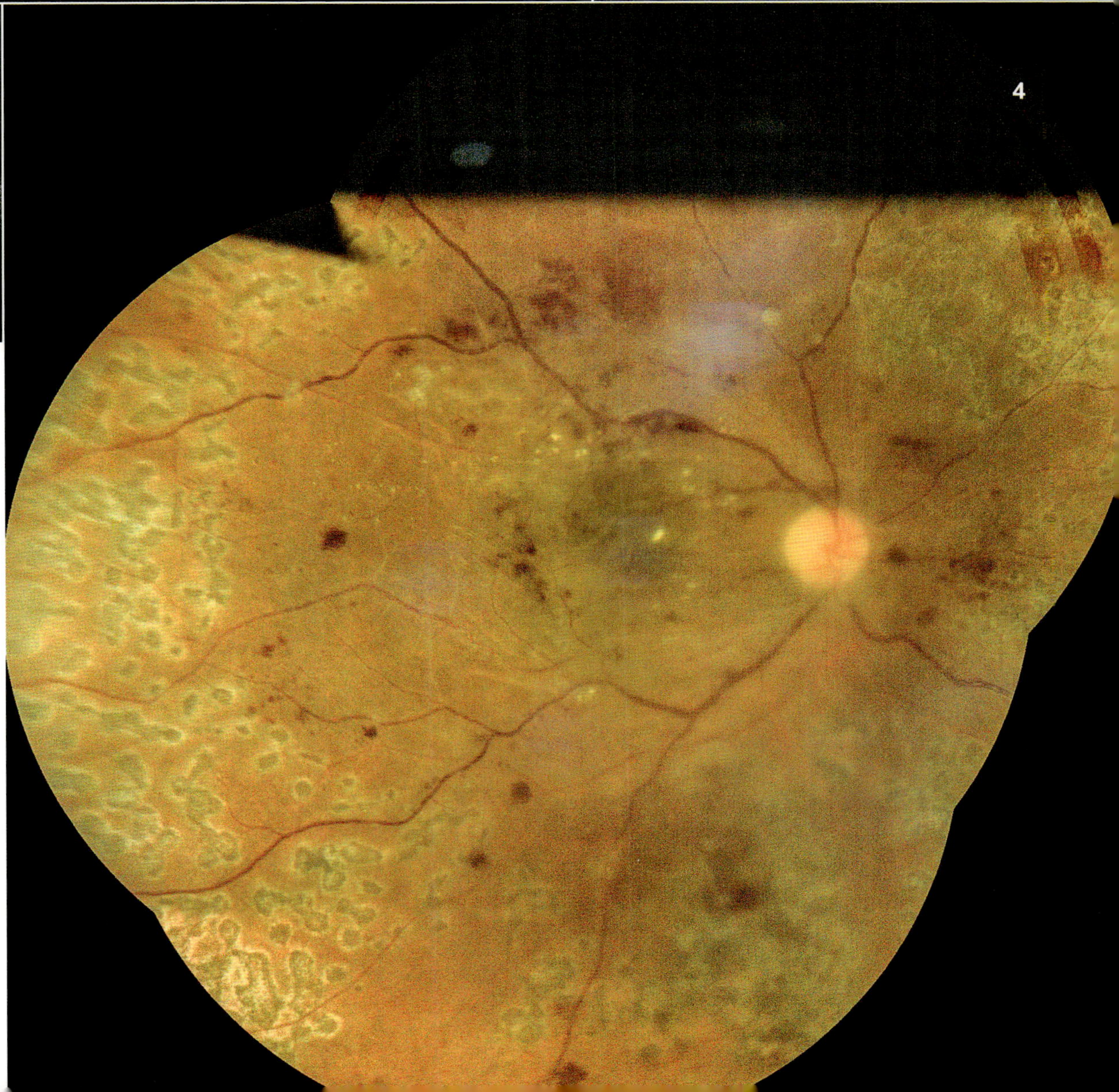


Figure 3

*25-gauge pars plana vitrectomy was performed in his right eye with intraocular gas tamponade. Three weeks postoperatively media clarity is grade 1 and 360 degree endolaser marks can be seen. Remaining gas bubble can be seen in superior part of retina which will eventually diffuse out. Best corrected visual acuity was 6/36.*

Figure 4

*Postoperative OCT scan shows total resolution of preretinal bleed, good signal strength from retinal layers with clear media. There was persistence of mild macular thickening in perifoveal area at 2 months.*□

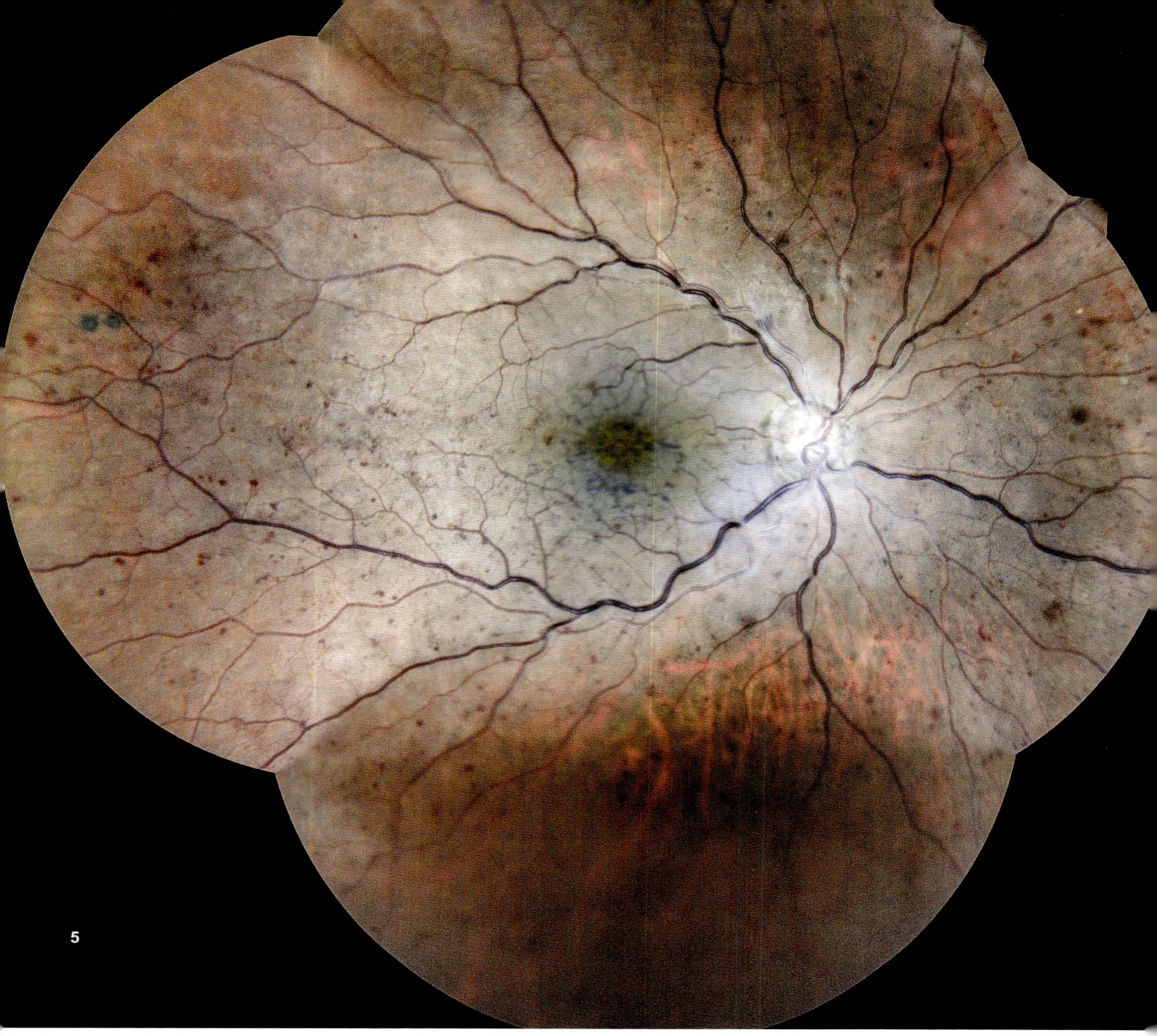

Figure 5 *Nonischemic variant of central retinal vein occlusion. Color fundus photograph of a case of nonischemic CRVO demonstrating intraretinal retinal hemorrhages in all four quadrants, minimal vascular tortuosity and macular thickening.*

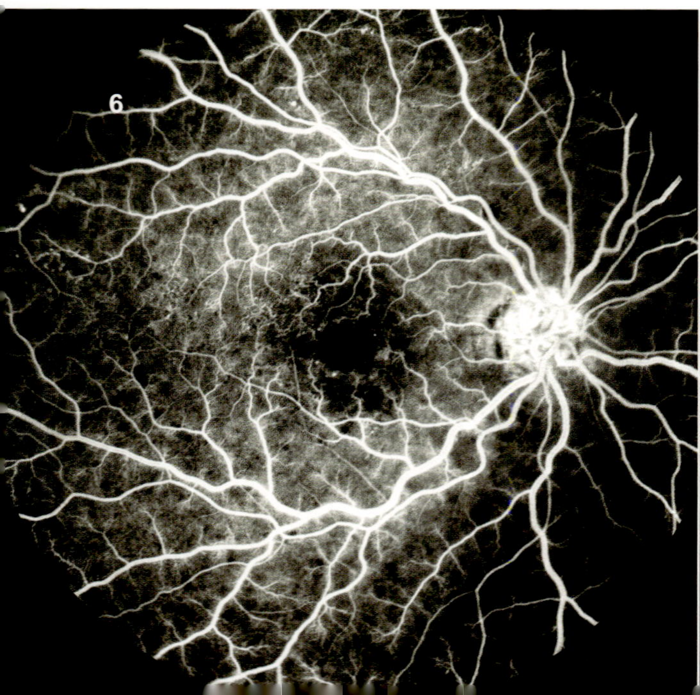

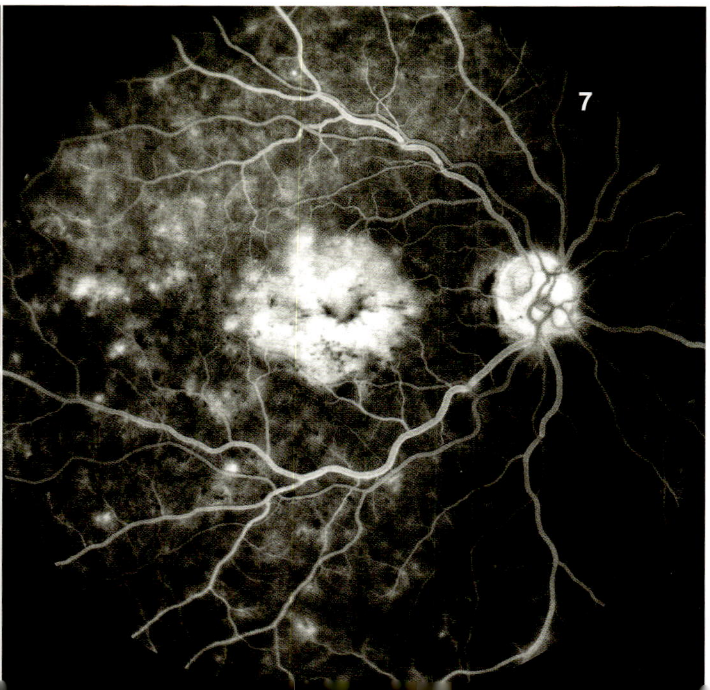

Figure 6

*Early frame of angiogram demonstrating multiple hypo-fluorescent dots as a result of blockage of fluorescein dye due to underlying retinal hemorrhages. Also note intact perifoveal capillary network highlighting good perfusion in a case of non-ischemic CRVO.*

Figure 7

*Late phase of fluorescein angiogram demonstrating petalloid leakage at the fovea due to cystoid macular edema.*

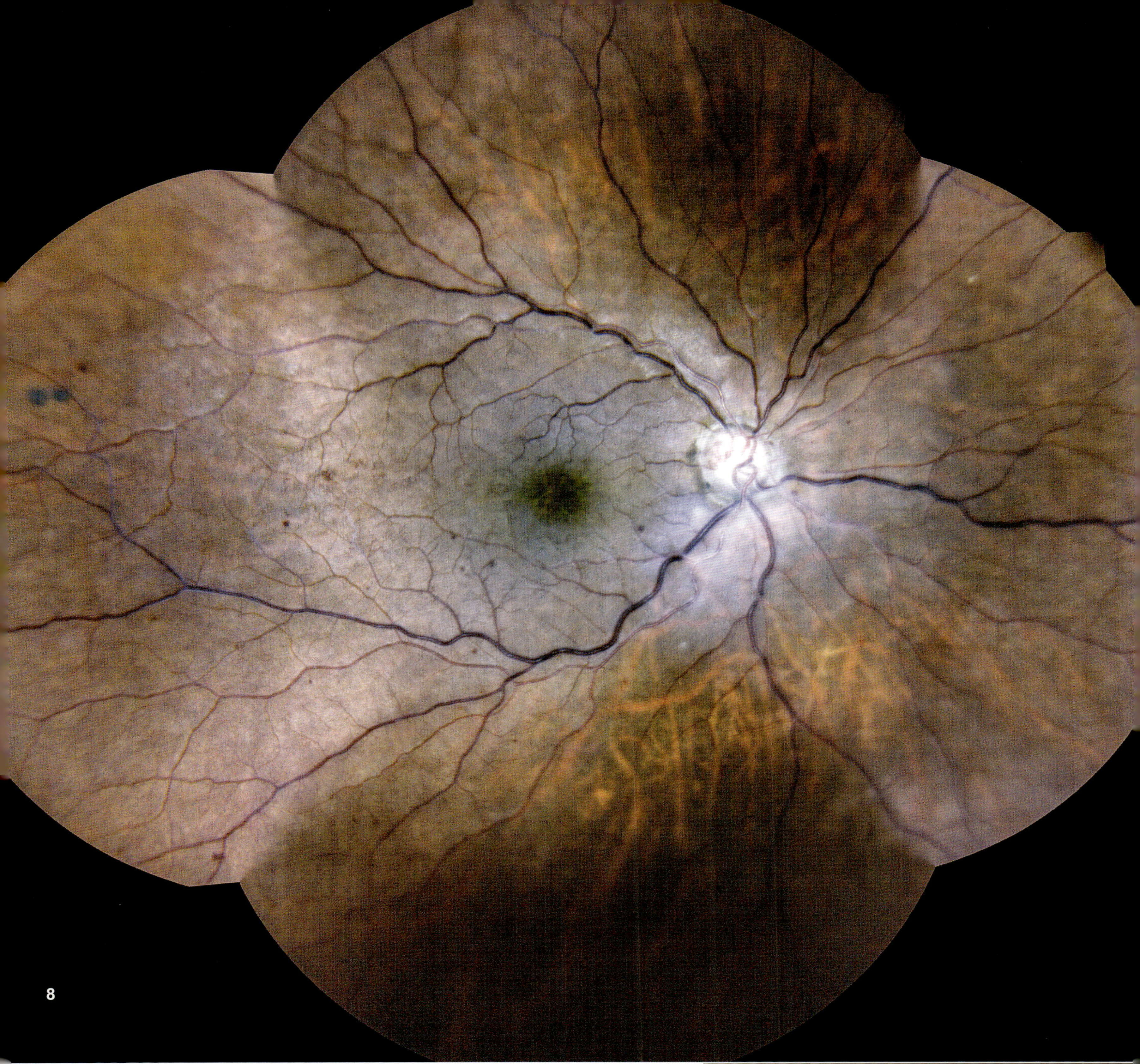

8

Figure 8 *Nonischemic variant of central retinal vein occlusion: 6 months after monthly intravitreal injections treatment.*

Figure 9 *Spectral domain OCT at the onset demonstrating intraretinal cystic fluid pockets due to macular edema associated with CRVO.*

Figure 10 *Spectral domain OCT demonstrating reduction in the retinal fluid, restoration of normal foveal contour 6 months later. Minimal intraretinal cysts are still persisting.*

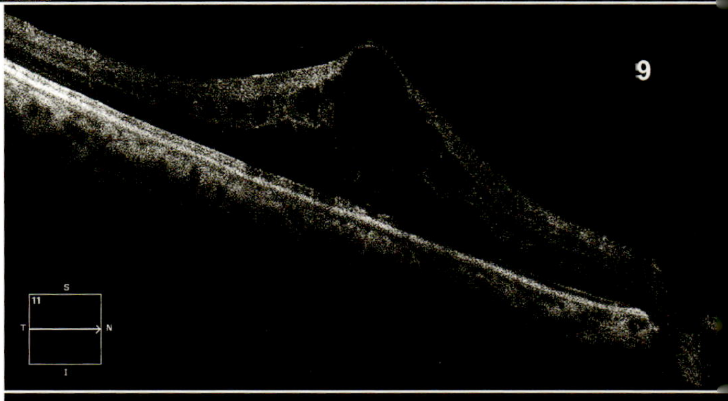

9

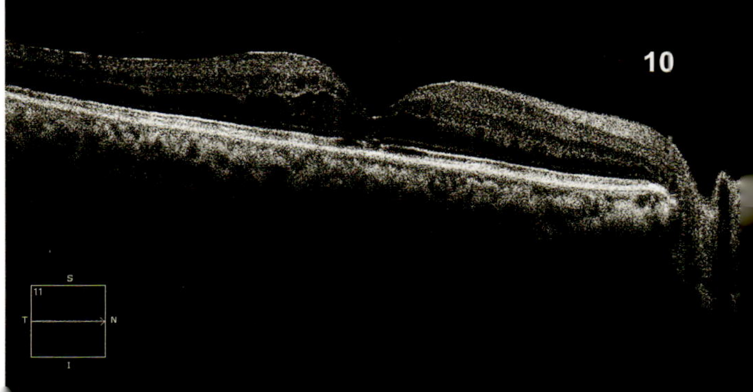

10

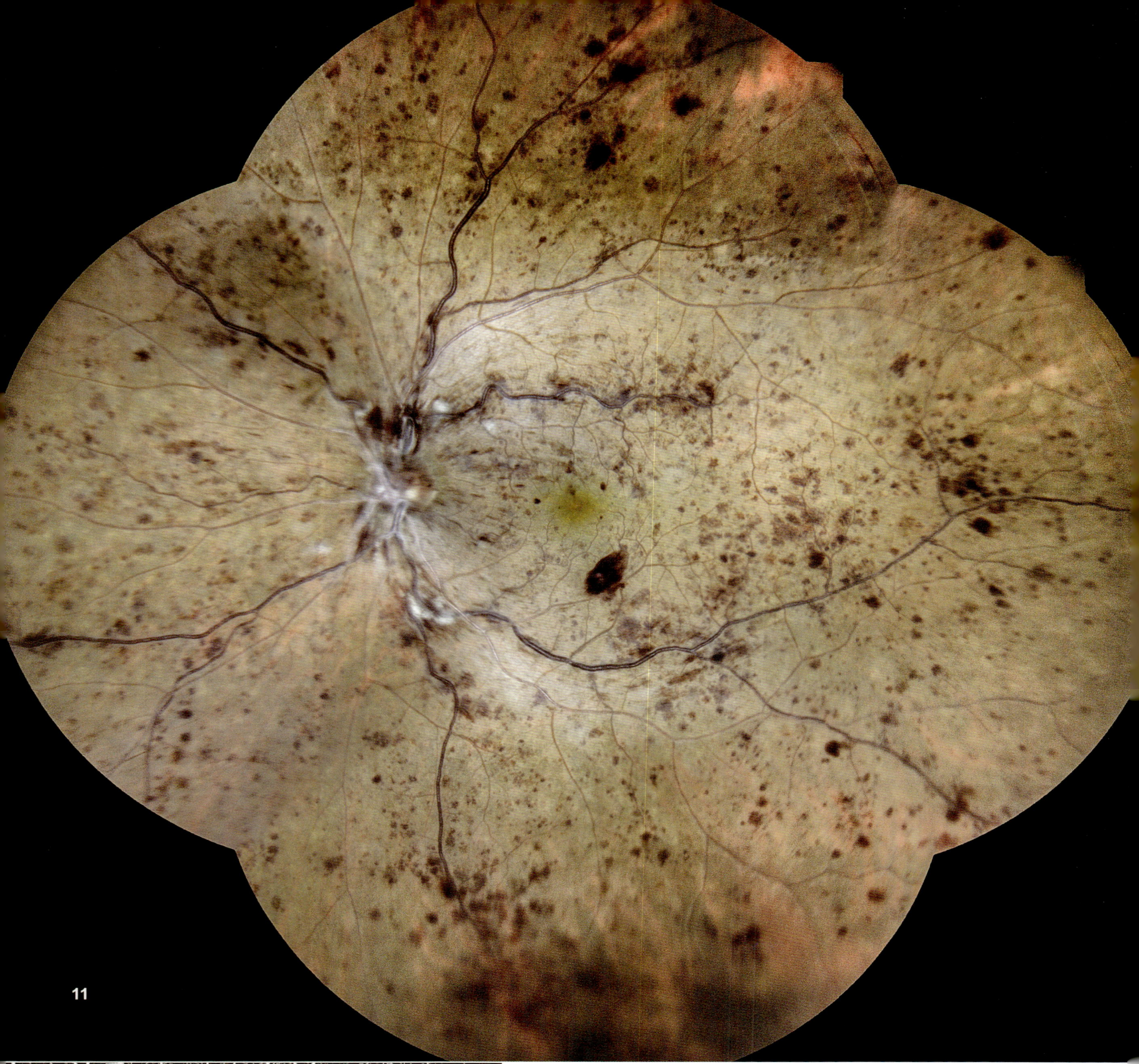

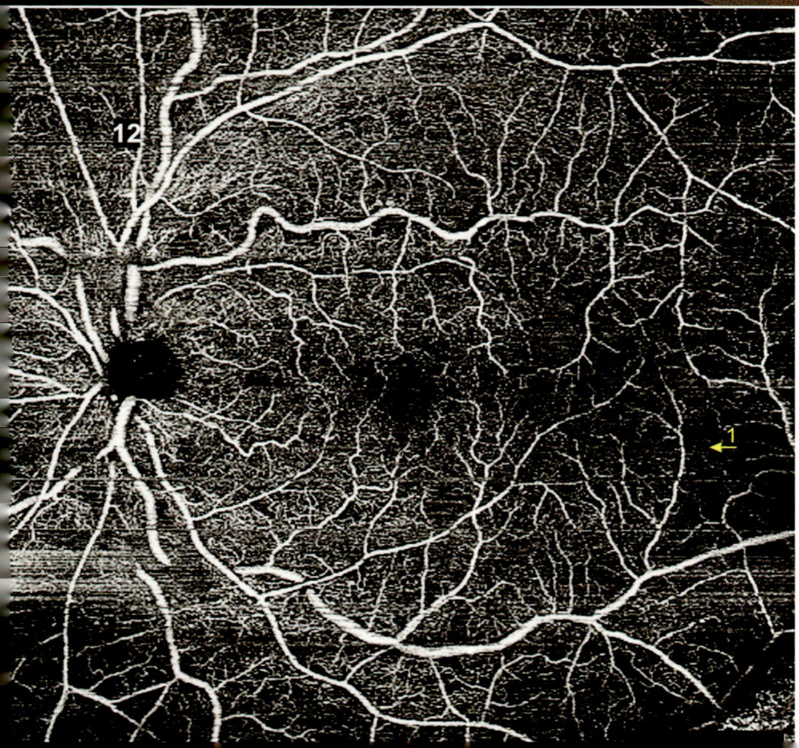

Figure 11 *Color fundus photograph of a nonischemic central retinal vein occlusion.*

Note the presence of multiple scattered intraretinal hemorrhages, tortuous vessels and few cotton wool spots.

Classification of CRVO into nonischemic and ischemic is essential because nonischemic CRVO is a relatively benign disease, with permanent central scotoma as a major complication from cystoid macular edema. There are functional (VA, RAPD) and morphological (fundus picture, FFA) tests to differentiate between ischemic and nonischemic.

Figure 12 *12 mm × 12 mm superficial slab of OCT angiography of central field shows few areas of nonperfusion (1).*

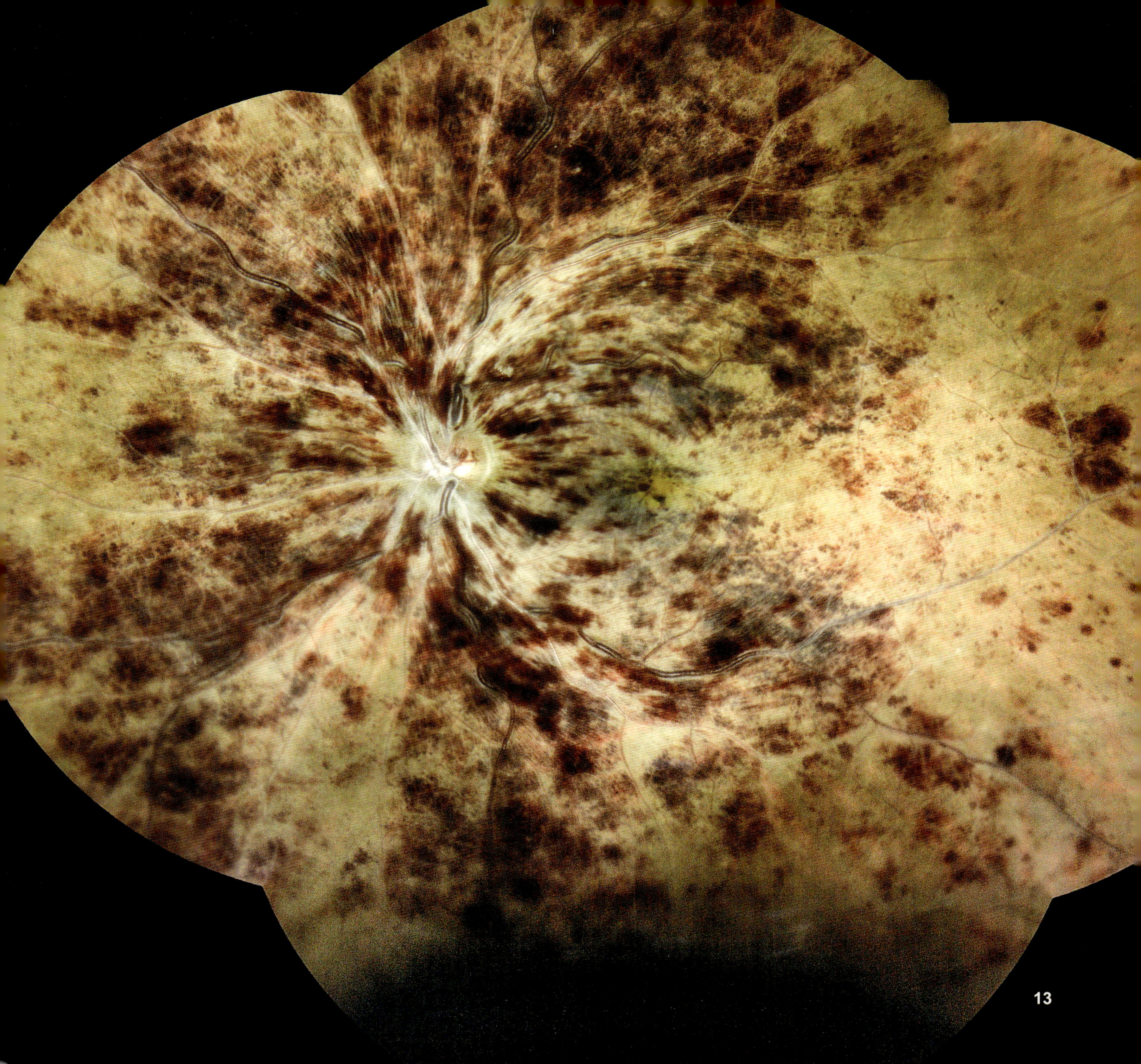

13

Figure 13 *Color fundus photograph demonstrating conversion to ischemic central retinal vein occlusion after 3 months.*

Note the presence of increase in the retinal hemorrhages, radiating from the optic disk in classic "blood and thunder" appearance. Landmark CVOS study has demonstrated cumulative chance of conversion of 13% within 18 months from baseline nonischemic CRVO at the onset to nonperfused ischemic CRVO. If there is a significant increase in the retinal hemorrhages it becomes necessary to assess retinal perfusion. But the major drawback of traditional FFA is that extensive hemorrhages will have a masking affect on retinal details. Such cases benefit from OCTA as it allows the retinal microvasculature to be visualized at various retinal depths.

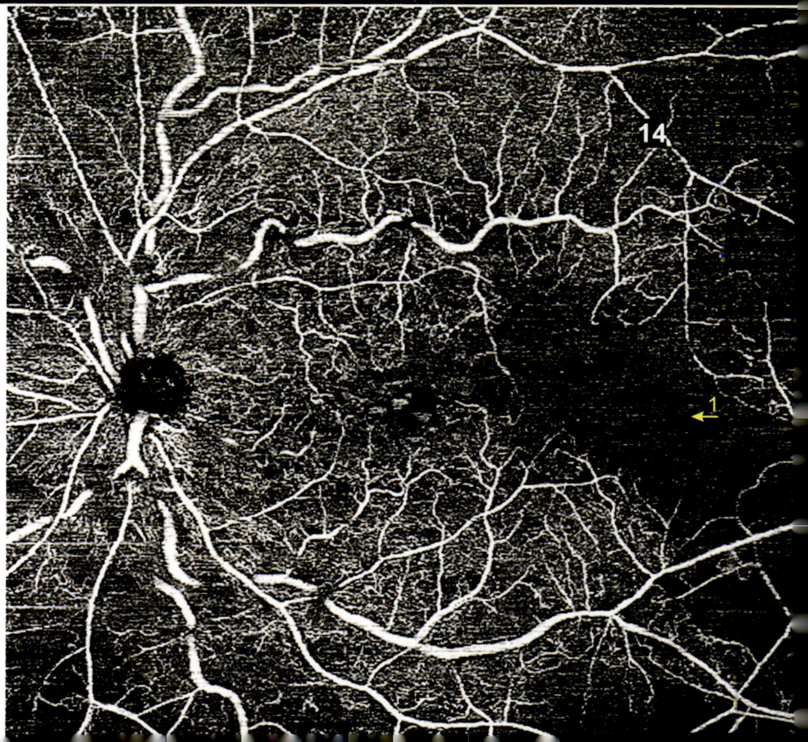


14

Figure 14 *12 mm × 12 mm OCT angiography image done 3 months later demonstrates a wider field of nonperfusion of retinal vasculature in the temporal macula, indicating progressive ischemic (1).* □

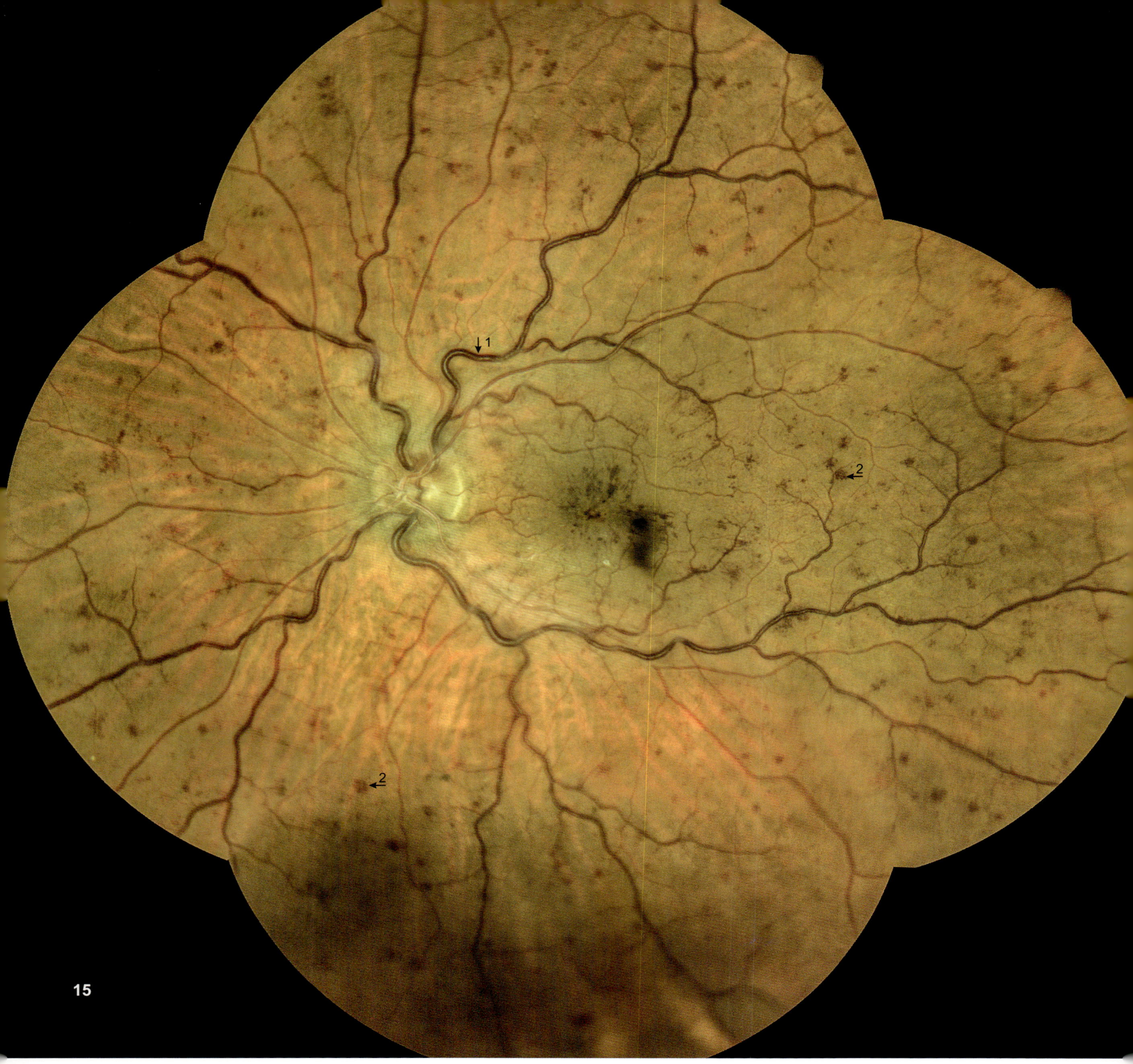


Figure 15 *Color fundus photograph of an eye with central retinal vein occlusion (CRVO) demonstrating typical features of venous tortuosity (1), macular thickening and intraretinal hemorrhages (2) in all four quadrants of the fundus.*

CRVO is a retinal vascular condition that is commonly seen in patients above 65 years. Diabetes, hypertension, hyperlipidemia and associated glaucoma are the common risk factors, although hypercoagulation hematological disorders and autoimmune vasculitis are also known causes especially in patients with younger age of presentation. It is usually a unilateral disease, however annual risk of developing any type of retinal vascular occlusion in the fellow eye is approximately 1% per year.

CRVO usually occurs due to thrombotic occlusion of central retinal vein. The most common symptom is sudden onset of painless blurred vision. With time, the extent of retinal hemorrhage may decrease or resolve completely with resultant retinal pigment epithelium alterations. The time course for resolution of the hemorrhages varies and is related on the amount of hemorrhages produced by the occlusion. Macular edema usually persists after resolution of hemorrhages. □

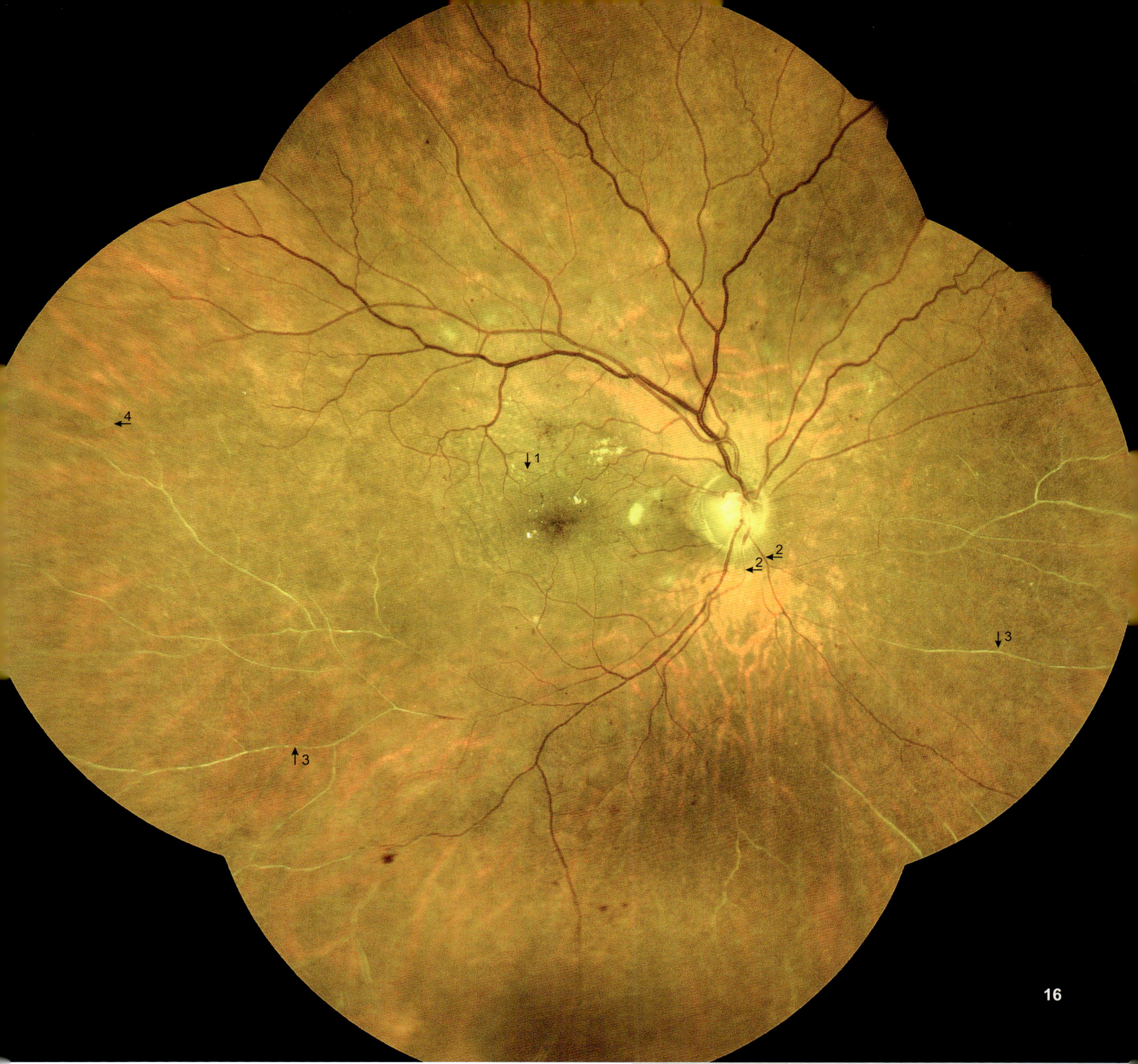

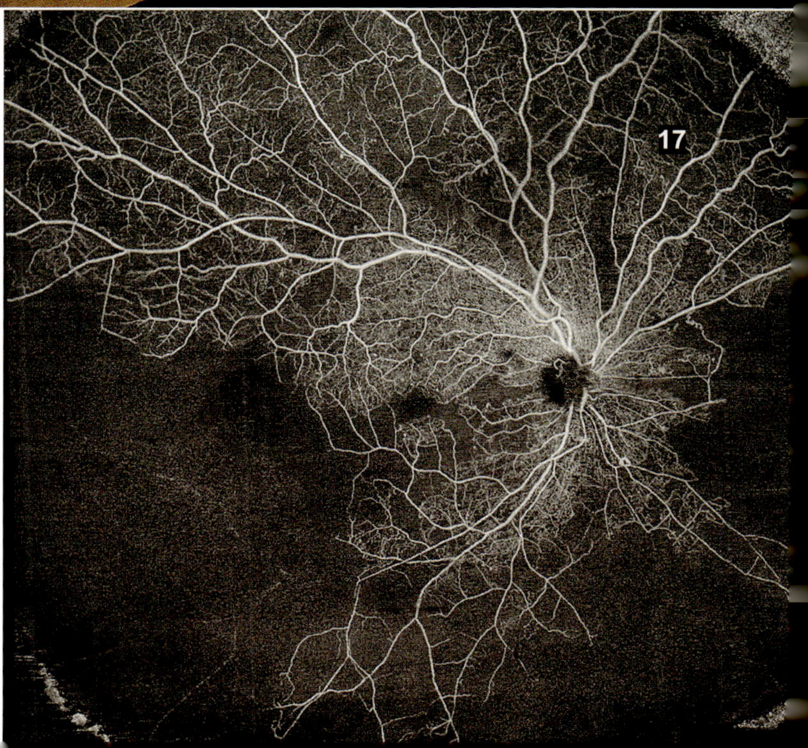

Figure 16 *Case of ischemic hemiretinal vein occlusion with moderate non-proliferative retinopathy and diabetic macular edema (treated with macular laser).*

Color fundus montage of a 65-year-old diabetic male with moderate non-proliferative diabetic retinopathy. He had been previously treated with macular grid laser. Macular laser scars (1) are seen at the posterior pole. There are a few resolving hard exudates and cotton wool spots. Retinal vascular caliber was normal in superior hemisphere. However generalized attenuation of artery and vein is seen as they originates from lower margin of the optic disk (2). Also note sclerosed retinal veins supplying the retinal periphery (3) with silent retinal mid-periphery due to massive capillary nonperfusion (4).

Figure 17 *12 mm × 12 mm OCT angiography at the level of superficial capillary plexus demonstrating loss of retinal vasculature due to nonperfusion of the inferior half of the retina.* □

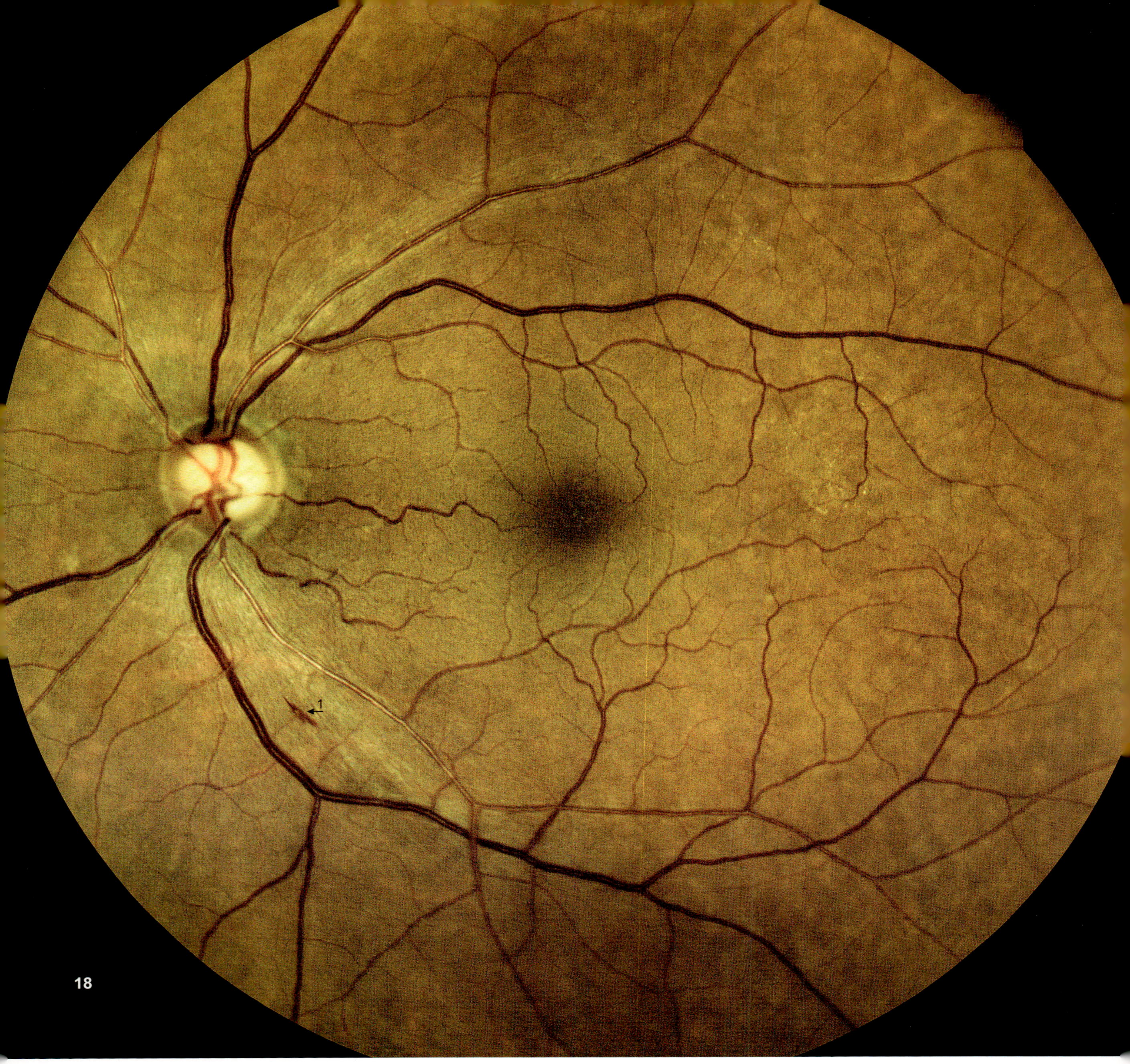


Figure 18 *A 75-year-old hypertensive male came for a regular follow-up. Color fundus photograph shows the presence of a single splinter hemorrhage along the inferotemporal vein (1). At this stage patient was advised blood pressure monitoring and observation.*

Figure 19 *Color fundus photograph at 1 month shows increase in the number of retinal hemorrhages. Clinical diagnosis was an incipient hemiretinal vein occlusion.*

Figure 20 *Color fundus photograph at 2 months from the onset shows further increase in the retinal hemorrhages which were distributed in inferior hemispheric retina and dilated and tortuous inferior retinal vein.*

Figure 21 *Color fundus photograph 3 months later demonstrates a classic hemiretinal vein occlusion with thickening of inferior part of macula. At this stage patient was advised intravitreal anti-VEGF injection.*

Figure 22 *Color fundus photograph 4 weeks after anti-VEGF injection demonstrates the drastic reduction in the amount of retinal hemorrhages and reduced vascular tortuosity.*

Figure 23 *Color fundus photograph 4 weeks after second intravitreal anti-VEGF injection: rapid reabsorption of retinal hemorrhages is noticeable.*

Figure 24 *Color fundus photograph 4 weeks after third intravitreal anti-VEGF injection: note that hemiretinal vein occlusion has almost completely reabsorbed with normal foveal reflex.*□

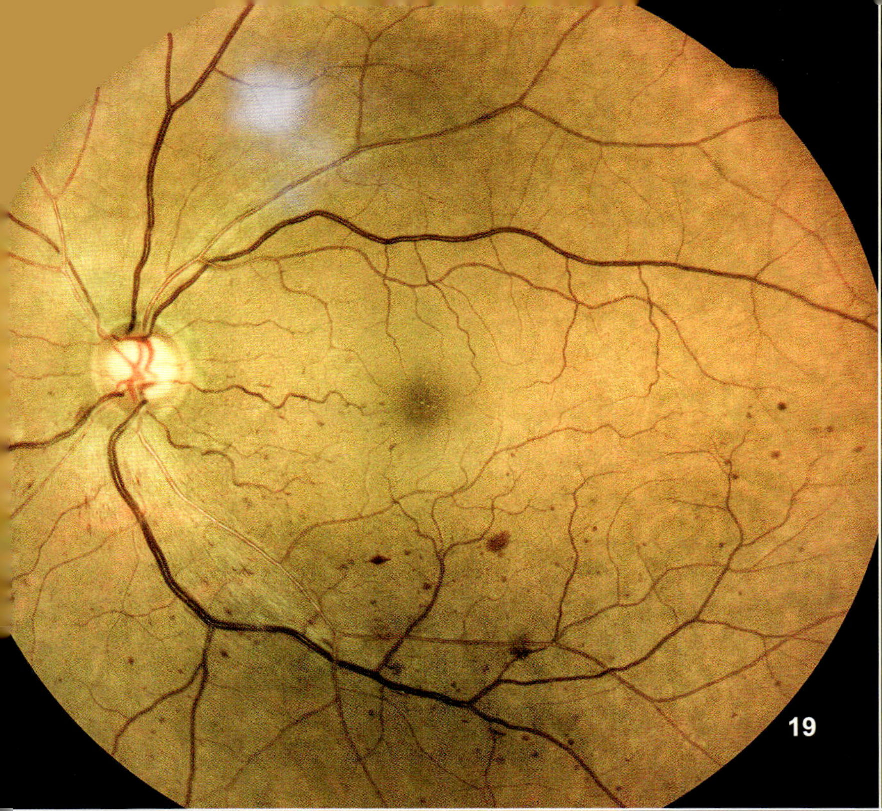

19

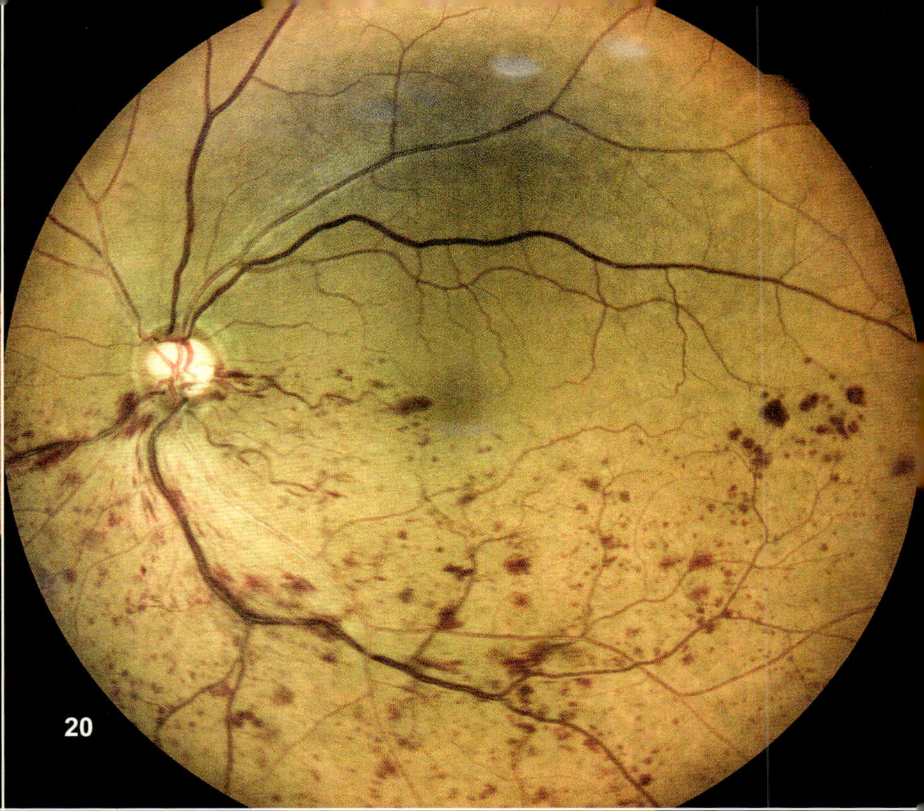

20

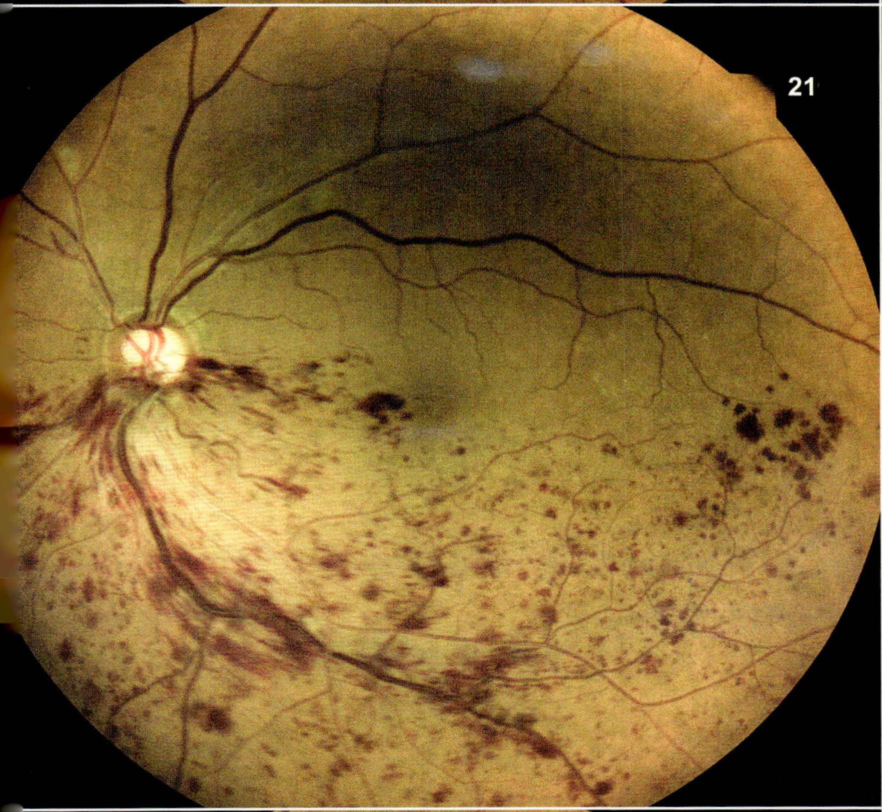

21

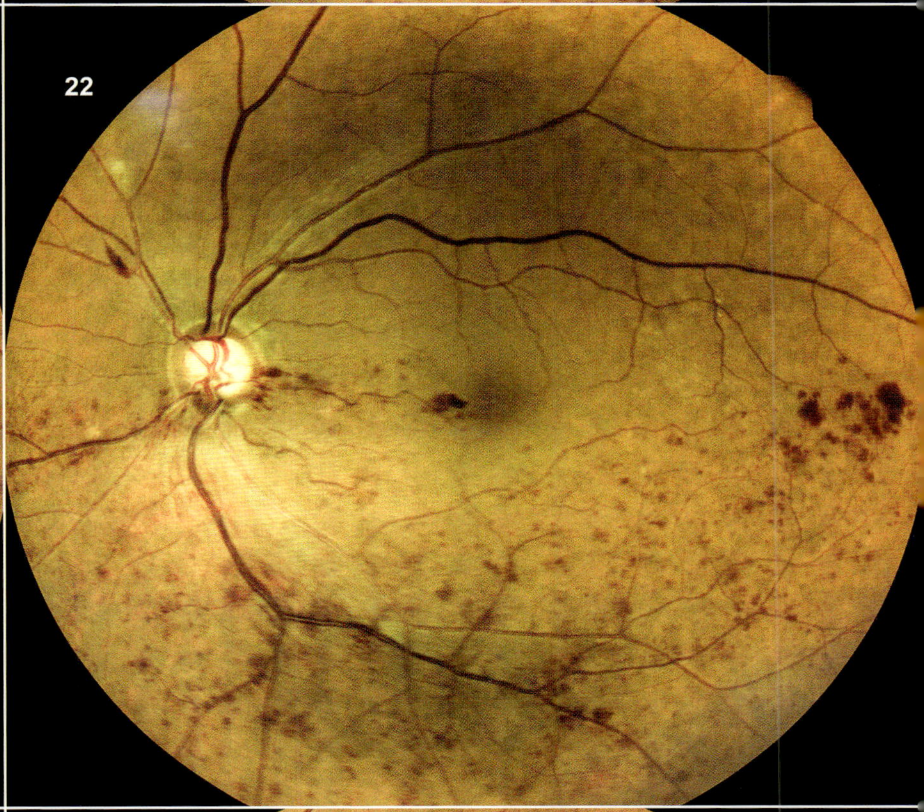

22

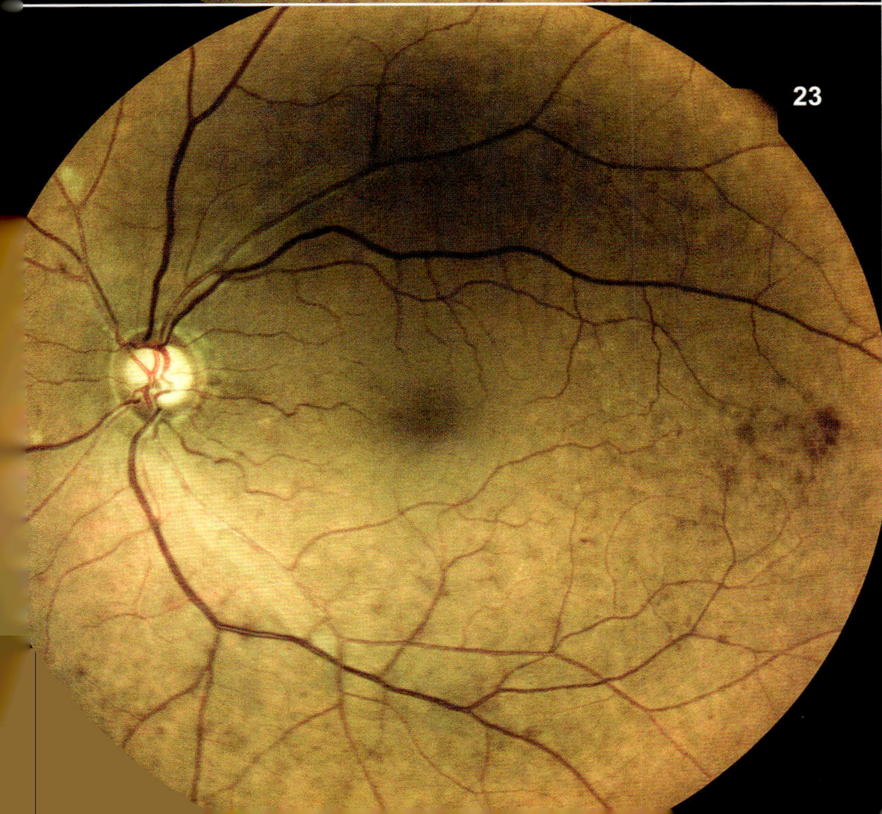

23

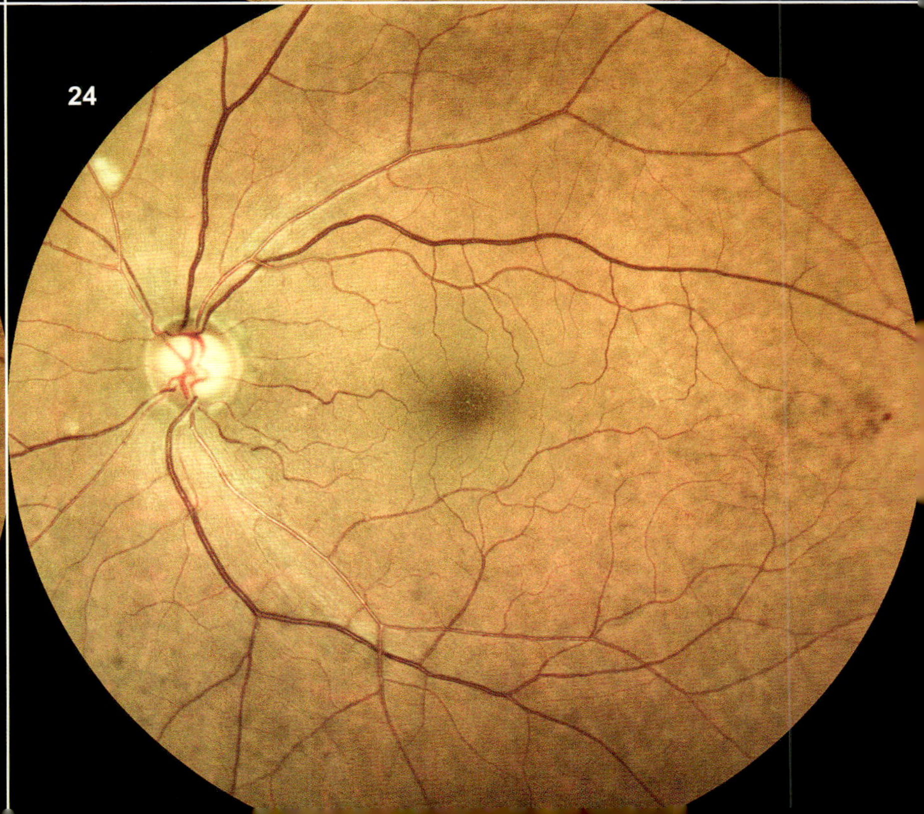

24

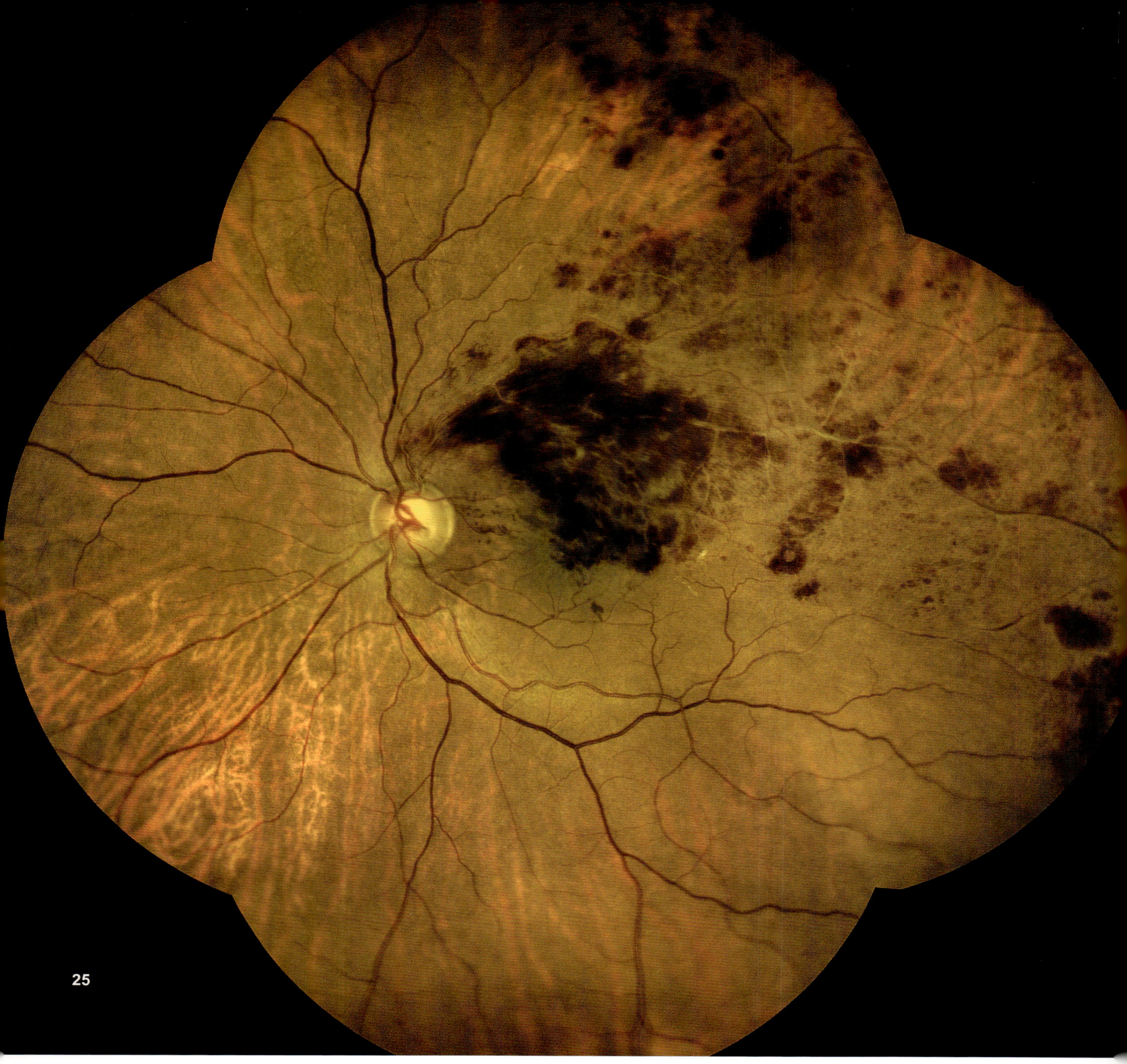

Figure 25 *Case of superotemporal branch retinal vein occlusion with peripheral ischemia.*

Fundus photograph of acute, superotemporal branch retinal vein occlusion demonstrating segmental pattern of intraretinal hemorrhage.

Location of the venous block determines the distribution of intraretinal hemorrhage. In this case, occlusion is peripheral to the optic disk, along the superotemporal vessel and hence segmental superotemporal distribution of retinal hemorrhages. Hemorrhages extend up to the foveal center and may reduce central visual acuity. Visual acuity may recover completely if there is no associated other cause for the visual loss, such as macular edema or macular ischemia.

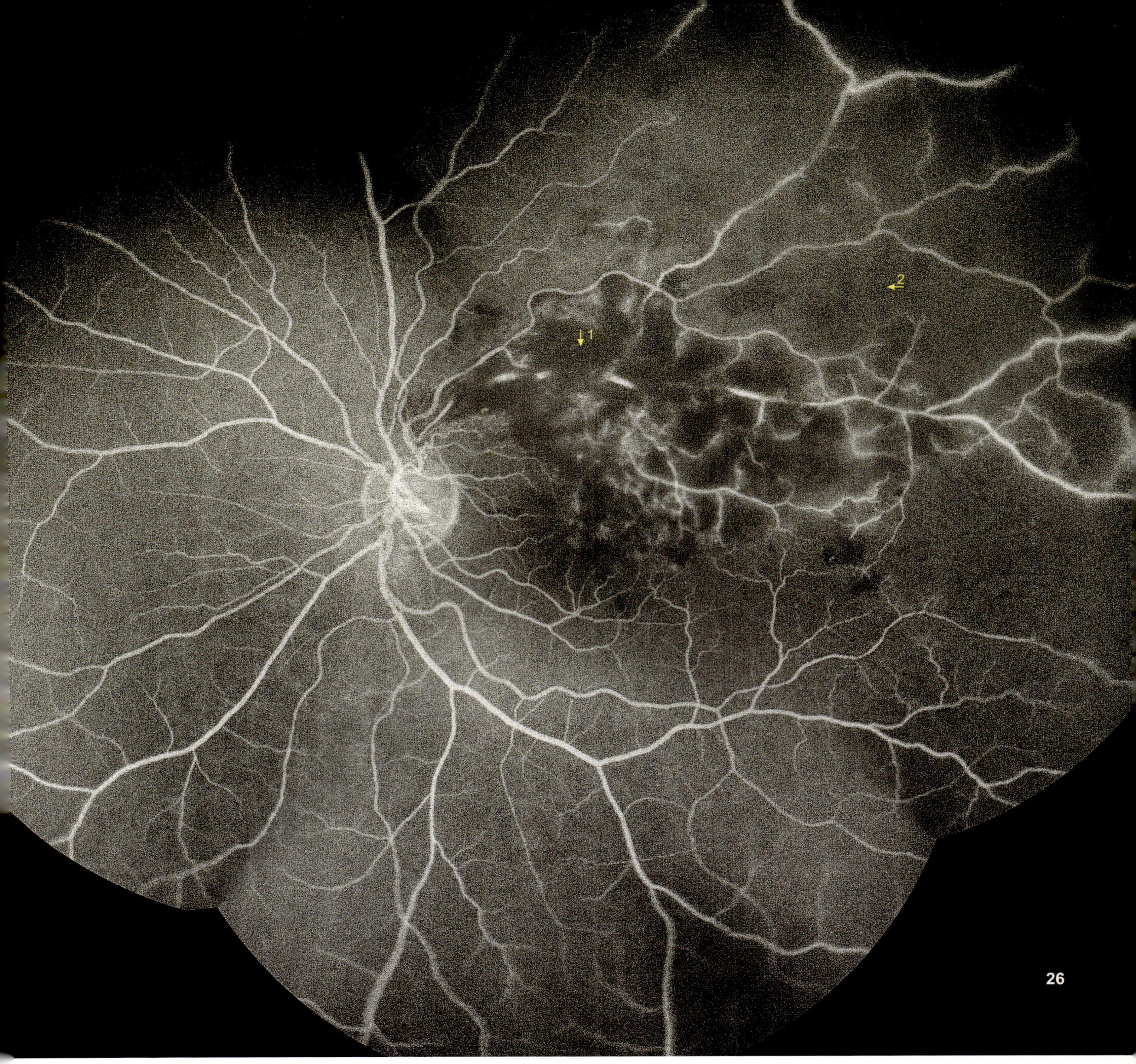


Figure 26 *FFA collage demonstrating blocked hypofluorescence due to underlying retinal hemorrhages (1). Also note presence of large area of capillary nonperfusion (2) in superotemporal periphery.*

Note the difference in type of hypofluorescence arising from the retina hemorrhages and nonperfusion retina. Hypofluorescence that originates from the masking affect of underlying retinal hemorrhages appears more darker, whereas the hypofluorescence that arises from the areas of non-perfusion appear slightly fainter. There is abrupt termination of retinal capillaries in the region of nonperfusion.

Fluorescein angiogram in the acute phase of retina vein occlusion usually fails to give complete information about the retina perfusion status and should be performed once retinal hemorrhages have reduced a bit. □

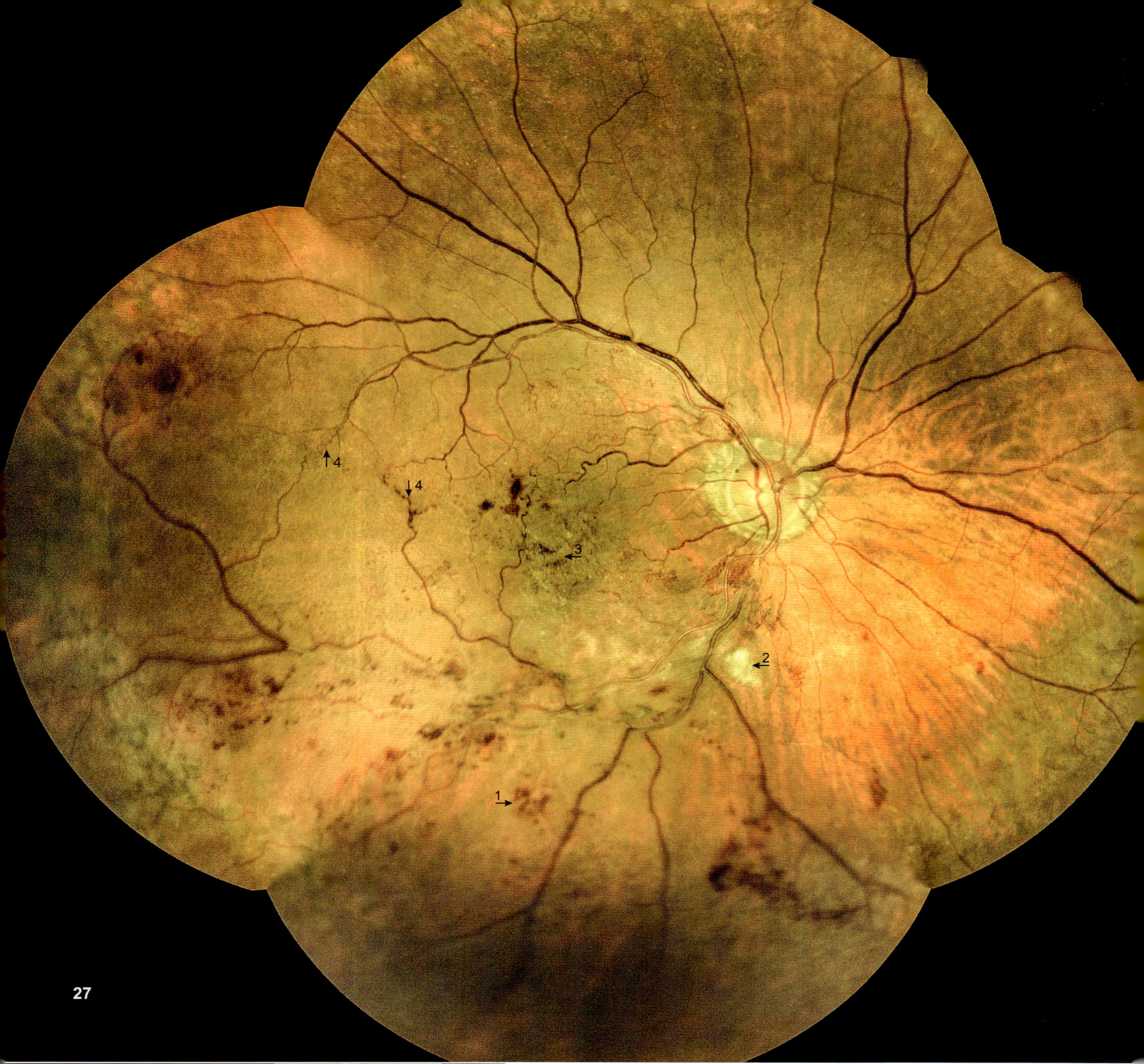


27

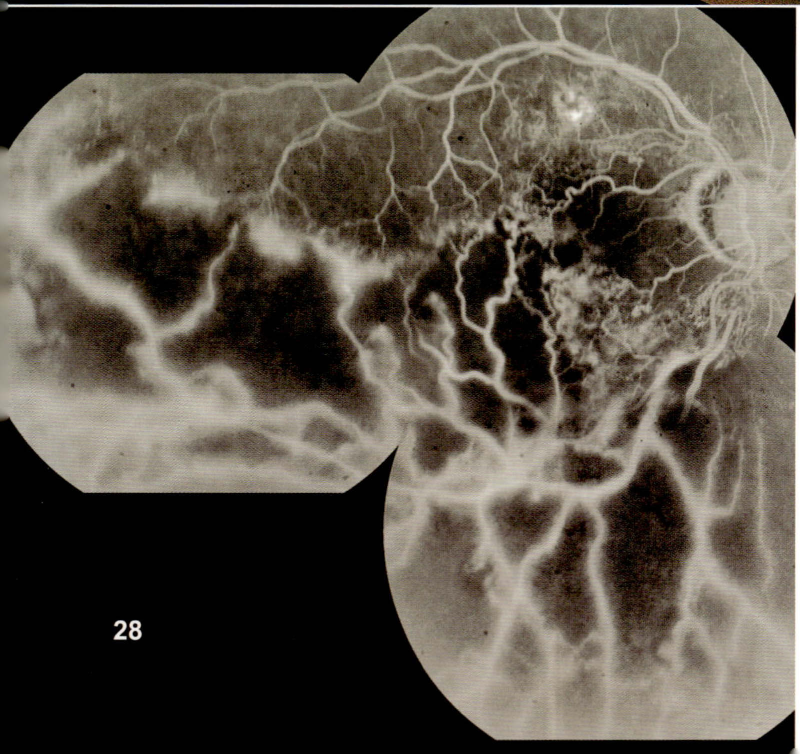

28

Figure 27 *Color fundus montage photo of a case of ischemic branch retinal vein occlusion. Note the presence of intraretinal hemorrhages in the inferotemporal quadrant (1), cotton wool spots (2), glistening reflex at the macula (3). There is presence of retinal vascular remodeling (4) and large area of silent looking retina, devoid of any vasculature in the temporal periphery suggestive of peripheral retinal ischemia.*

Landmark BRVO study has demonstrated that eyes which shows larger areas of retinal capillary nonperfusion (greater than 5 disk diameters) are at the increased risk of neovascularization and subsequent vitreous hemorrhage. it concluded that if sector laser photocoagulation is applied in eyes with nonperfusion, incidence of NV can be reduced from about 40% to 20%.

Figure 28 *FFA montage image demonstrates vessel staining, perifoveal capillary dropout and enlarged irregular foveal avascular zone with large area of capillary nonperfusion.*

29

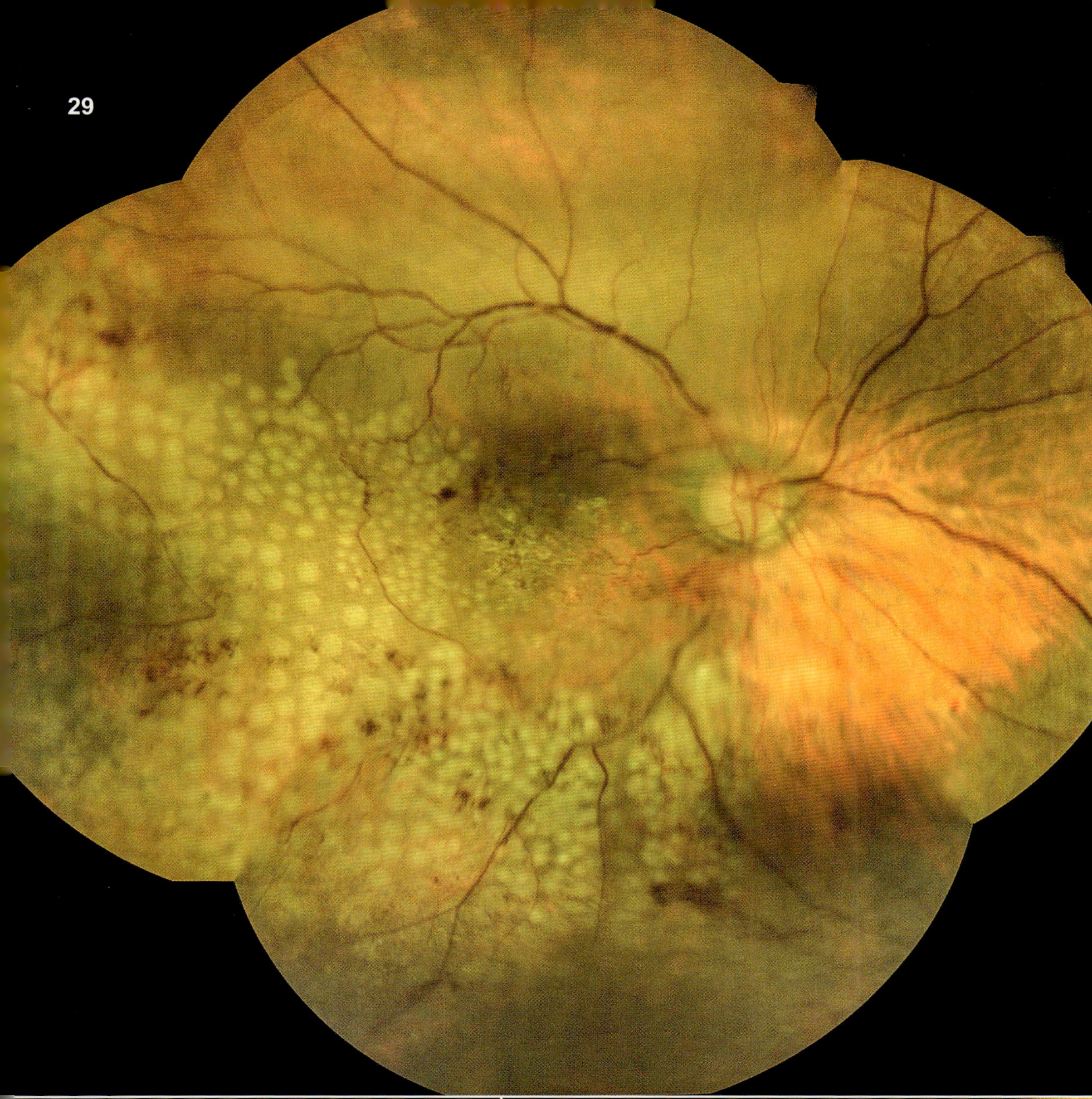

Figure 29

*Immediate post-treatment fundus photograph showing pattern of peripheral scatter laser photocoagulation to area of nonperfusion and grid laser to the macula.*

Figure 30

*OCT scan at presentation shows large amount of intraretinal cystic fluid spaces involving the fovea. There is a fine epiretinal membrane.*

30

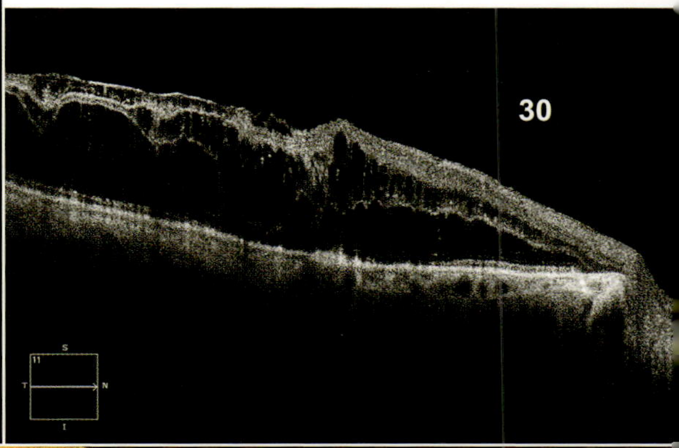

31

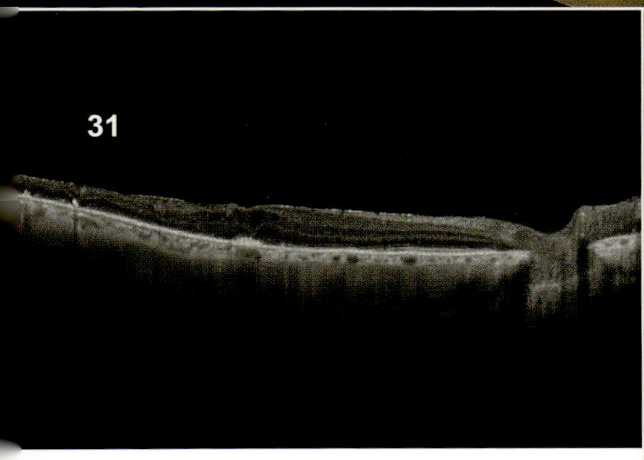

Figure 31

*OCT scan 1 month post anti-VEGF injection and sector laser photocoagulation. There is drastic reduction in the retinal fluid spaces. Note the areas of disorganized inner retinal layers (DRIL) in the temporal macula that signifies inner retinal ischemia.*

Figure 32

*Color fundus photograph done 1 month post a single anti-VEGF injection and sector laser photo-coagulation.*

32

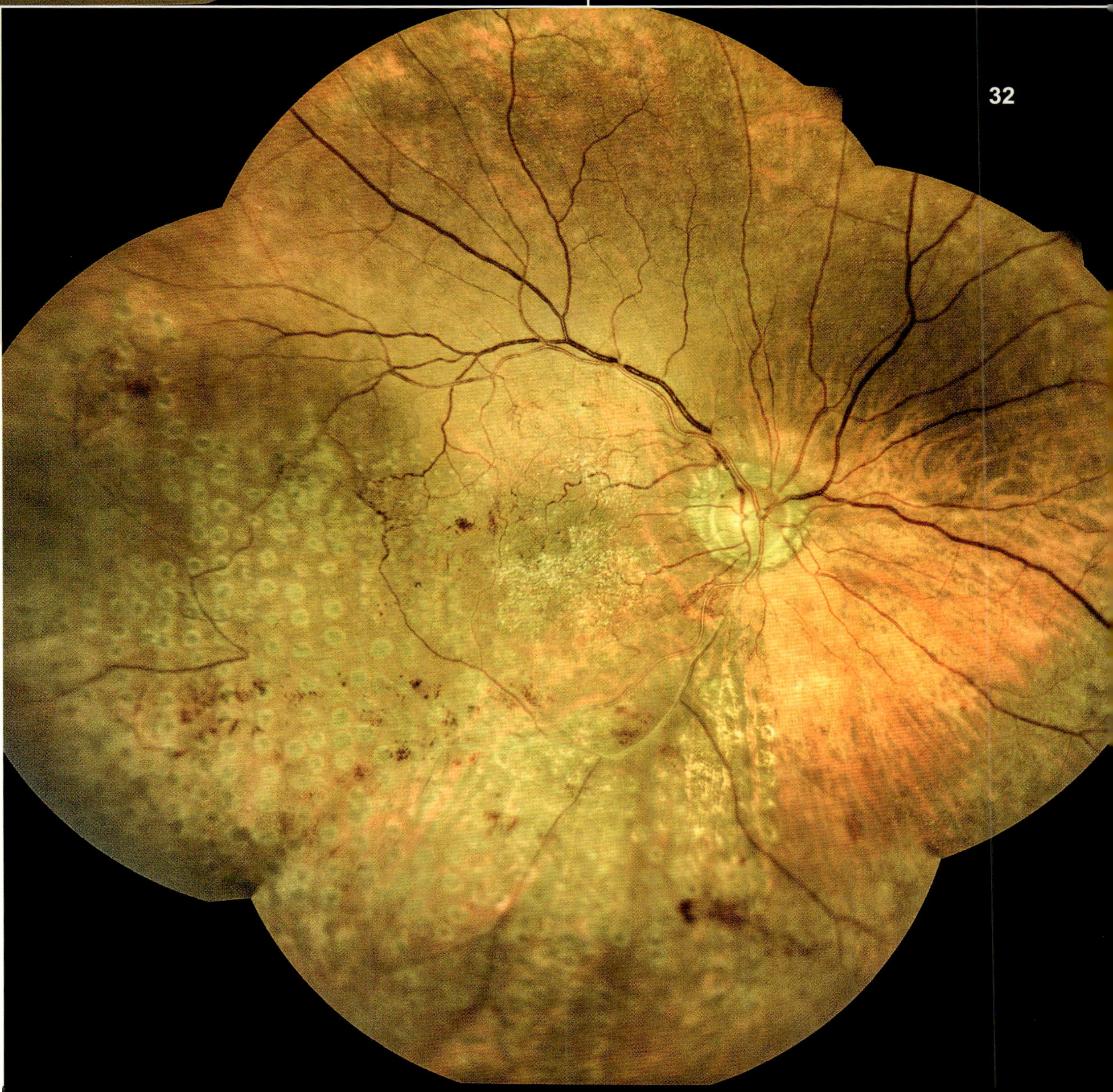

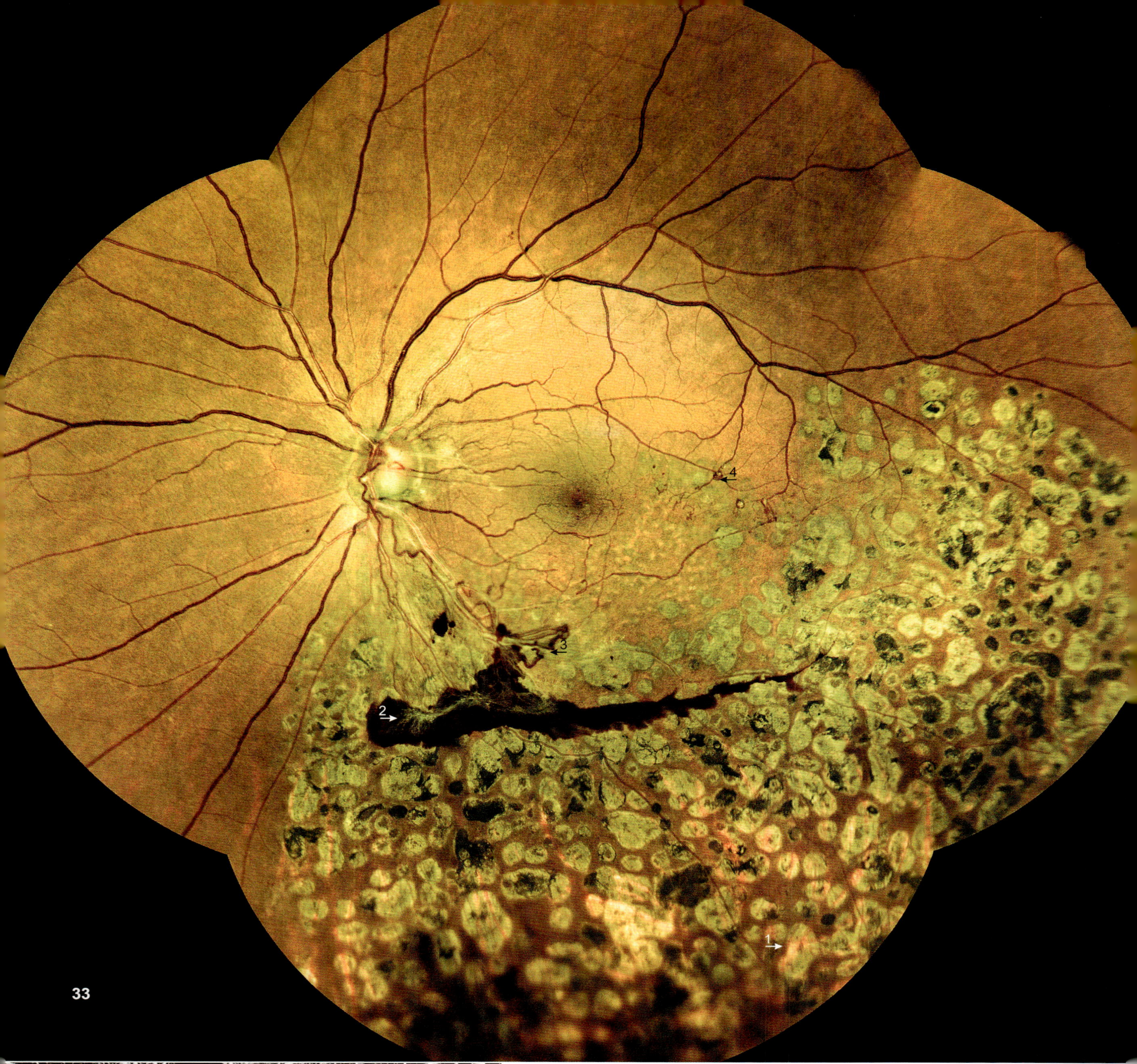


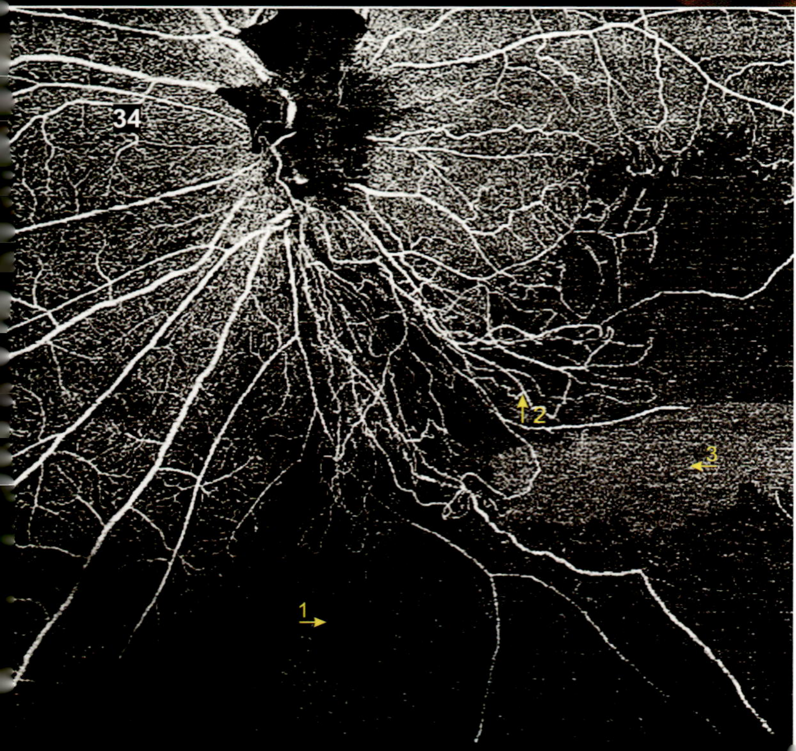


Figure 33 *Case of old branch retinal vein occlusion with fresh neovascularization and preretinal hemorrhage.*

A 54-year-old hypertensive female with previous history of retinal laser and intravitreal injections treatment for branch retinal vein occlusion presented to us with recent and sudden onset floaters. Note the presence of old laser scars along the inferotemporal arcade (1) and fresh preretinal hemorrhage (2) associated with a frond of neovascularization (3). Also note the presence of small capillary aneurysms in temporal macula (4 ).

Figure 34 *OCT angiography slab at the level of superficial capillary plexus demonstrates hyporegion in the inferotemporal macula due to capillary nonperfusion (1) and exuberant vascular proliferation (2). Preretinal hemorrhage has a blockage affect on the underlying retinal vascular details (3).*

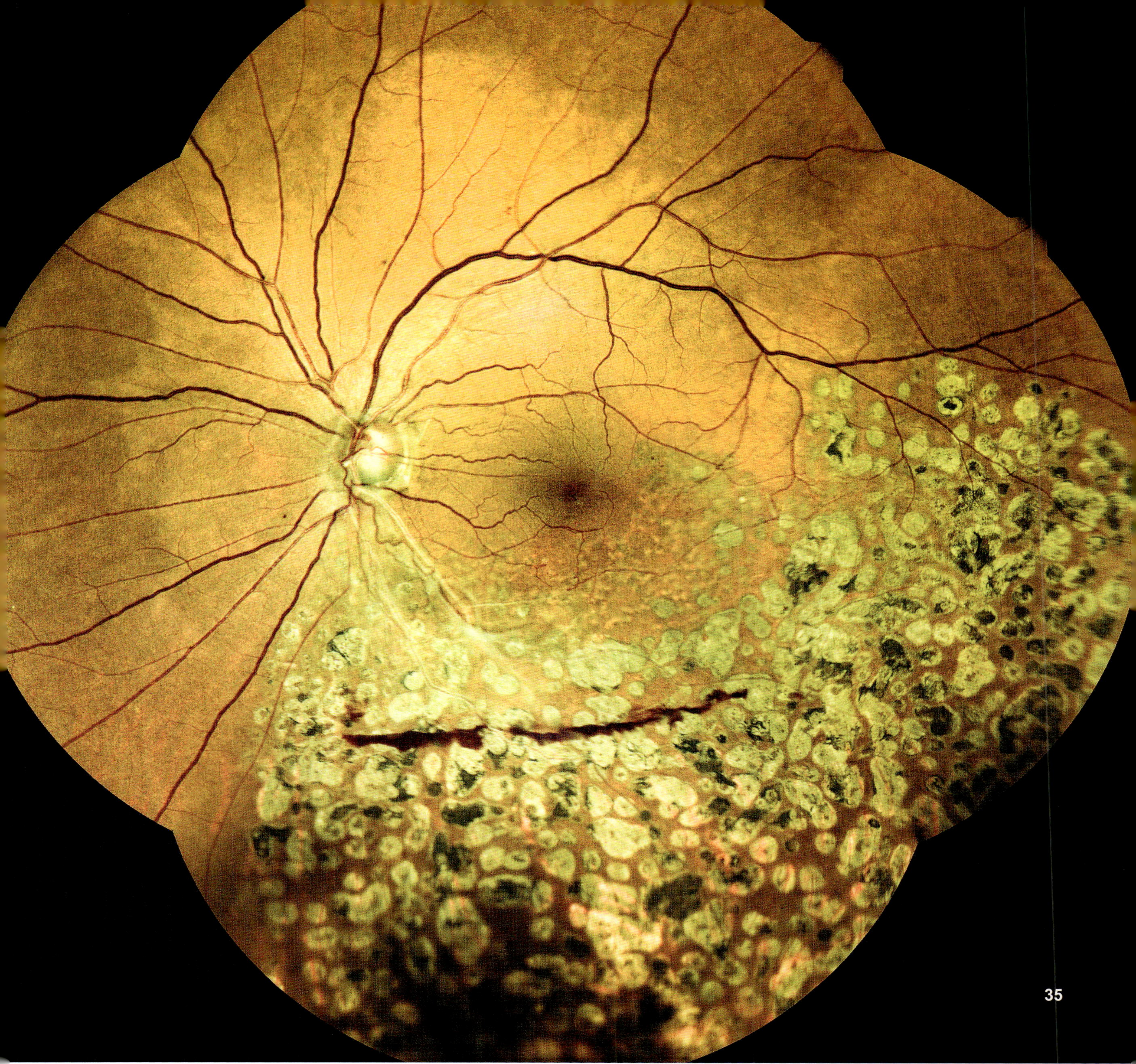


Figure 35 *Color fundus photograph at 1 month post-treatment. Note rapid regression of neovascularization frond, partial resolution of preretinal hemorrhages and disappearance of capillary aneurysms.*

Intravitreal anti-VEGF injections are a useful treatment option in cases with recurrent neovascular bleeds where laser has been done adequately. She is a 54-year-old female hypertensive patient for few years and has been previously treated for ischemic BRVO. At presentation her visual acuity was 6/6 as her fovea was not involved and floaters were as a result of preretinal bleed. Since there was an active neovascularization frond, laser was adequate. A single intravenous injection of anti-VEGF was adequate.

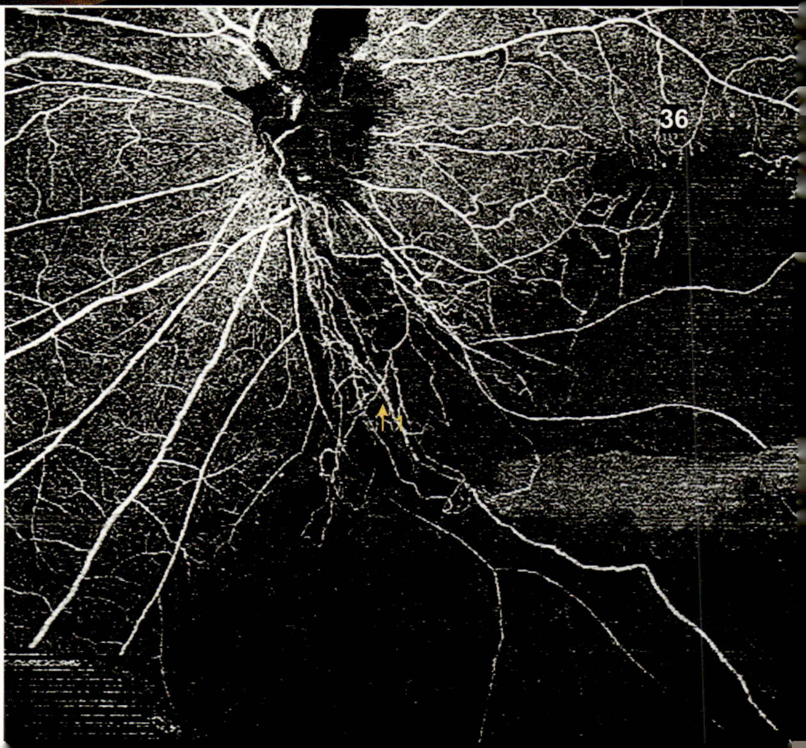


Figure 36 *OCT angiography superficial capillary plexus slab 1 month after anti-VEGF injection: Note the pruning of the abnormal vasculature with reduction in its caliber and size (1).*□

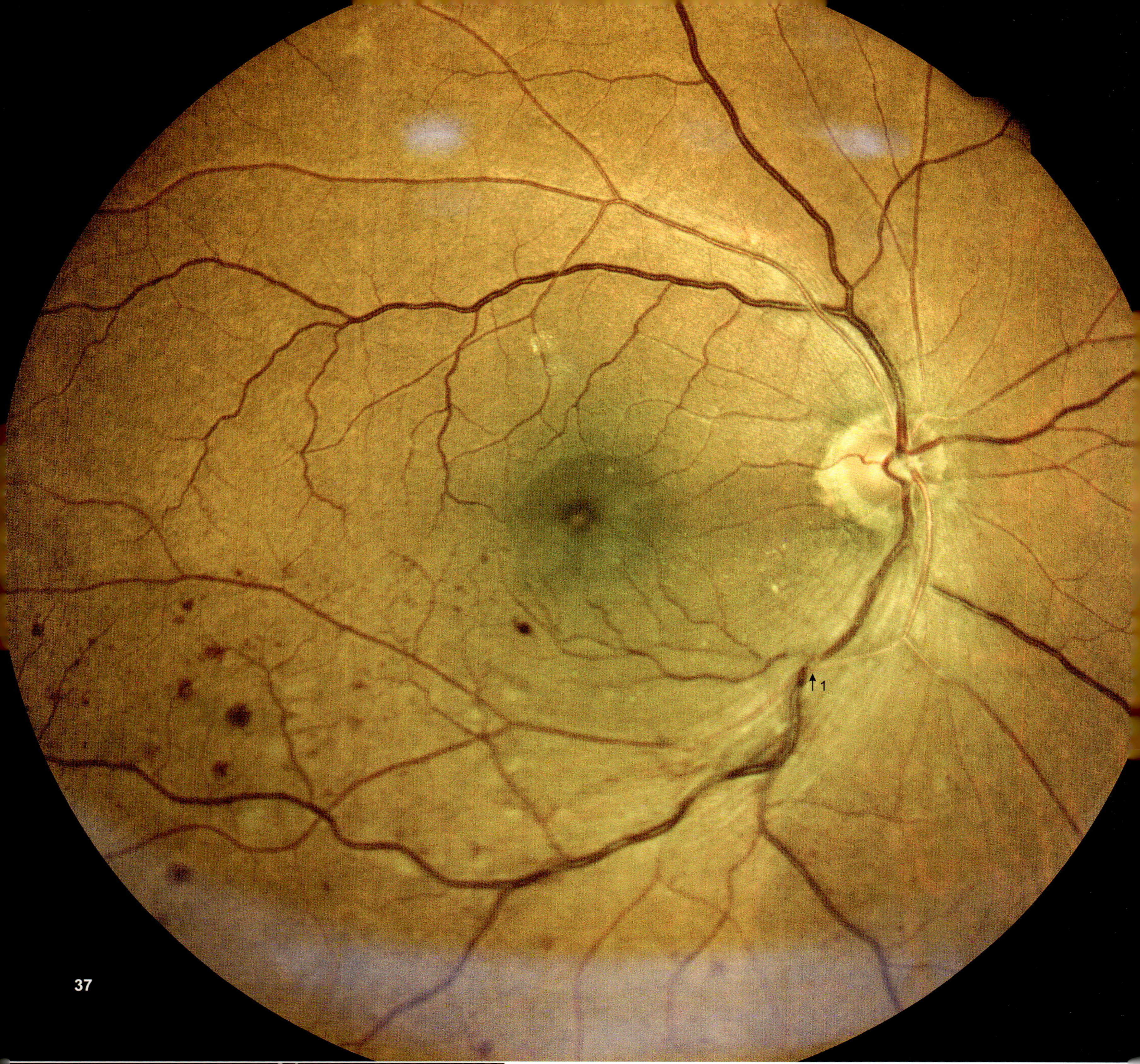


37

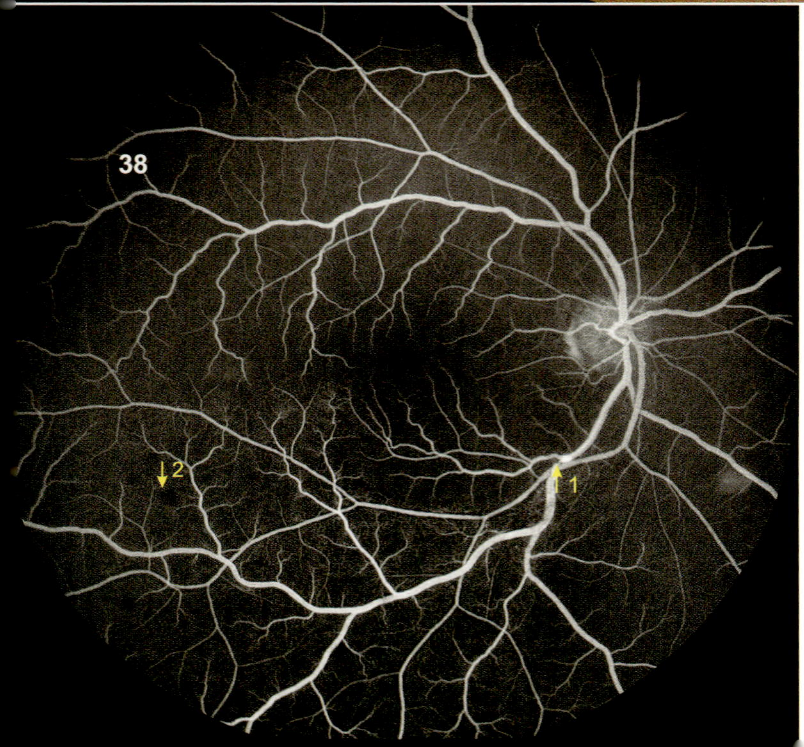


38

Figure 37 *Recent onset inferotemporal branch retinal vein occlusion with macular edema.*

Fundus photograph of a 65-year-old hypertensive who presented with sudden onset of blurred vision in right eye. Note the segmental distribution of retinal hemorrhages and cotton wool spots in the inferotemporal quadrant. The site of venous obstruction (1) at the arteriovenous crossing resulting in inferotemporal retinal vein occlusion is clearly evident. Macula is elevated due to leakage of fluid into the intraretinal layers from distended capillaries following vein obstruction.

Figure 38 *Early frames of fundus fluorescein angiography demonstrated hyperfluorescent plaque within the retinal vein at the site of AV blockade suggestive of a thrombus (1). Few scattered patches of blocked fluorescence due to retinal hemorrhages (2) are visible.*

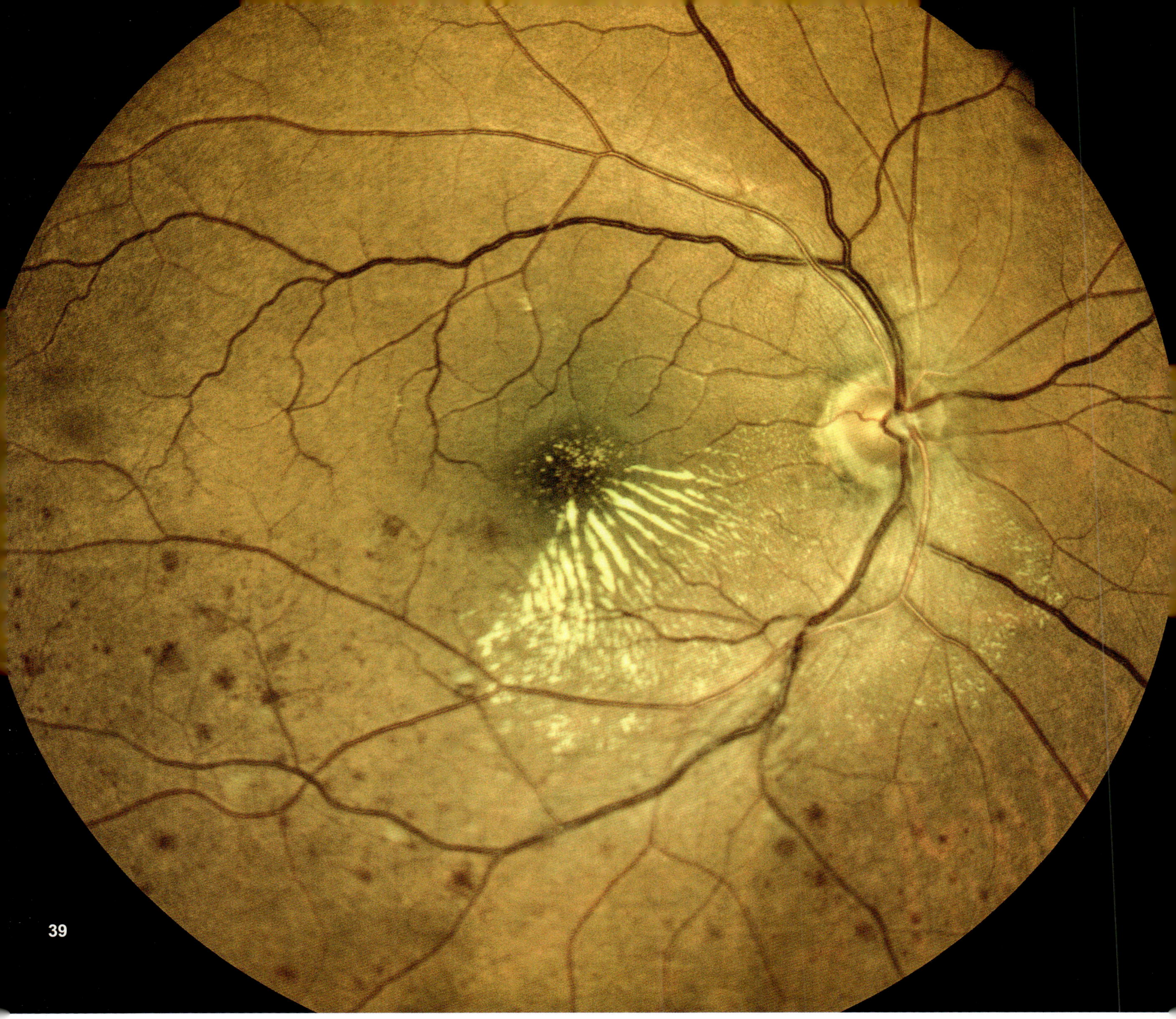


Figure 39 *Inferotemporal BRVO with circinate retinopathy at 1 month following treatment. Note significant reduction in macular thickness at 1 month post anti-VEGF injection, however there is development of circinate retinopathy.*

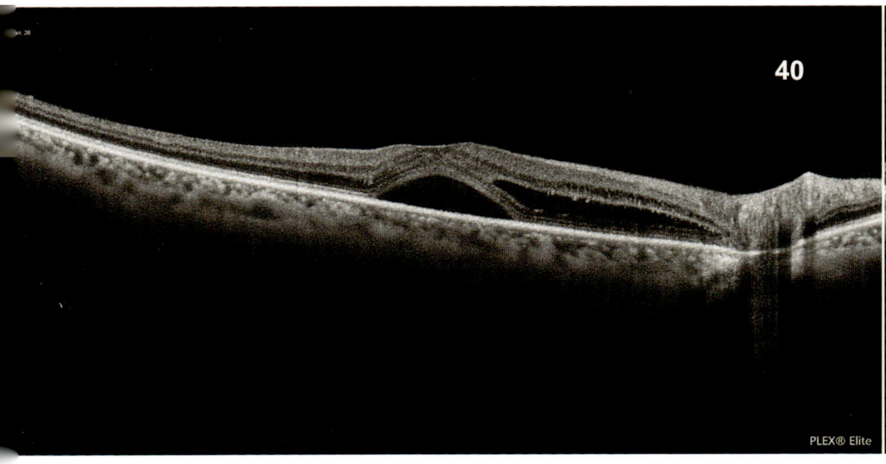


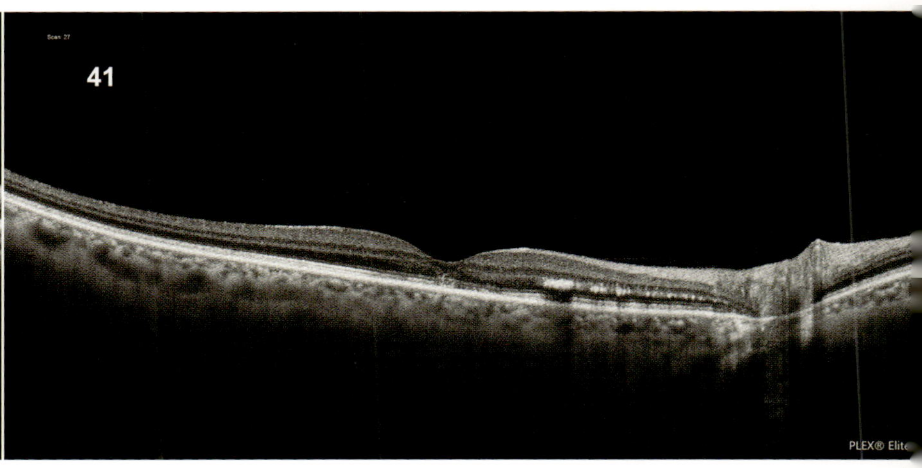


Figure 40 *SS-OCT at the time of presentation shows serous macular detachment at the fovea with presence of intraretinal fluid in the outer retinal layers.*

Figure 41 *SS-OCT scan done 1 month after single anti-VEGF injection shows complete reabsorption of subretinal and intraretinal fluid. Hyper-reflective dots were seen in the OPL layer due to lipid deposition.* □

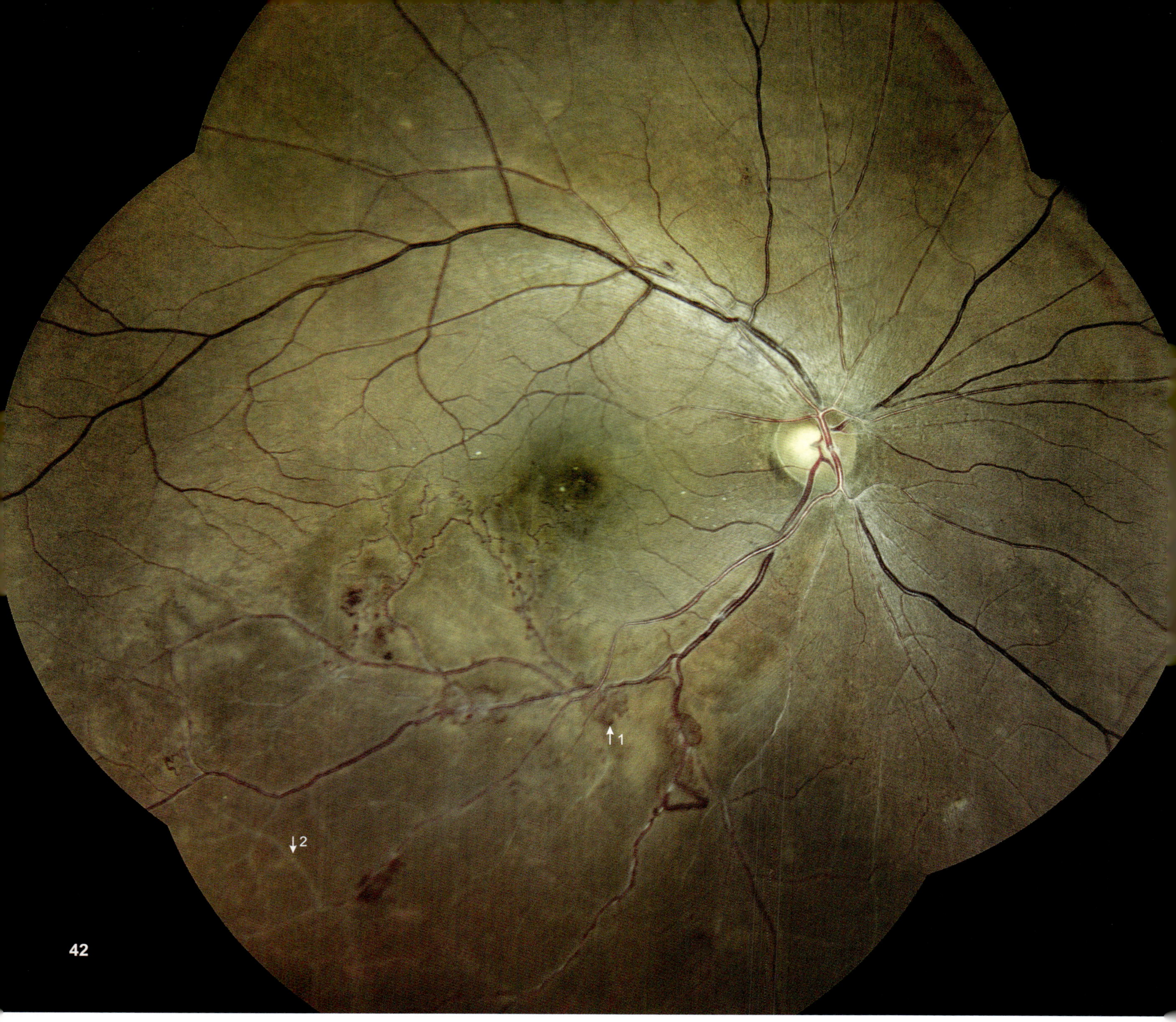


Figure 42 *Color fundus montage photograph demonstrating retinal neovascularization in a case of branch retinal vein occlusion.*

Note neovascular fronds arising from the inferotemporal retinal vein (1) silent looking retina in the inferotemporal quadrant and ghost vessels in the periphery due to peripheral ischemia (2).

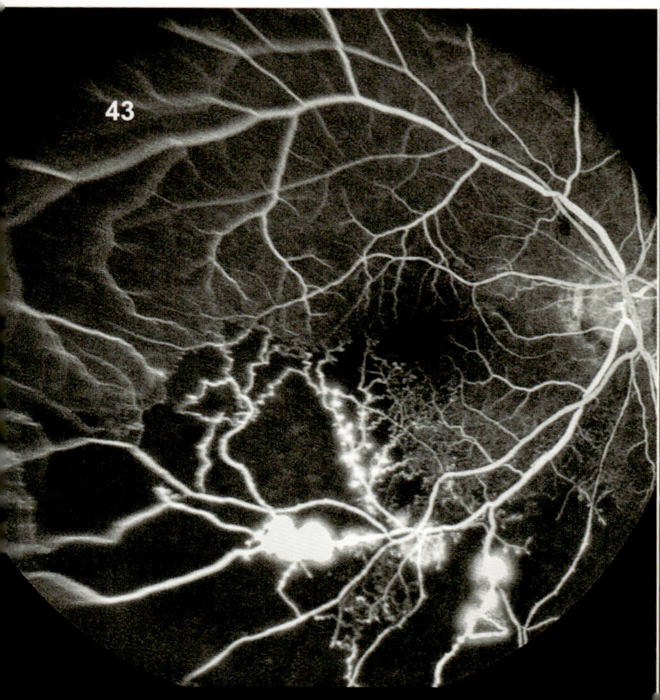


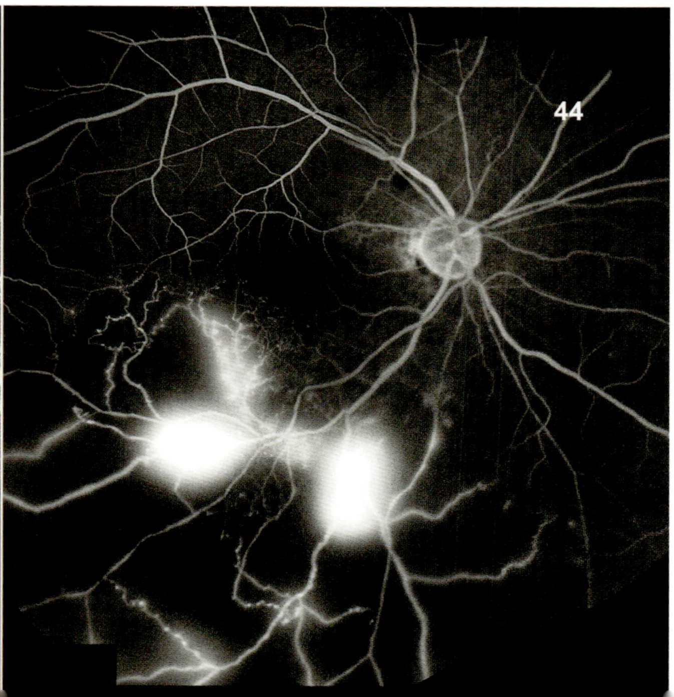


Figure 43

*Early frame of FFA demonstrates irregular perifoveal capillary network, large hypofluorescent area of capillary nonperfusion in the inferotemporal macula with early hyperfluorescence from underlying retinal neovascularization.*

Figure 44

*FFA montage at the late phase of dye demonstrating increasing hyperfluorescence due to leakage from NVEs and extensive capillary nonperfusion extending till the periphery of interior retina.*□

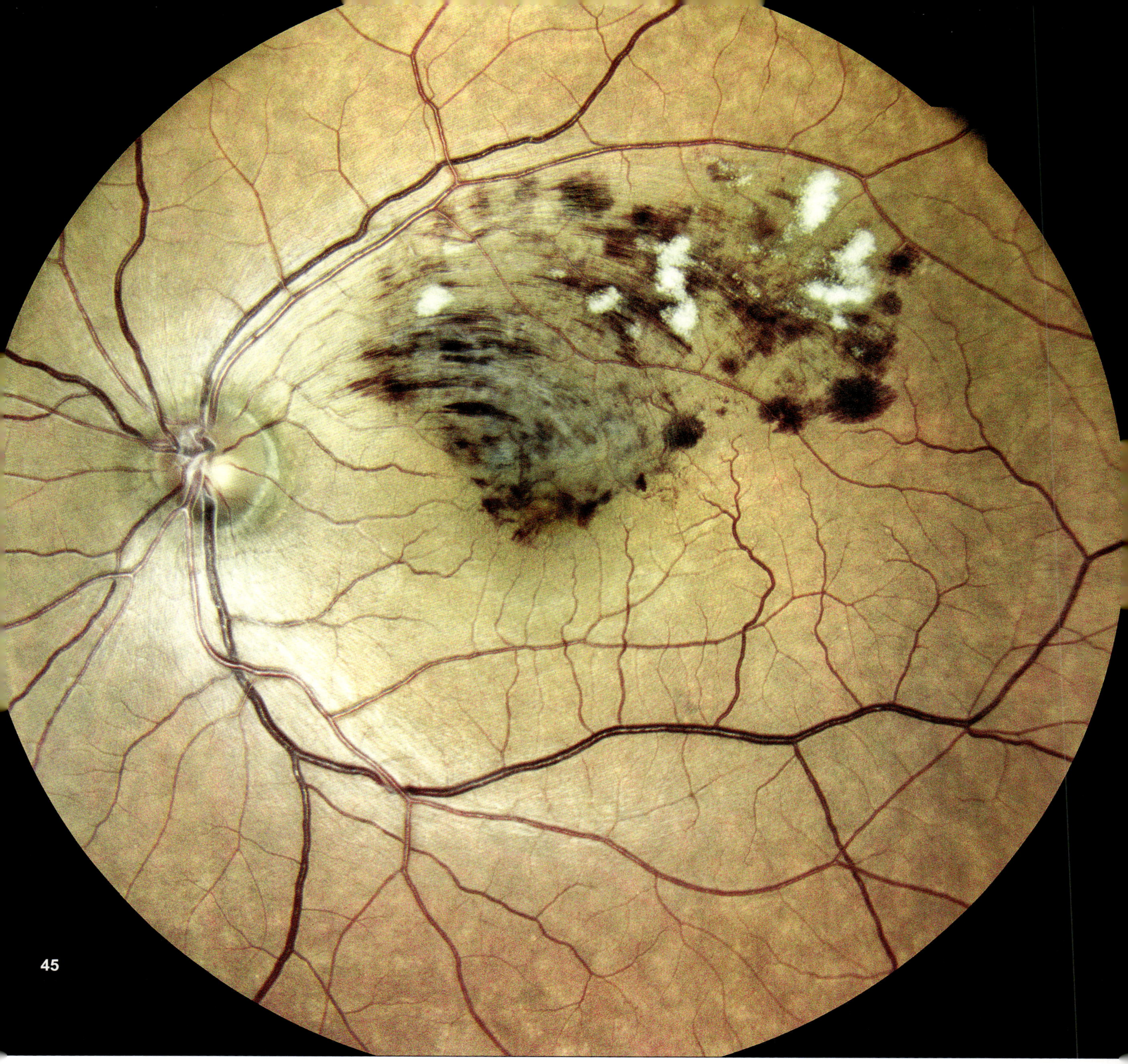


Figure 45 *A case of macular branch retinal vein occlusion.*

Color fundus photograph shows multiple scattered superficial hemorrhages and cotton wool spots distributed between fovea and superior temporal vascular arcade. Note the presence of macular thickening and macular hemorrhages. Branch retinal vein occlusion has a sudden onset. The patient presents with blurred vision or a field defect. Fundus examination reveals segmental distribution of intraretinal hemorrhages. Intraretinal hemorrhages are less marked when the occlusion is perfused or nonischemic and more marked when the occlusion is nonperfused or ischemic or associated with retinal capillary nonperfusion. Intravitreal anti-VEGF injections are indicated in cases with macular edema. Presence of retinal neovascularization or vitreous hemorrhage is an indication for sector pan retinal photocoagulation. Pars plana vitrectomy is needed for nonresolving vitreous hemorrhage or complicated retinal tractional detachment.□

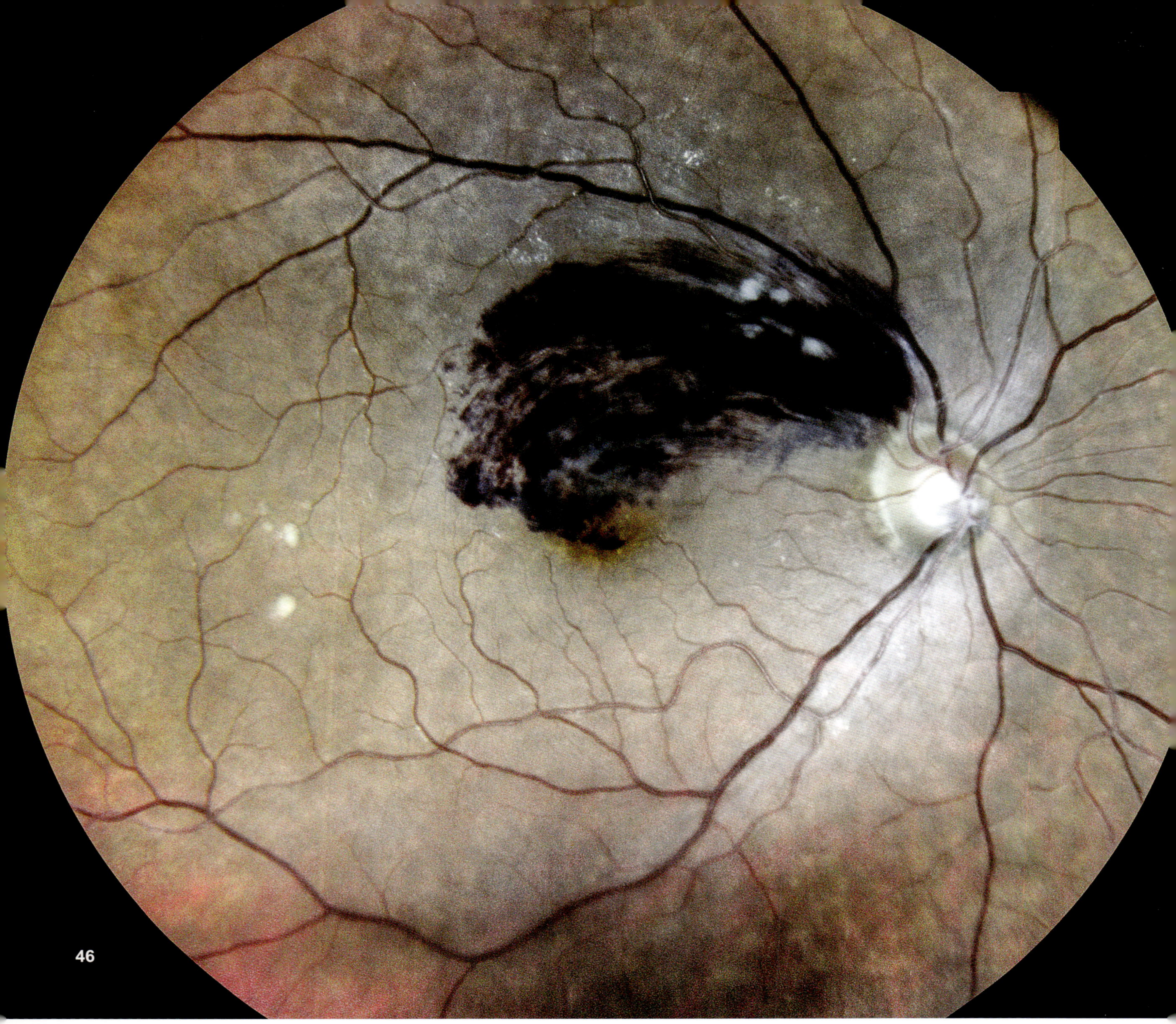

Figure 46 *Color fundus photograph demonstrating a macular branch retinal vein occlusion. If venous blockage involved a tributary draining the macula, it results in segmental distribution of intraretinal hemorrhages in the draining area only as seen in this case of superotemporal macular BRVO.*

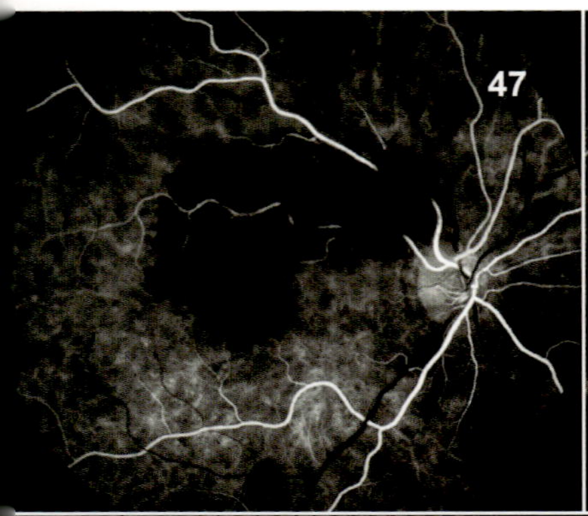

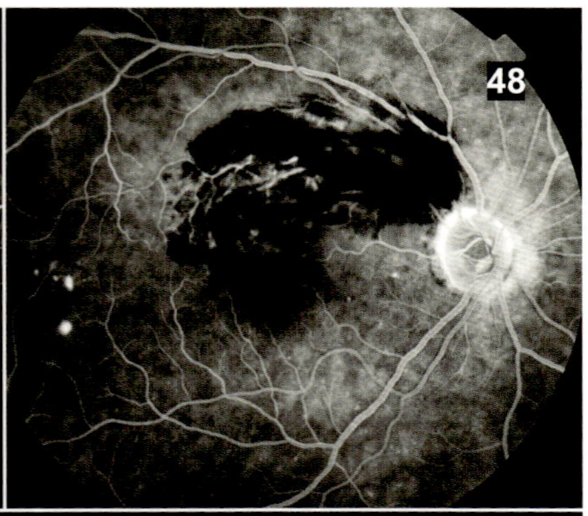

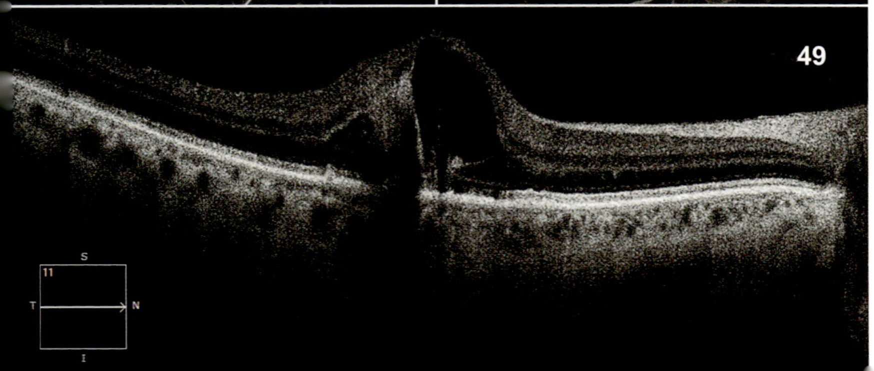

Figure 47 *Early frame of angiogram demonstrating hypofluorescence in the area of retinal hemorrhage. Foveal perfusion status could not be ascertained at this stage due to presence of retinal hemorrhage.*

Figure 48 *Late phase of angiogram shows rest of the retina is well-perfused except superotemporal macular region. There is cystoid leakage at the fovea.*

Figure 49 *Spectral domain OCT scan passing through the fovea demonstrates large foveal cyst with surrounding hyper-reflectivity in the inner retinal layers due to retinal hemorrhage.* □

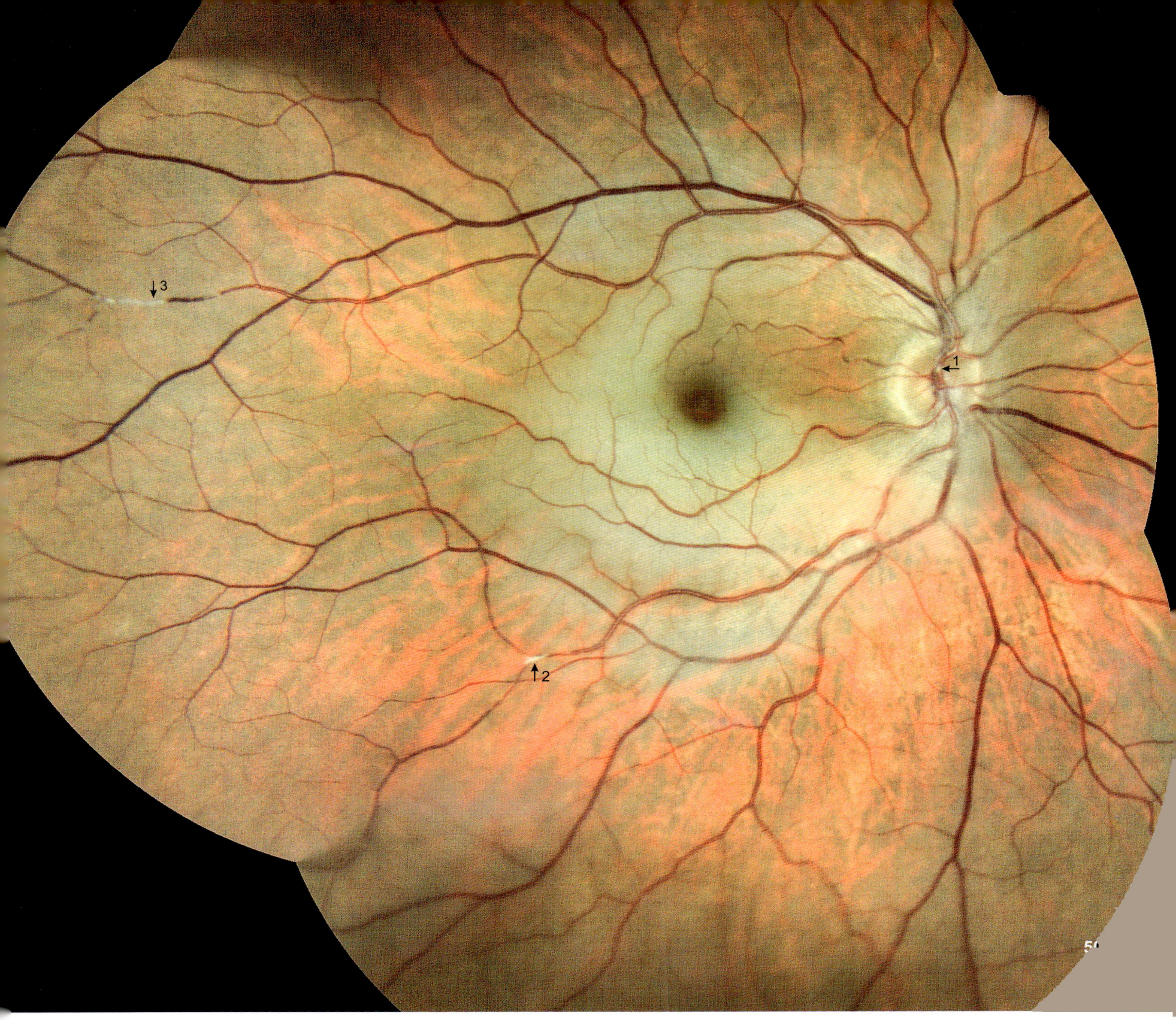


Figure 50 *Case of acute central retinal artery obstruction. Whitening or opacification of the superficial retina is characteristic appearance of infarcted retina. A cherry red spot can be seen centrally. The retinal opacification is more pronounced in the perifoveal retina where retina in the thickest. Note the presence of multiple intra-arterial glistening patches (1, 2, 3) seen due to retinal emboli.*

Figure 51

*Fundus fluorescein angiogram at 41 seconds after dye injection shows poor filling of retinal vasculature.*

Figure 52

*Late phase of angiogram at 7 minutes after dye injection: The leading edge of dye is abnormal in the areas of emboli (1). There is segmental patchy dye filling of the peripheral arteries (2).* □

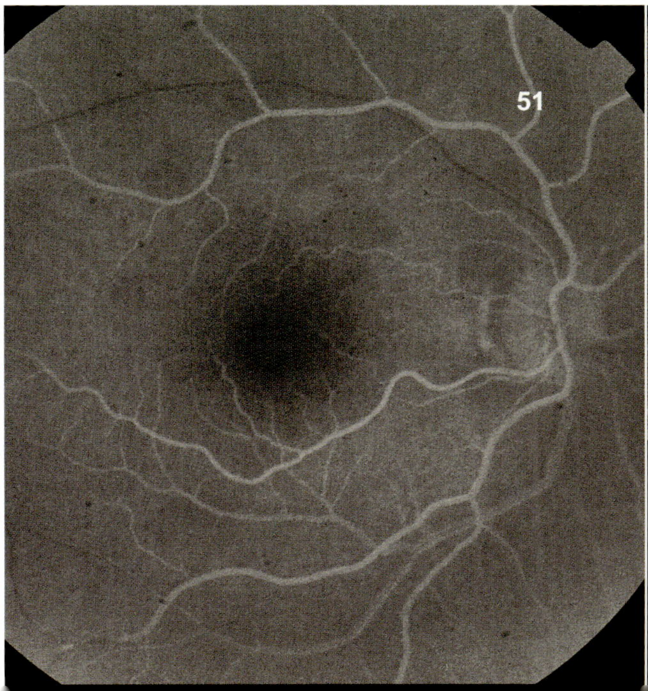


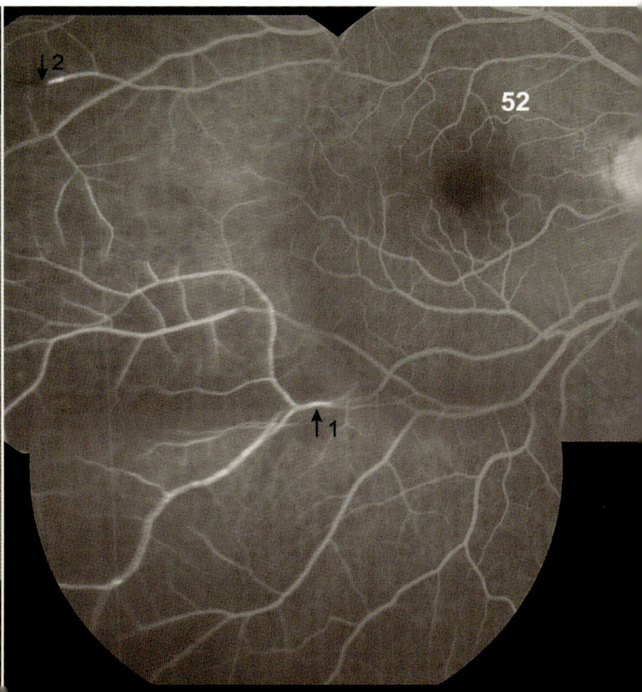

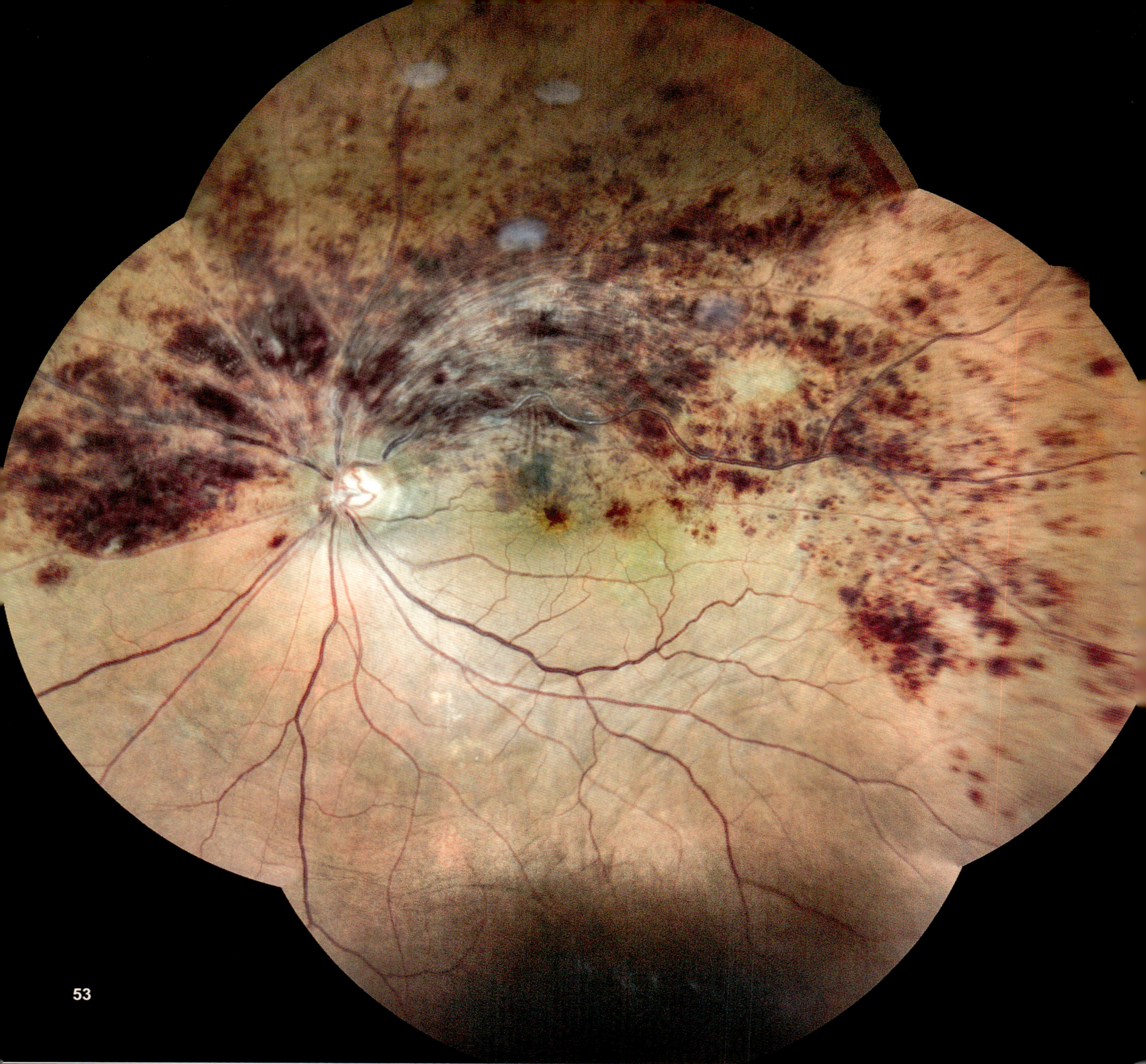

53

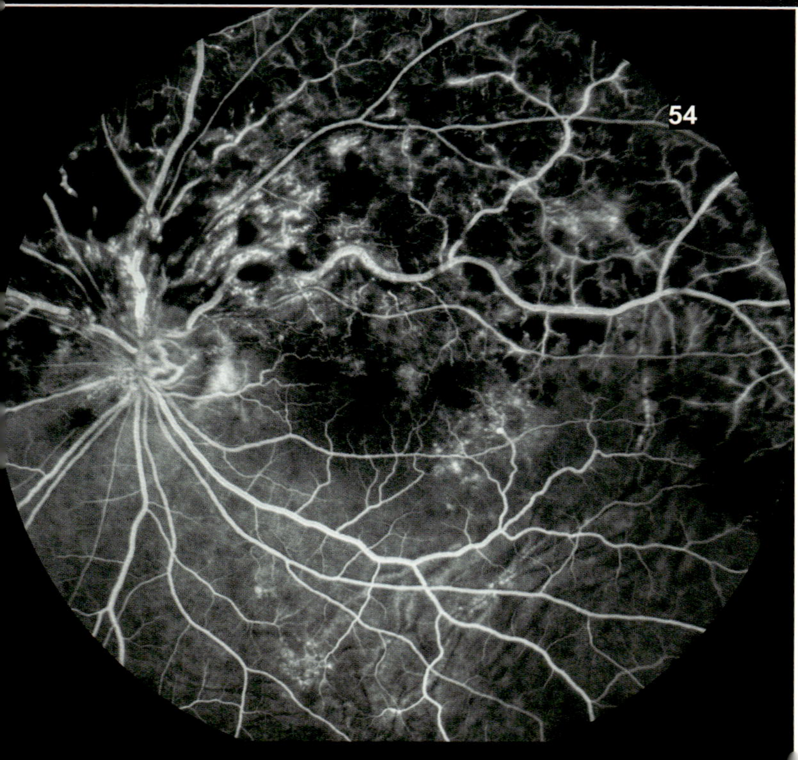

54

Figure 53 *Case of superior hemispheric retinal vein occlusion in a patient with known history of glaucoma.*

Multiple scattered superficial hemorrhages are noticeable in the superior hemispheric retina. Inferior of retina is remarkably normal. Retinal veins appears slightly tortuous. Macular hemorrhages are also seen involving the fovea. Optic disk is glaucomatous.

Figure 54 *Early frame of FFA demonstrating blocked hypofluorescence from retinal hemorrhages.*

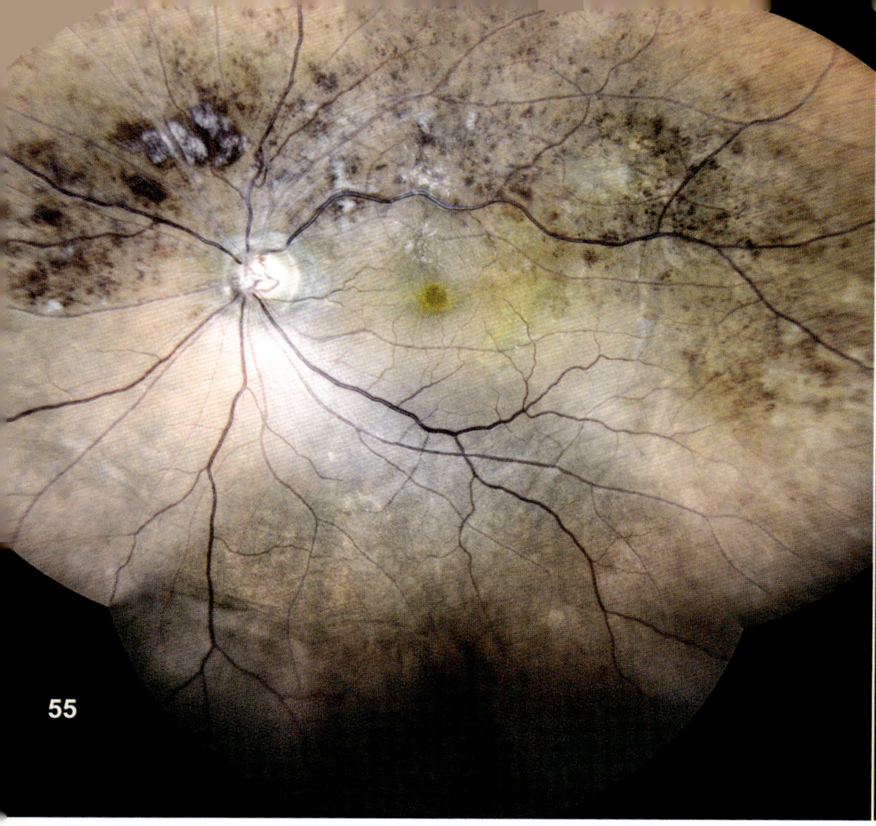


Figure 55 *Color fundus montage 3 months after anti-VEGF injection given at four weekly interval. Retinal hemorrhages have reduced. Appearance of fovea is normal. Few cotton wool spots are visible now.*

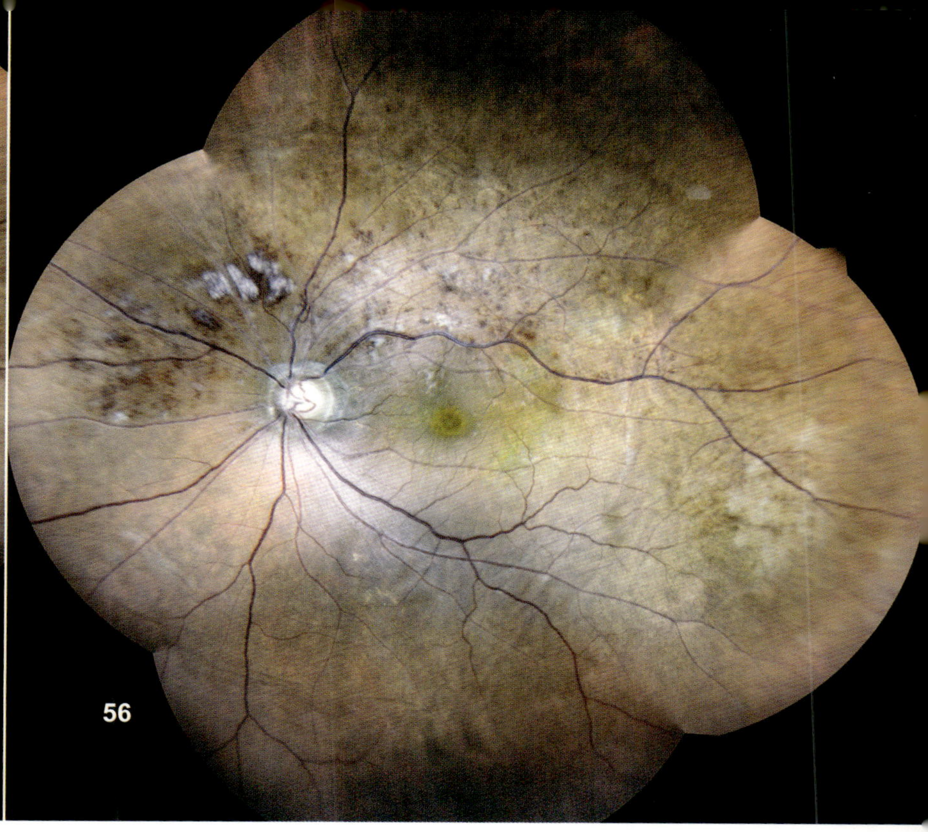


Figure 56 *Color fundus montage 6 months later. Note further reduction in the hemorrhages.*

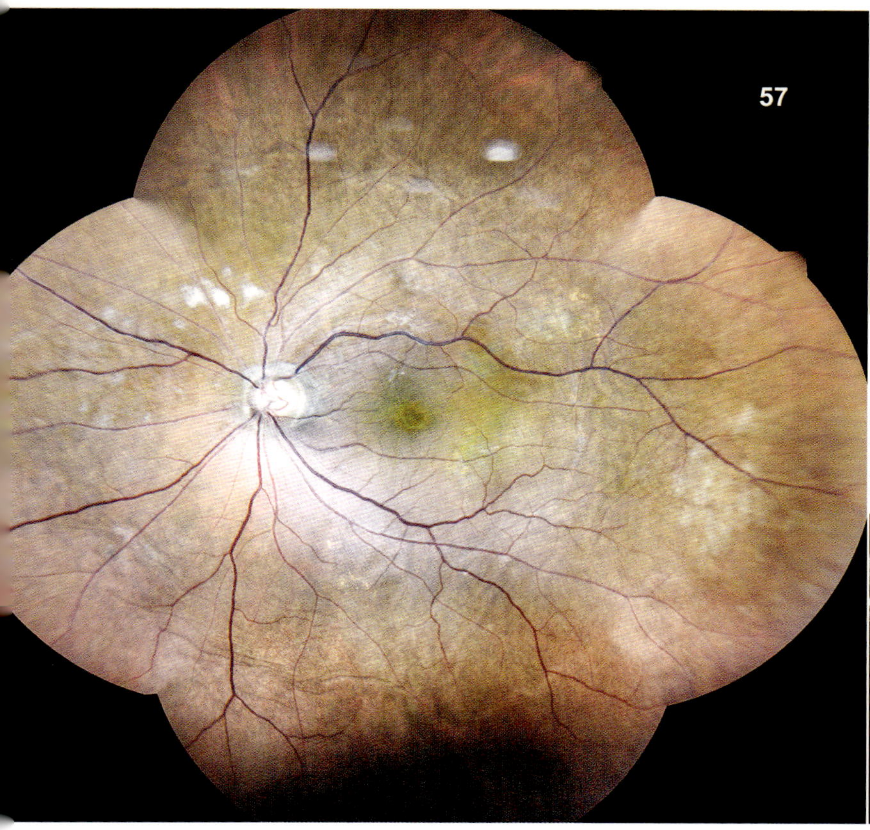


Figure 57 *Color fundus montage 9 months later showing resolved HRVO. Patient continued to receive an anti-VEGF injection on pro rata basis throughout these 9 months.*

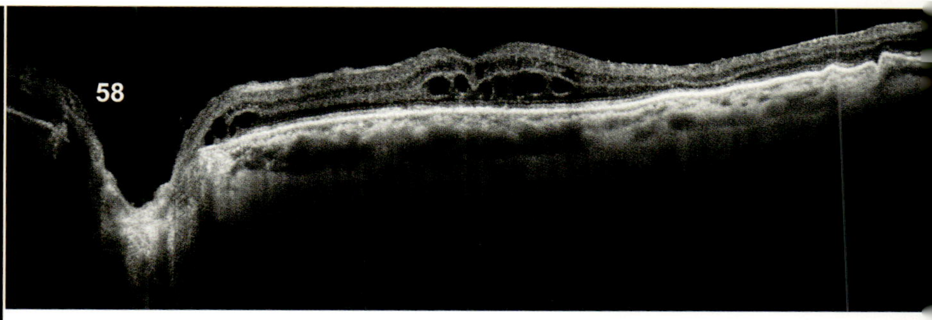


Figure 58 *Optical coherence tomography scan image at presentation demonstrating cystoid macular edema.*

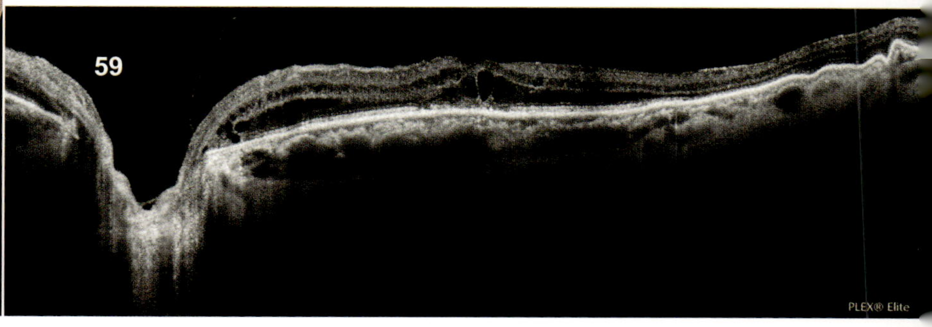


Figure 59 *Optical coherence tomography scan at 3 months demonstrating reduction in macular edema.* □

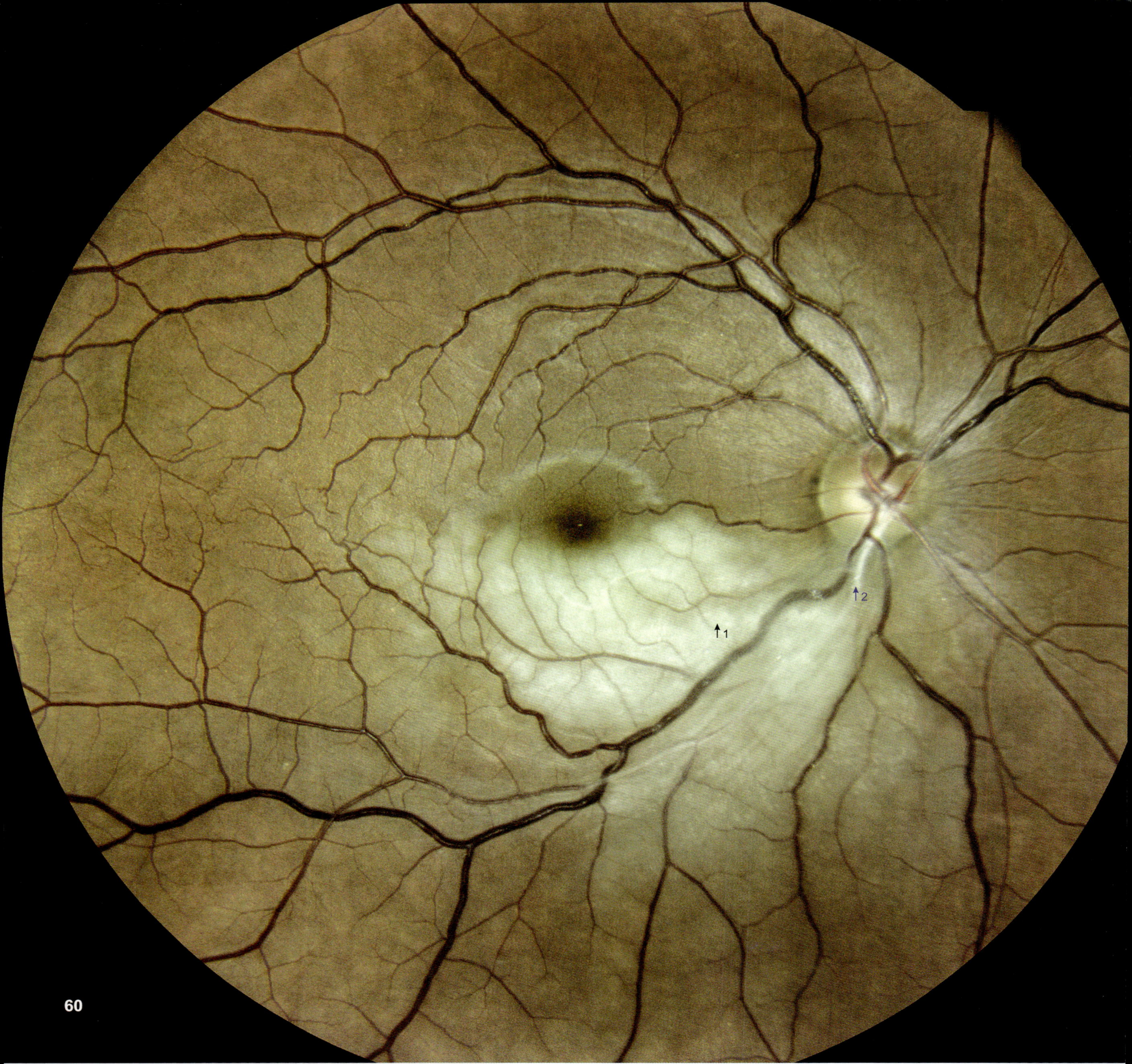


60

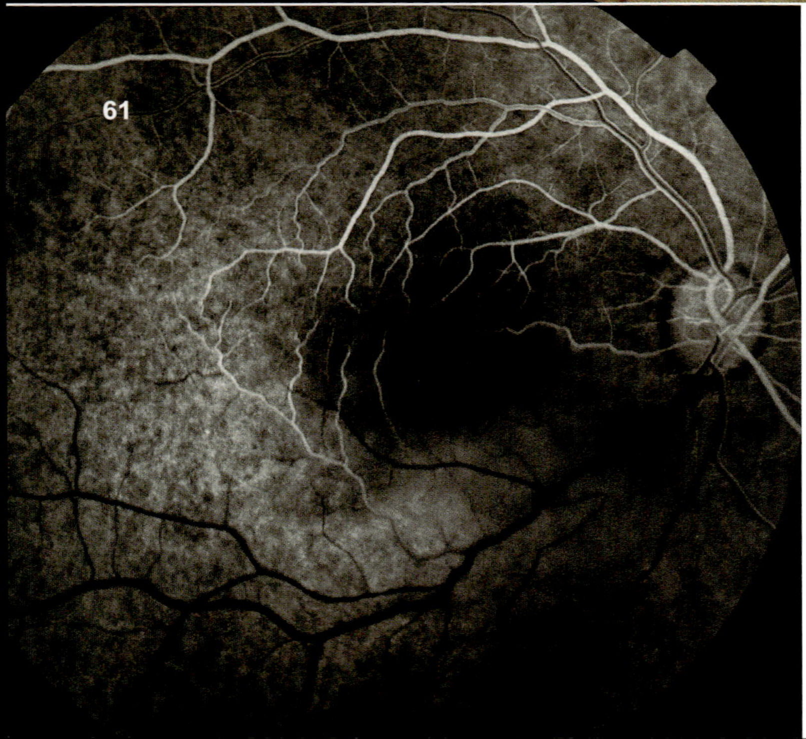

61

Figure 60 *Color fundus photograph of 45-year-old female with branch retinal artery occlusion: Note a localized region of retinal opacification in the inferotemporal macula (1) along the distribution of obstructed inferotemporal retinal artery (2).*

Retinal whitening probably occurs secondary to blockage of axoplasmic flow in the nerve fiber layer as it reaches the hypoxic retina.

Over 90% of branch retinal artery obstructions involve temporal retinal vessels. Visual prognosis is usually good unless the fovea is completely surrounded by whitening. About 80% of the eyes eventually improve to 6/12 or better, although residual field defects usually remain. Complete hematological and cardiology check up is a must in a case of BRAO.

Figure 61 *Early arteriovenous frame of angiogram shows delay in the filling of inferotemporal artery and vein whereas normal flow of dye was observed in the superior retinal artery and laminar flow is seen in the superotemporal vein.*

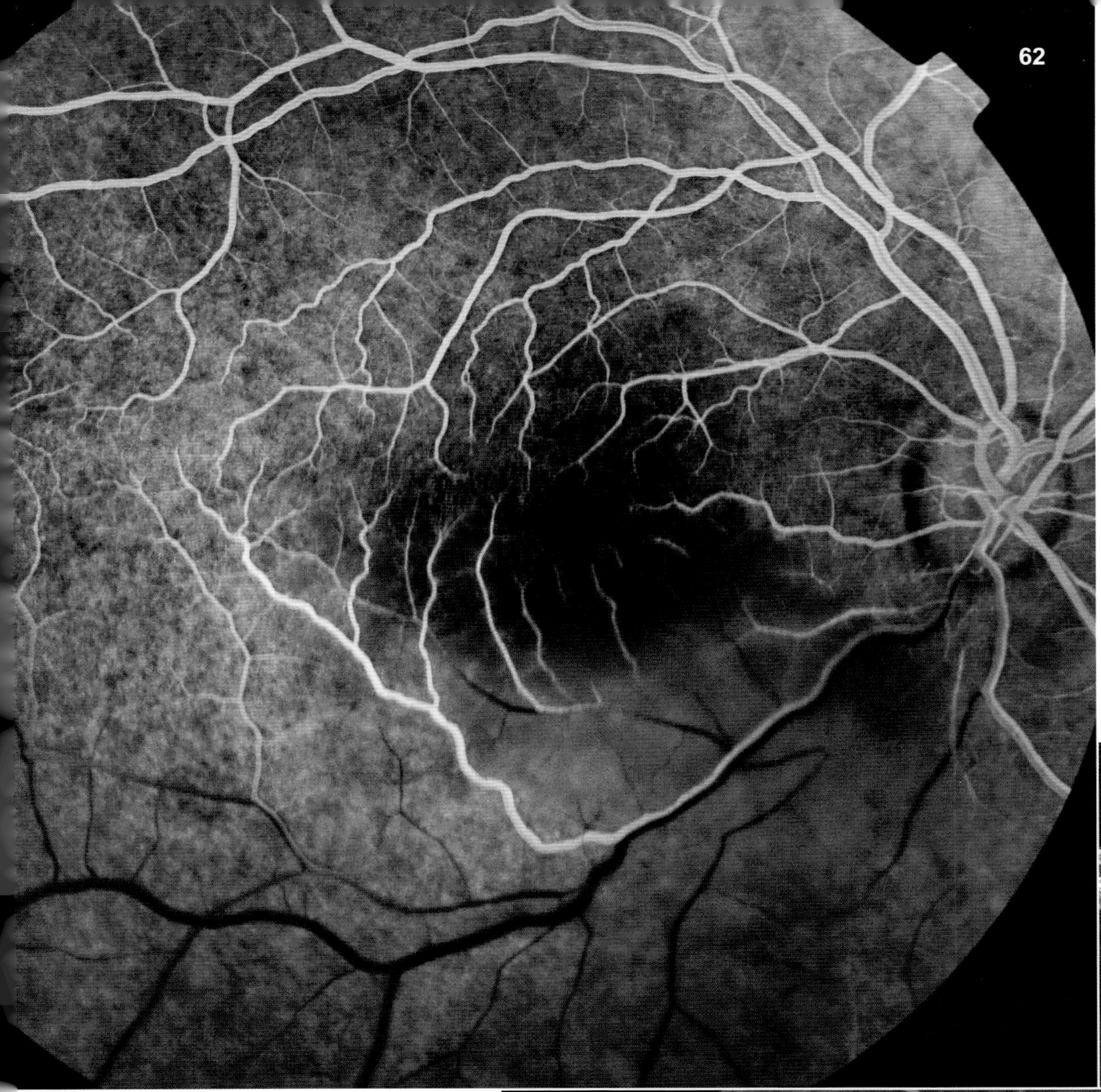


Figure 62

*Mid-phase of angiogram depicts retrograde filling of the inferotemporal vein, and slow patchy flow along the inferotemporal artery.*

Figure 63

*SD OCT scan passing through the area of artery occlusion shows opacification of the inner retinal layers with loss of architectural details.*

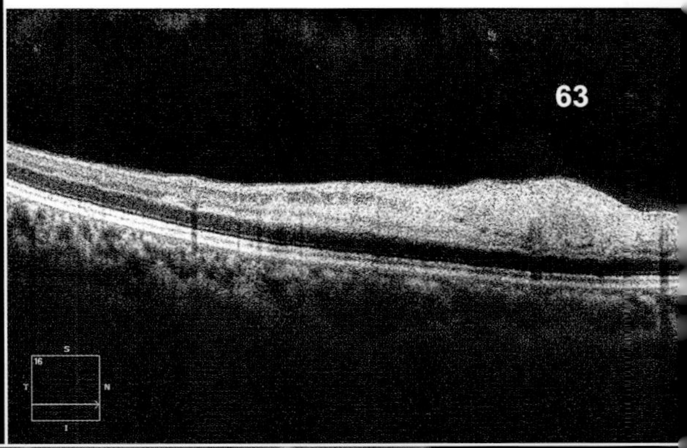


Figure 64

*Late phase of angiogram demonstrating minimal staining of retinal venules and capillaries and incomplete filling of retinal artery with fluorescein dye.* □

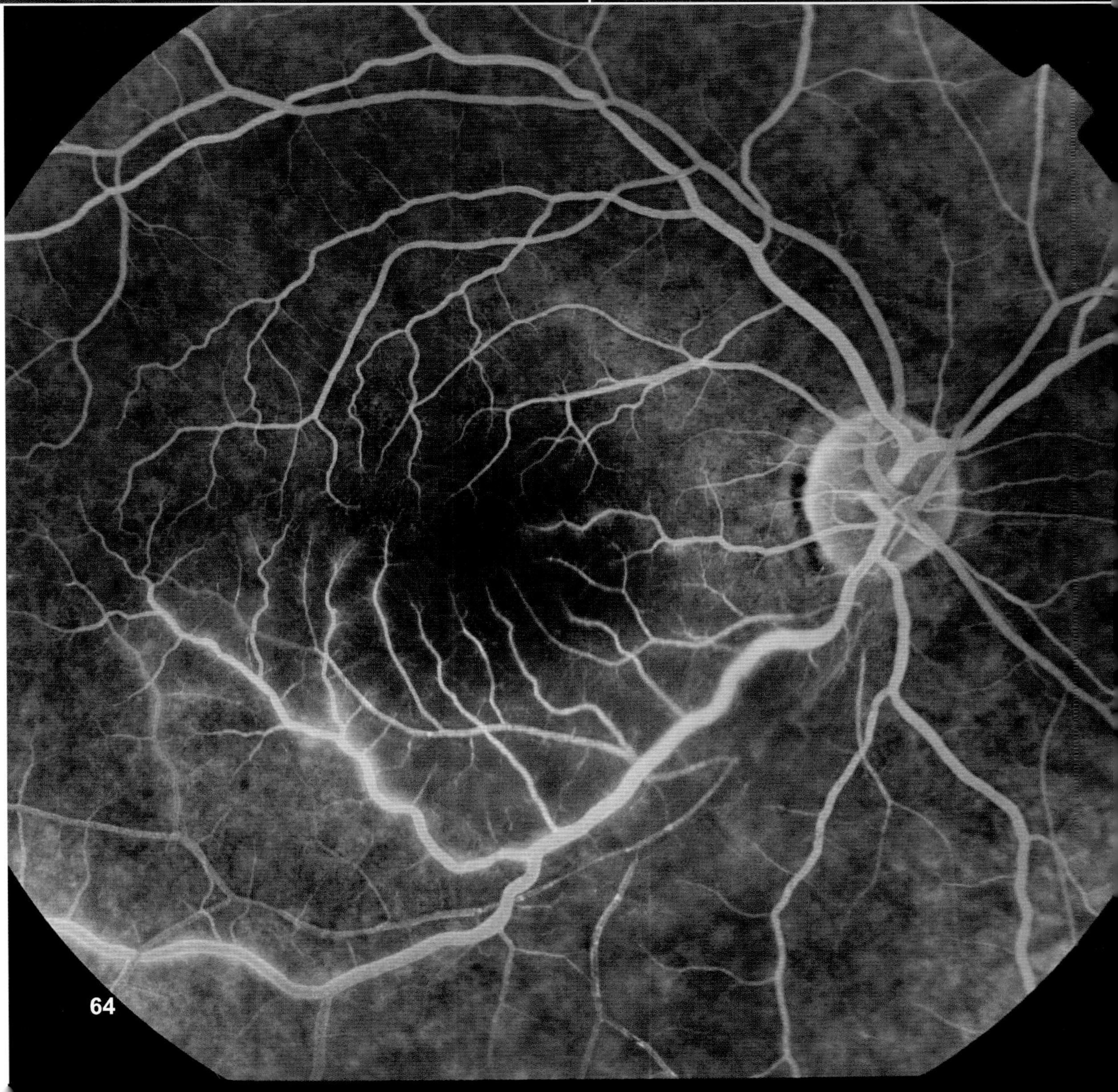

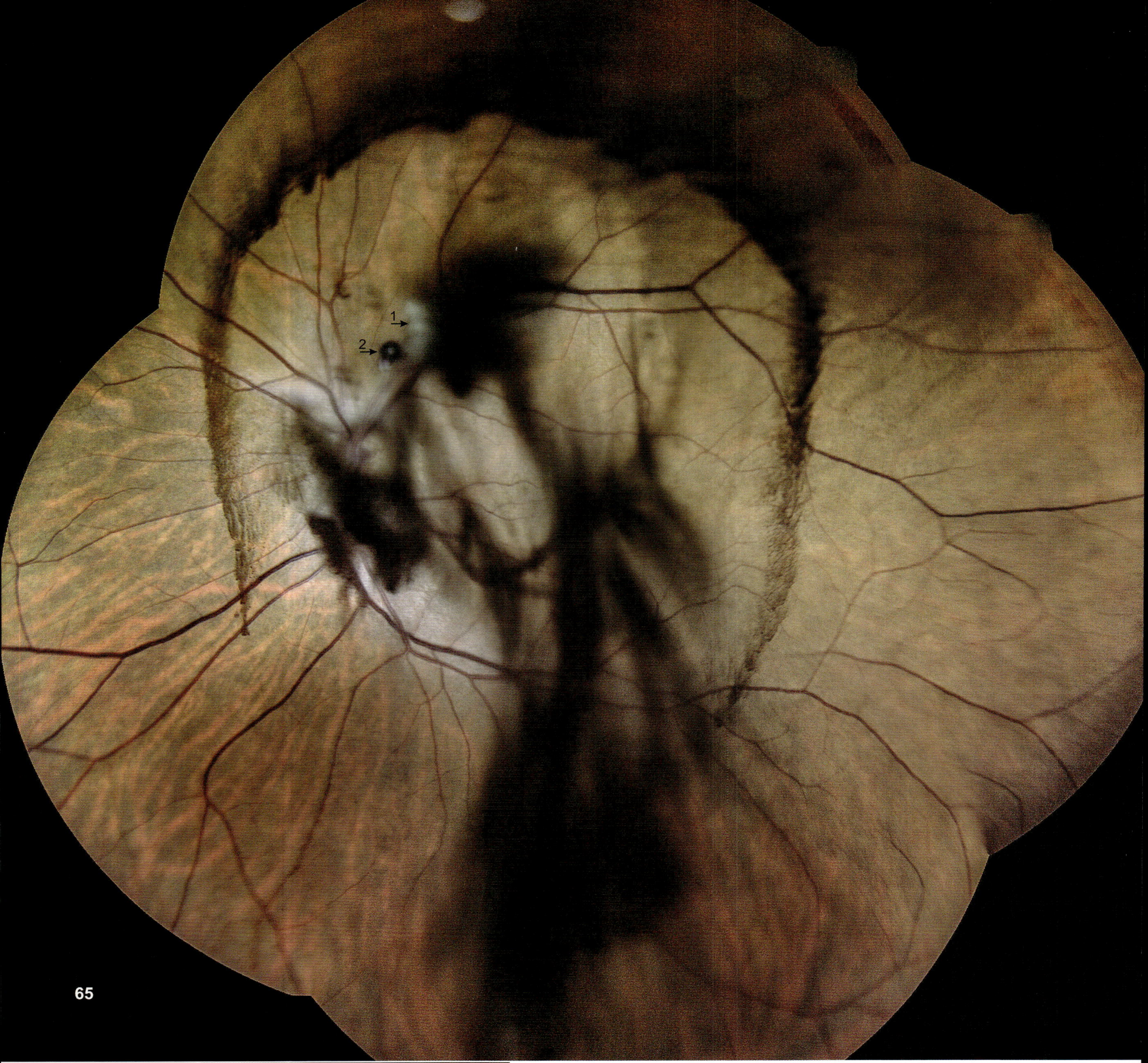


65

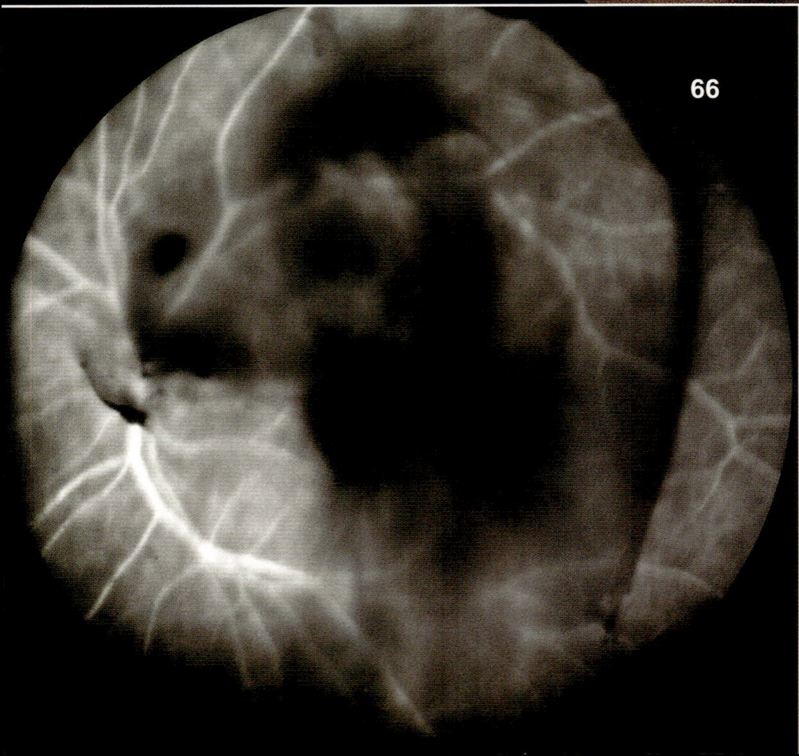

66

Figure 65 *Acquired retinal artery microaneurysms (RAM) associated with vitreous hemorrhage. Color fundus photograph shows small cotton wool spot (1) adjacent to an oval patch of retinal hemorrhage associated with a microaneurysms (2) and dark red opacity anterior to the retina due to vitreous hemorrhage.*

Vitreous hemorrhage is a serious complication that happens due to rupture of retinal artery microaneurysms. Approximately 2% of all vitreous hemorrhages are caused by RAM lesions. Occasionally microaneurysms may not be detected because of the overlying hemorrhages, therefore careful follow-up is needed in such cases. At times vitreous hemorrhages may be absorbed spontaneously, but other cases may need pars plana vitrectomy to remove the hemorrhage.

Figure 66 *FFA demonstrates that the details of underlying microaneurysms are obscured in the concerned area, due to masking affect of associated retinal hemorrhage and vitreous hemorrhage.*

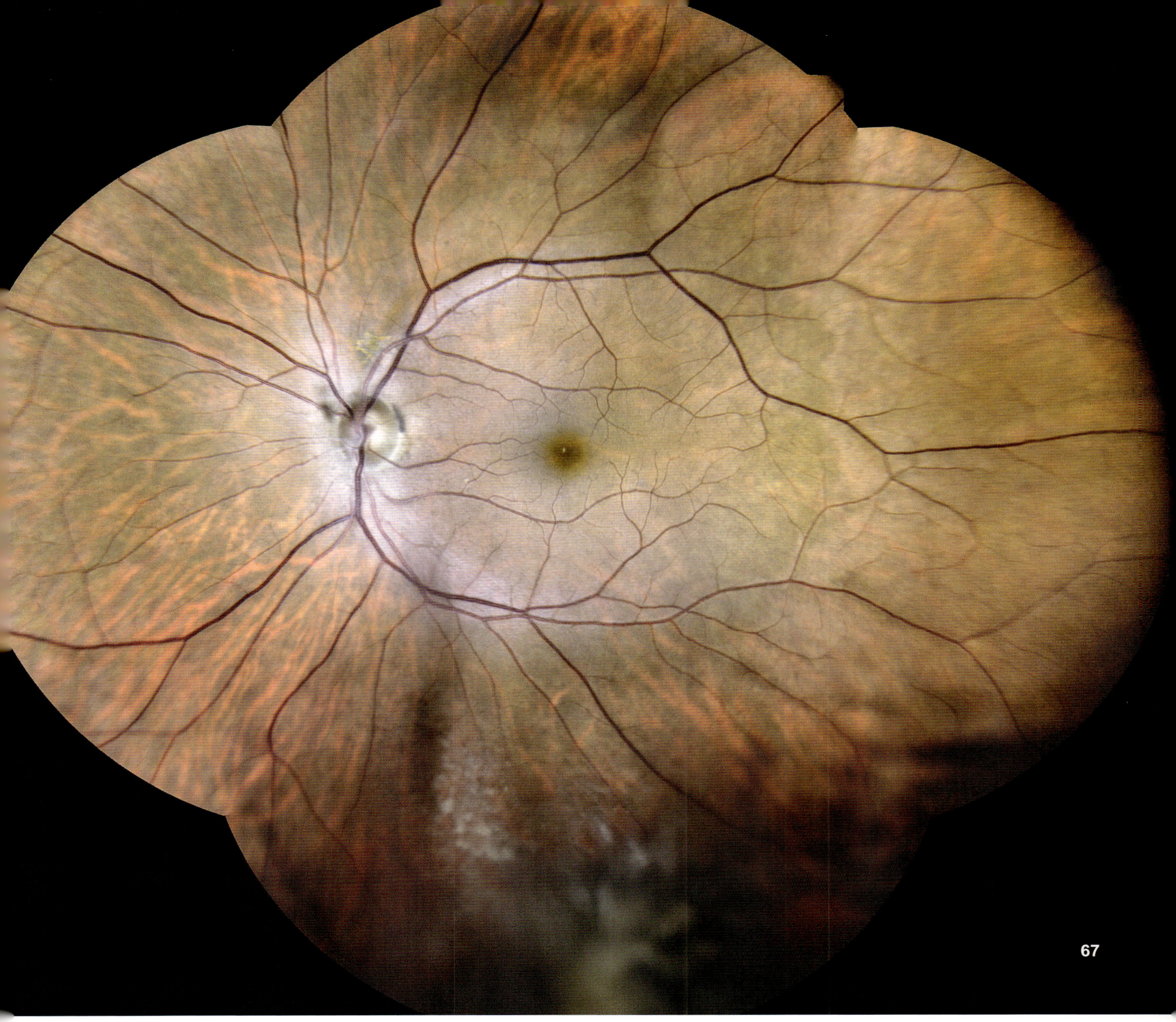


Figure 67 *Case of retinal artery microaneurysms associated with vitreous hemorrhage: Color fundus image 3 months after laser treatment.*

Patient underwent direct laser photocoagulation to the Retinal artery microaneurysms using yellow laser. While attempting direct photocoagulation one has to be careful as retinal artery obstruction in a known complication of such treatment. Note grayish colored old vitreous hemorrhage is still visible in the inferior periphery. Posterior pole of the retina is normal now and laser scars were seen at the site of RAM.

Figure 68 *Spectral domain OCT scan passing through the area of RAM: Note the presence of large oval-shaped dilated retinal vessel in the superficial retina with underlying shadowing of deeper retinal architecture and a vitreous opacity.* □

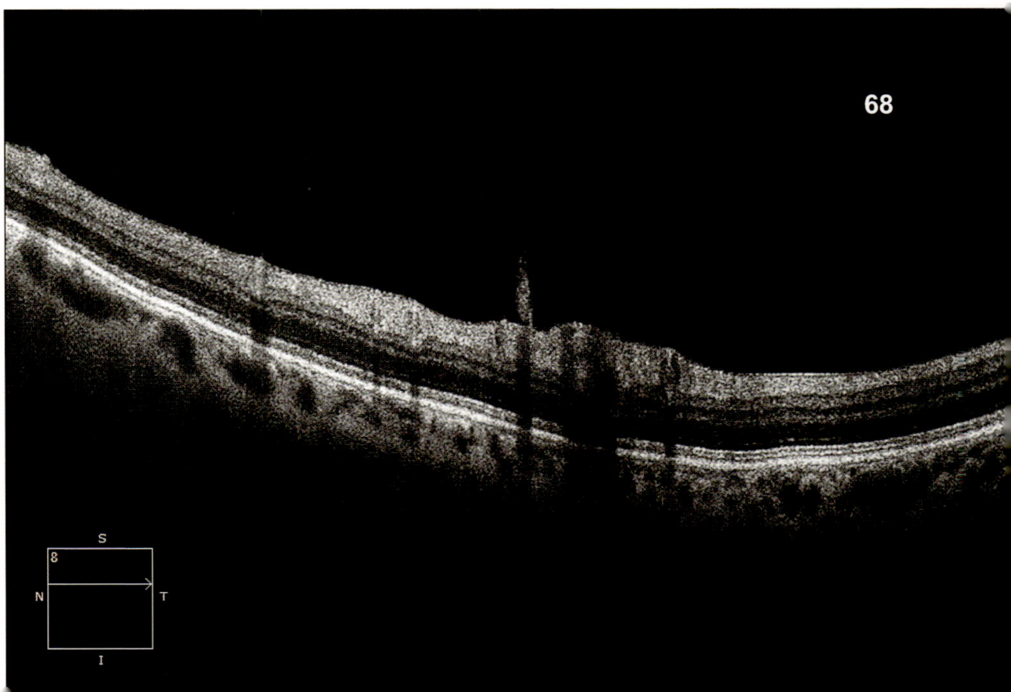

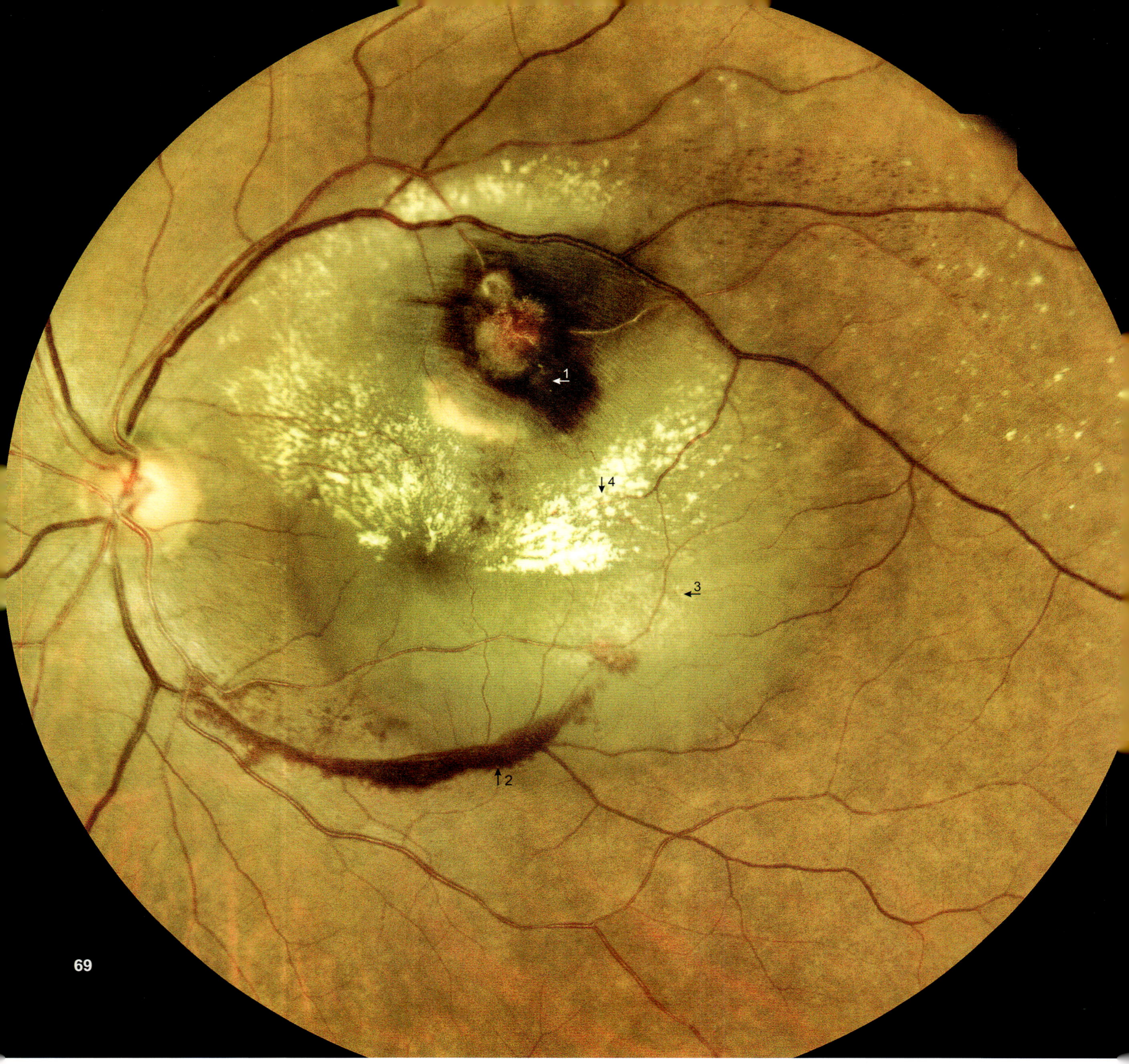


Figure 69 *A 62-year-old female with hypertension had subretinal hemorrhage (1), preretinal bleed (2), massive retinal exudation (3) with lipid deposition (4) associated with retinal artery macroaneurysm (RAM).*

RAM appears as a fusiform dilation of retinal arteriole, arising most commonly from superotemporal retinal artery.

Retinal artery macroaneurysm affects patients in sixth and seventh decades of life. Often associated are vascular problems such as hypertension and general arteriosclerotic cardiovascular disease. Often they are located at the site of an arteriolar bifurcation or an arteriovenous crossing. The superotemporal artery is the most commonly reported site of involvement because patient with such involvement are more likely to have visual impairment. Women make-up majority of reported cases. Most cases are unilateral, while 10% may be bilateral.

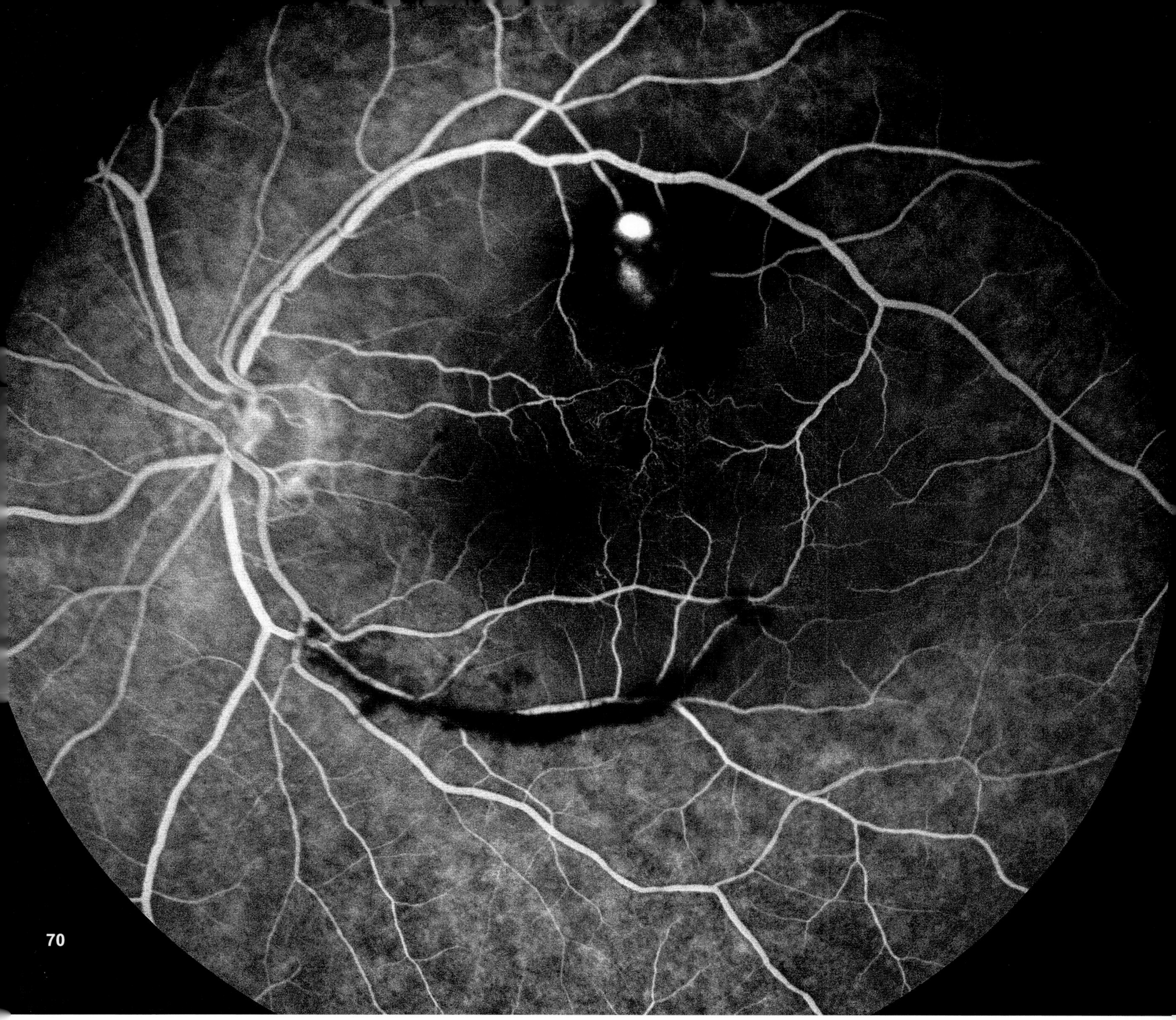

Figure 70 *The fluorescein angiogram demonstrates round well-defined area of hyperfluorescence in the early phase of the angiogram from the acquired macroaneurysm. Preretinal bleed and subretinal bleeds have a masking hypofluorescent effect.*

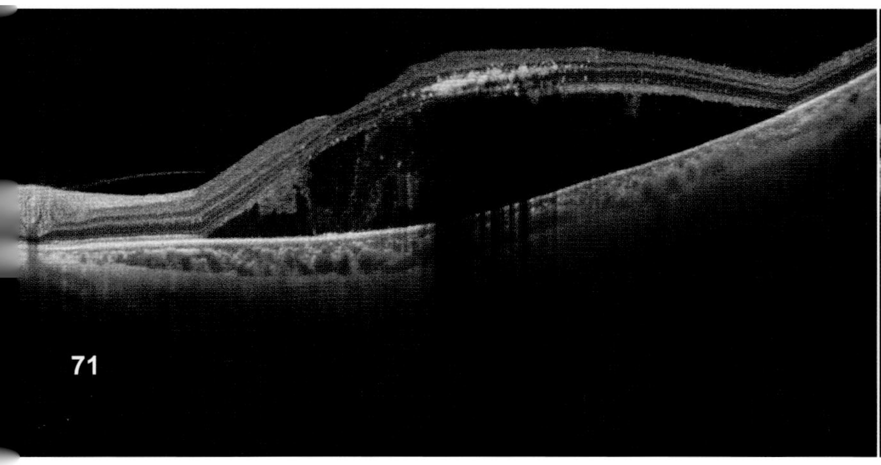

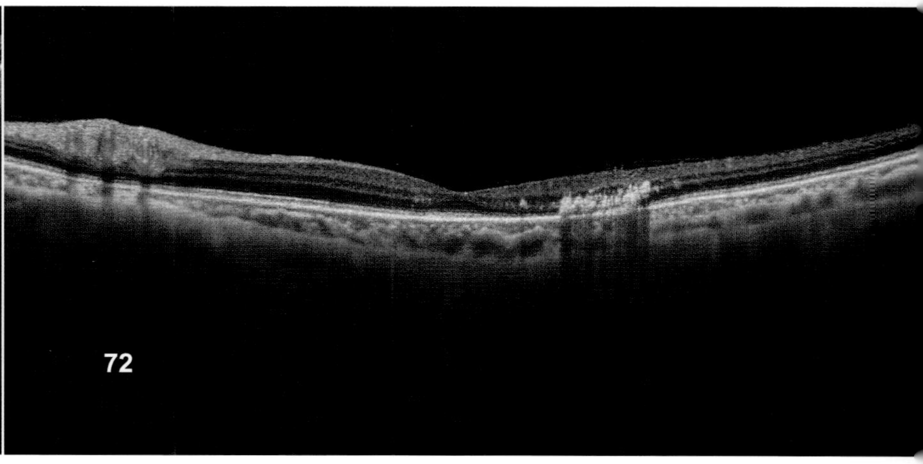

Figure 71 *Optical coherence tomography scan at baseline shows massive subretinal fluid involving the fovea. Also note the presence of retinal hard exudates.*

Figure 72 *Optic coherence tomography scan after treatment demonstrating hyper-reflective hard exudates in the outer plexiform layer and complete resolution of the subretinal fluid.*

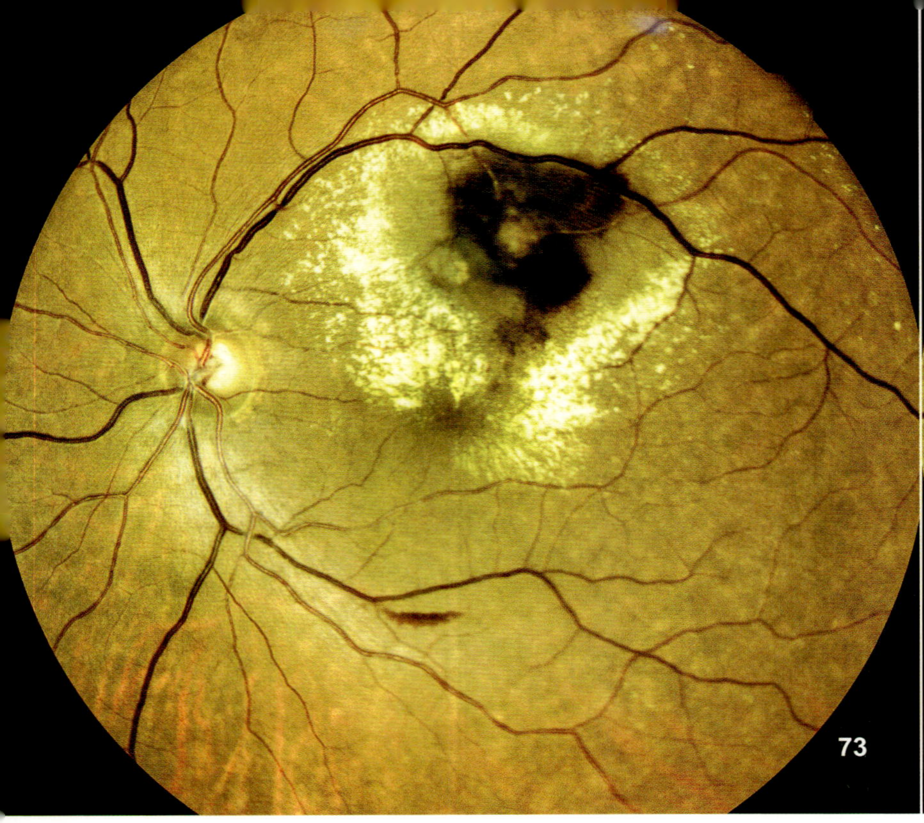


Figure 73 *Color fundus photograph 2 months later: Patient received 2 intravitreal anti-VEGF injections at 4 weekly interval resulting in resolution of retinal edema at the fovea to a larger extent, although there is persistent lipid exudation around the superotemporal fovea. At this stage laser photocoagulation was advised.*

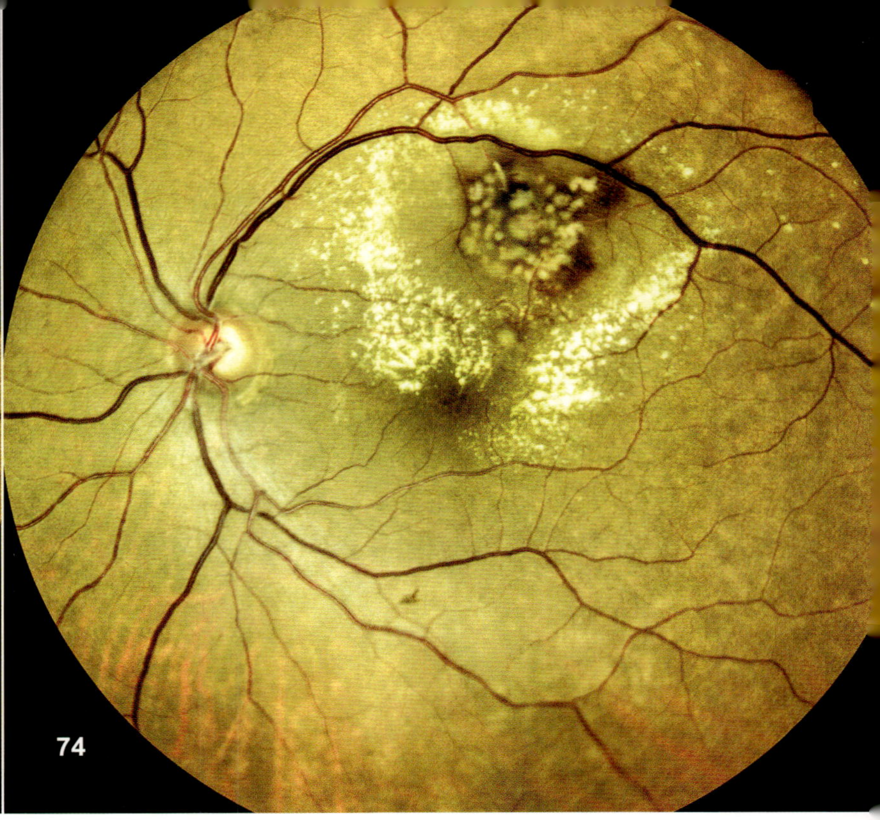


Figure 74 *Color fundus photograph immediately after laser photocoagulation using area centralis lens, spot size 100 microns, with long duration, low intensity burns.*

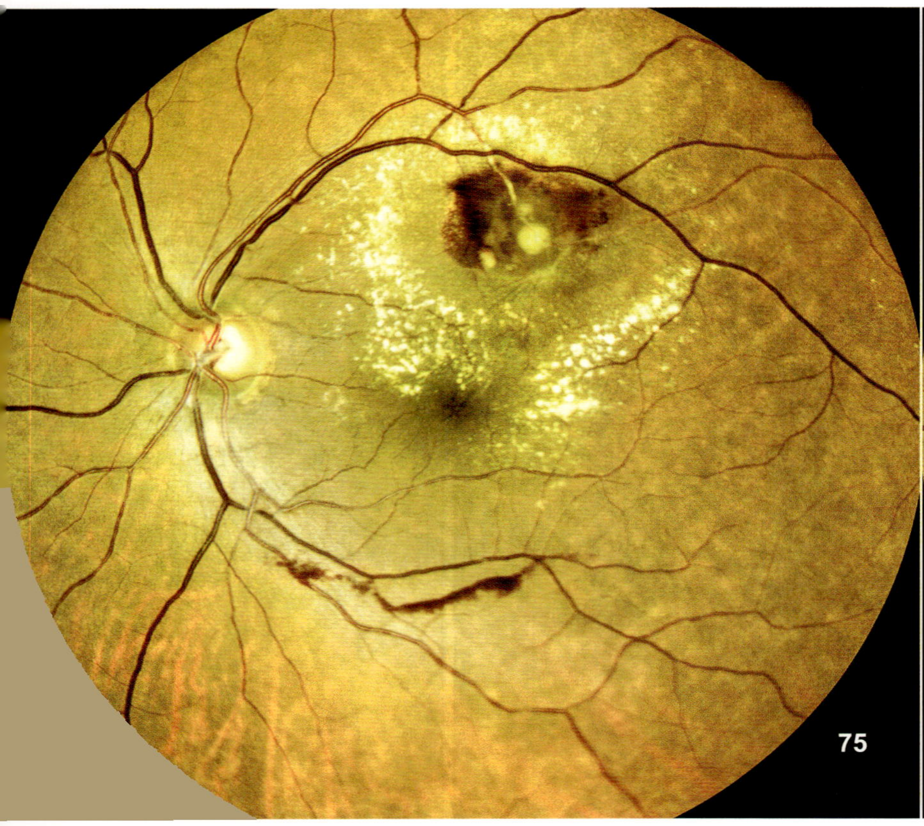


Figure 75 *Color fundus photograph 1 month postlaser shows further reduction in lipid exudation, reduction in the subretinal hemorrhage and thrombosed macroaneurysm.*

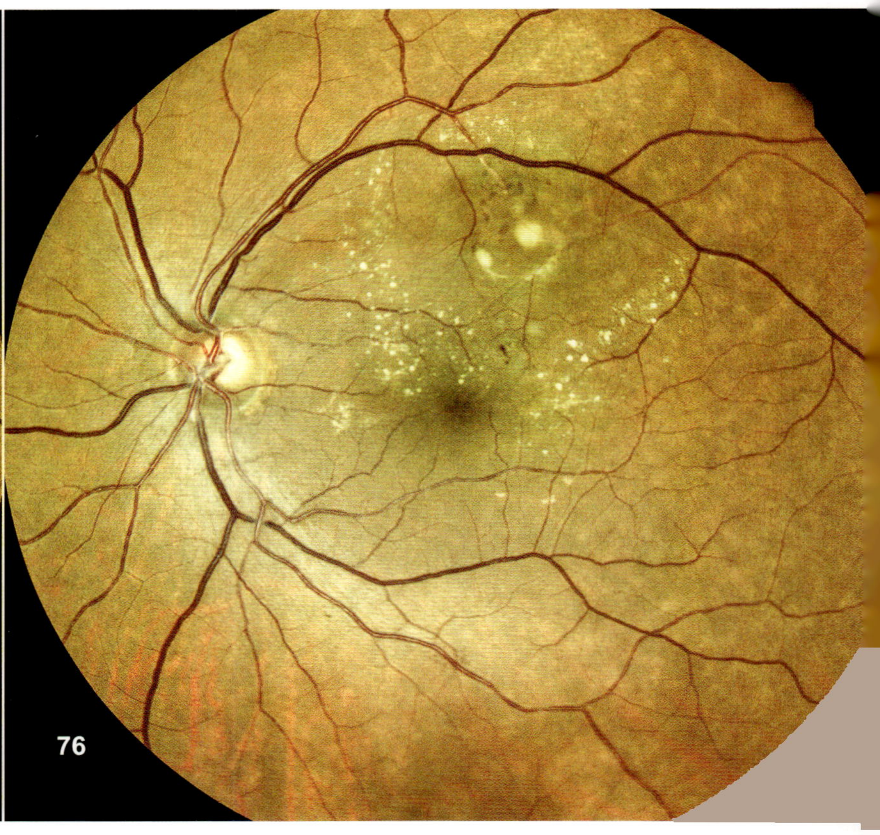


Figure 76 *Color fundus photograph 3 months postlaser treatment. Complete resolution of retinal bleed and further reduction in the hard exudates is appreciated with thrombosed RAM.* □

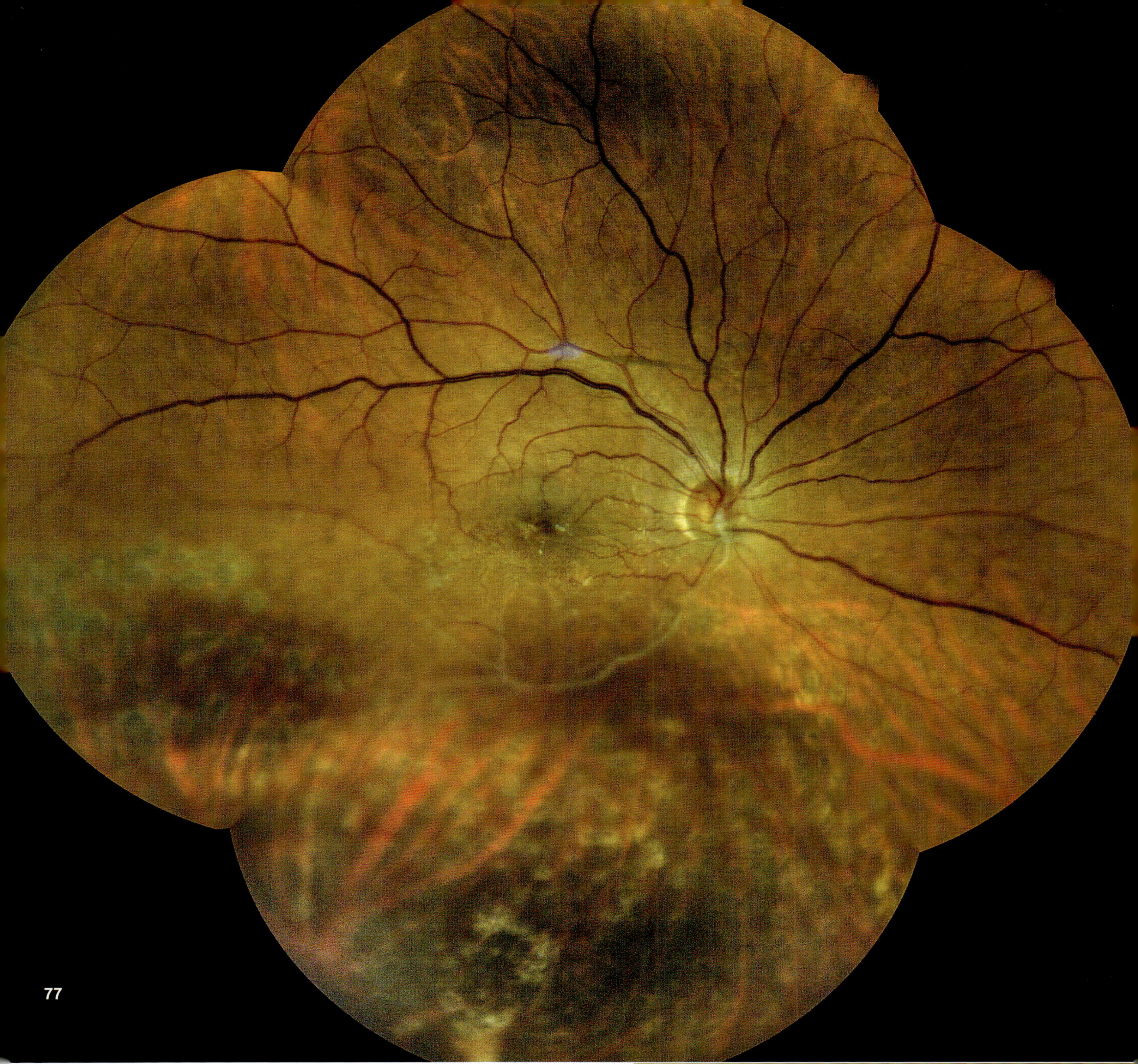


Figure 77 *A case of retinal vein occlusion with vitreous hemorrhage managed with 25-gauge pars plana vitrectomy.*

He underwent 25-gauge pars plana vitrectomy, inferotemporal branch retinal vein occlusion (BRVO) with neovascularization elsewhere was identified as etiology of hemorrhage. Endolaser marks were applied in a scatter pattern inferotemporally.

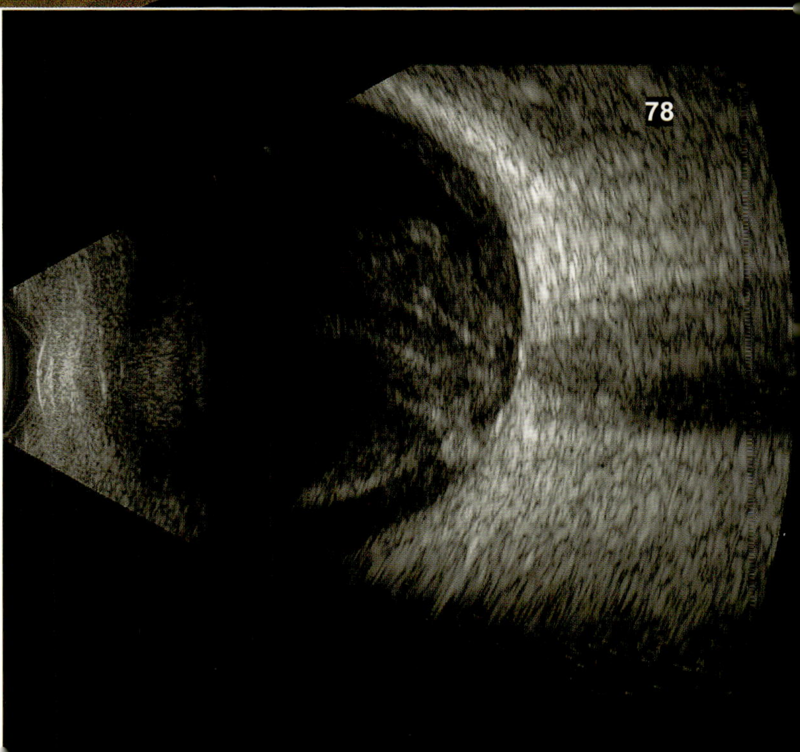


Figure 78 *A 66-year-old male presented with complaints of decrease vision in left eye since 2 weeks, with sudden onset of floaters. He gave history of hypertension. Media clarity was grade 4 with no view of fundus. Ultrasound demonstrated dense moderate amplitude echoes in vitreous cavity suggestive of vitreous hemorrhage.*□

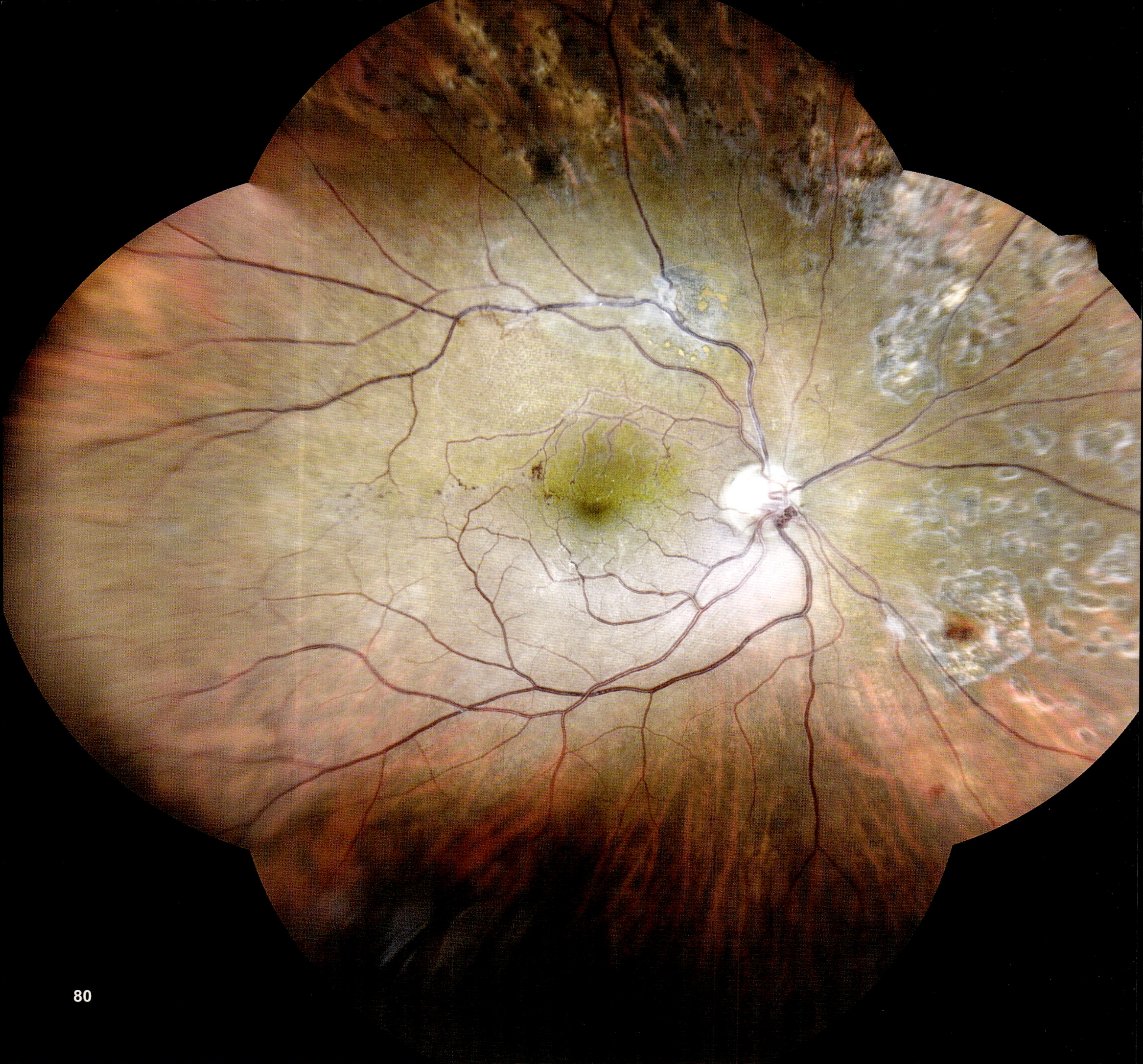

80

79

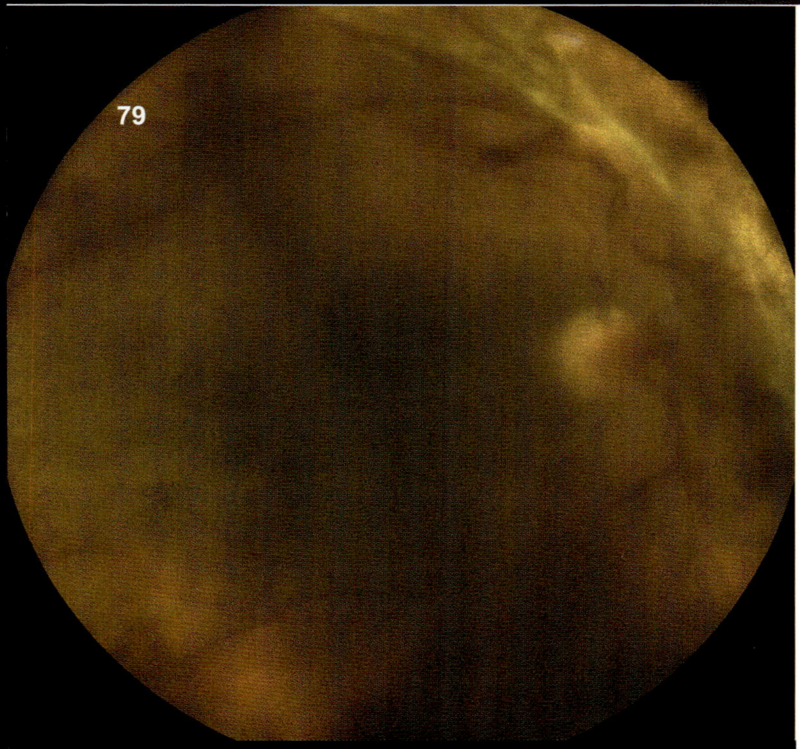

Figure 79 *A 67-year-old female presented with sudden appearance of black spots in front of her right eye for the past 5 days. Her best corrected visual acuity was counting fingers in right eye. She was a known case of glaucoma on topical medications. She was also known hypertensive with poor control on single oral antihypertensive. Fundus photo shows dense vitreous hemorrhage obscuring most of the fundus details, however the disk can be seen faintly as also a few retinal vessels. Whitish fibrovascular proliferation along the nasal and superior aspect of retina can also be seen.*

Figure 80 *Six weeks postoperatively BCVA improved to 6/18, media clarity improved to grade 1. Fundus photo shows scatter laser marks around the area of branch retinal vein occlusion superiorly and nasally. Regressing neovascularization can be seen nasally, which will need follow-up with serial fundus fluorescein angiography. Residual fibrous tissues can be seen along the blood vessel nasally which was too adherent to peel.*

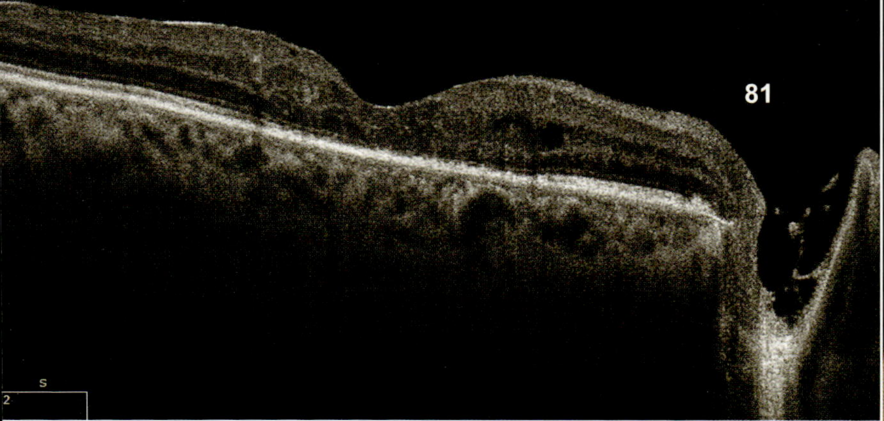


Figure 81 *SS-OCT scan was performed postoperatively shows attached neurosensory layer of retina with few residual hyporeflective spaces nasally. There was diffuse atrophy of outer retinal layers.*

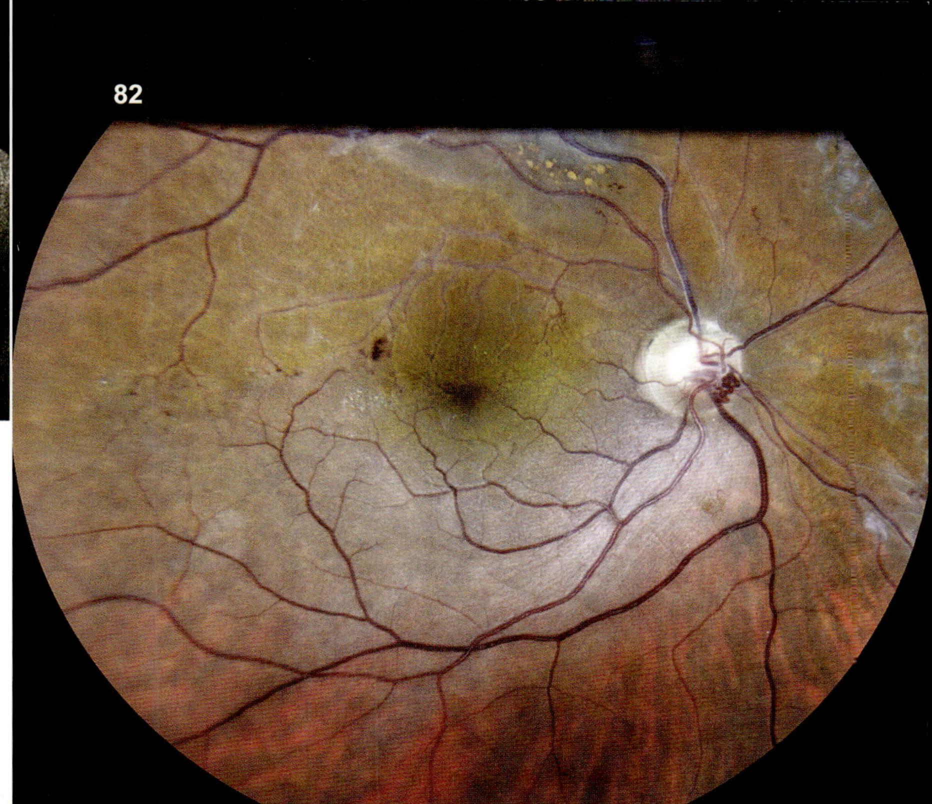


Figure 82 *25-gauge PPV was done, after complete release of vitreous traction, pneumatic reattachment was performed, followed by transvitreal laser photocoagulation. Sulfur hexafluoride (SF6) was injected to provide postoperative tamponade. Two weeks around 25% of gas still remains in the eye, however macular details can be seen more clearly. Some collateral can also be identified on the disk.*

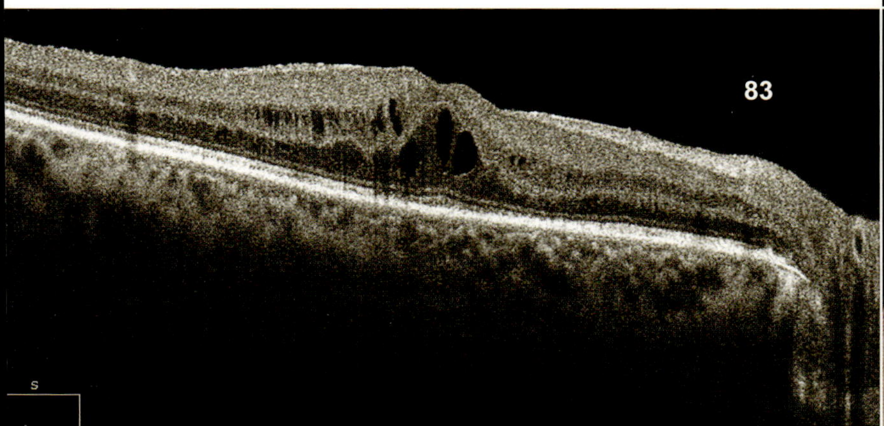


Figure 83 *SS-OCT shows large hyporeflective vertically elongated cyst like spaces at the fovea suggestive of cystoid macular edema.*

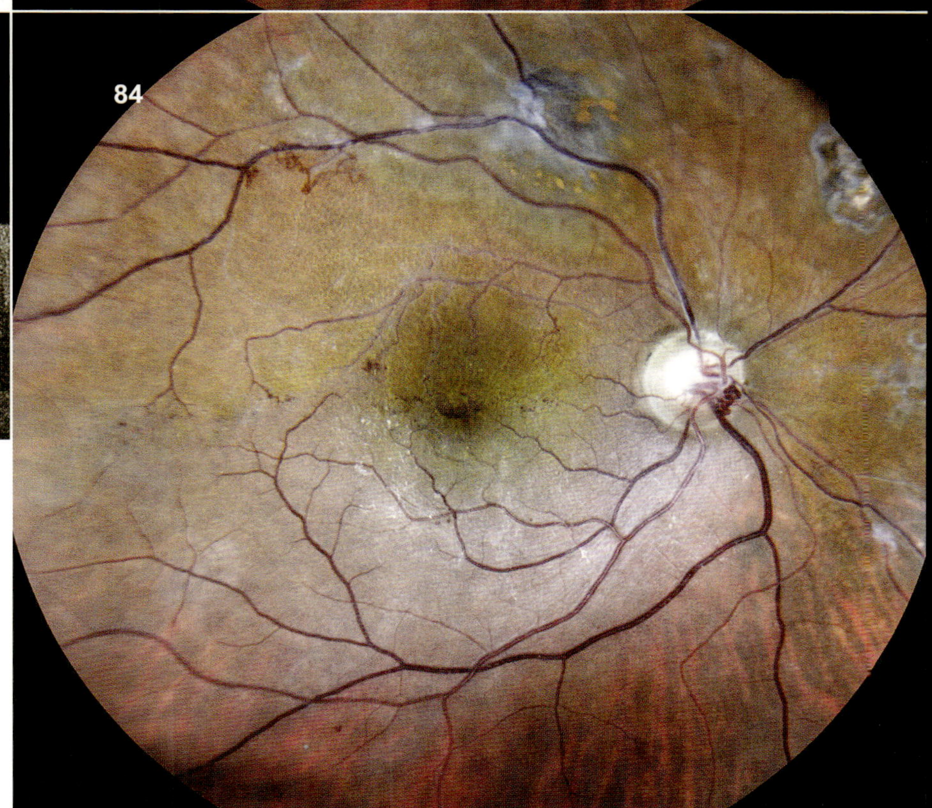


Figure 84 *Six weeks postoperatively BCVA improved to 6/18, media clarity improved to grade 1. Fundus photo shows scatter laser marks around the area of branch retinal vein occlusion superiorly and nasally. Regressing neovascularization can be seen nasally.*

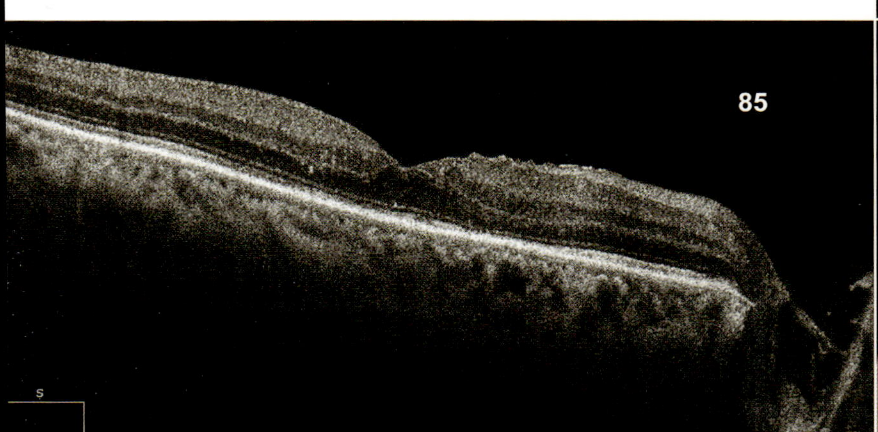


Figure 85 *SS-OCT also confirms resolution of hyporeflective cystoid spaces. The macular edema resolution has corresponding gain in visual acuity.*

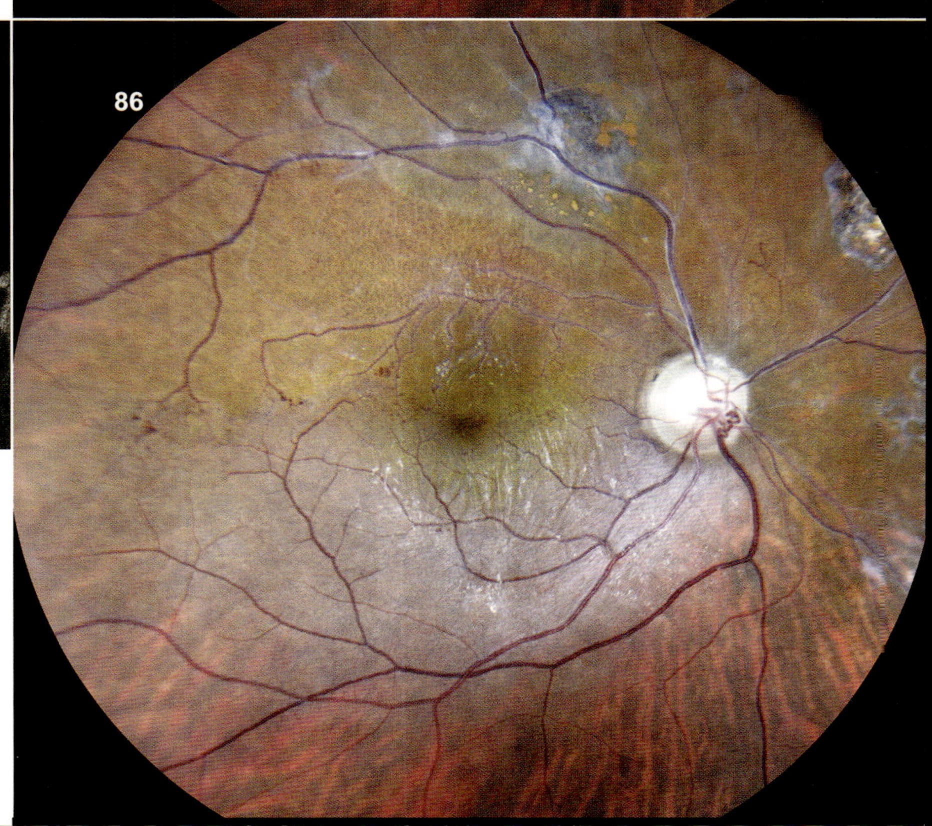


Figure 86 *She was given intravitreal anti-VEGF injection in her right eye. Three weeks later, fundus photo shows regression of neovascularization and reduction of cyst-like spaces. Best corrected visual acuity improved to 6/18.* □

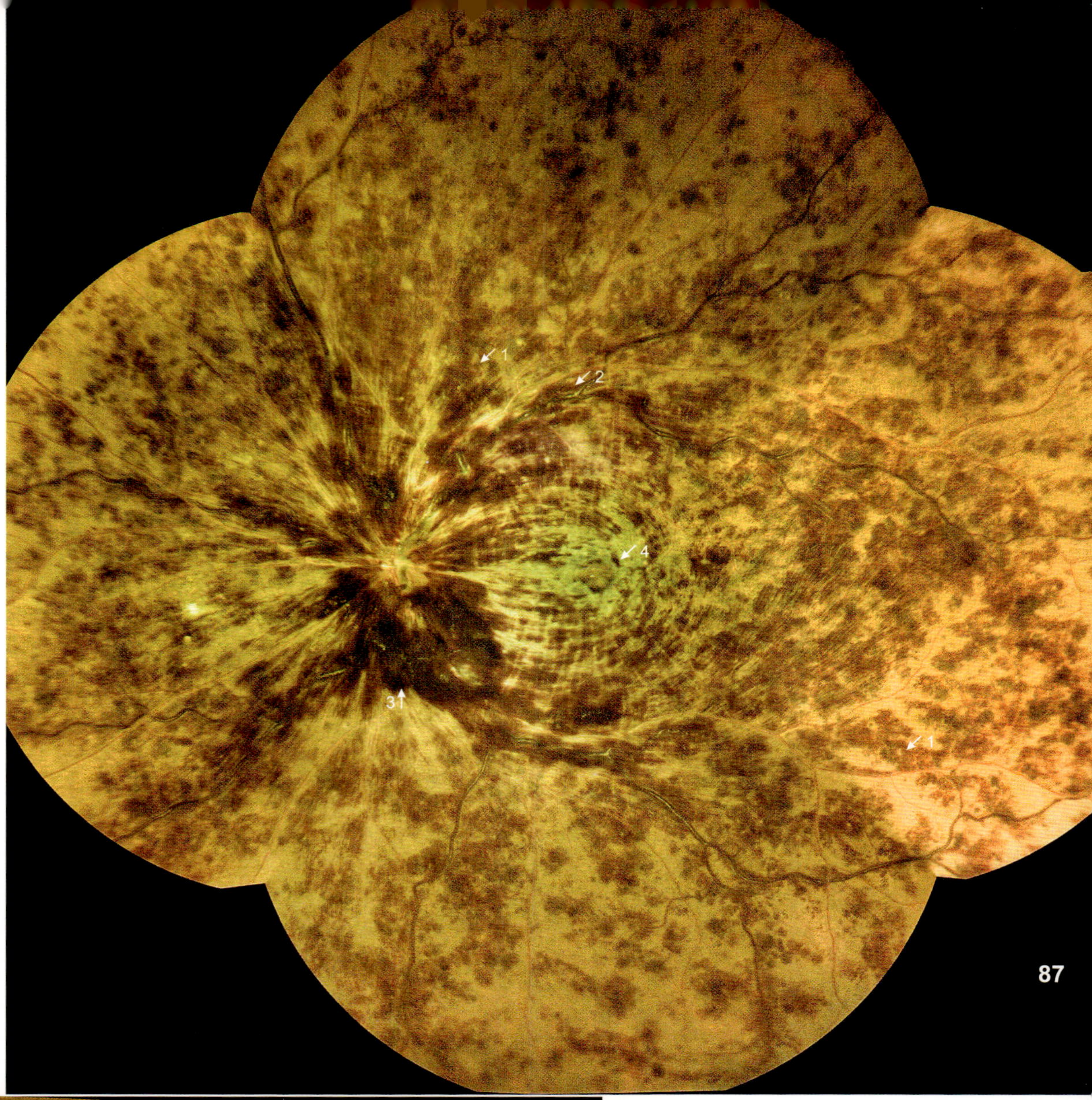

87

Figure 87

*Color fundus montage image of left eye in a case of recent onset central retinal vein occlusion. Classic "blood and thunder" appearance is seen in the left fundus image. Multiple flame-shaped retinal hemorrhage scattered in all 4 quadrats of retina, (1) dilated tortuous retinal vein, (2) disk swelling with peripapillary hemorrhages (3) and edematous macula (4).*

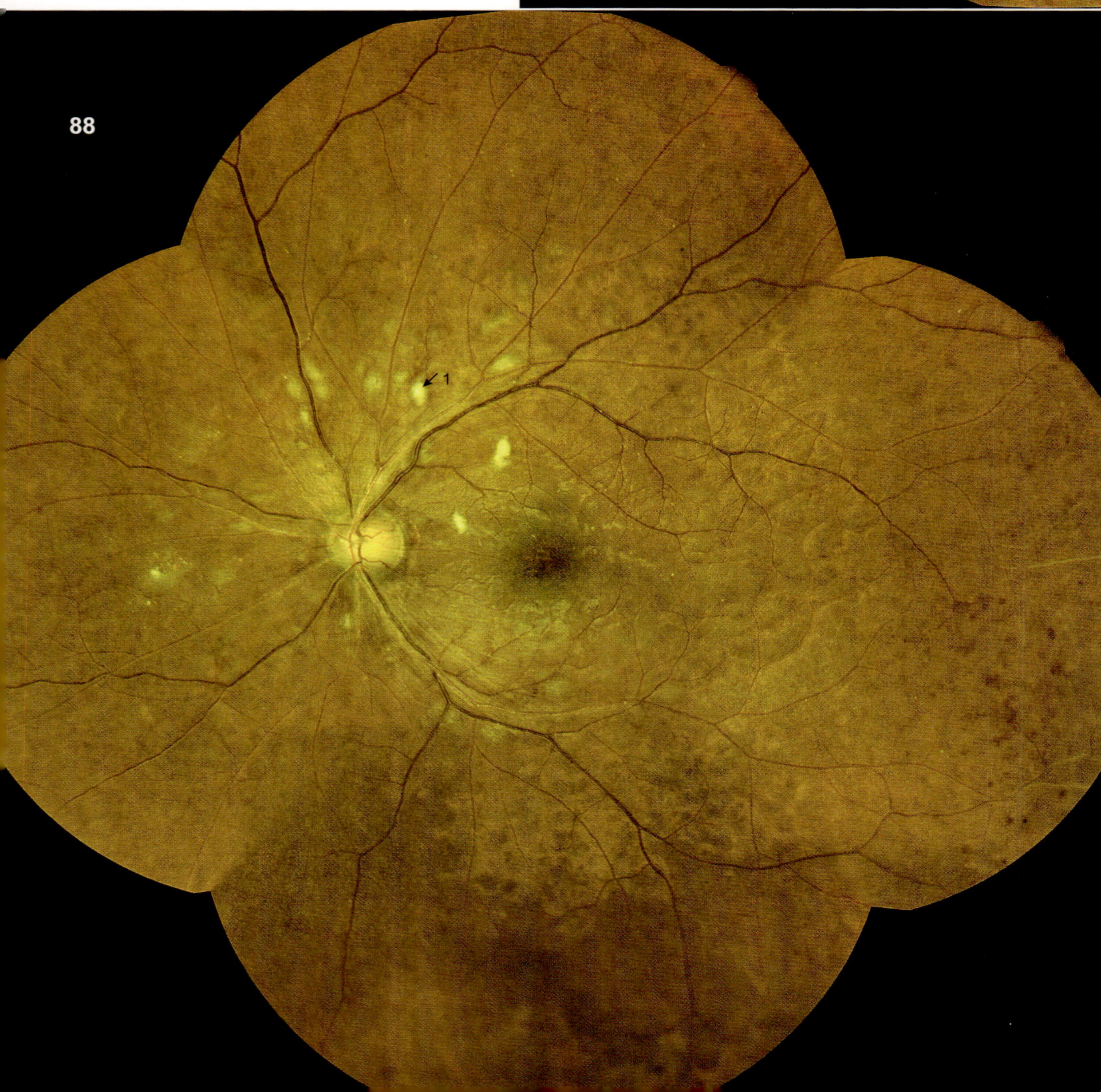

88

Figure 88

*Color fundus montage image of same patient after 5 months of treatment with 4 weekly intravitreal anti-VEGF injections demonstrates almost complete resolution of retinal hemorrhages optic disk and retinal vessel appears normal but few cotton wool spots were seen in the superior retina (1).*

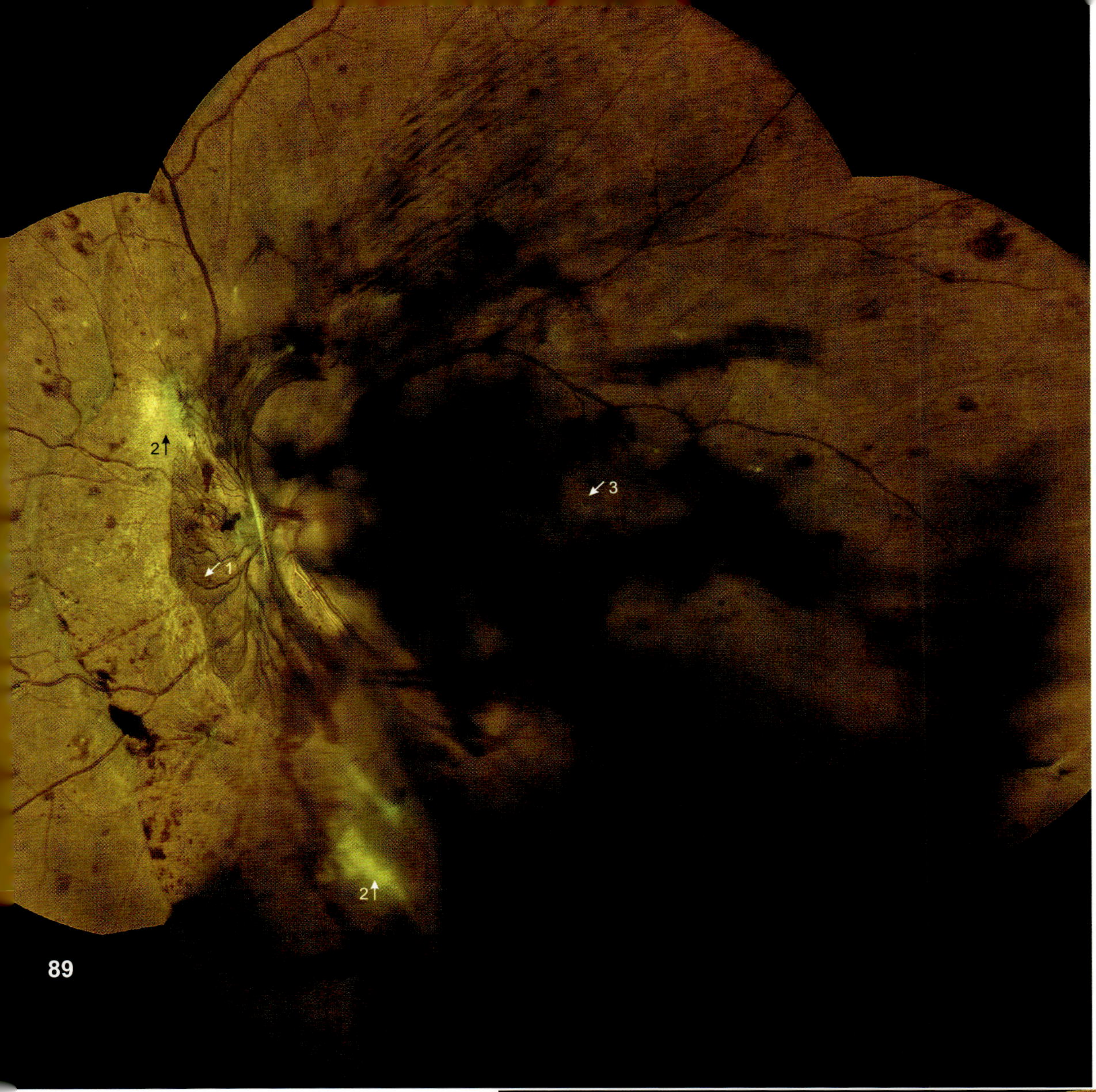


Figure 89

*Color fundus montage image of left eye of the same patient 1 year later (he was lost to follow-up). Patient has developed retinal neovascularization (1) with traction (2) and vitreous hemorrhage grade 2 (3).*

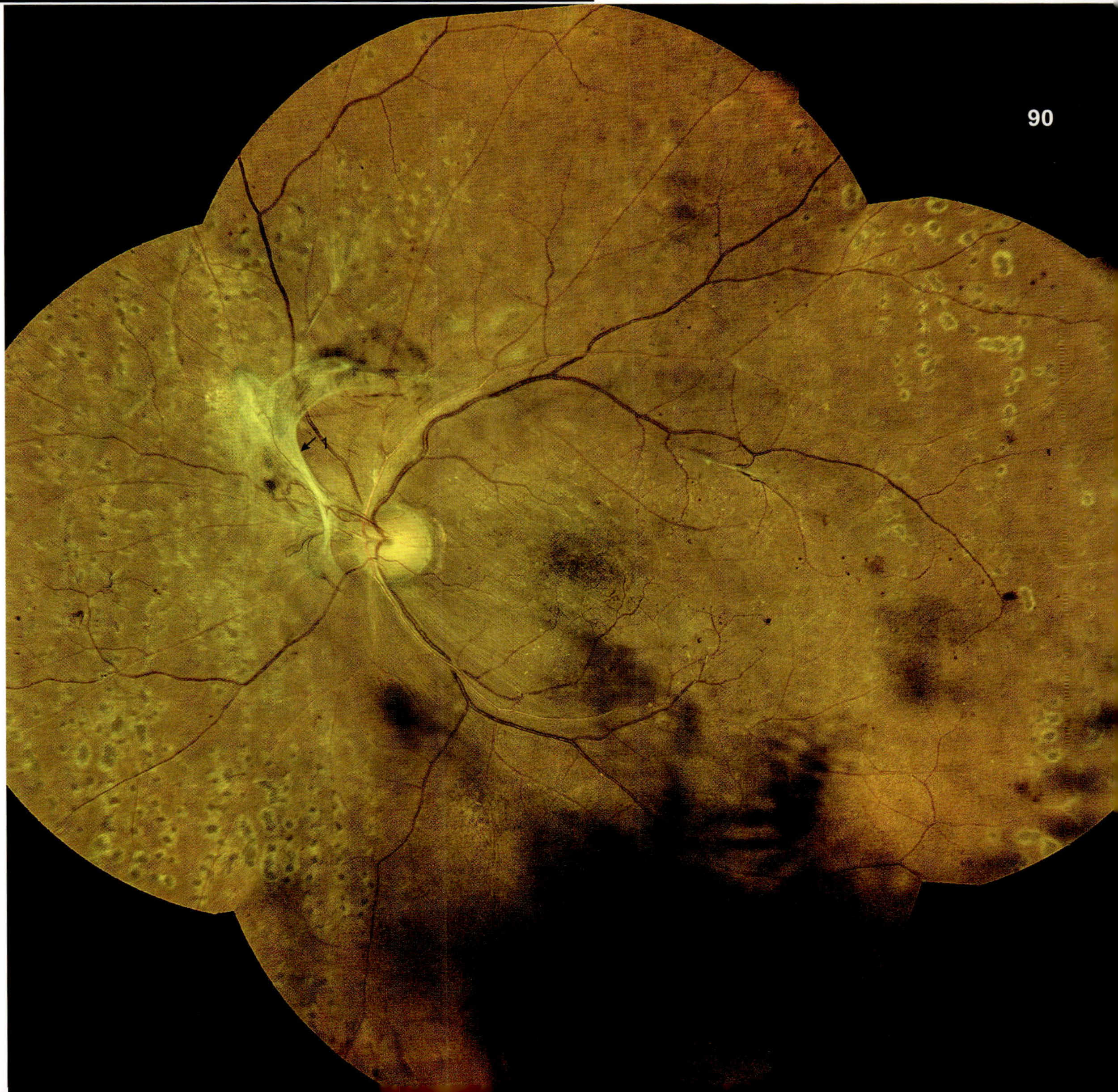


Figure 90

*Color fundus montage after treatment with anti-VEGF injection and panretinal photocoagulation. Fibrovascular traction bond from the disk to nasal retina is visible (1) NVD has repressed completely and vitreous hemorrhage has repressed from posterior pole. Multiple PRP scars are seen in the mid-periphery of retina.*

Our case highlights the importance of regular treatment and follow-ups on retinal vascular disease. Although risk of development of anterior segment neovascularization is more commonly seen in ischemic CRVO at 3–7 months but late development of retinal NV can lead to vitreous hemorrhage. Hence, similar follow-ups at 3–4 months are advisable for at least 2 years.

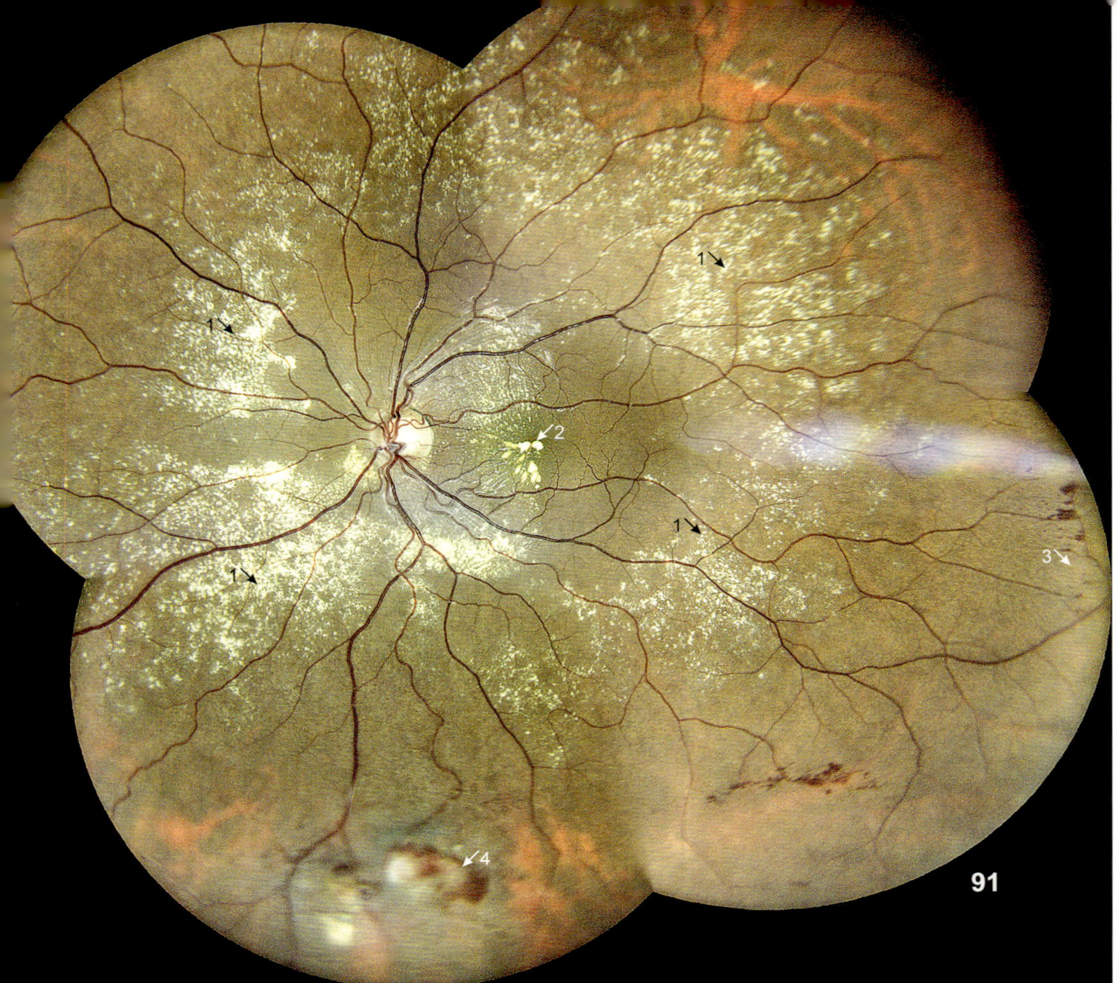

Figure 91

*Color fundus montage image of a young adult male demonstrating typical features of Coats disease (stage 2B). Multiple hard exudates (lipid deposits) could be seen in all 4 quadrants (1) with foveal exudation (2). Dilated tortuous capillaries aneurysm are seen in the temporal periphery (3), fusiform arterial dilation ("light bulb" aneurysms) could be seen in inferior periphery (4).*

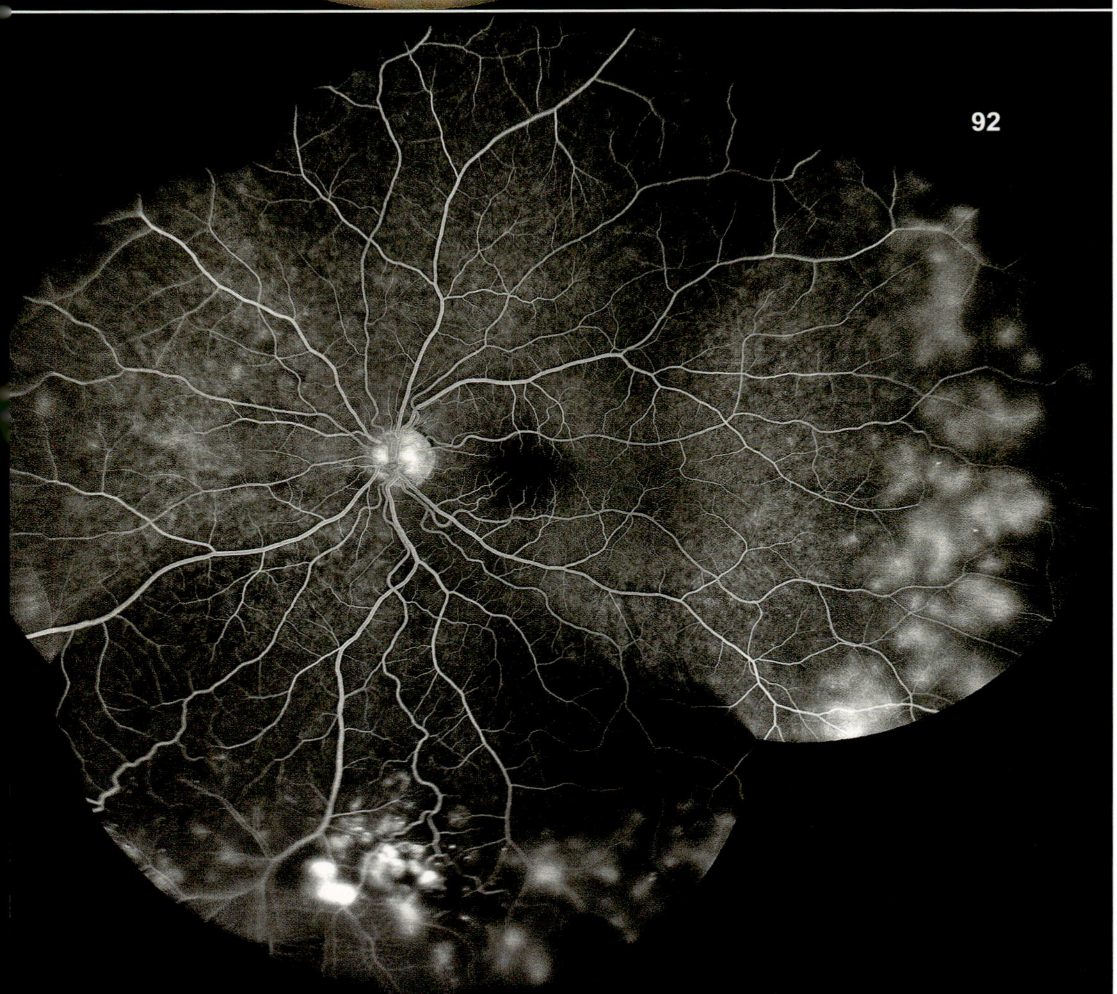

Figure 92

*Fundus autofluorescence montage: Multiple patches of hyperfluorescent leakage points could be seen all along the temporal and inferior retinal periphery arising from the vascular abnormalities in Coats disease.*

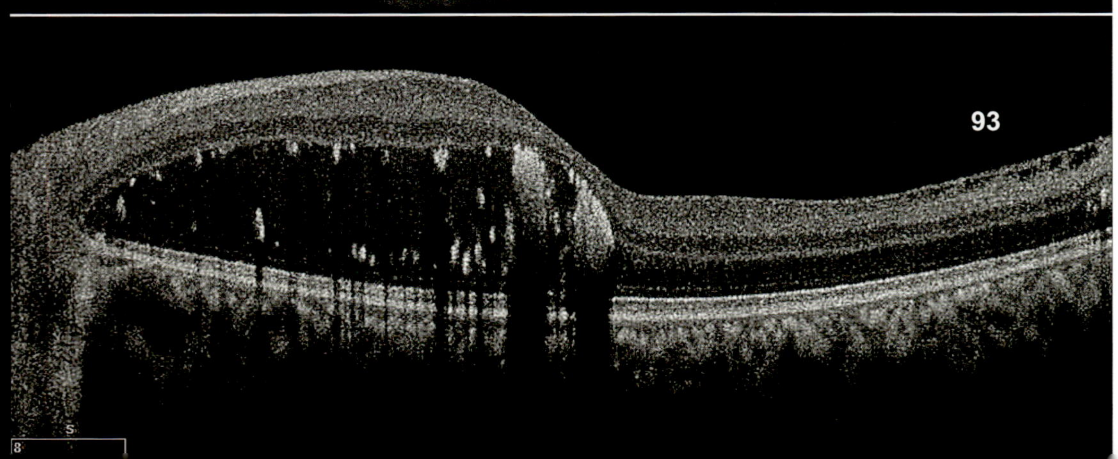

Figure 93

*SD-OCT shows macular edema secondary to foveal exudates in Coats disease. Increased retinal thickening, increase hyporeflectivity is seen in OPL and ONL layers along with multiple hyper-reflective dots representing lipid exudation.*

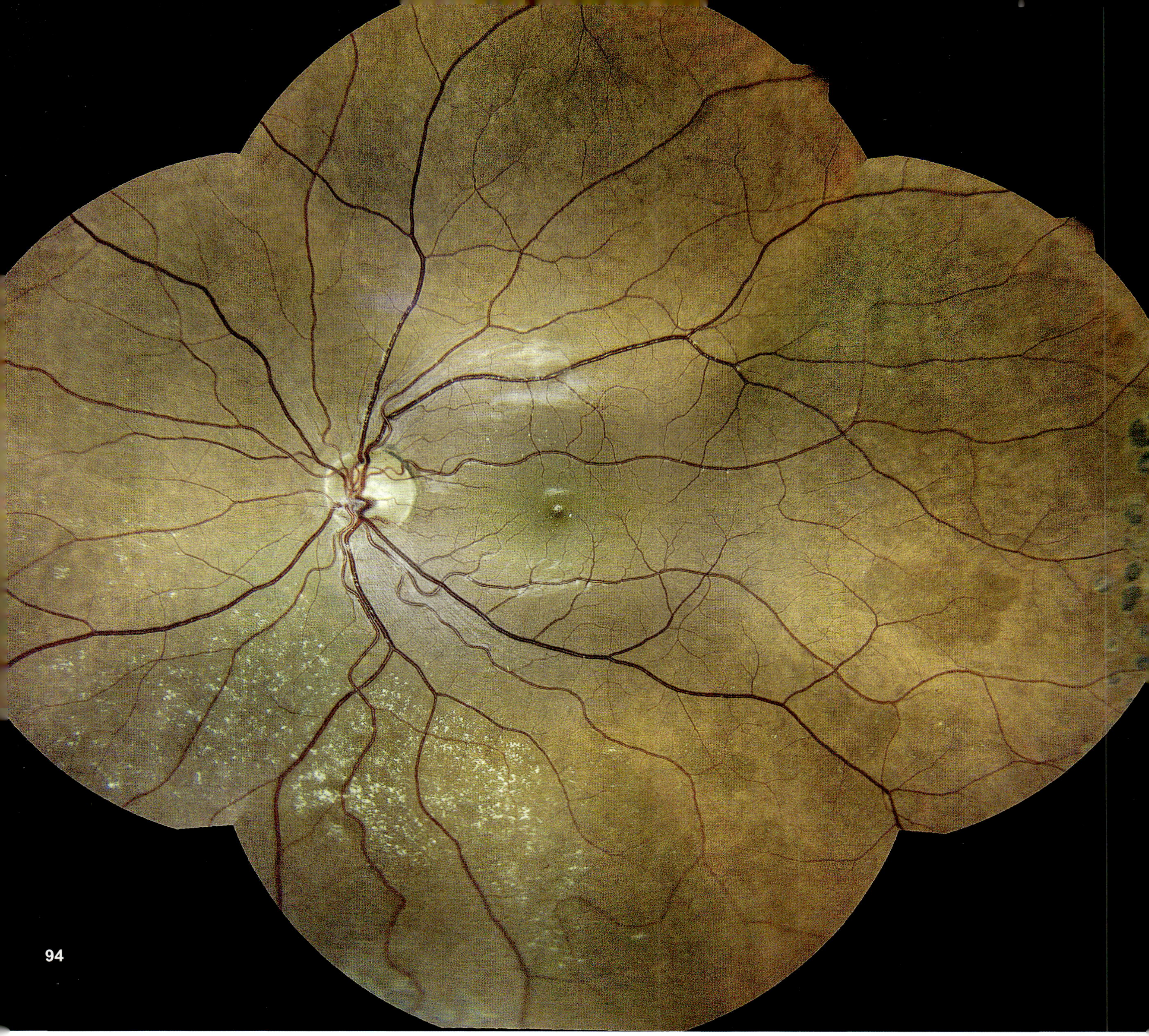


Figure 94 *Color fundus montage of same patient with Coats disease—6 months after treatment with anti-VEGF injections and scatter laser photocoagulation demonstrates significant reduction in lipid exudation at fovea and mid-peripheral retina.*

Figure 95 *OCT scan image of Coats disease demonstrating significant reduction in macular edema following treatment with anti-VEGF injections and scatter laser.* □

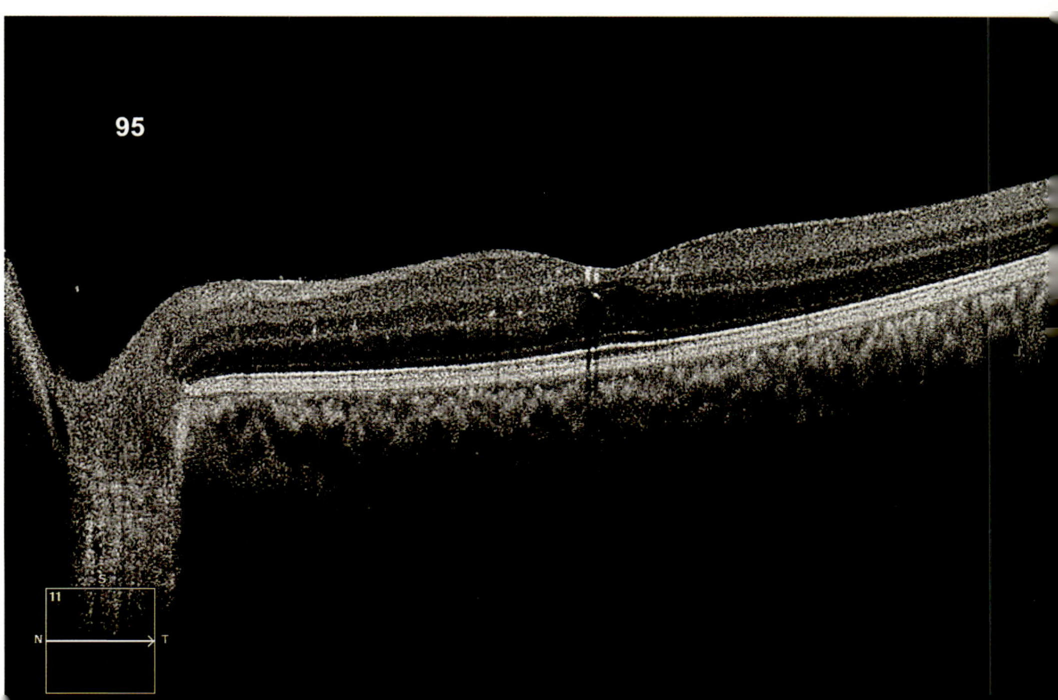

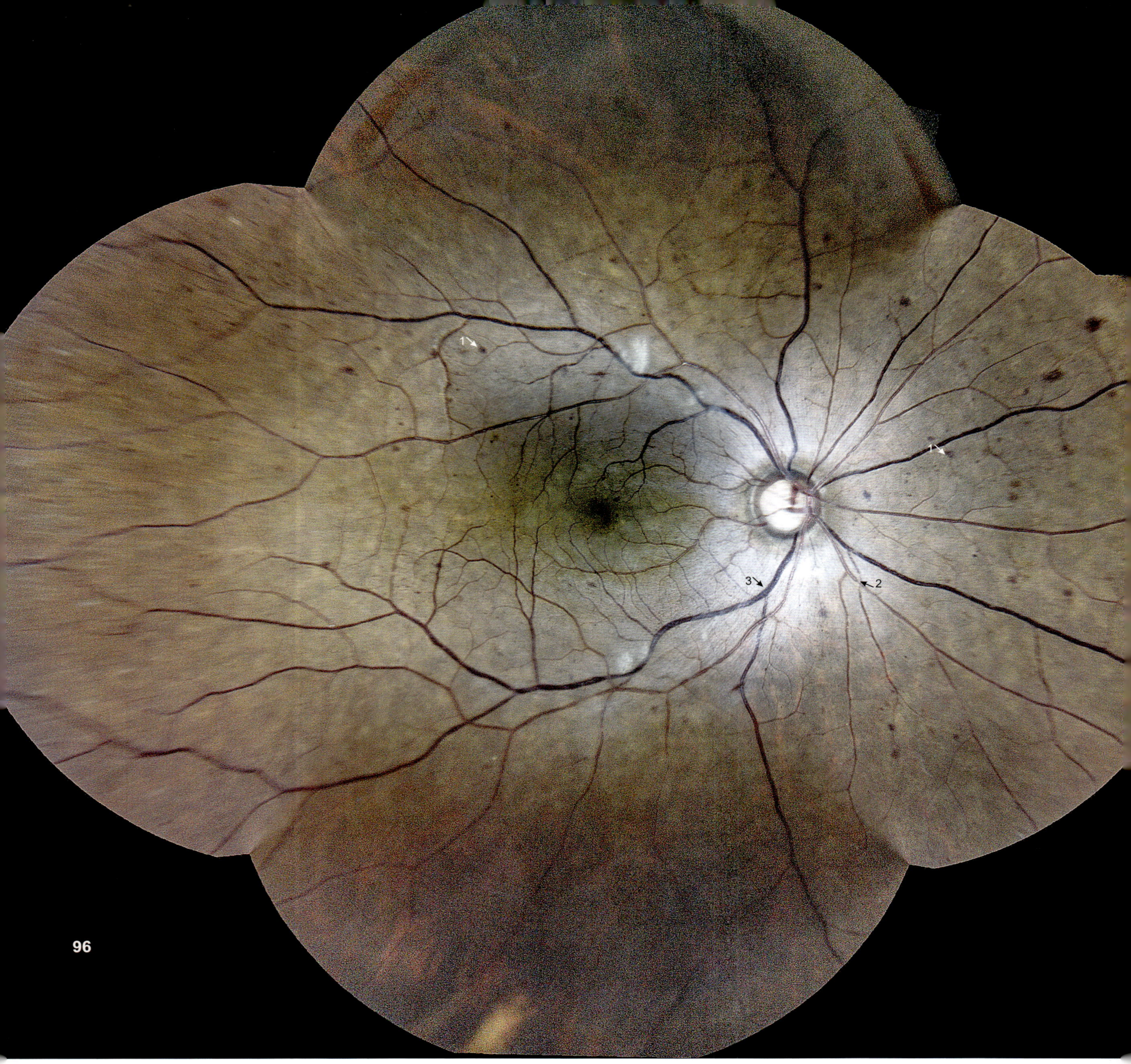


96

Figure 96 *A case of ocular ischemic syndrome (OIS): Color fundus montage image shows deep intraretinal dot blot, round, red retinal hemorrhages scattered in the mid-peripheral retina and posterior pole (1) also note narrowing of retinal arteries (2) and dilated but not tortuous retinal veins (3).*

Figure 97 *FFA image at 16 seconds after dye injection demonstrating nonfilling of choroid suggestive of delayed choroidal filling in a case of OIS.*

Figure 98 *FFA image at 30 seconds after dye injection showed choroidal hyperfluorescence (1) and patchy early filling of retinal arteries (2). This demonstrates prolonged time aim to retina time suggestive of OIS.*

Figure 99 *FFA image taken at 53 seconds demonstrating delayed arteriovenous transit time. At 53 seconds after dye injection there is incomplete patchy filling of retinal veins.*

Figure 100 *FFA image, at 1:30 seconds demonstrating dye circulate in arteries and veins except infero-temporal vein is still not filled with dye.*

Figure 101 *Late phase of fundus fluorescein angiography demonstrating hyperfluorescence optic disk staining and late arteriocular staining and leakage suggestive of chronic hypoxic endo-thelial ischemia.*

Figure 102 *Swept source OCT scan in a case of ocular ischemic syndrome shows thin choroid (1) and retina! specification linear patches in the OPL/INL layers of retina (2).* □

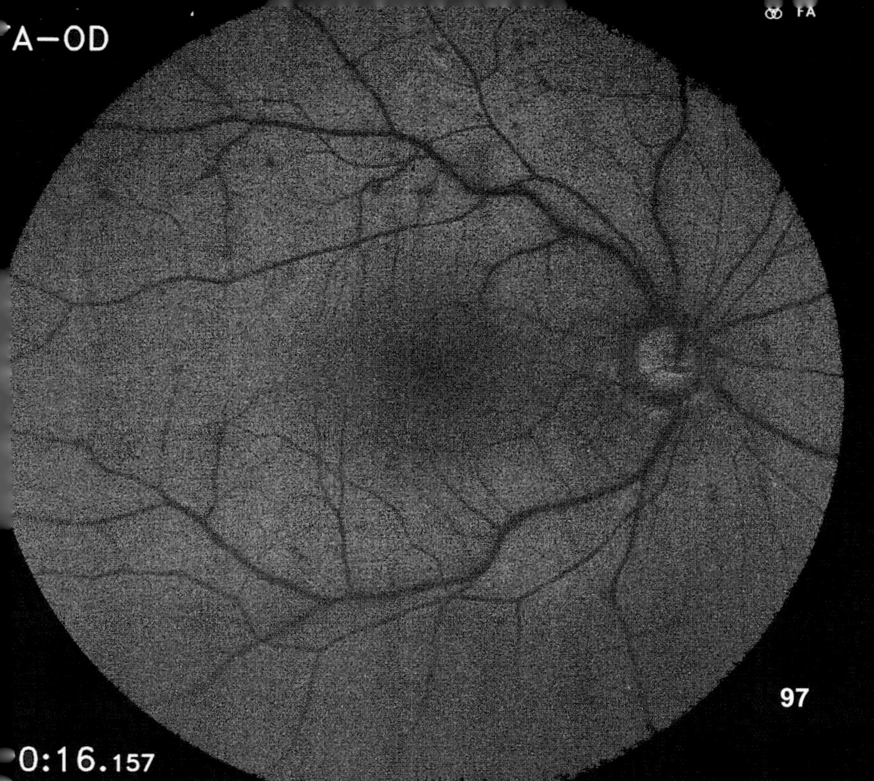
A-OD
FA
97
0:16.157

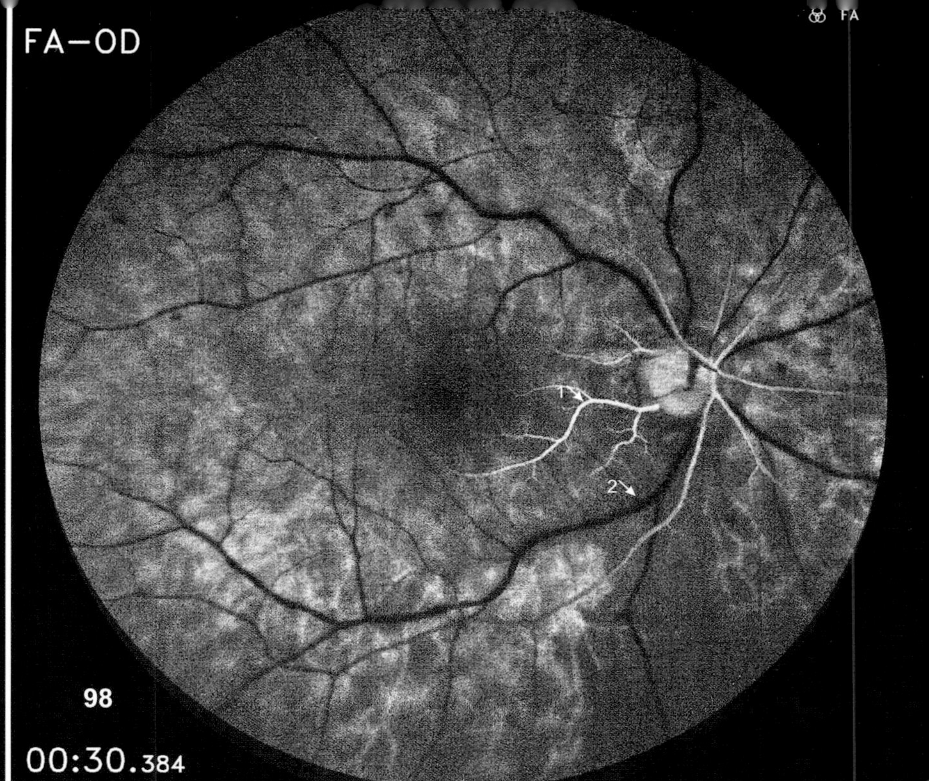
FA-OD
FA
1
2
98
00:30.384

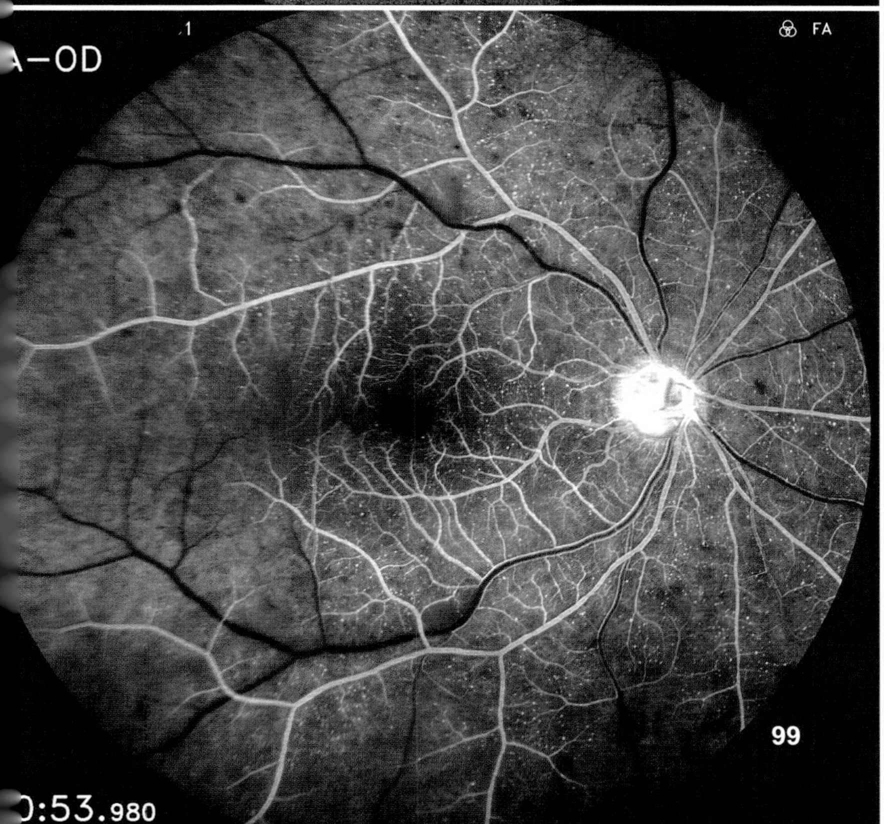
A-OD
FA
99
0:53.980

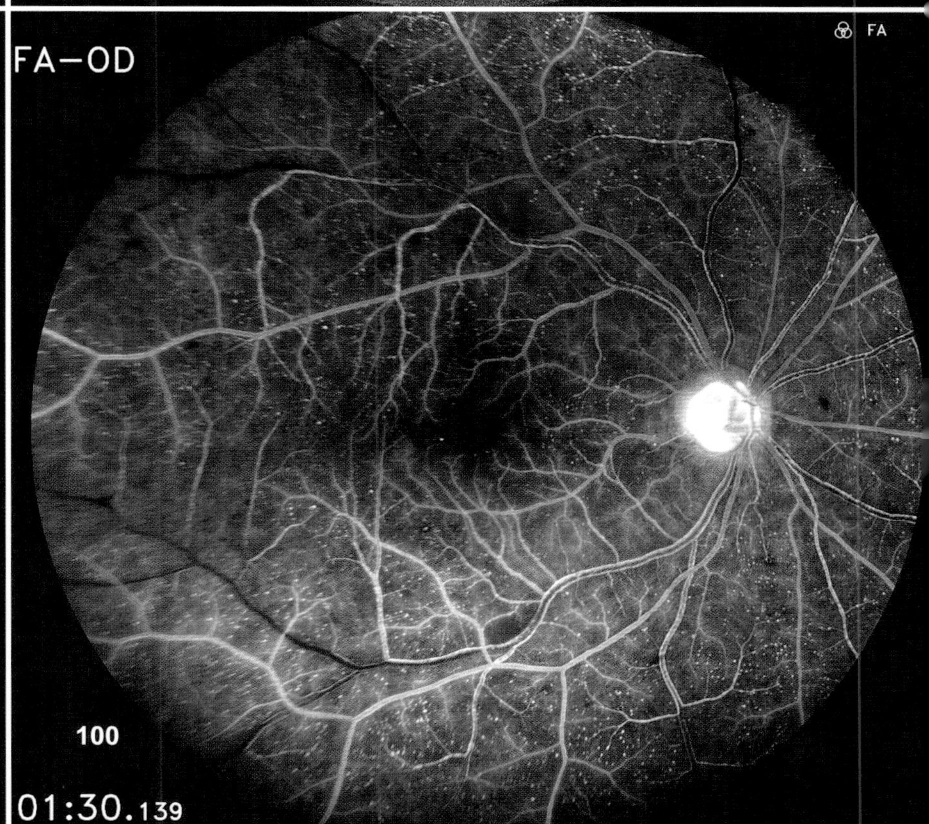
FA-OD
FA
100
01:30.139

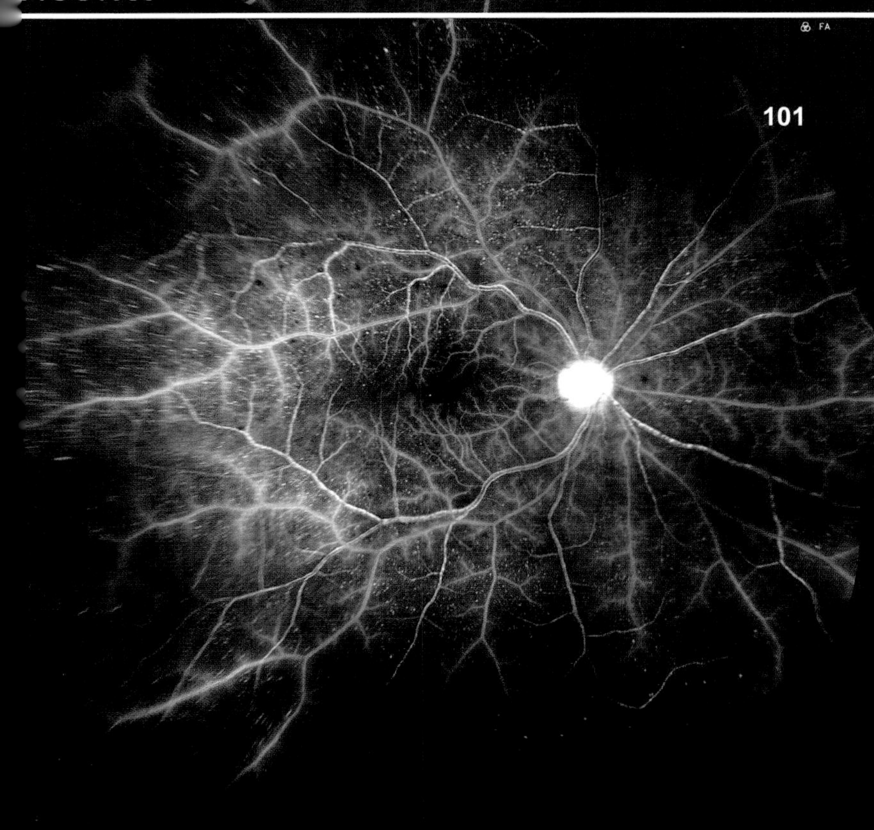
FA
101

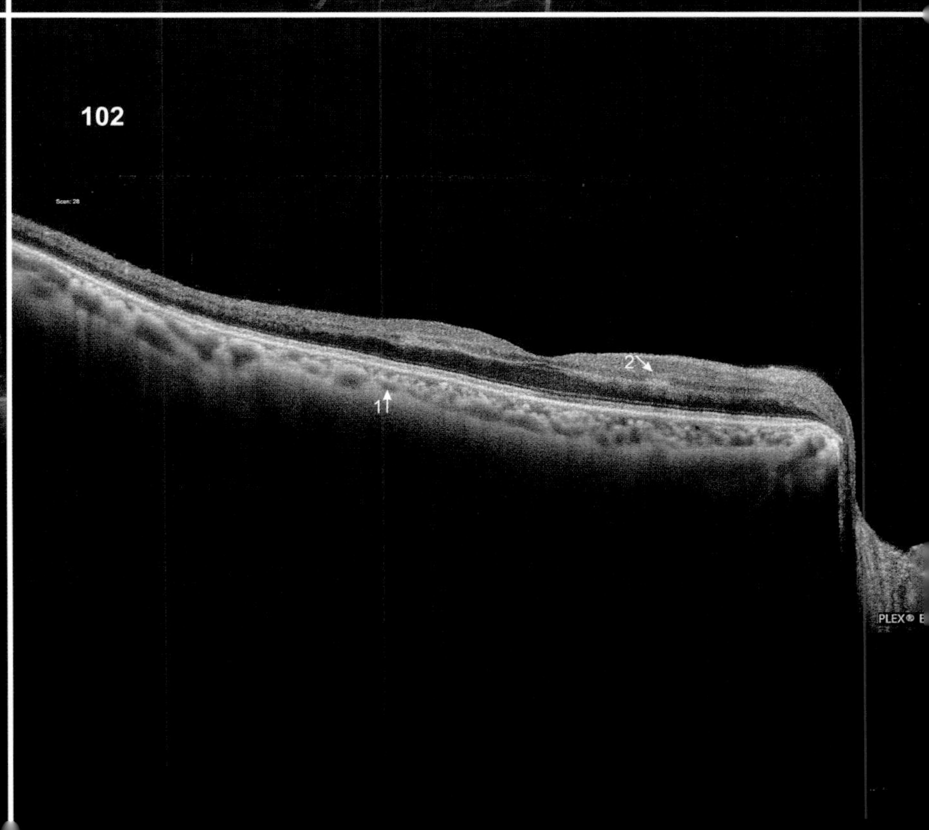
102
2
1

Figure 103

*Anemic retinopathy: Color fundus montage image demonstrating subhyaloid bleed at fovea (1) and multiple Roth spots (2) in a patient with anemic retinopathy secondary to severe ulcerative colitis.*

Figure 104

*Spectral domain OCT scan demonstrating subhyaloid bleed at the fovea in a case of anemic retinopathy.*

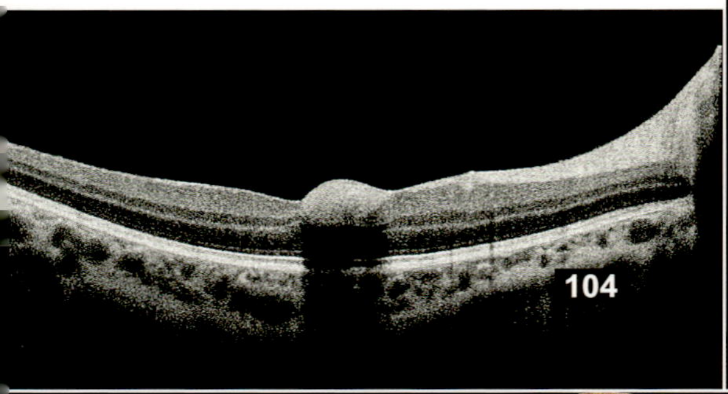


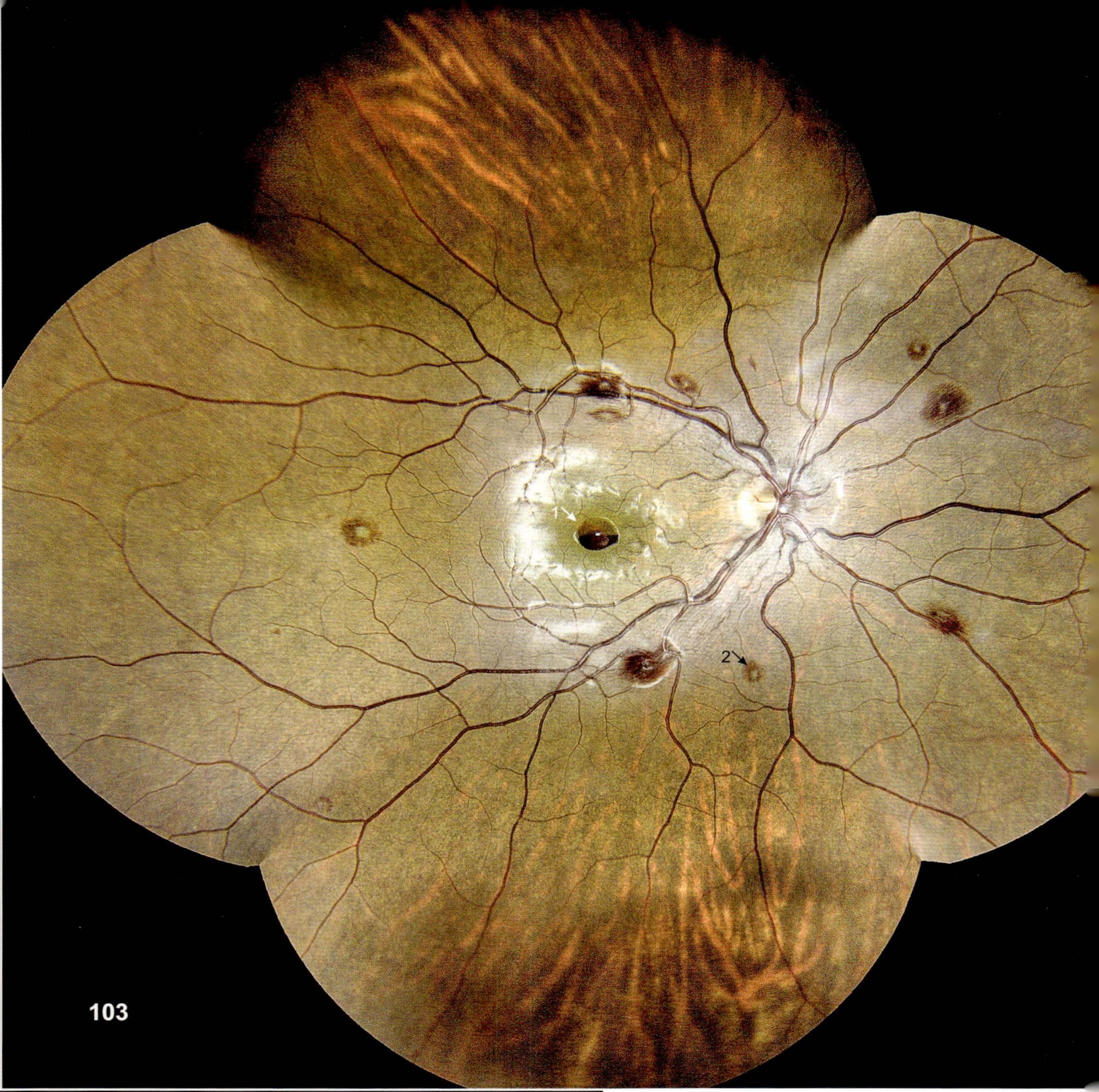


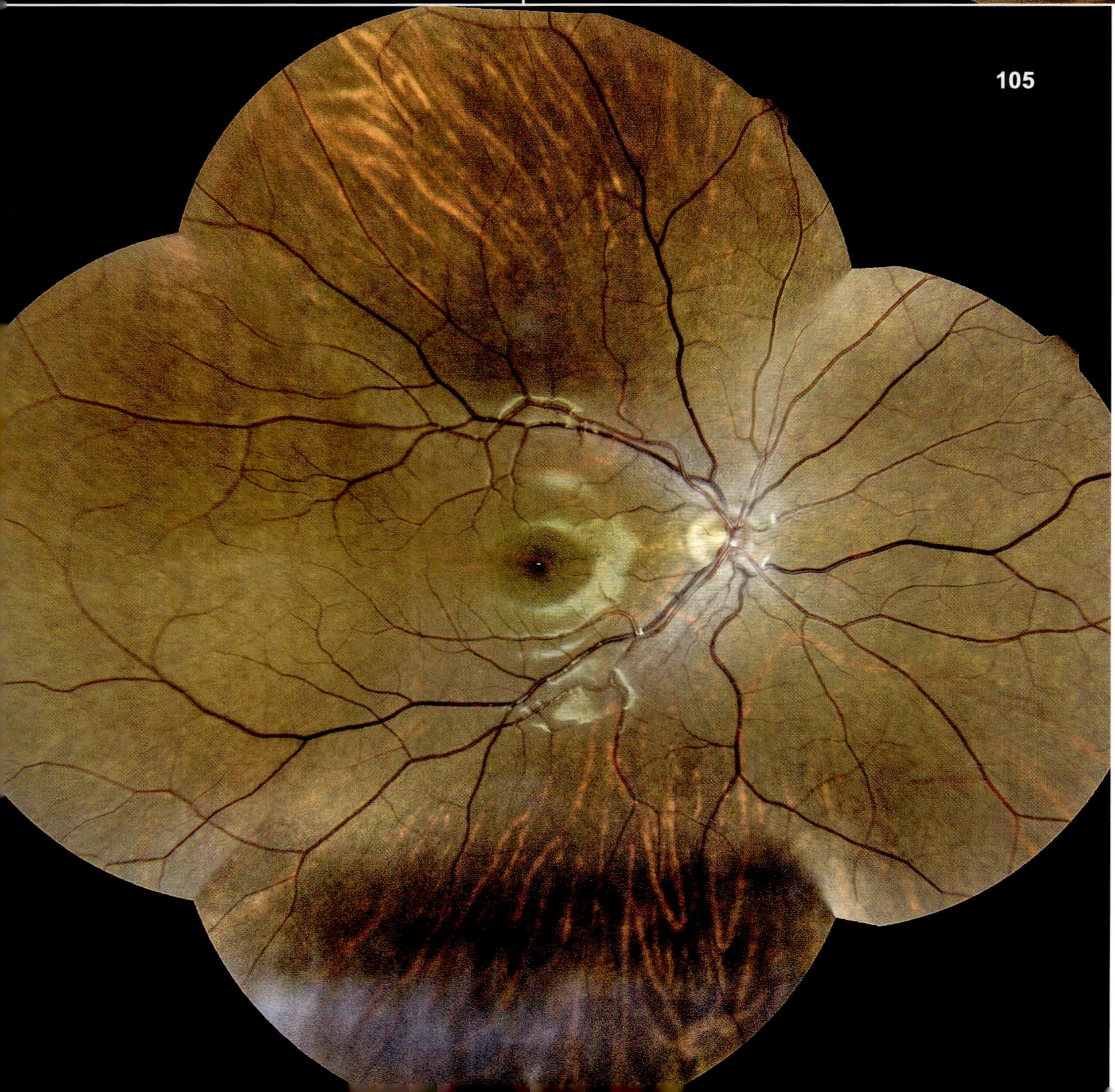


Figure 105

*Color fundus montage image of same patient with anemic retinopathy 6 weeks later shows complete resolution of all retinal hemorrhages. Patient had received 2 units of blood transfusion, no ocular treatment was indicated.*□

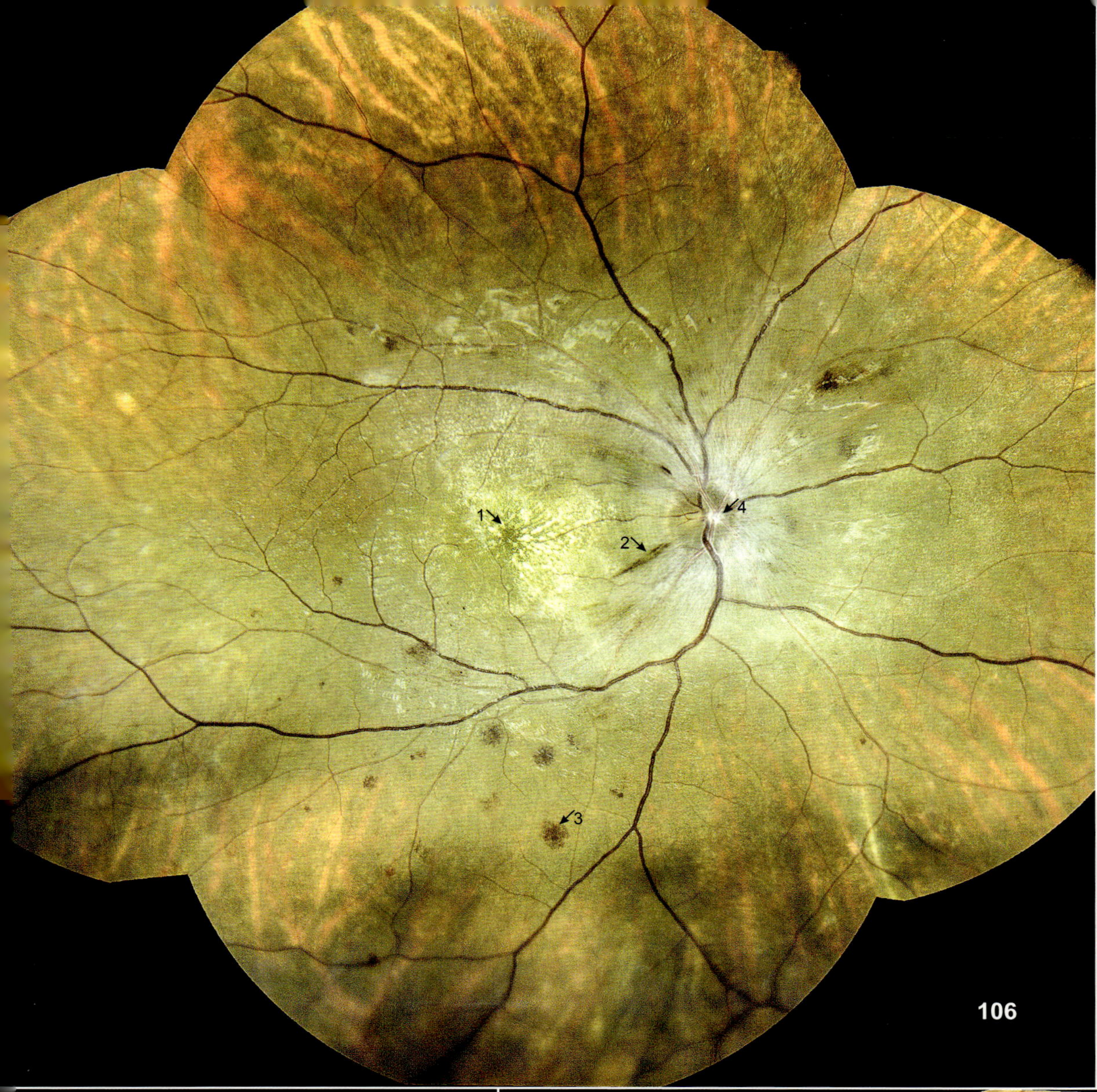


Figure 106

*Hypertensive retinopathy with macular star. Right eye wide field fundus montage image in a young 25-year-old female with recent kidney transplant secondary to hypertension. Note the presence of yellow retinal exudate at fovea, perifoveal region (1), splinter-shaped peripapillary hemorrhage (2) and few round deep intraretinal hemorrhages (3). Optic disk appears edematous (4).*

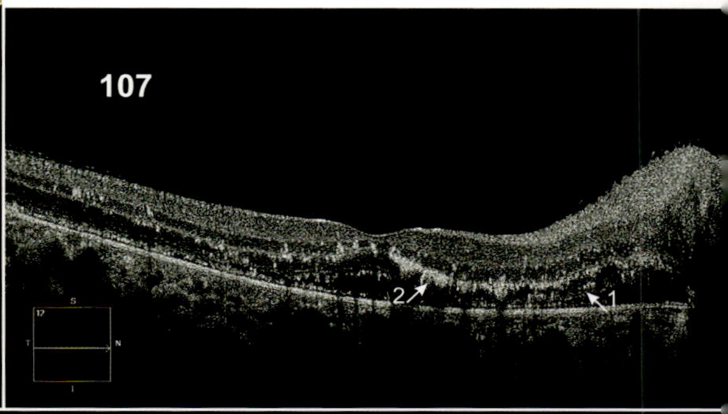


Figure 107

*Spectral domain OCT scan in a case of hypertensive retinopathy. Note the diffuse increased hyporeflectivity of outer nuclear and outer plexiform layers (1). Multiple tiny hyperreflective dots (2) represents retinal lipid exudation. Also note diffuse thickening of the peripapillary optic disk region representing optic disk edema.*

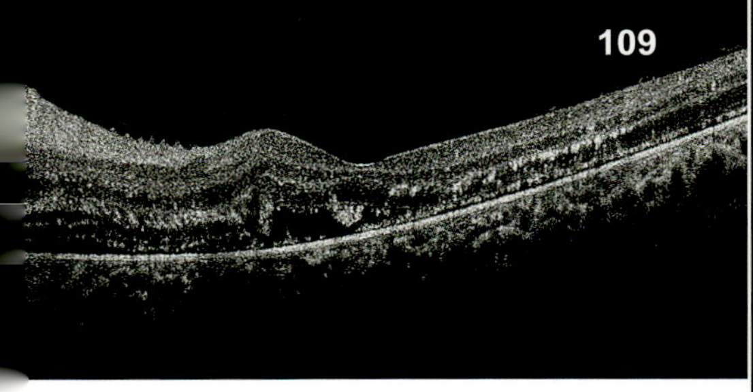


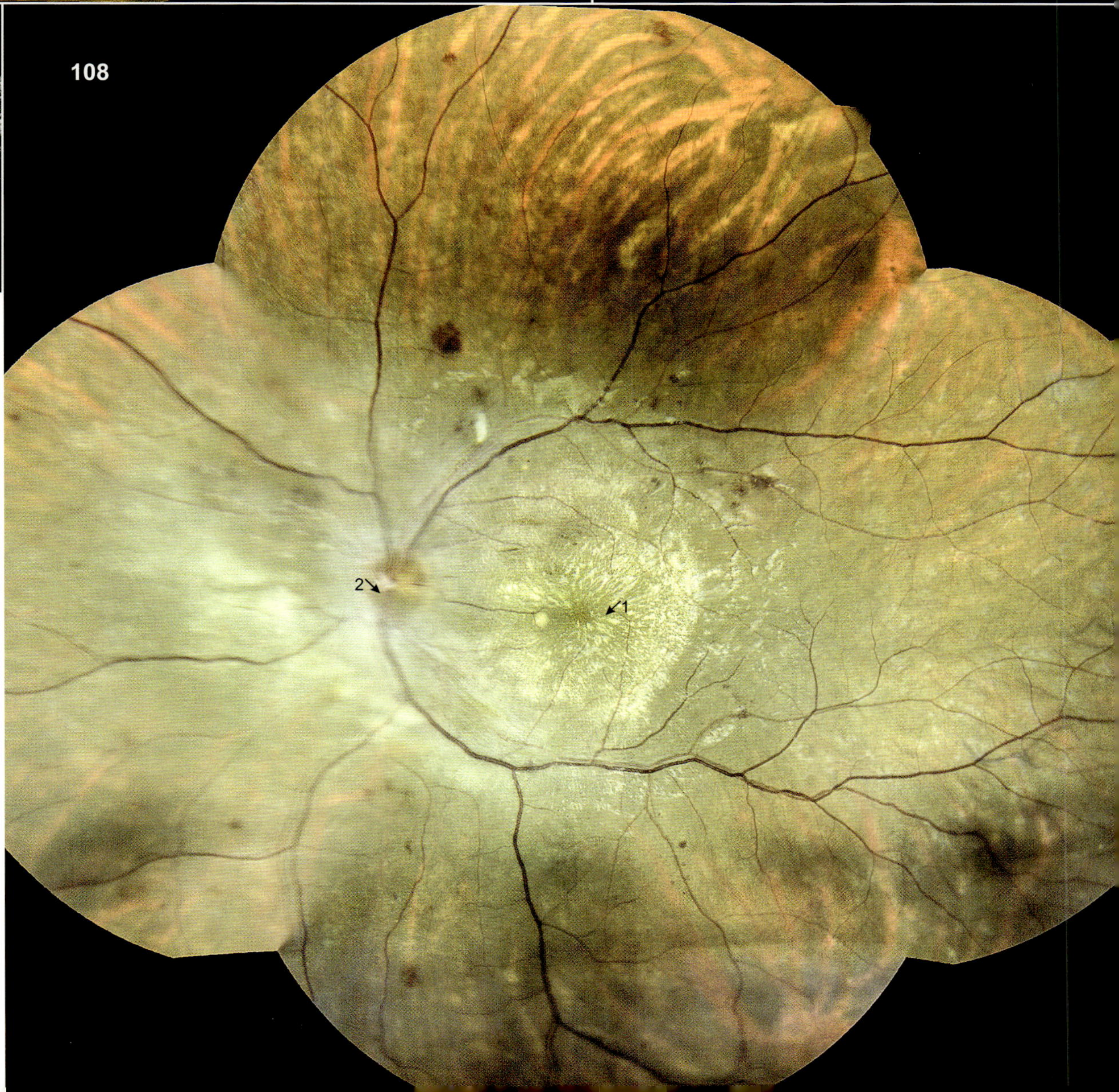


Figure 108

*Color fundus montage image of left eye of same patient with hypertensive retinopathy. Note the bilaterally symmetrical retinal findings of macular star (1) and optic disk edema (2).*

Figure 109

*SD-OCT scan of left eye of same patient with macular star secondary to hypertensive retinopathy.*

*Note:* Hypertensive retinopathy is usually a self-limiting condition and does not require any local treatment. Priority should be given to urgent control of hypertension and patient should be referred to local physician for management of hypertension. □

A case of malignant hypertension.

Figure 110

*Color fundus image demonstrating papilloedema (1) multiple splinter hemorrhages (2) whitish fluffy cotton wool spots (3) and few intraretinal hemorrhage (4).*

Figure 111

*SD-OCT scan demonstrating serous macular detachment (1) and peripapillary retinal edema (2) in a case of malignant hypertension.*

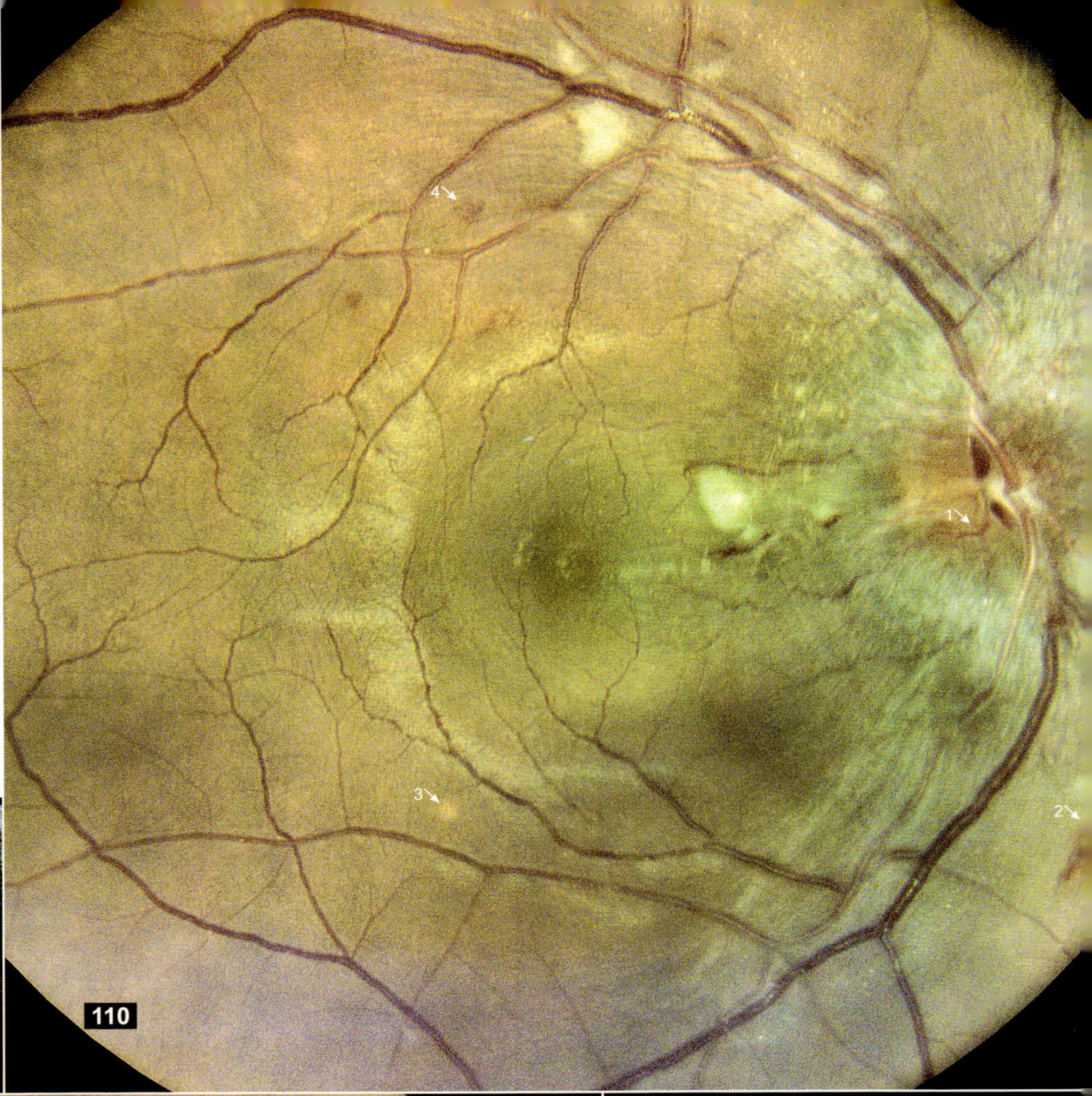


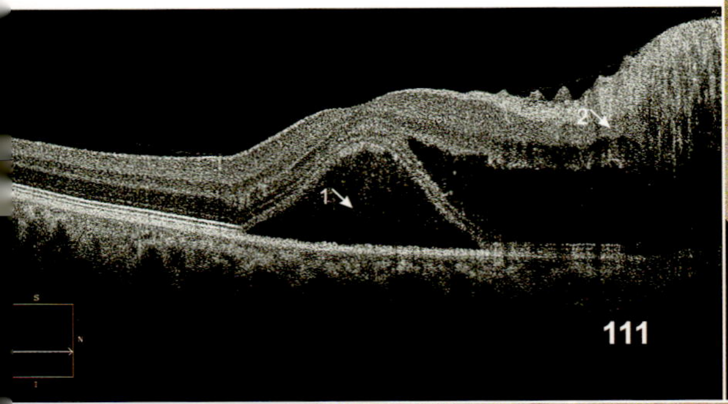


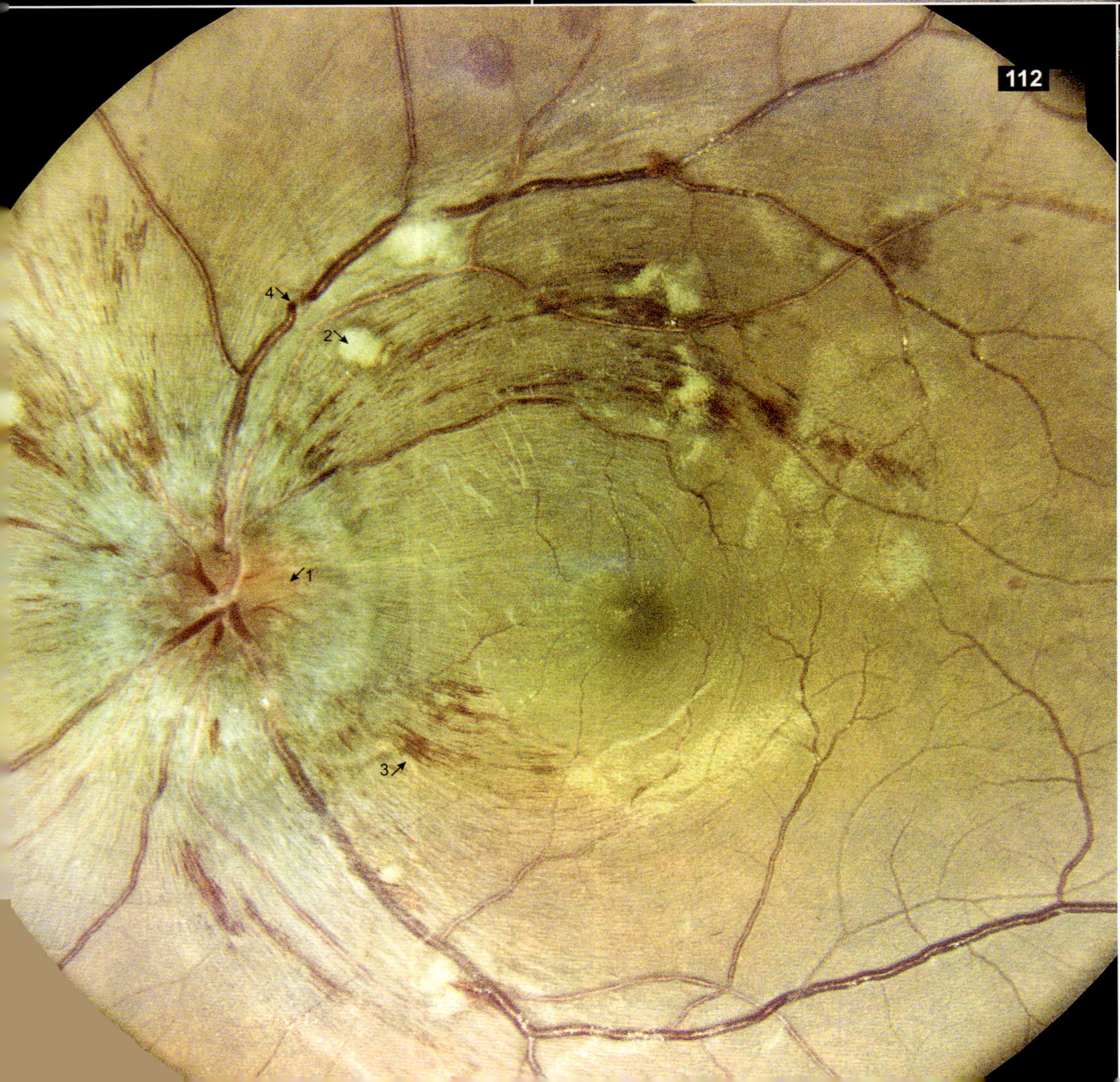


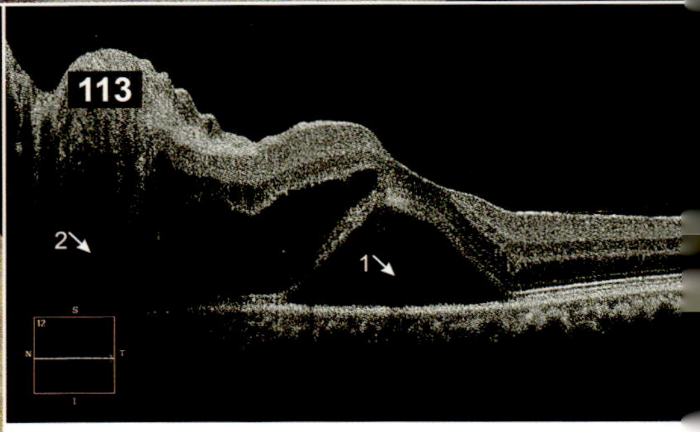


Figure 112

*Color fundus image of left eye of same patient with malignant hypertensio demonstrates bilateral symmetrical clinica findings—optic disk has sign grade papilloedema with blurred margin (1) dis hyperemia elevated along with cotton woo spots (2) splinter hemorrhages (3). Als note venous tortuosity with nicking (4).*

Figure 113

*SD-OCT scan of left eye of the same patien with malignant hypertension. Peripapillar intraretinal edema (1) and serous fluid a fovea (2) can be seen.* □

# CHAPTER 4

## MACULA

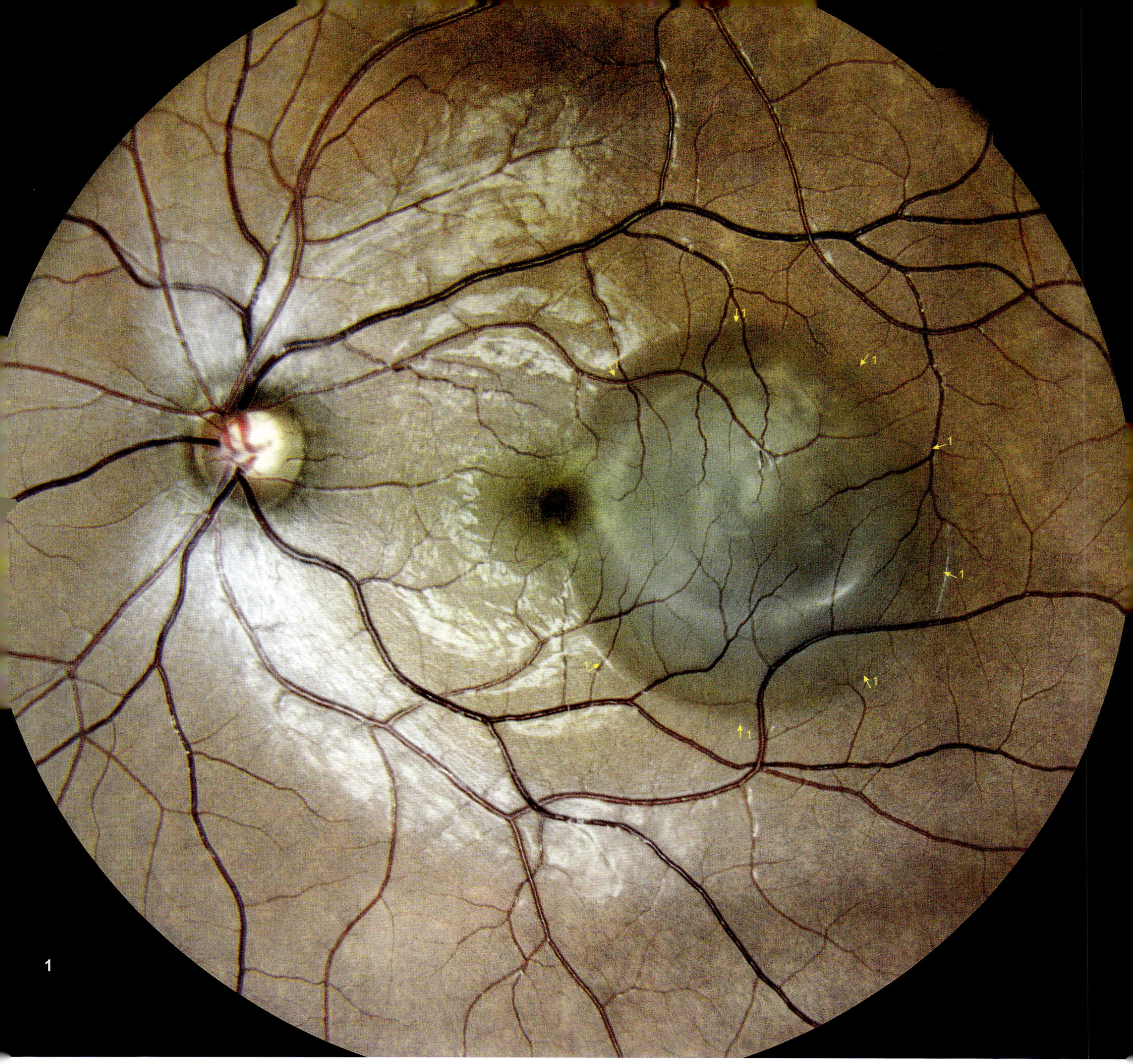


Figure 1 *The color fundus photograph shows a well-defined round elevated grayish lesion in the temporal macula suggestive of localized neurosensory detachment (1) in patient with central serous chorioretinopathy. In the central part of neurosensory detachment, there is a ring-like yellowish subretinal nodular deposits consistent with fibrin deposition (1).*

Central serous chorioretinopathy (CSCR) is an idiopathic condition associated with stress and intake of steroids that usually affects young adult males. It causes visual impairment due to leakage of fluid in the macula. The acute form usually resolves within 3 months sometimes leaving color vision and contrast discrimination difficulties in a few patients.

In many patients it is a recurrent problem where the fluid builds up in the macula but resolves spontaneously. If the conditions persist beyond 3 months it is then called chronic CSR. The shallow subretinal fluid persists in the retina causes permanent RPE damage leading to irreversible visual loss. OCT scan helps in diagnosing CSR as it identifies subretinal fluid in the fovea. FFA helps to confirm the diagnosis by identifying the characteristic leakage pattern. The treatment options available for non-resolving CSCRs are usually focal laser to the extrafoveal leakage points. Oral mineralocorticoids for example eplerenone has been used successfully.

Chronic CSR are difficult to treat, photodynamic therapy, micropulse laser treatment and anti-VEGF injections have been used with varying results. □

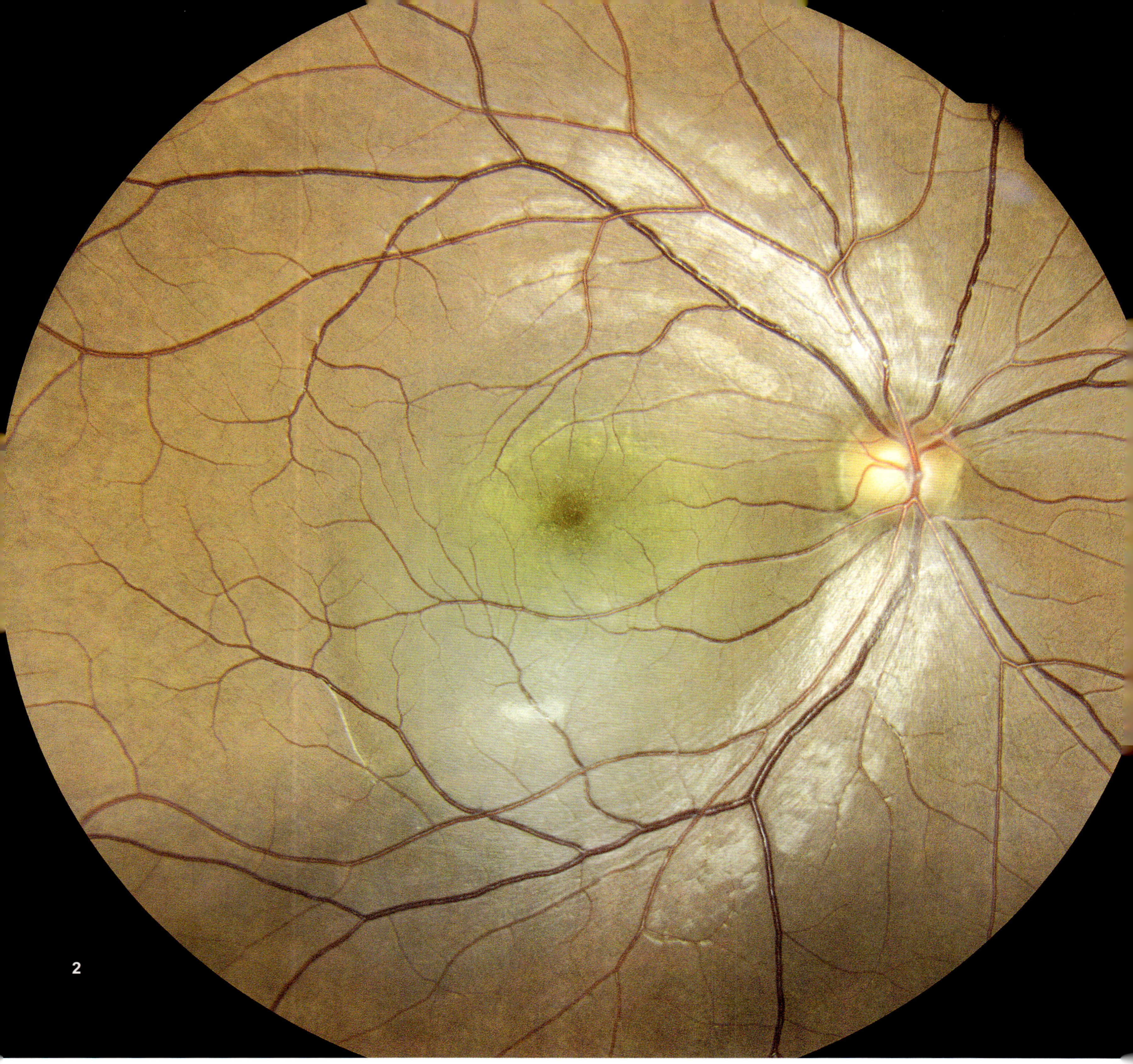


Figure 2 *Case of central serous chorioretinopathy: Color fundus photograph shows neurosensory detachment suggestive of CSR.*

A 35-year-old young male presented to the clinic with complaints of blurred vision in his right eye persisting for the last few days. Visual acuity at presentation was recorded to be 6/12. Patient underwent fluorescein angiogram and OCT scans to confirm the diagnosis of CSR, identify site of leak and to rule out the presence of choroidal neovascular membrane. Since the duration of symptoms was less than a month, he was advised observation alone as 90% cases of acute CSR are known to resolve spontaneously. He was advised to avoid stress and not to use of steroids in any form.

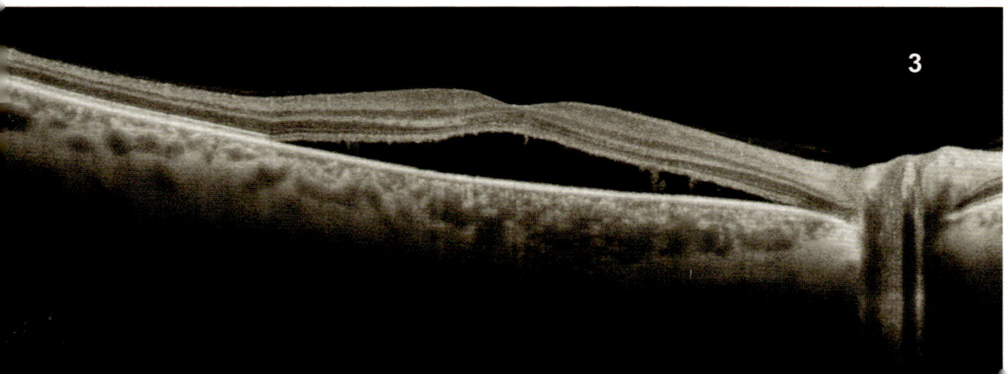


Figure 3 *Swept source optical coherence tomography photograph demonstrating sensory detachment of macula.*

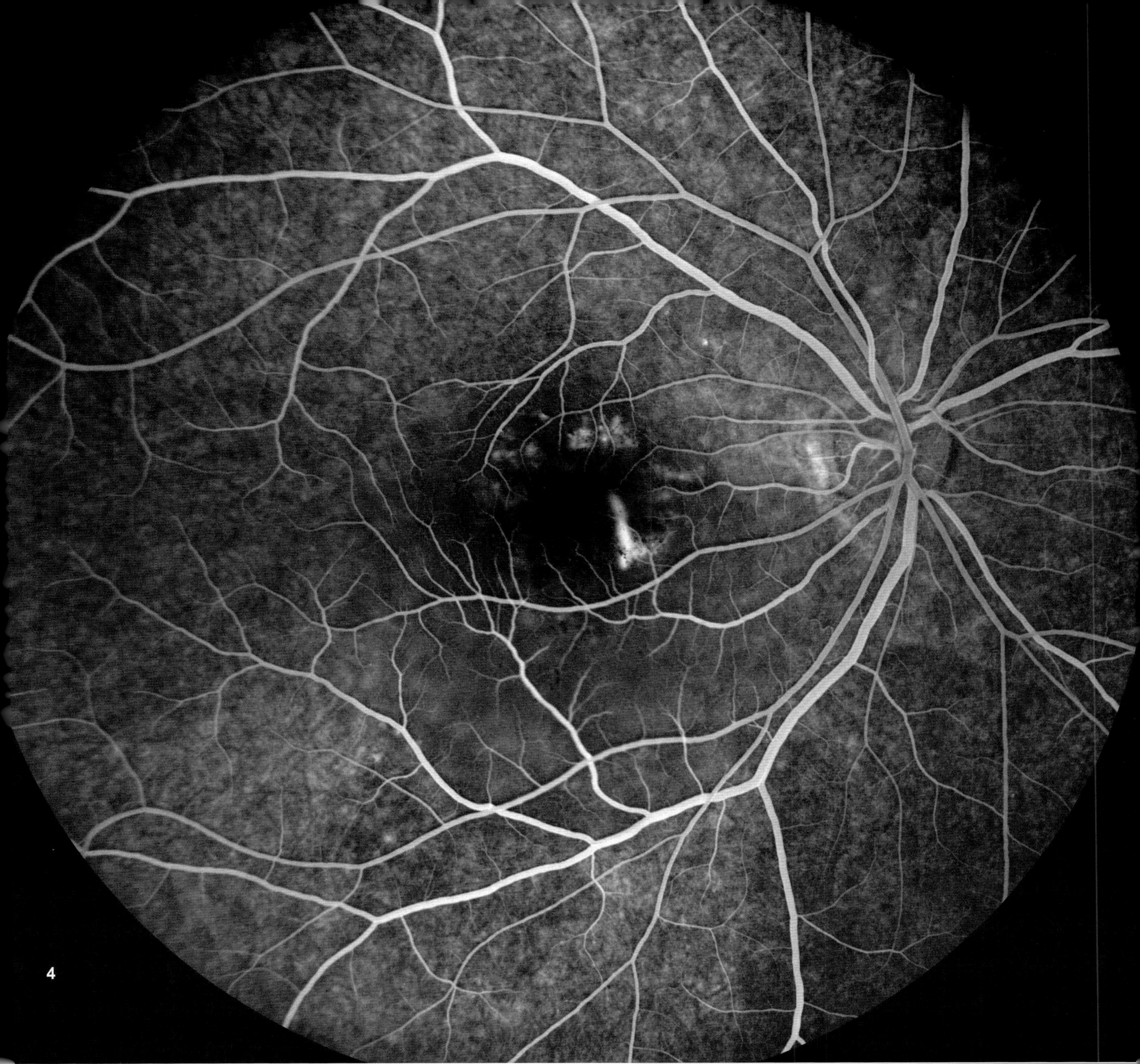


Figure 4 *FFA identified a hyperfluorescent RPE point leakage in the early phase that rises in a smokestack pattern.*

Fluorescein angiogram in a patient of CSR helps to confirm the diagnosis. As the site of leakage is juxtafoveal, focal laser is contraindicated. Such patients may need micropulse laser therapy or half fluence photodynamic therapy if the disease has not shown spontaneous resolution after 3 months.

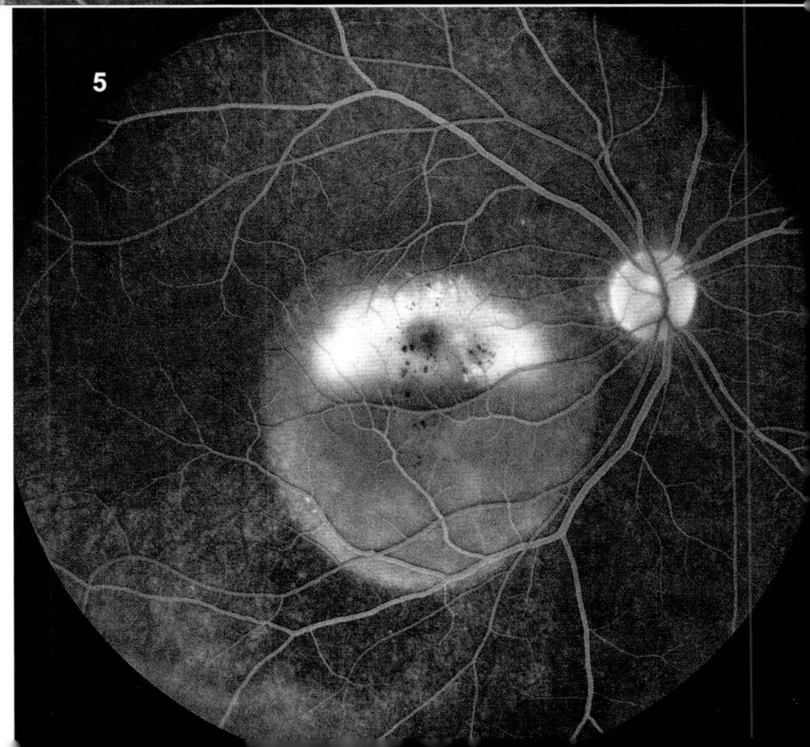


Figure 5 *Late fluorescein angiogram shows pooling of dye in the area of sensory detachment as angiogram progresses.* □

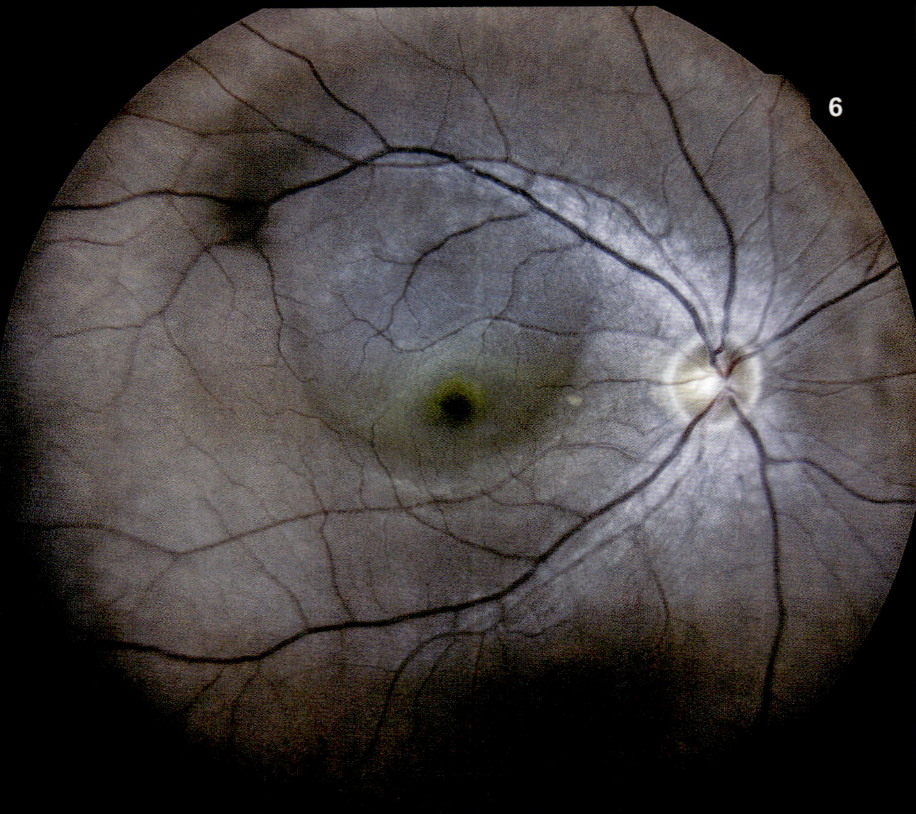

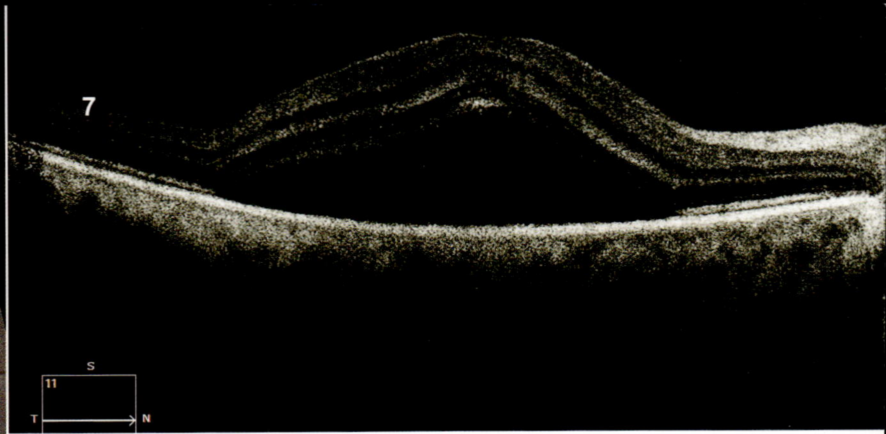


Figure 6 *Central serous chorioretinopathy: Color fundus photograph shows an area of neurosensory detachment in the superior macula, also involving the center of fovea.*

Figure 7 *OCT of the right macula shows subretinal fluid including the subfoveal area at presentation.*

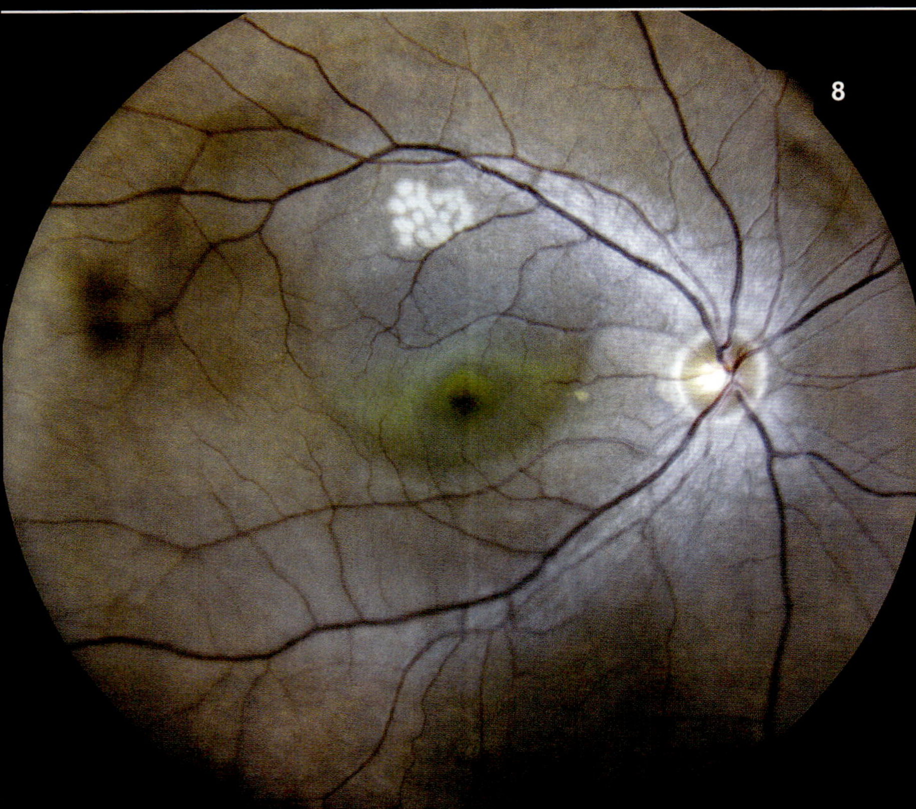

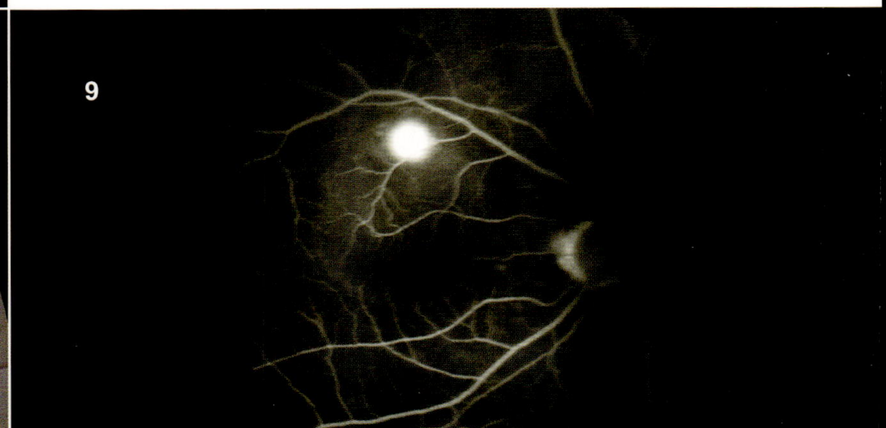

Figure 8 *Color fundus photograph immediately after laser photocoagulation. As the point of RPE leakage was extrafoveal so the patient underwent a yellow focal laser (low intensity long duration burns) to the point of leak.*

Figure 9 *The fluorescein angiogram shows ink blot pattern of leakage in the extrafoveal region.*

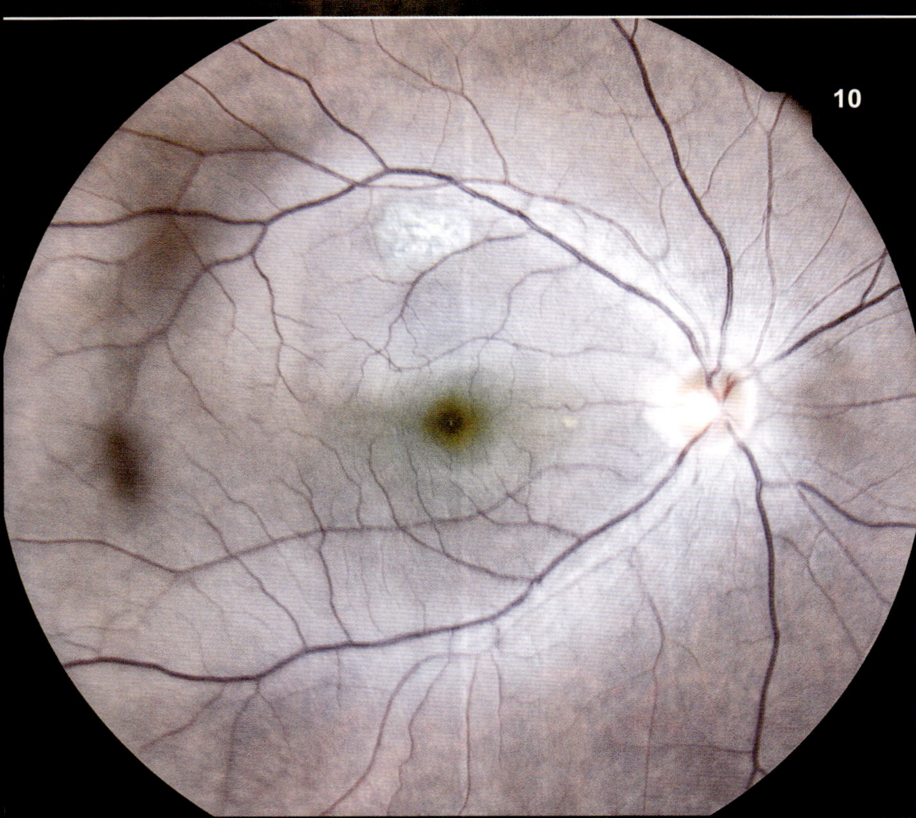

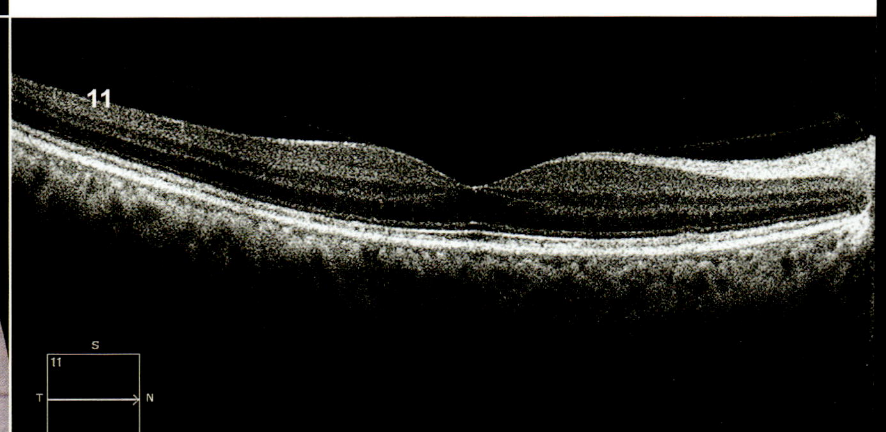


Figure 10 *Color fundus photograph 6 weeks postlaser treatment demonstrating laser scars at the superior macula.*

Figure 11 *OCT scan done at 6 weeks postlaser treatment demonstrates normal foveal profile.* □

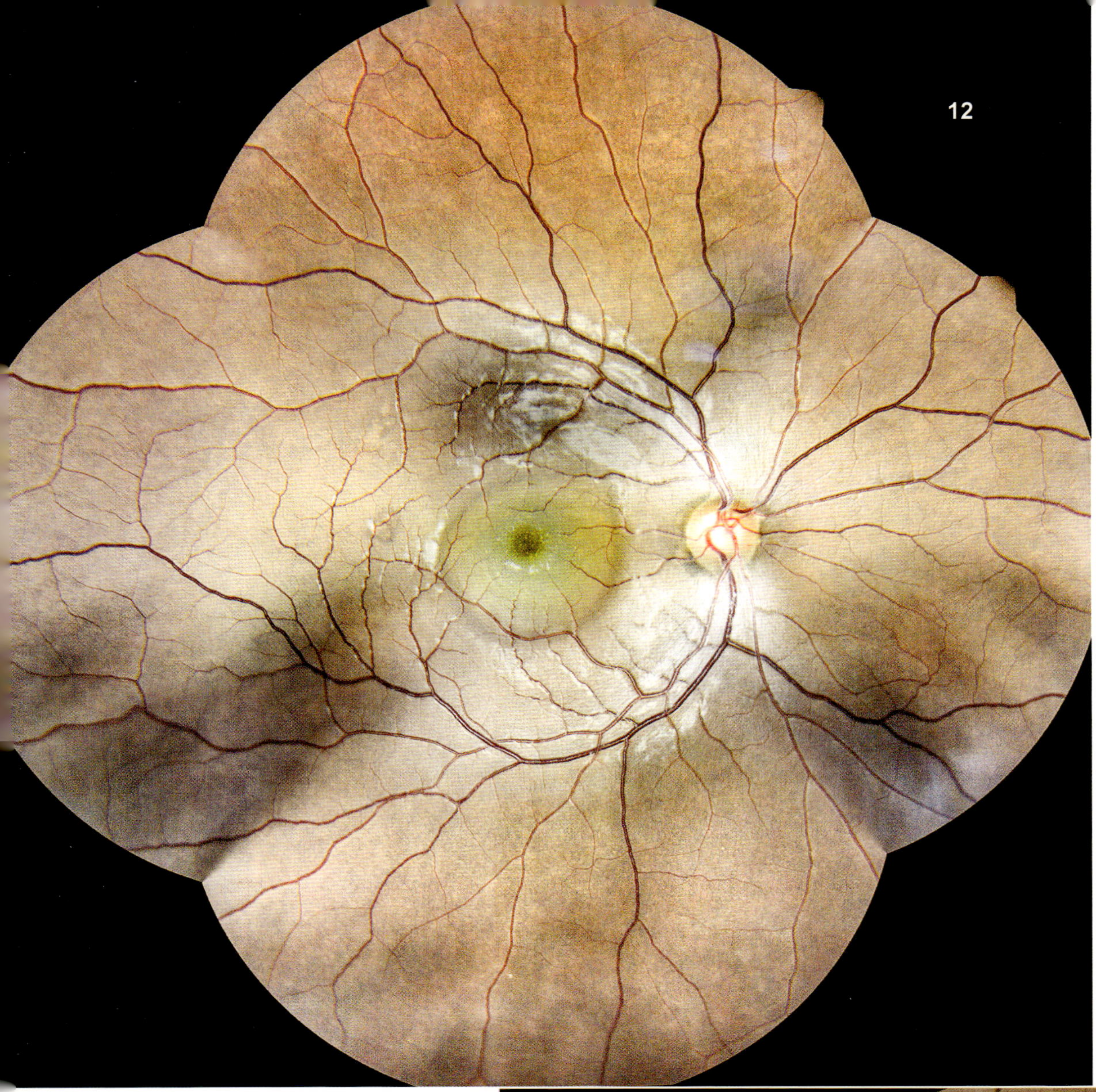


Figure 12

*Case of central serous chorioretinopathy with typical neurosensory detachment at the fovea.*

Young Indian male presented with sudden onset blurred vision in his right eye. Visual acuity at presentation was 6/12 and clinical diagnosis of central serous chorioretinopathy (CSCR) was made. Left eye was asymptomatic with visual acuity of 6/6.

Figure 13

*Extramacular variant of central serous chorioretinopathy: Left fundus photograph of the same patient: macula was normal but nasal midperiphery (1) shows round area of neurosensory detachment.*

Even though the hallmark of CSCR is the presence of serous detachment of neurosensory retina in the posterior pole, but at times episodes may be limited to extramacular region that usually go undetected as they are asymptomatic. Note the large bullous serous detachment in the upper nasal quadrant with discrete edges. □

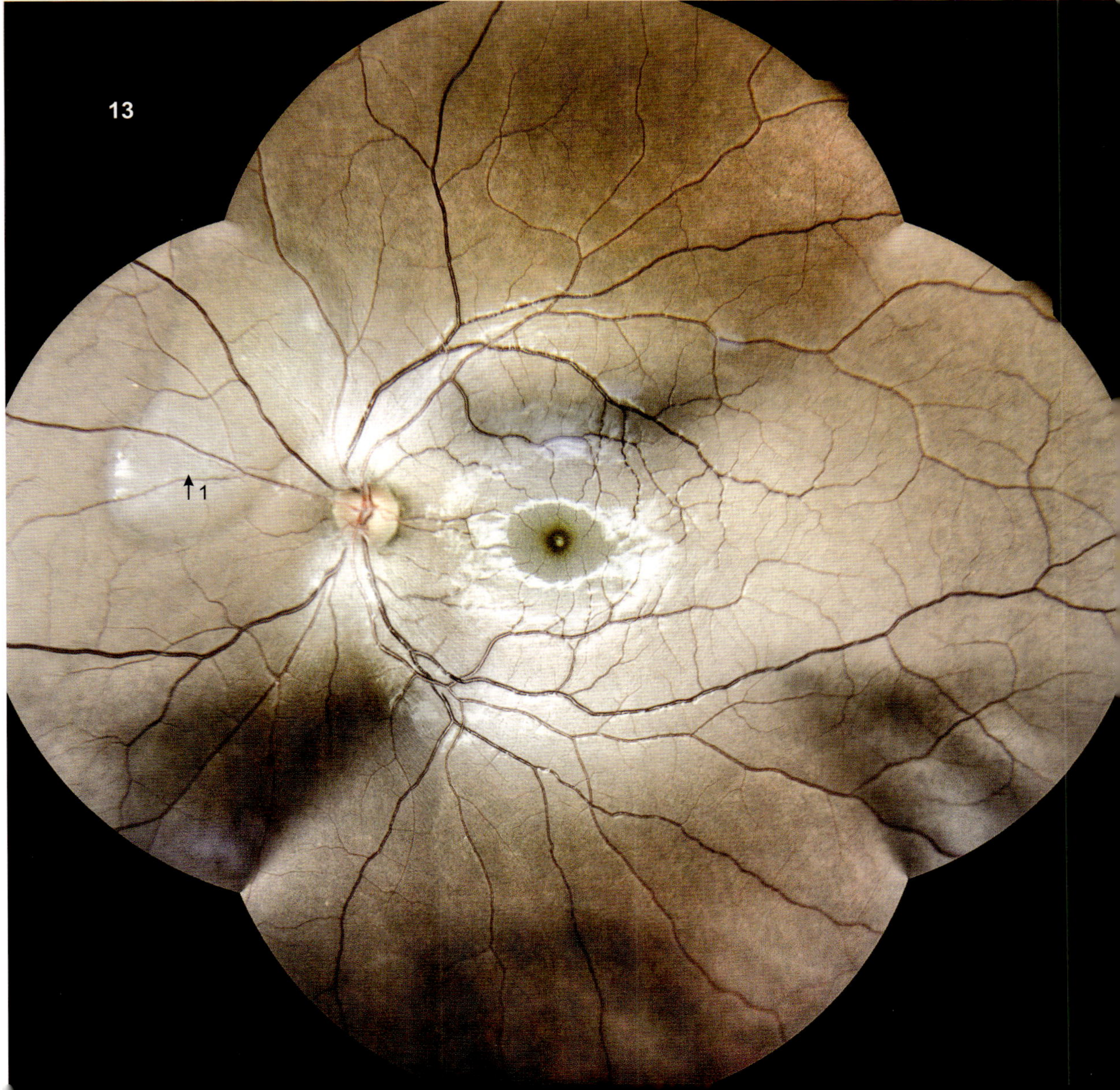

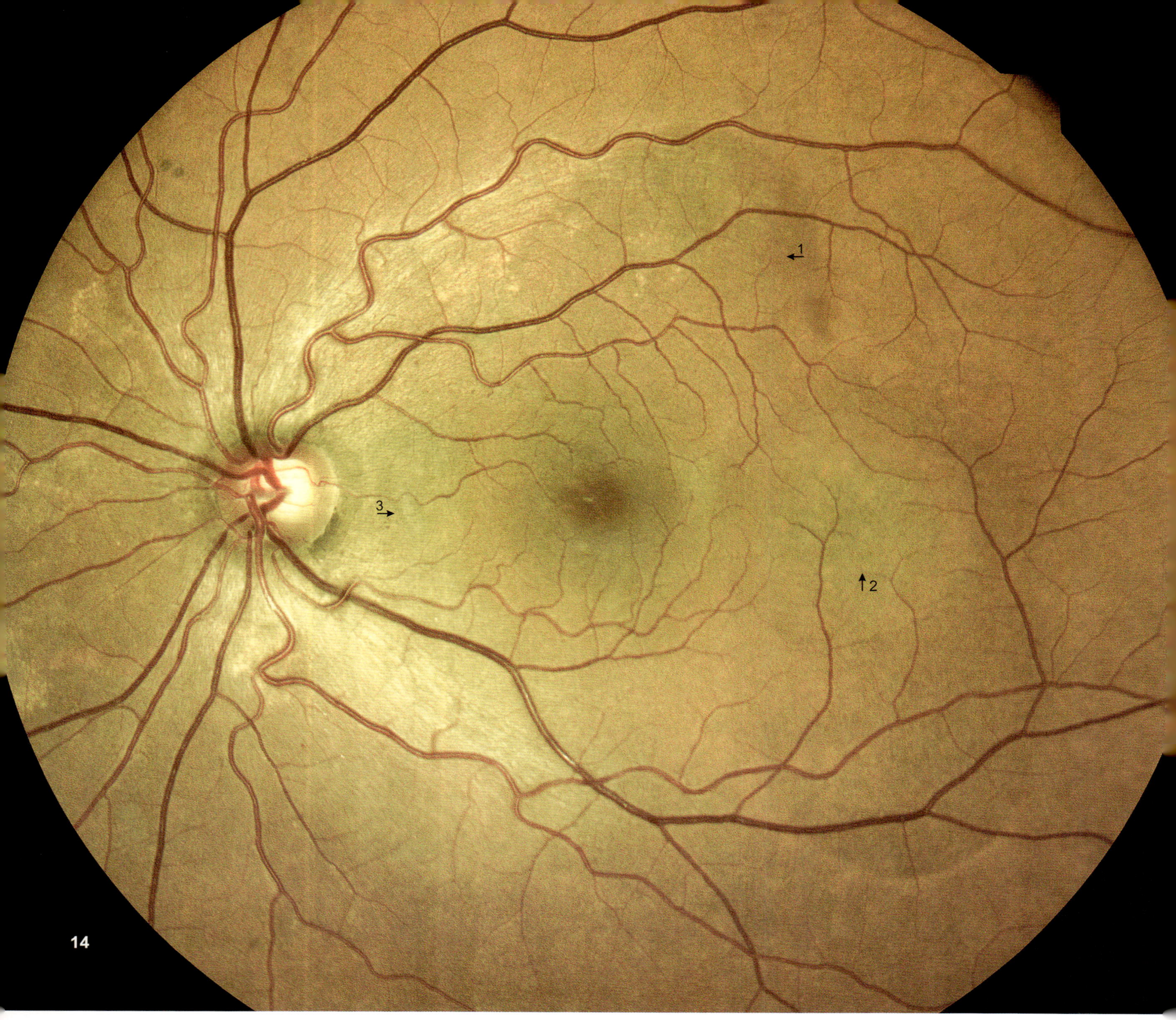


Figure 14 *Color fundus photograph of a case of multifocal central serous chorioretinopathy. Three scattered patches of retinal elevation were seen at the posterior pole (1, 2, 3).*

Multifocal CSR is a rare variant characterized by accumulation of subretinal fluid at the posterior pole of the fundus causing multiple areas of serous retinal detachment. inflammatory disorder VKH is a common differential. Clinical history (absence of headaches/pain/tinnitus), absence of inflammatory cells on slit-lamp examination and fluorescein angiogram help to differentiate a CSR from VKH.

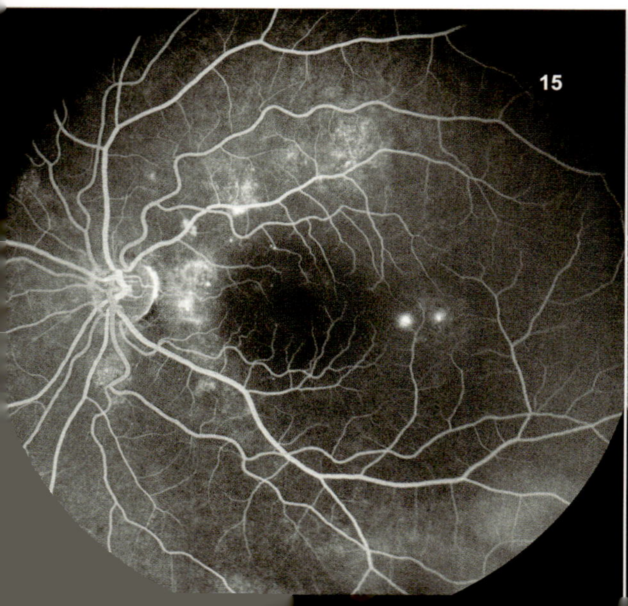


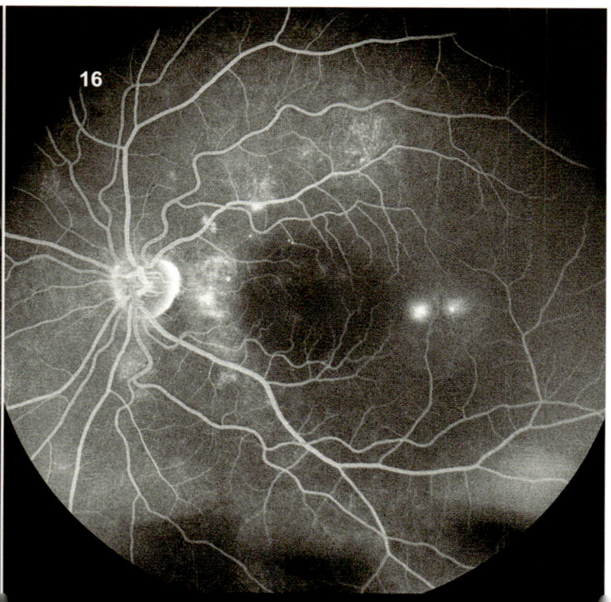


Figure 15 *FFA was suggestive of multiple RPE pinpoint leaks all along the posterior pole. Note the optic disk is normal.*

Figure 16 *Late phase of angiogram demonstrating increasing fluorescence from these RPE leaks in an ink blot pattern.*

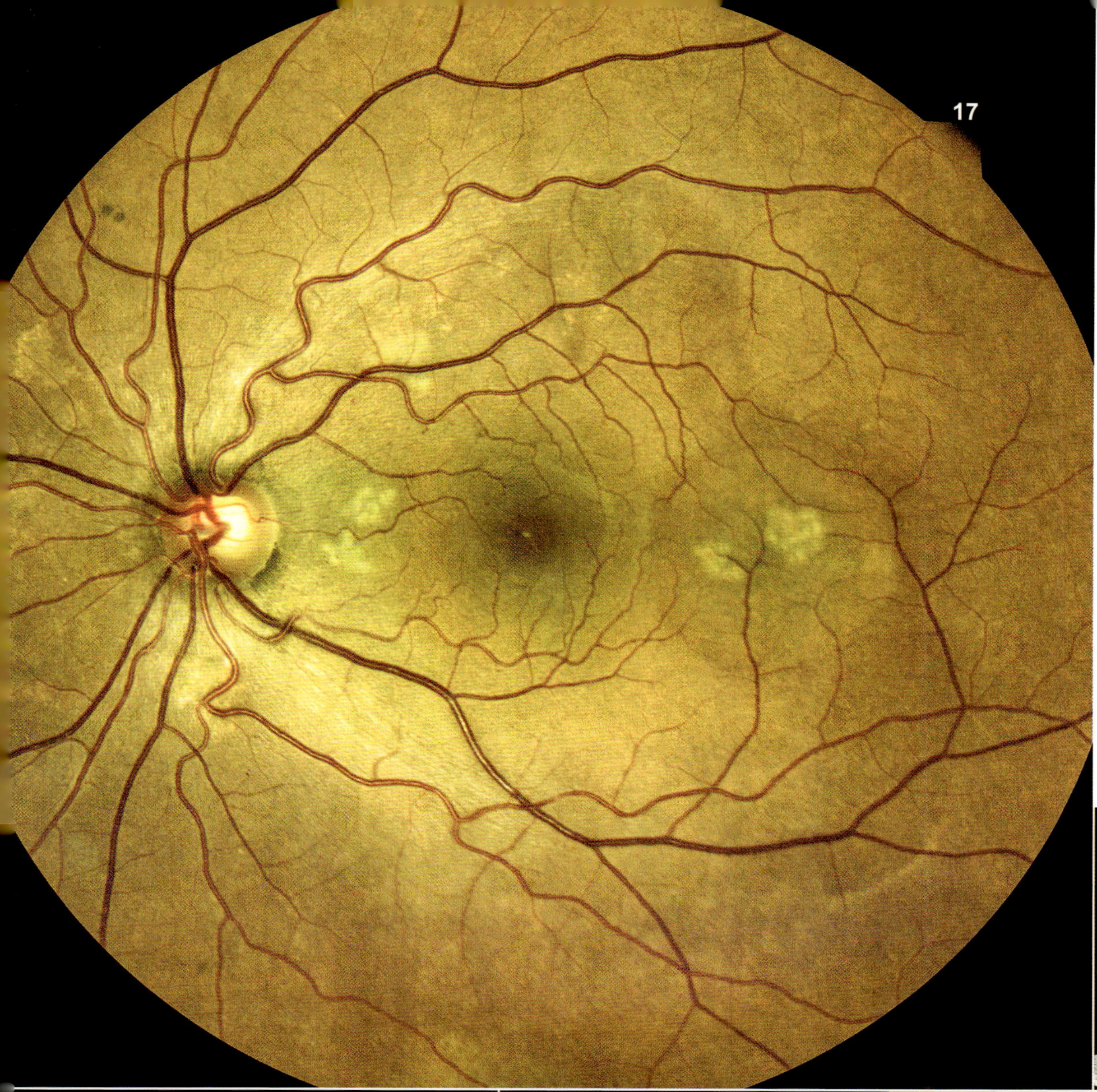


Figure 17

*Color fundus photograph immediately after focal laser photocoagulation.*

Figure 18

*Baseline OCT scan shows presence of subretinal fluid at the nasal and temporal edge of the macula.*

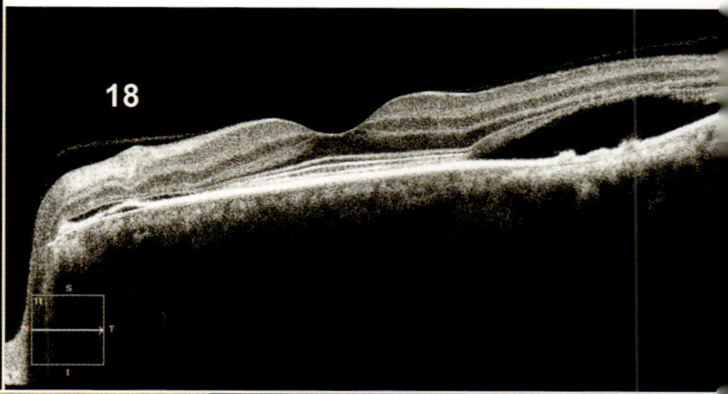


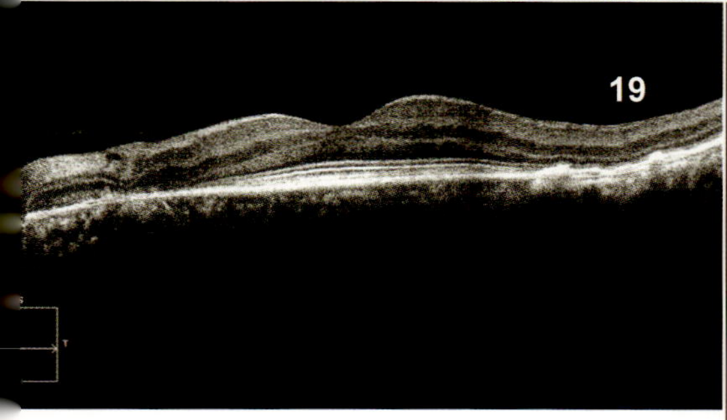


Figure 19

*OCT scans postlaser treatment show resolution of subretinal fluid with areas of RPE atrophy at the temporal edge.*

Figure 20

*Color fundus photograph 3 months post-treatment demonstrating disappearance of sensory detachments with flattening of the posterior pole. Small patch of RPE atrophy is seen at the temporal macula (1).* □

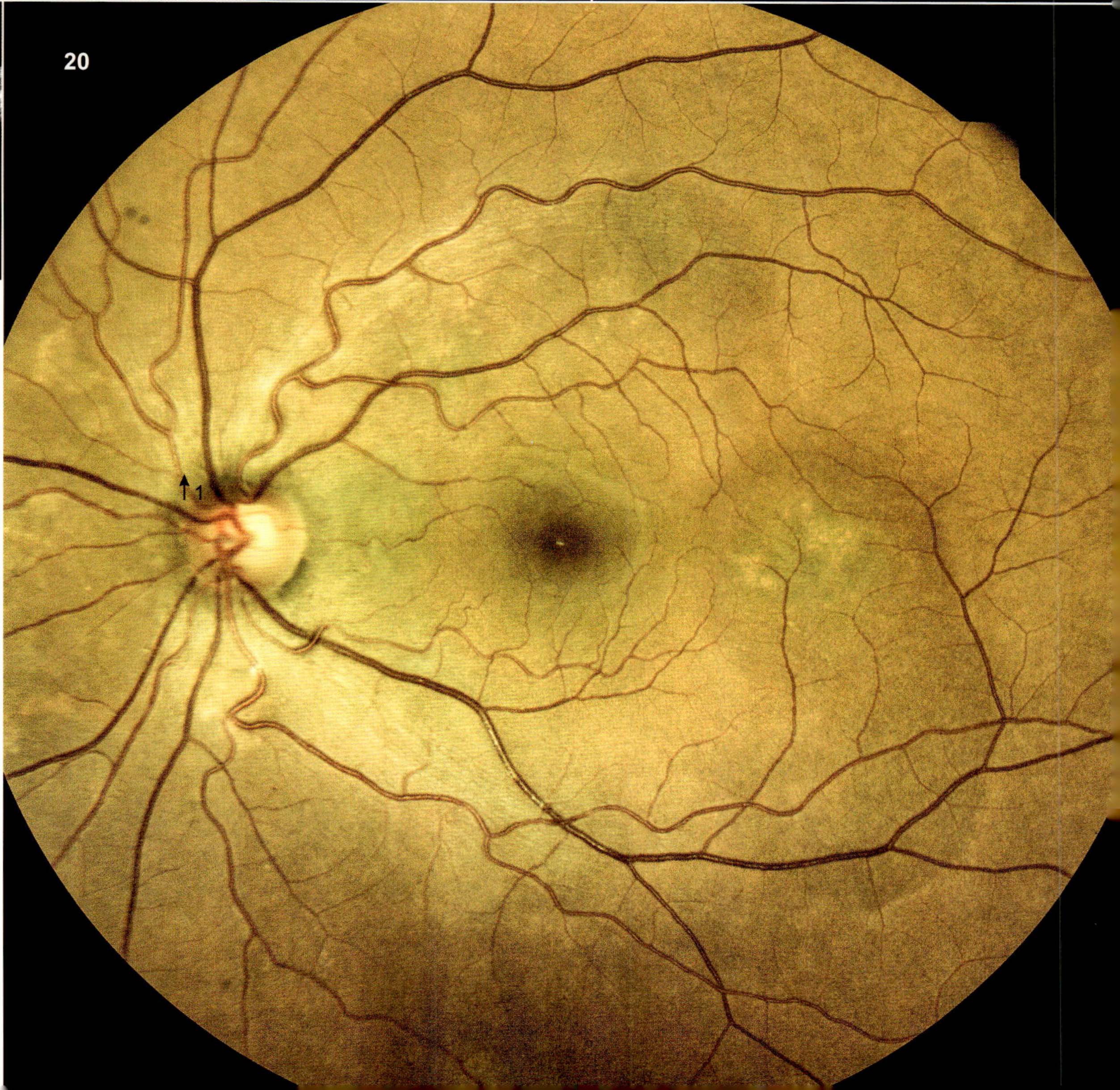

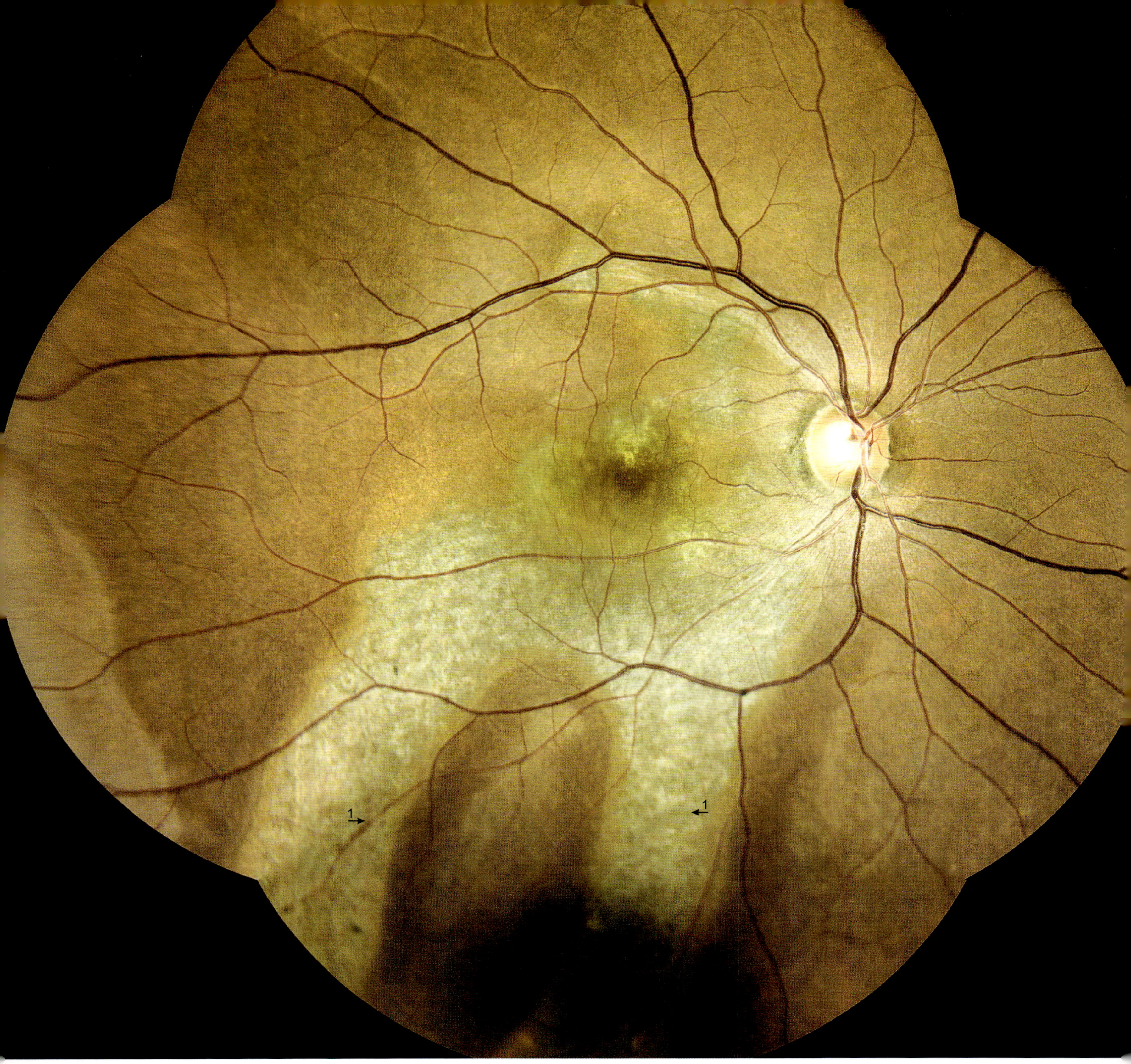


Figure 21 *Case of chronic central serous chorioretinopathy demonstrating inferior retinal tracts (diffuse retinal pigment epitheliopathy).*

Colored fundus photograph of a 52-year-old male with a chronic CSCR reveals diffuse RPE changes in the macula. Note the atrophic RPE tract expanding inferiorly (1).

Chronic CSR has distinct morphological features as compared to acute persistent CSR of more than 3 months duration. Chronic CSCR is characterized by widespread RPE changes, pigment clumping and RPE atrophy with chronic shallow subretinal fluid best seen on OCT. These RPE changes are referred to as diffuse retinal pigment epitheliopathy. Some chronic CSR patients develop gravitational descending tracts in inferior retina with RPE changes due to long standing accumulation of subretinal fluid. There is also an increase in risk of CNVM in cases of chronic CSR.

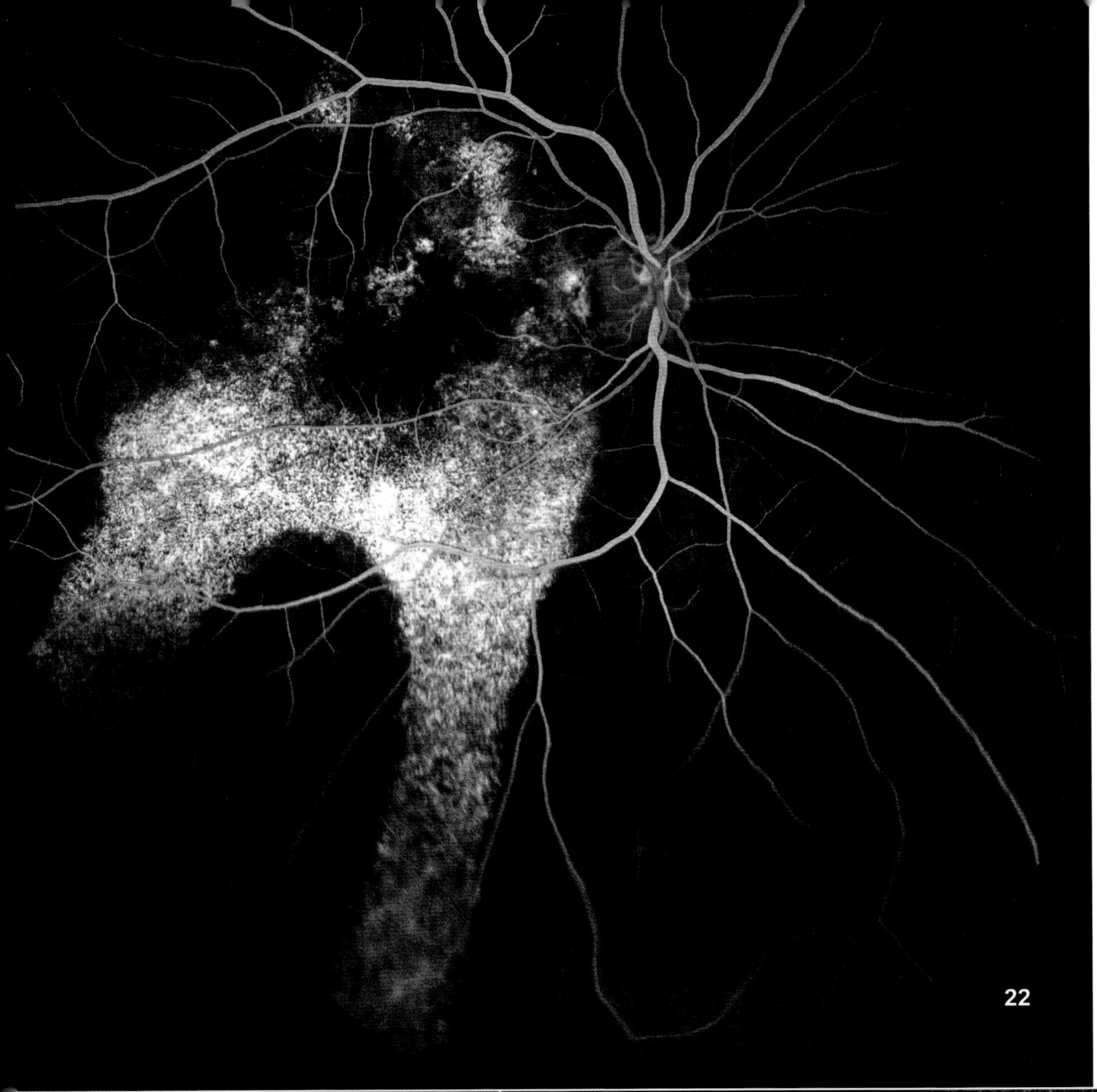

Figure 22

*FFA shows multiple pinpoint leaks at the level of RPE suggestive of chronic CSCR along with an inferior tract of hyperfluorescent RPE staining.*

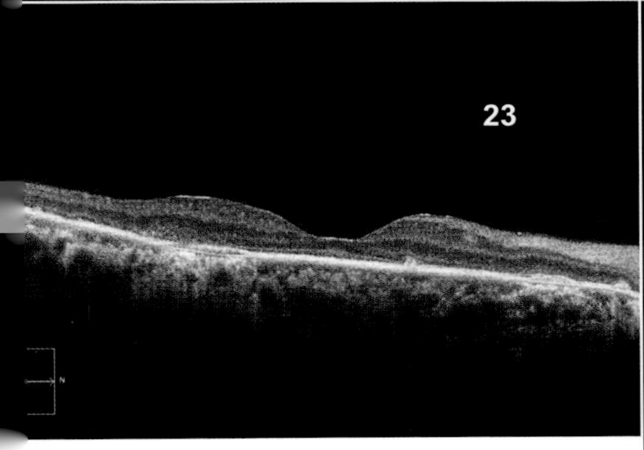

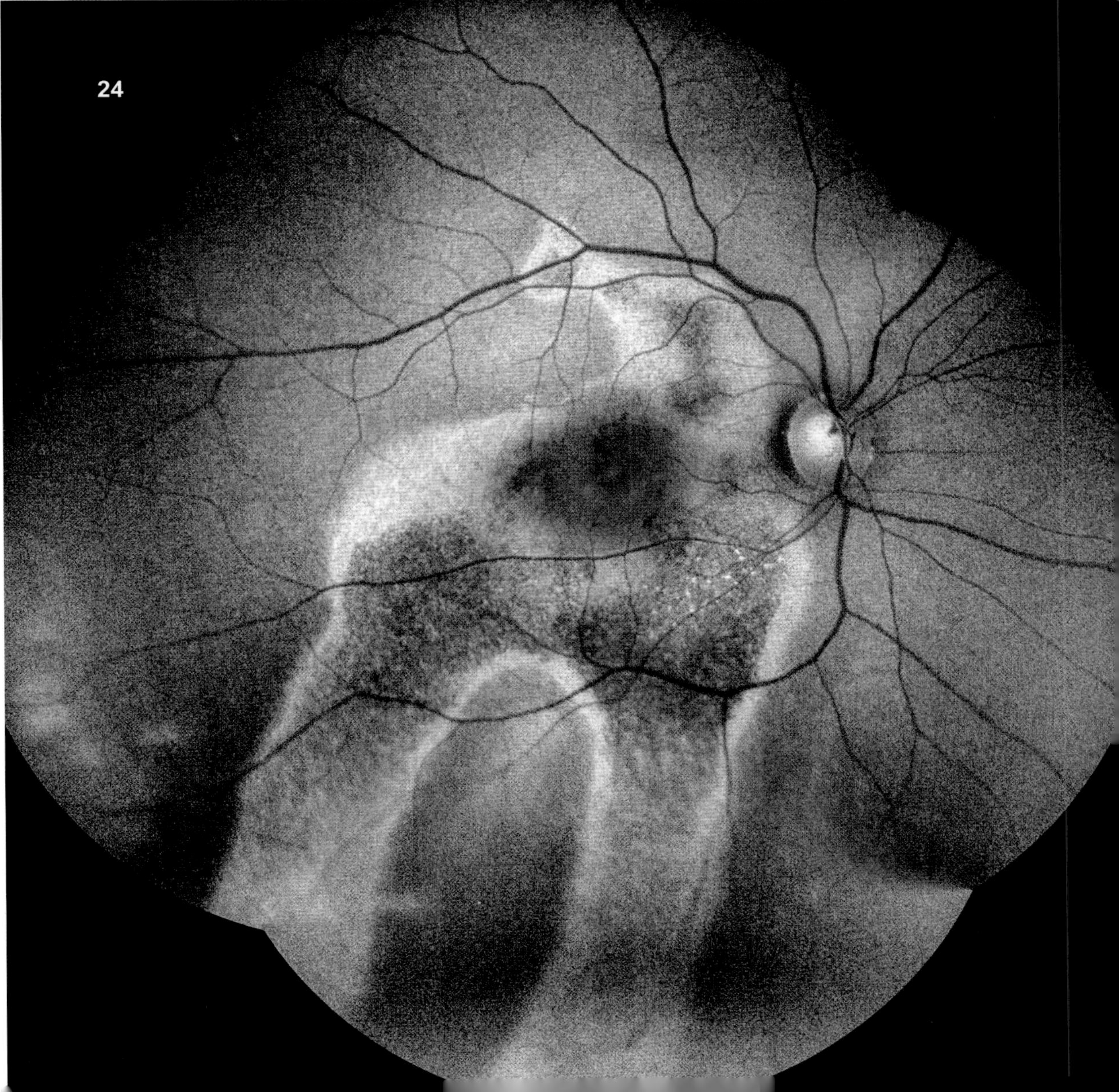

Figure 23

*On OCT there is an outer retinal damage as evident by the loss of photoreceptor layers and irregular RPE layer. There is no subretinal fluid seen.*

Figure 24

*Fundus autofluorescence of a descending tract in CSCR: Marked hypoautofluorescence suggests chronic disease and irreversible RPE damage surrounded by a hyperautofluorescent ring.* □

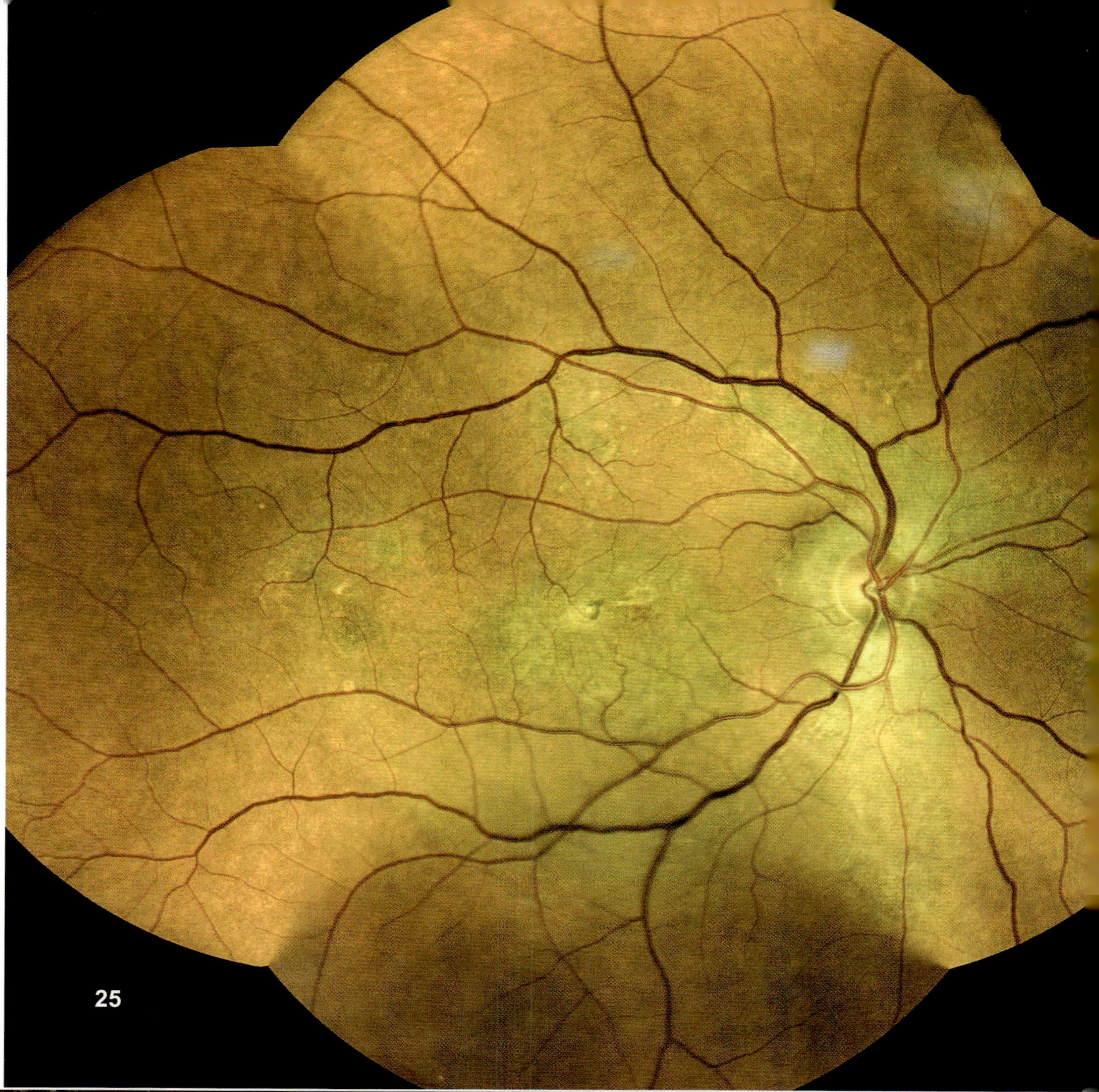

Figure 25

*Case of chronic central serous chorio-retinopathy.*

Color fundus photograph shows diffuse retinal pigment epithelium atrophic changes involving the posterior pole including the fovea and peripapillary region.

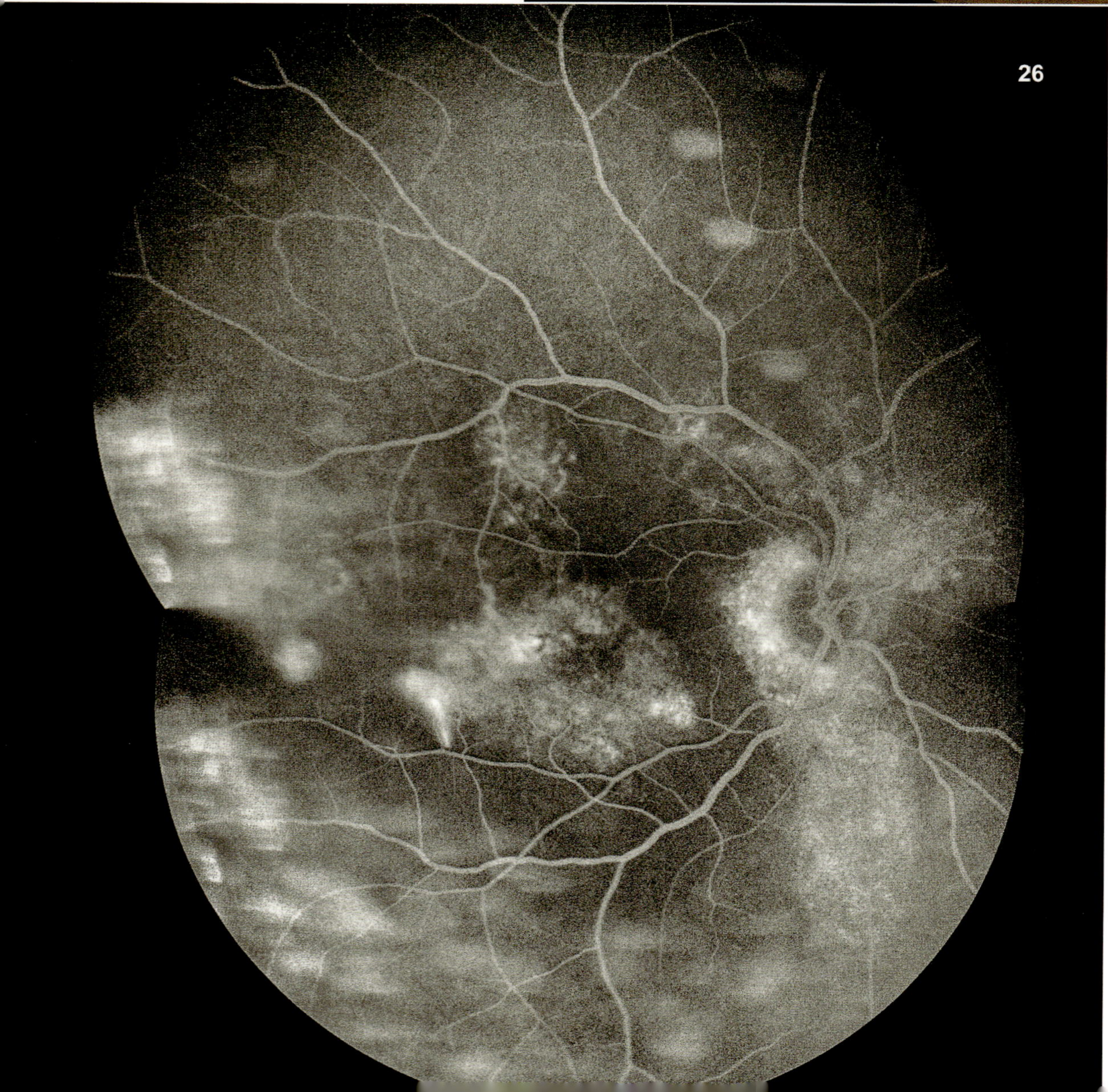

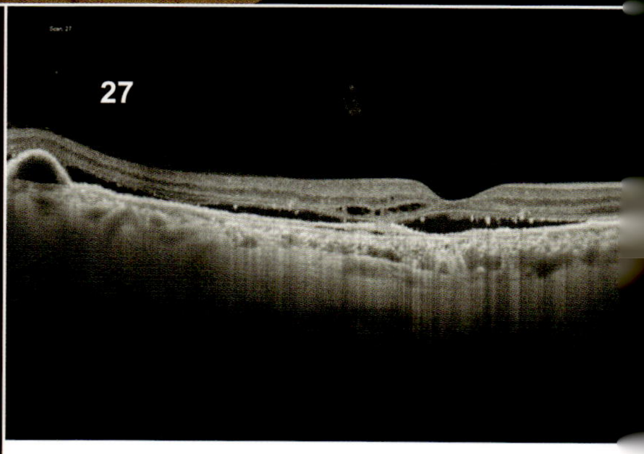

Figure 26

*Fluorescein angiogram demonstrating hyperfluorescent RPE staining. Also note multiple pinpoint RPE leaks near the fovea.*

Figure 27

*Swept source OCT scan demonstrating shallow subretinal fluid, few intraretinal cystic fluid pockets are also present due to chronicity of the disease condition.* □

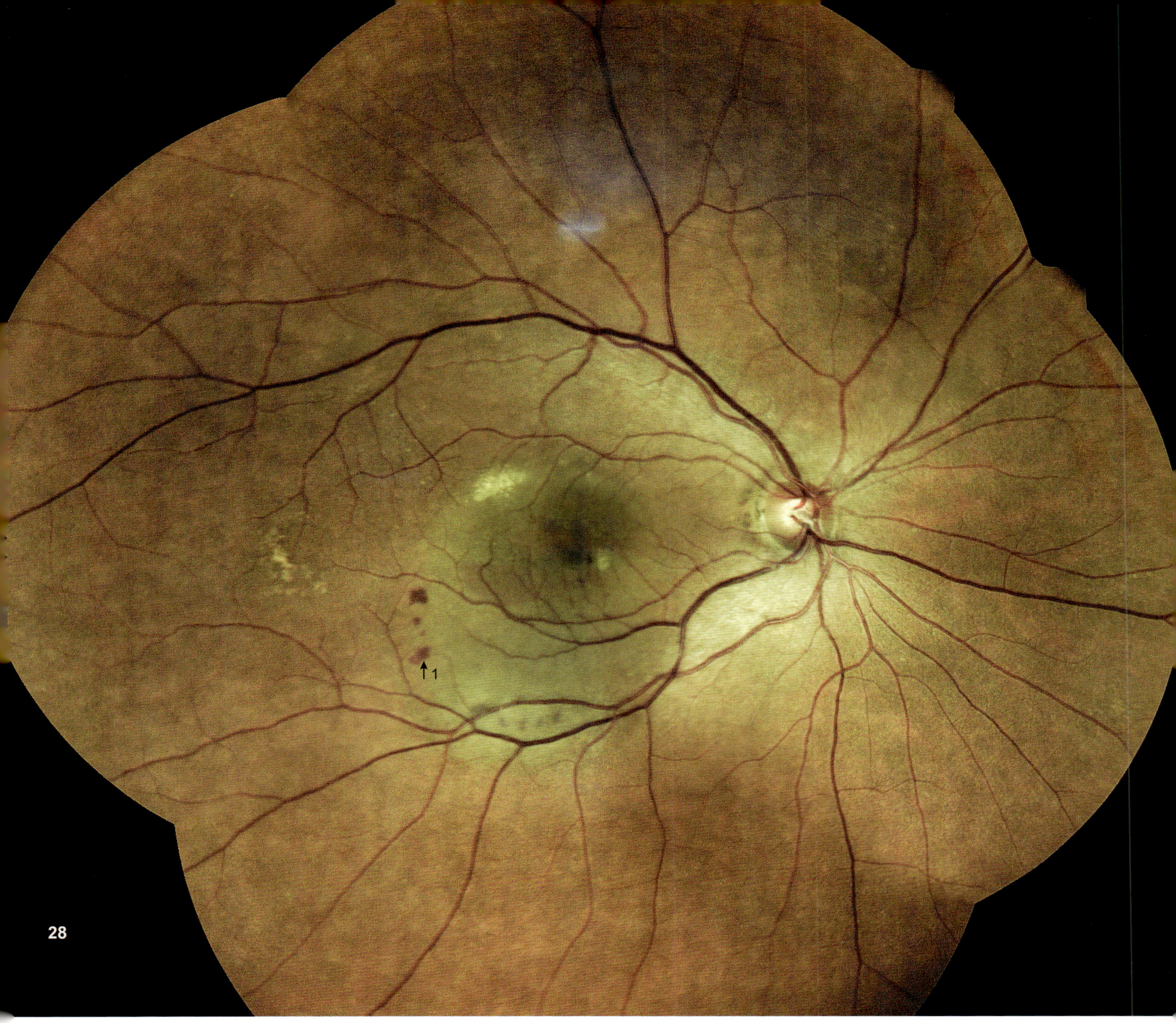


Figure 28 *Central serous chorioretinopathy associated with choroid neovascular membrane. The color fundus photograph shows an area of neurosensory detachment in the inferior macula. Note: Tiny retinal hemorrhages are seen (1), suggestive of an underlying CNVM.*

Figure 29 *FFA findings are consistent with the combined pathology of CSR and CNVM. The early FFA demonstrates a pinpoint RPE leak (1) and a vascularized PED (2) is seen inferior to the RPE leak confirming the presence of an associated CNVM.*

Figure 30 *Late phase of the angiogram shows increasing hyperfluorescence in an ink blot pattern from the RPE leak (1) and pooling of the dye in the area of vascularized PED.*

Figure 31 *Swept source OCT shows fibrovascular pigment epithelial detachment (PED) with adjacent subretinal fluid at baseline.*

Figure 32 *Swept source OCT scan at 4 weeks after intravitreal injection of Aflibercept demonstrated regression of SRF with persistent PED.* □

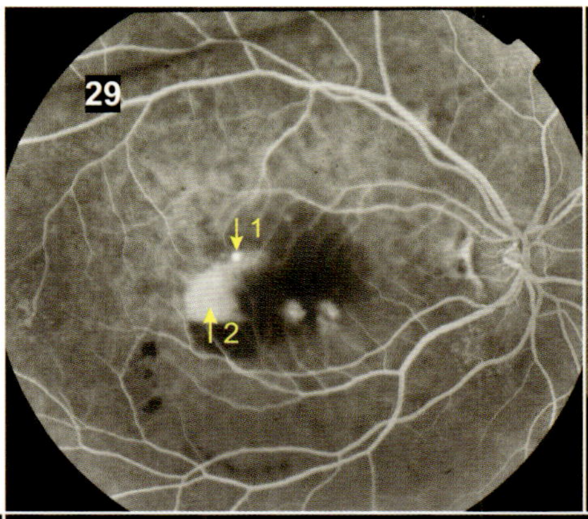


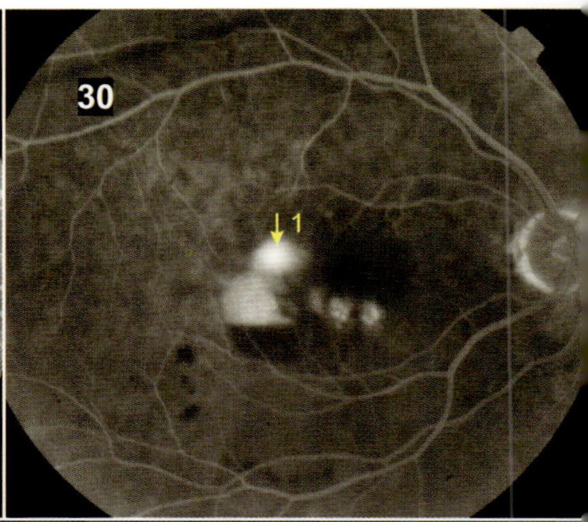


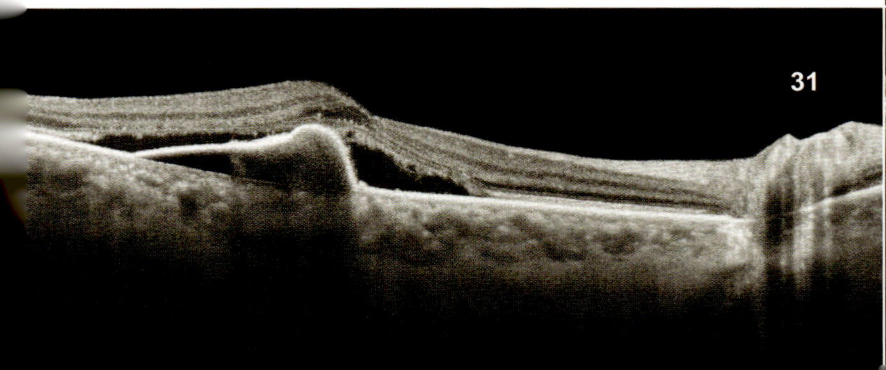


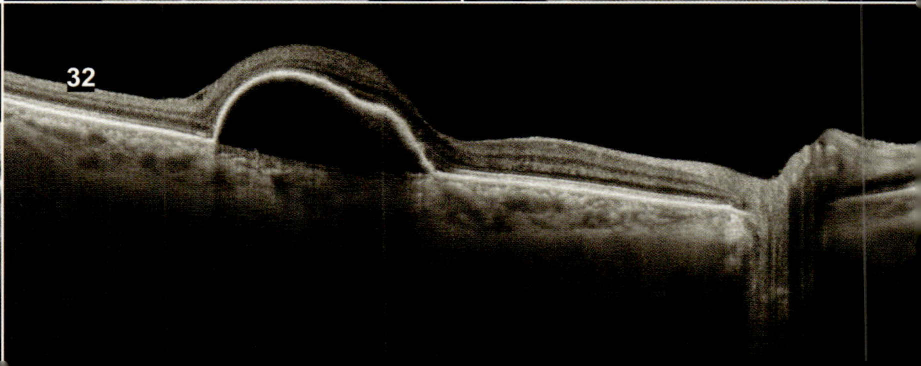

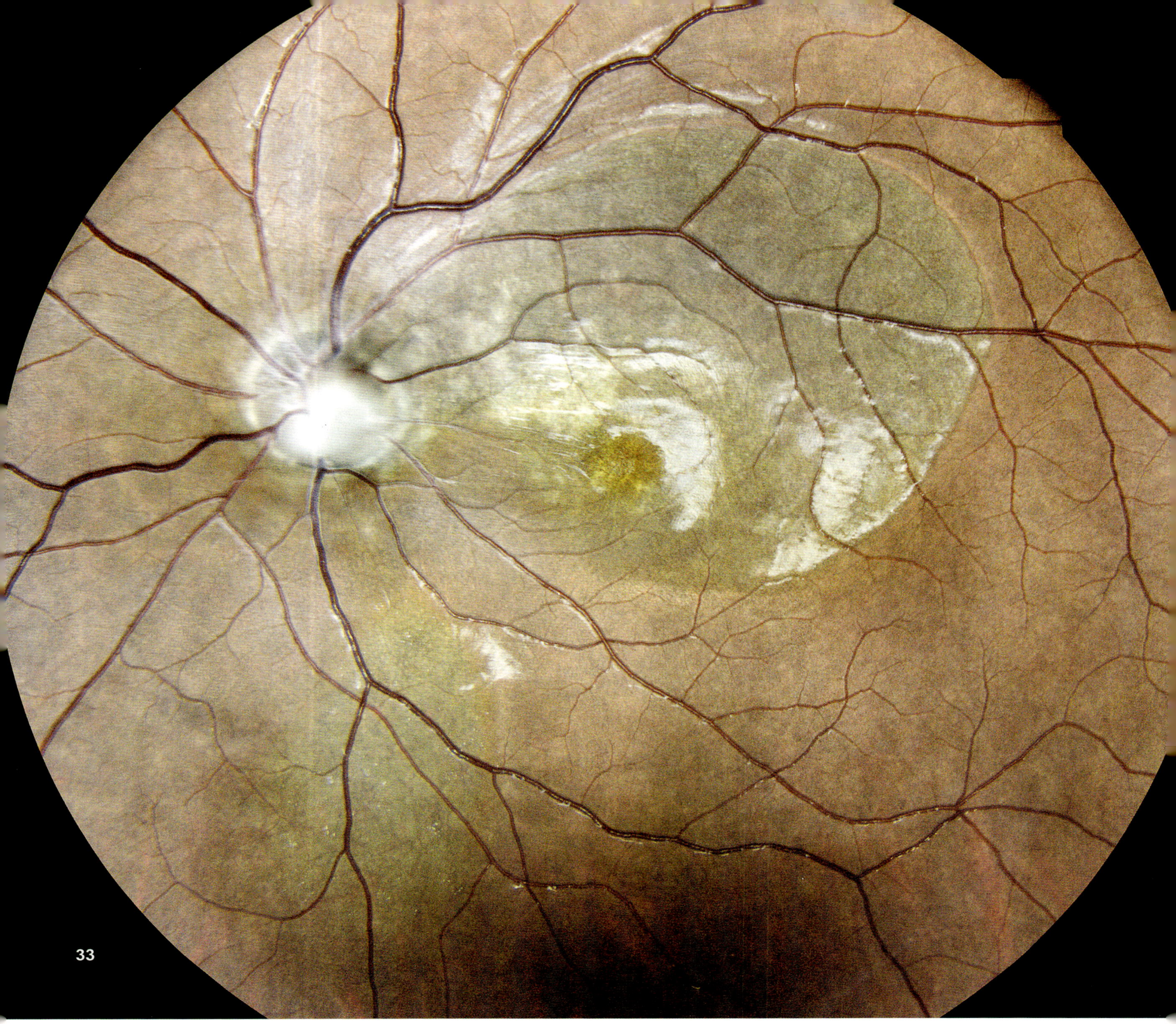


Figure 33 *Optic disk pit with maculopathy simulating central serous chorioretinopathy. Color fundus photograph shows an area of macular elevation extending up to the optic disk.*

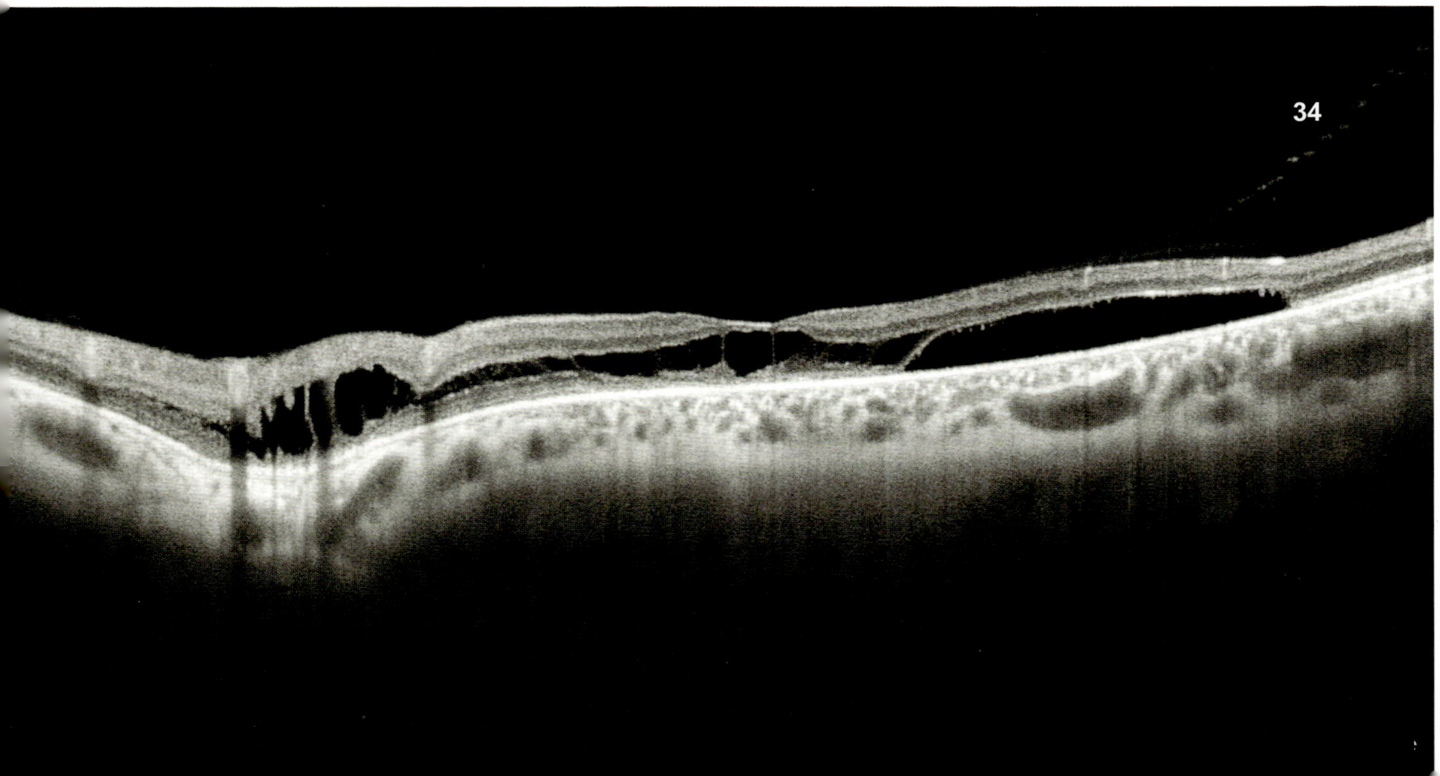


Optic disk has an abnormal congenital pit. Optic nerve pit with serous macular detachment simulates a CSCR but the OCT scan helps to differentiate the optic pit associated subretinal fluid from CSR-related SRF.

Figure 34

*Swept source optical coherence tomography scan shows schisis-like separation of the internal layers of retina extending from the disk to the fovea.*□

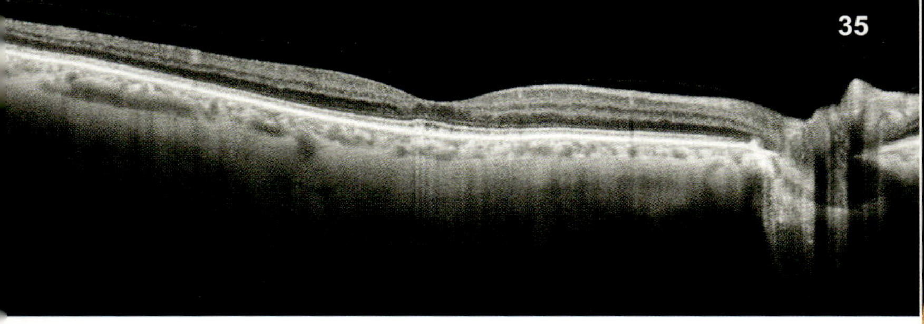



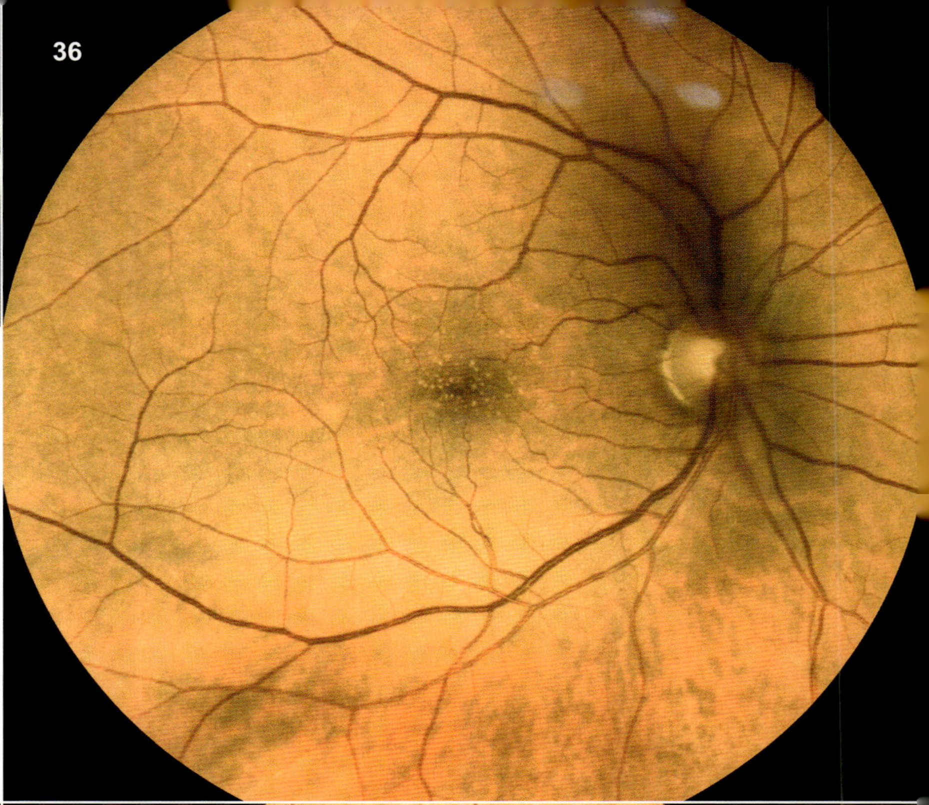



Figure 35

*Swept source OCT scan shows small RPE alterations suggestive of presence of drusen in a case of early nonexudative age-related macular degeneration.*

Figure 36

*Early stage of nonexudative ARMD: Few small scattered hard drusen were seen at the macula. An eye is considered to have the early stage of nonexudative AMD if there are few (approximately less than 20) medium sized drusen (63–124 μm) or pigment abnormalities and no other stage of AMD. No treatment is indicated at this stage.*

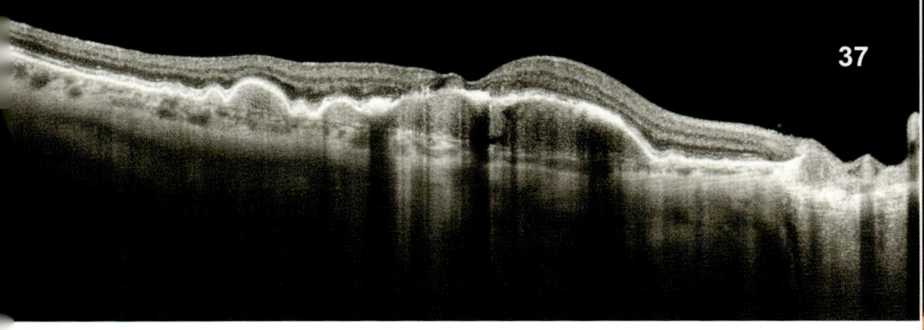



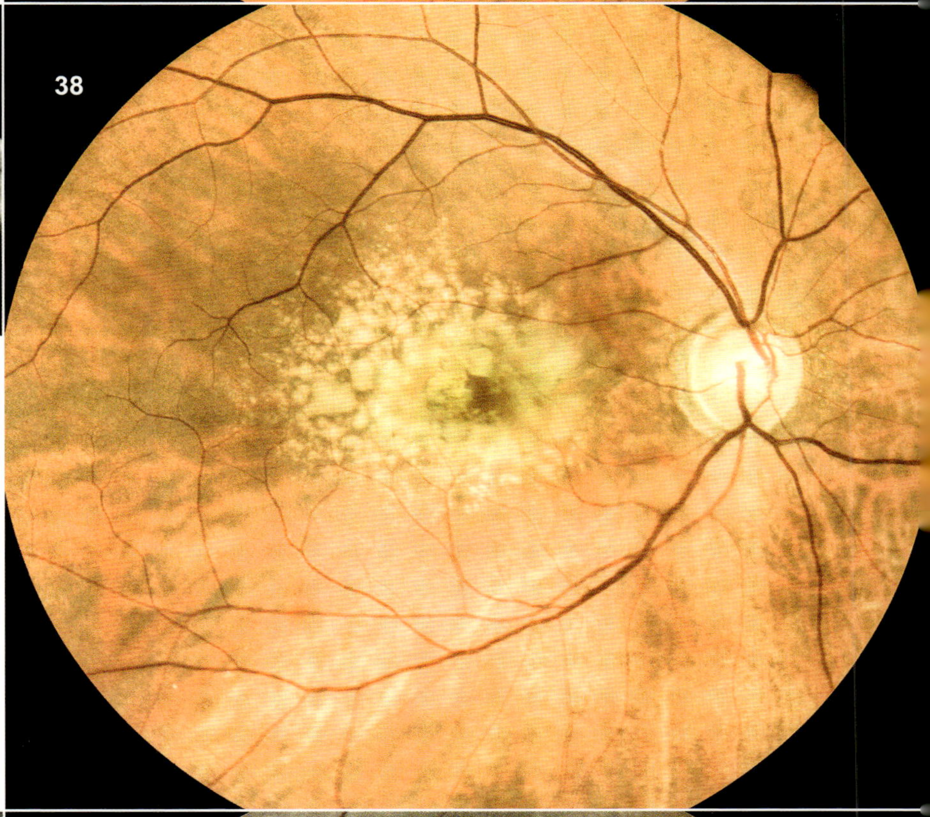



Figure 37

*Swept source OCT demonstrating multiple drusen and large area of RPE elevation at the fovea as a result of drusenoid pigment epithelial detachment.*

Figure 38

*Intermediate stage of ARMD: Note the presence of numerous soft, yellow drusen of solid appearance in the right eye of 75-year-old. If intermediate stage of ARMD is noted in at least one eye, then the individual should consider taking dietary supplement such as that used in AREDS.*

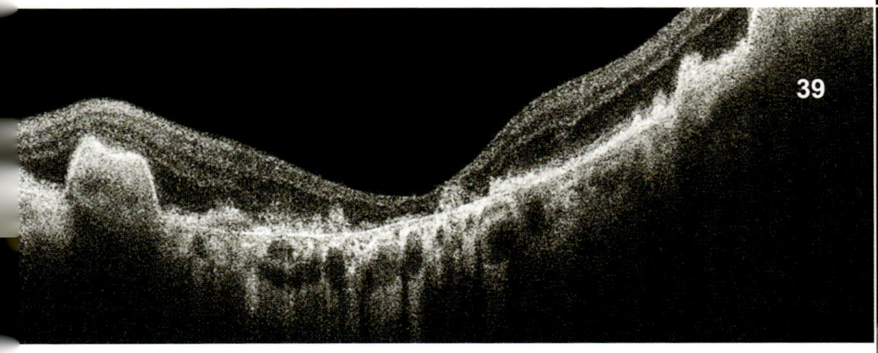



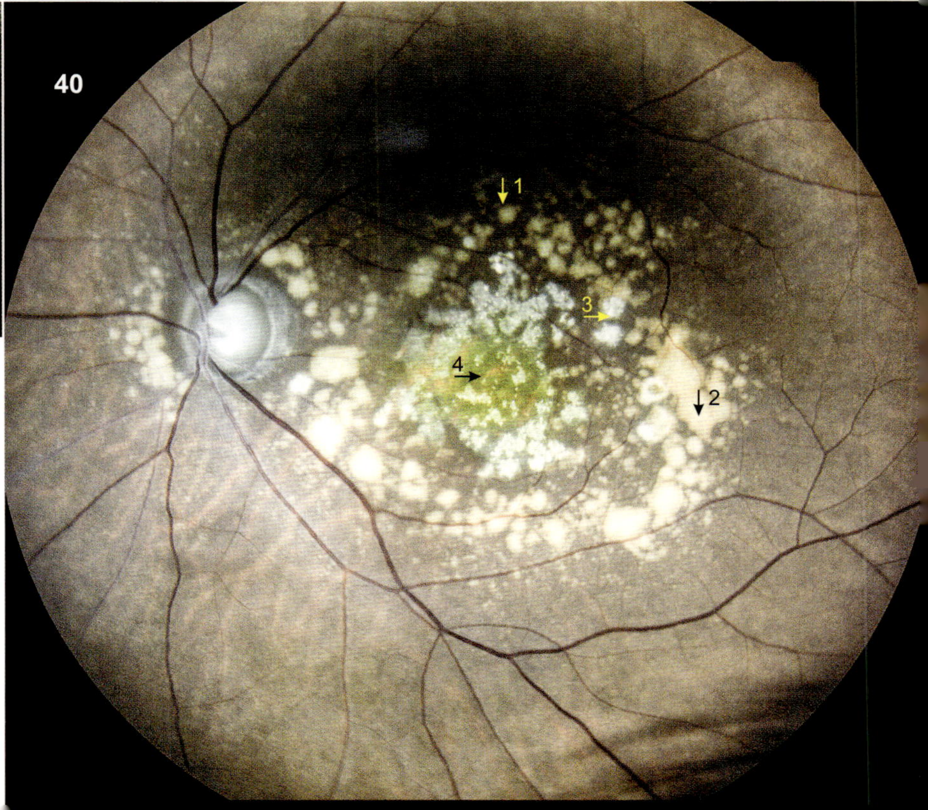



Figure 39

*Spectral domain OCT scan demonstrates outer retinal atrophy with increased choroidal transmission due to geographic atrophy involving the fovea with surrounding multiple RPE elevations as a result of underlying drusens.*

Figure 40

*Advanced stage of nonexudative ARMD-geographic atrophy (GA): Note the presence of multiple hard drusen (1), soft drusen (2) and few refractile drusen (3). Refractile drusen are a potential marker for development of GA. Also note drusen are fading centrally in an area of incipient atrophy of RPE (4) with visibility of underlying large choroidal vessels.* □

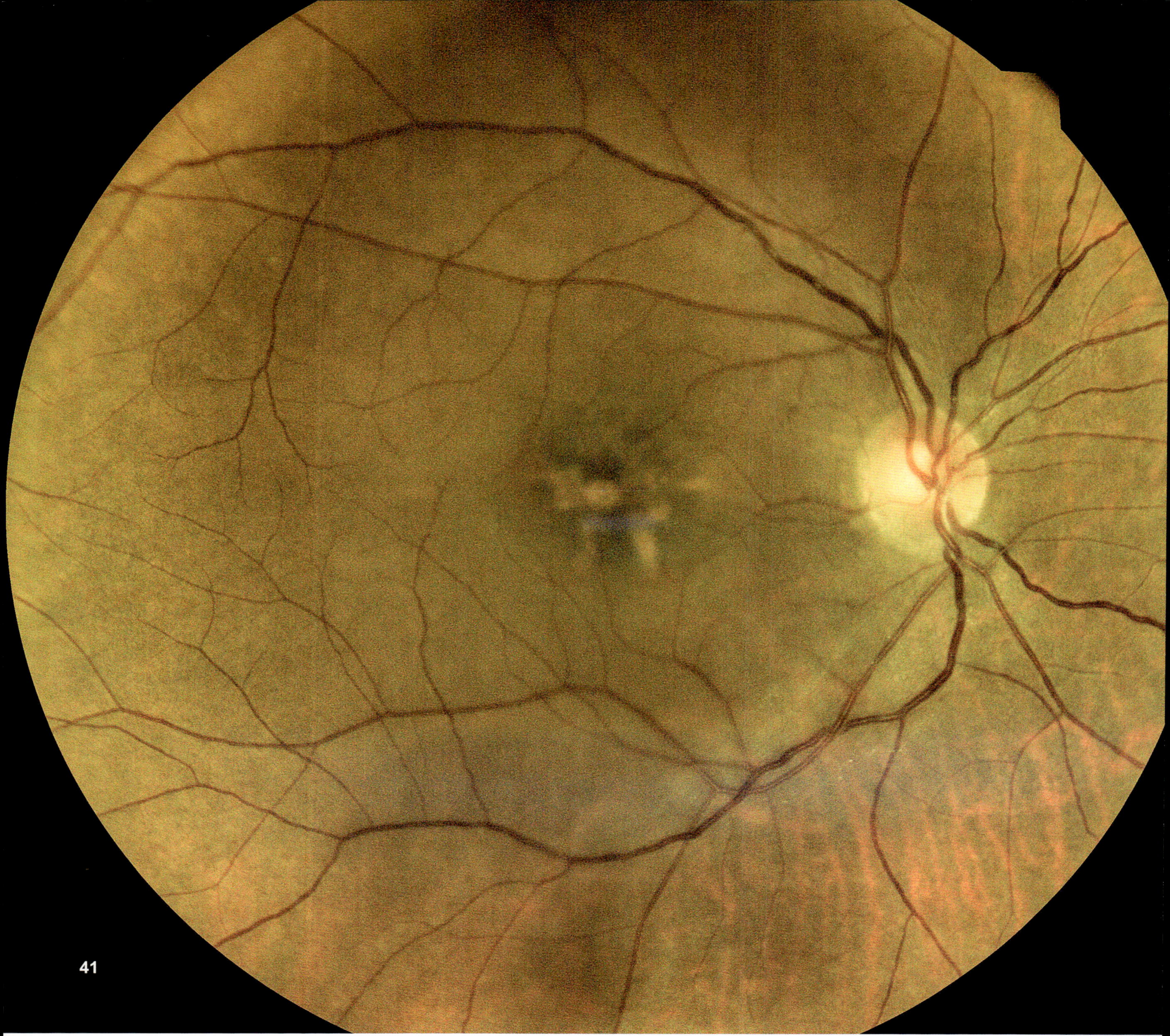

Figure 41 *Adult onset vitelliform macular degeneration: Color fundus photograph shows yellowish area of RPE pigmentary changes at the fovea.*

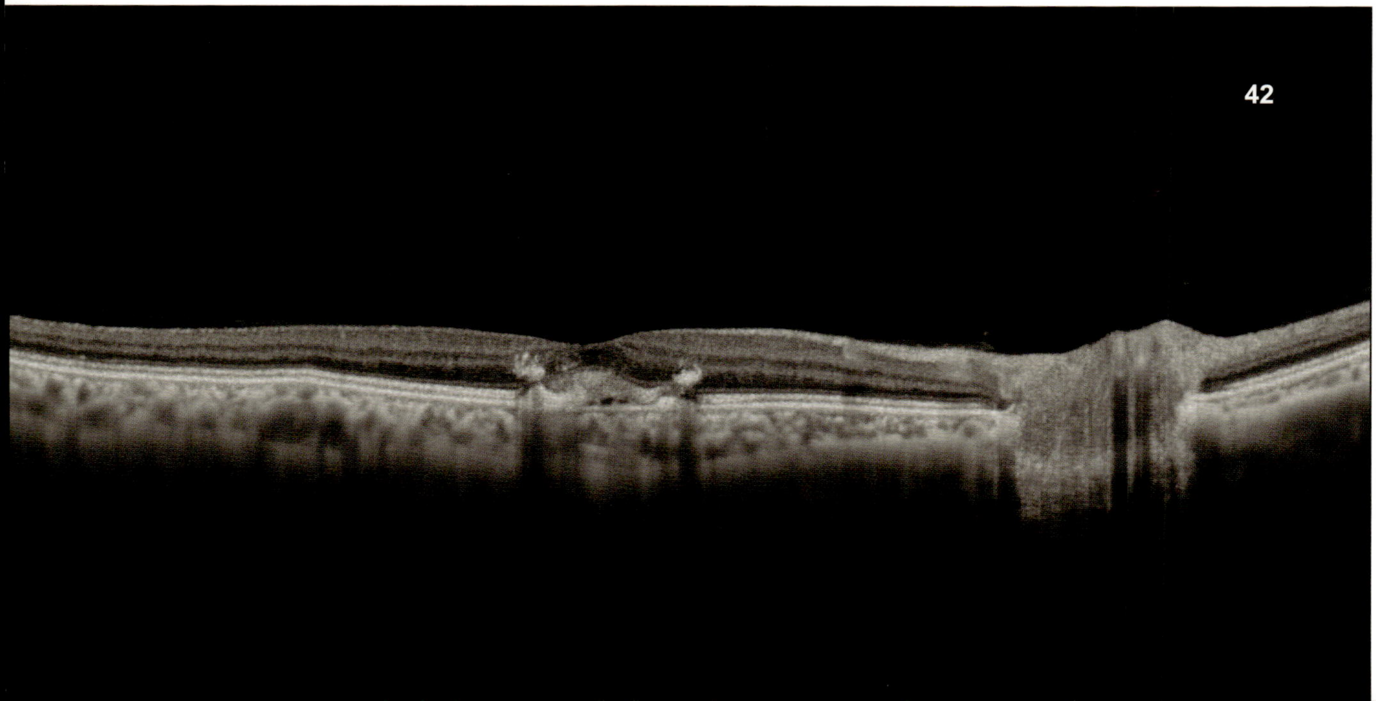

Figure 42 *Swept source OCT demonstrating a vitelliform lesion at the fovea. Note the absence of intraretinal and subretinal fluid.*

Adult onset vitelliform macular degeneration is a retinal disease characterized by round yellowish deposit found beneath the central retina. It is a mild disease, that may cause visual distortion in its advanced stages. It is important to differentiate this condition from neovascular ARMD as this condition does not require treatment with intravitreal injections. Making this distinction can avoid unnecessary interventions and risks associated with intravitreal treatment.

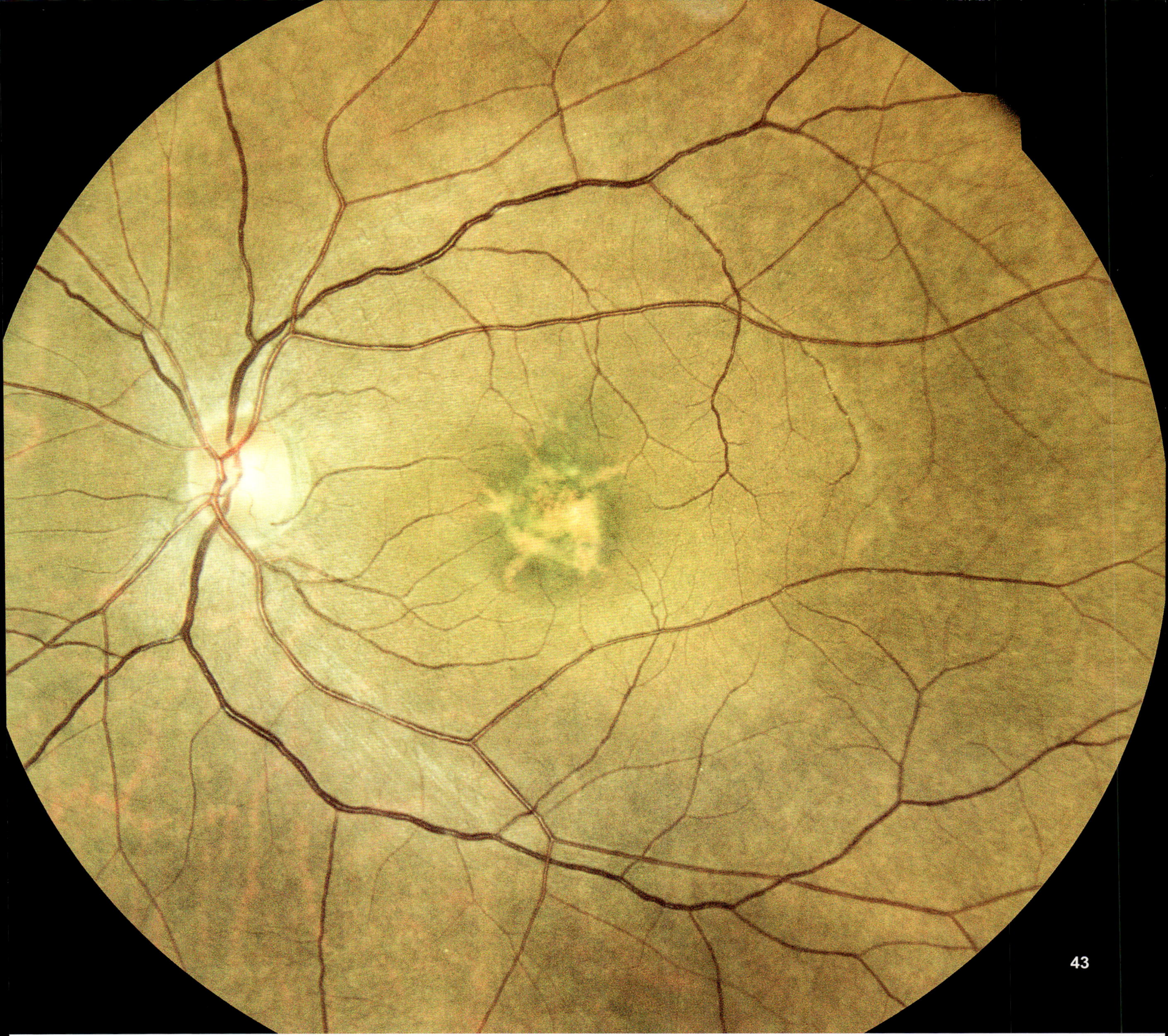

43

Figure 43 *Case of adult onset vitelliform macular degeneration demonstrating pseudo egg-yolk appearance.*

Figure 44 *Swept source OCT scan shows a hyper-reflective zone at the fovea demonstrating vitelliform material deposited in the macula.*

Adult onset vitelliform macular degeneration (AOVMD) has some clinical features similar to hereditary vitelliform macular dystrophy. AOVMD (BEST disease) usually occurs in age group of 40-50 years unlike BEST disease that has an onset in childhood and has an autosomal dominant pattern of inheritance. EOG is characteristically abnormal in patients with BEST disease, whereas in adult onset vitelliform macular degeneration, EOG is normal.□

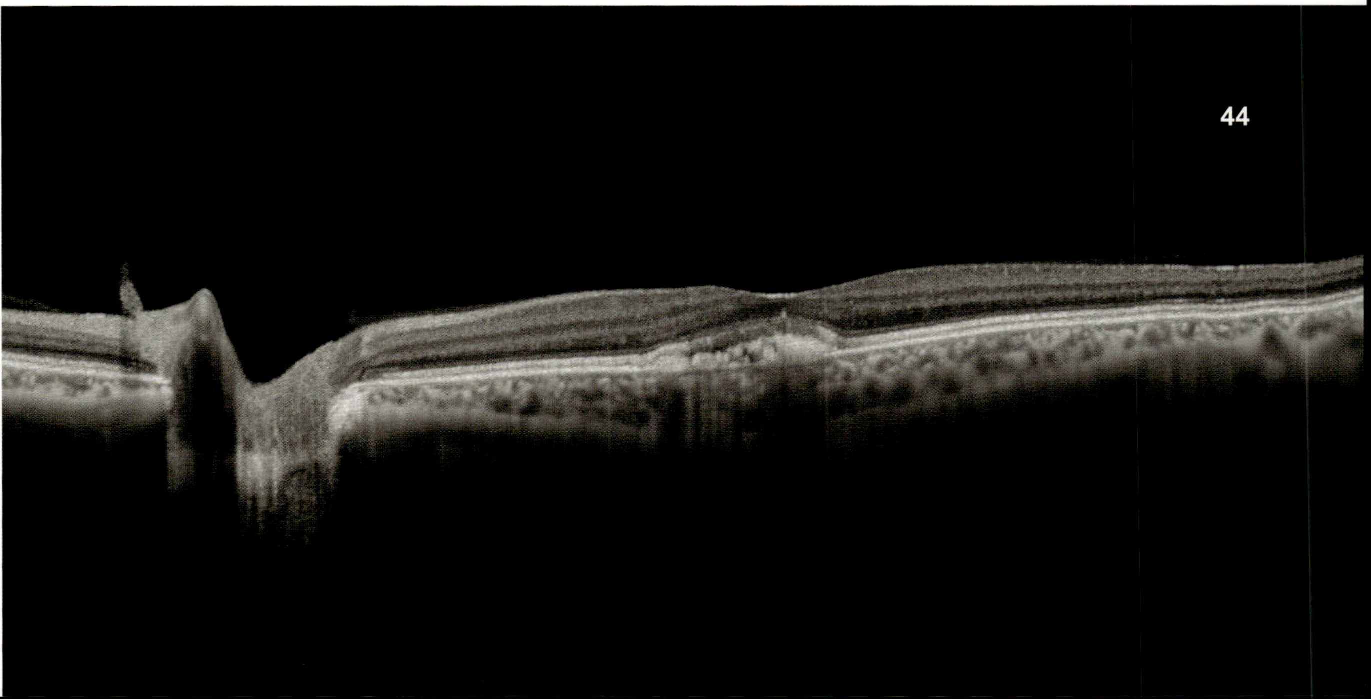

44

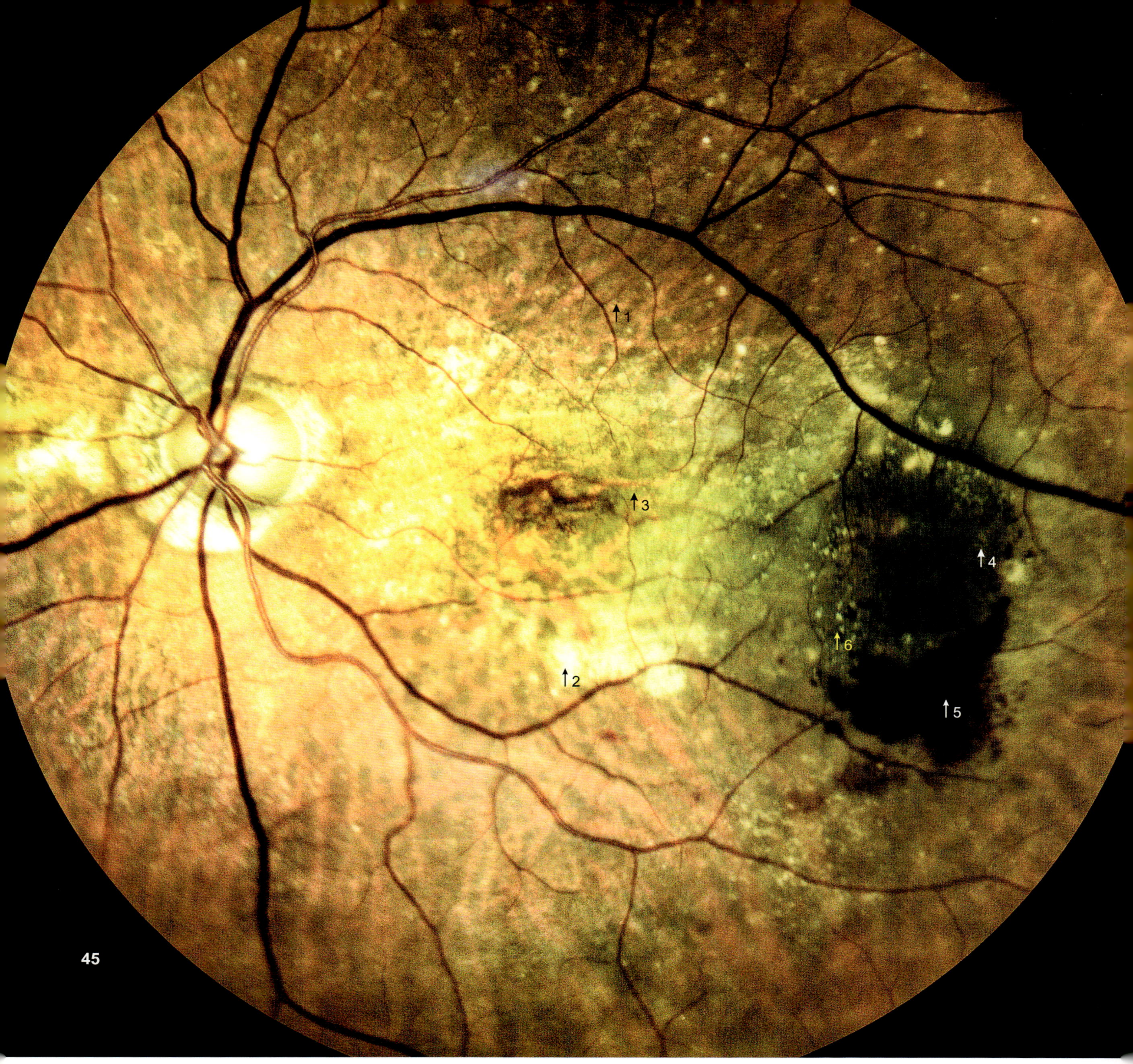


Figure 45 *Case of age-related macular degeneration: Color fundus photograph shows multiple small (1) large (2) scattered yellowish subretinal deposits of drusen all around the posterior pole with diffuse RPE irregularities/thickenings at the fovea (3). Note: Area of subretinal hemorrhage with fresh red blood (4) and slightly darker altered blood (5), intraretinal lipid exudates (6) and an area of neurosensory detachment (white arrow) at the temporal edge of macula suggesting underlying choroid neovascular membrane.*

Choroid neovascular membrane (CNVM) is characterized by the growth of abnormal blood vessels that grow in the choroid, break through the blood barrier between choroid and retina and then they cause severe vision loss. It may occur as an idiopathic entity but is most commonly seen in association with exudative age-related macular degeneration. It is also found in patient with pathological myopia, angioid streaks, trauma/choroidal rupture and inflammatory diseases of choroid and retina.

FFA, ICGA and OCT have been the standard diagnostic modalities to identify the CNVM and monitor the treatment response. Recently noninvasive OCTA has been used extensively to diagnose CNVM.

CNVMs are classified into type 1 (occult), type 2 (classic) and type 3 (RAP) depending on the origin of the neovascular complex. They are also classified based on the location of the membrane into three subtypes—subfoveal, juxtafoveal and extrafoveal. The mainstay of treatment of active CNVM is intravitreal antivascular growth factors injections (anti-VEGF) that are usually given every 4–6 weeks interval. Laser photocoagulation and photodynamic therapy has also been used in few selected cases. □

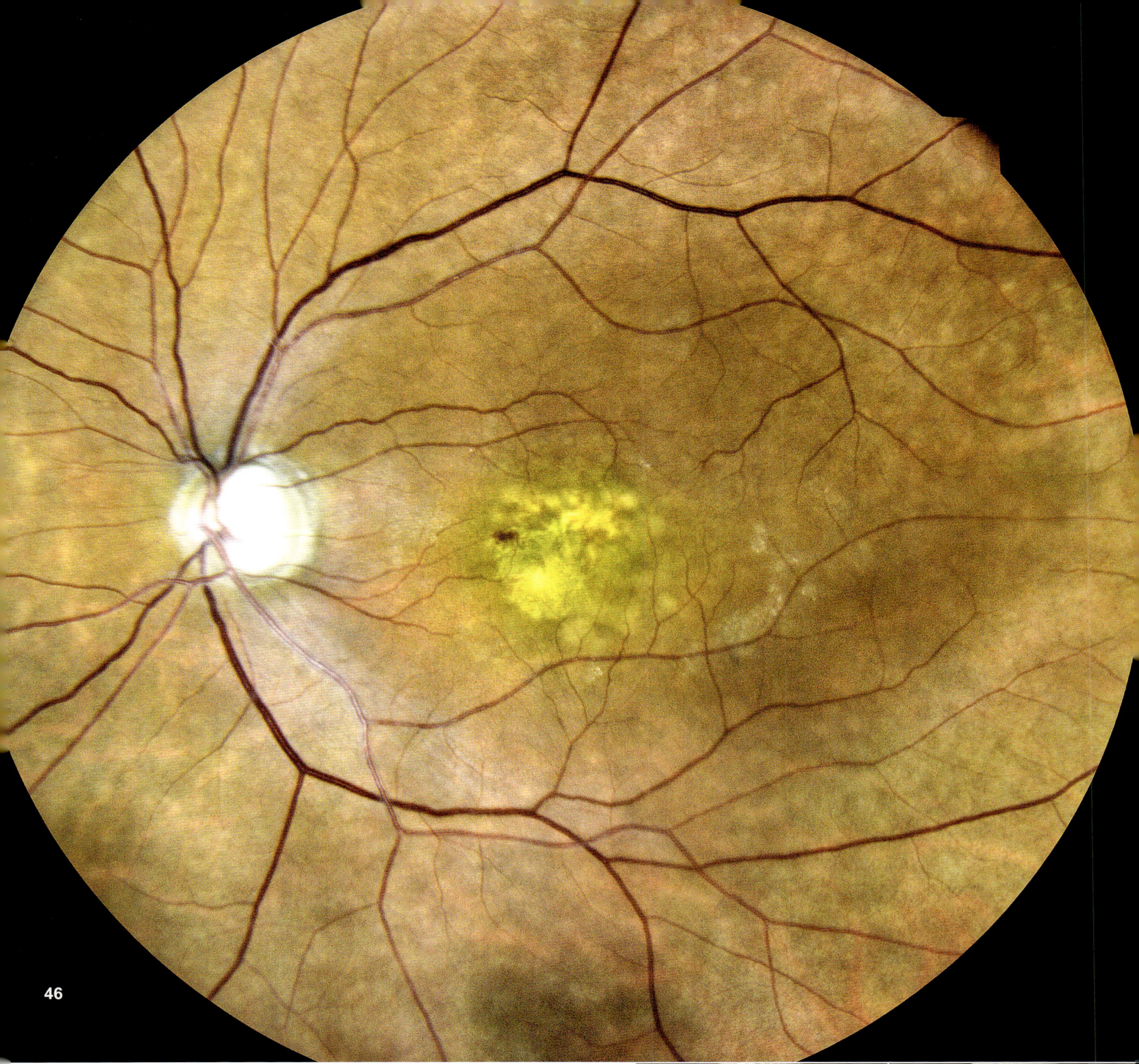

46

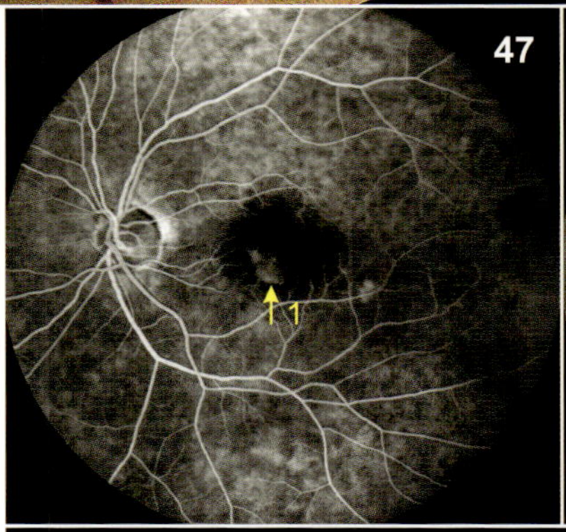

47

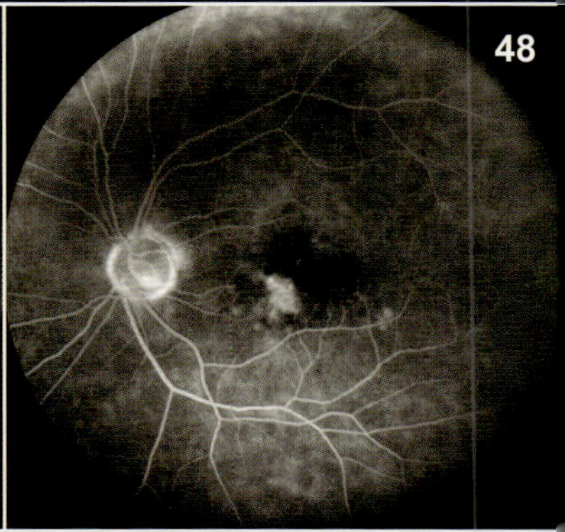

48

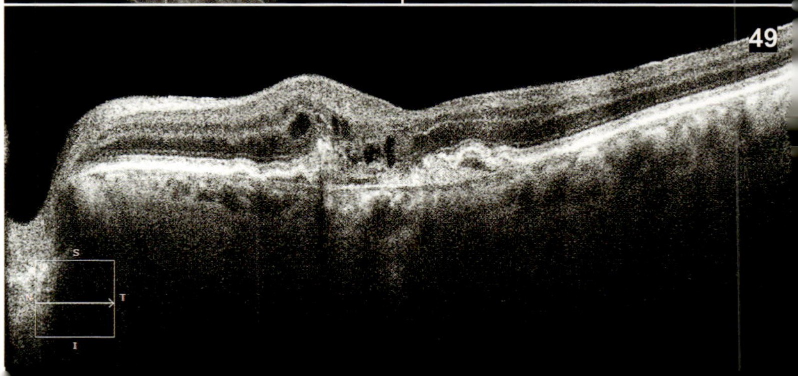

49

Figure 46 *Case of exudative age-related macular degeneration with choroidal neovascularization.*

Color fundus photograph of a 75-year-old shows RPE pigmentary changes at macula with grayish elevated lesion at nasal edge of fovea and a tiny retinal hemorrhage. Age-related macular degeneration is the most common cause of development of CNVM. CNVM are new abnormal blood vessels that grow beneath the retina and when they leak, they cause vision loss.

Figure 47 *Early frame of FFA shows well-defined lacy pattern of hyperfluorescence suggestive of classic choroid neovascular membrane (1).*

Figure 48 *Late frame of FFA shows increasing hyperfluorescence at the site of lesion suggestive of active CNVM.*

Figure 49 *Spectral domain OCT shows fibrovascular PED subretinal hyper-reflective material suggestive of type 2 CNVM and presence of intraretinal cystoid spaces.* □

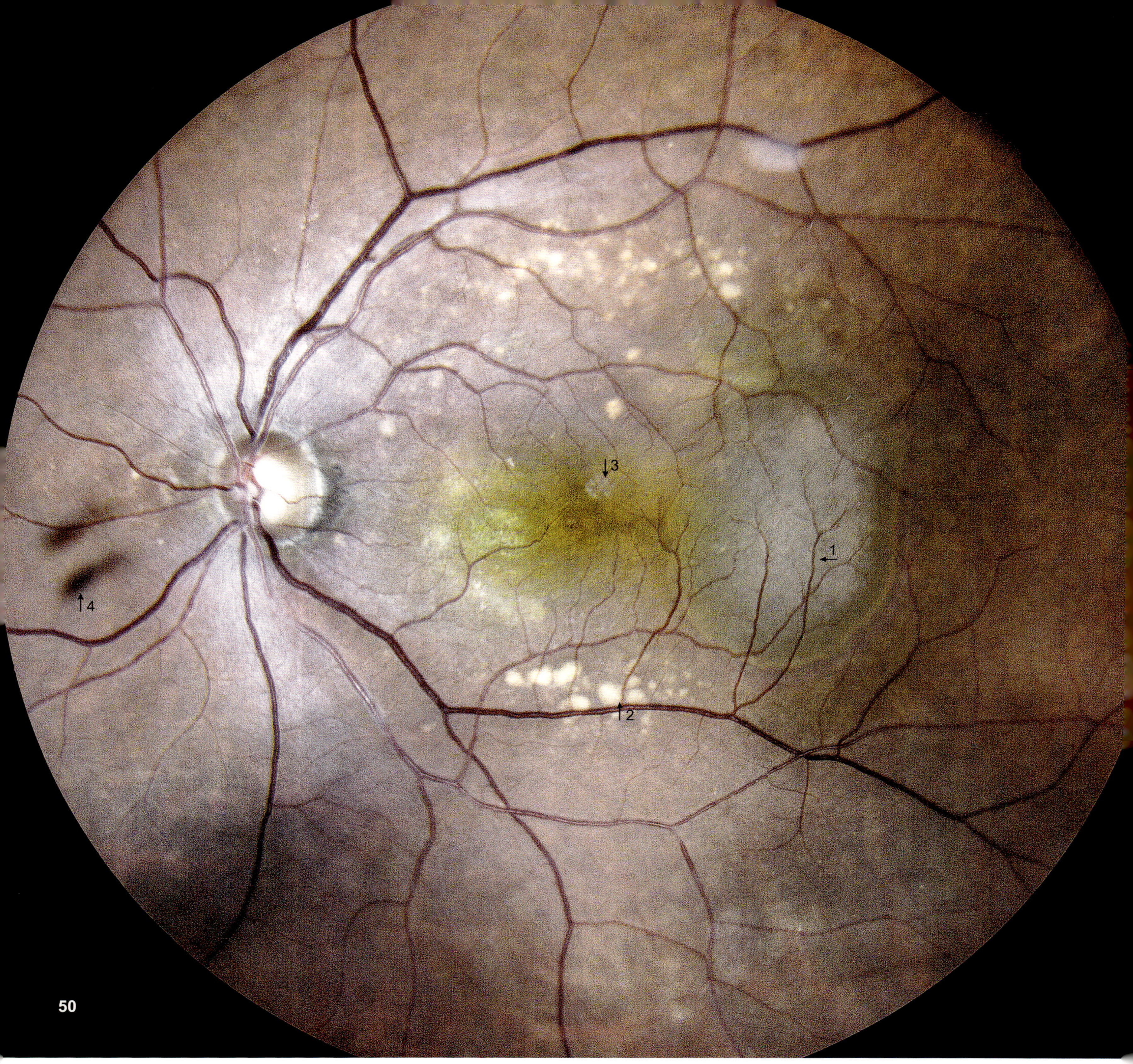


Figure 50 *Oval, distinct dome-shaped grayish area of detachment of RPE and overlying neurosensory retina with smooth surface is seen in temporal macula (1). Also note, soft drusenoid deposits, scattered at the posterior pole (2) and RPE irregularities (3) and presence of vitreous opacity due to posterior vitreous detachment (4).*

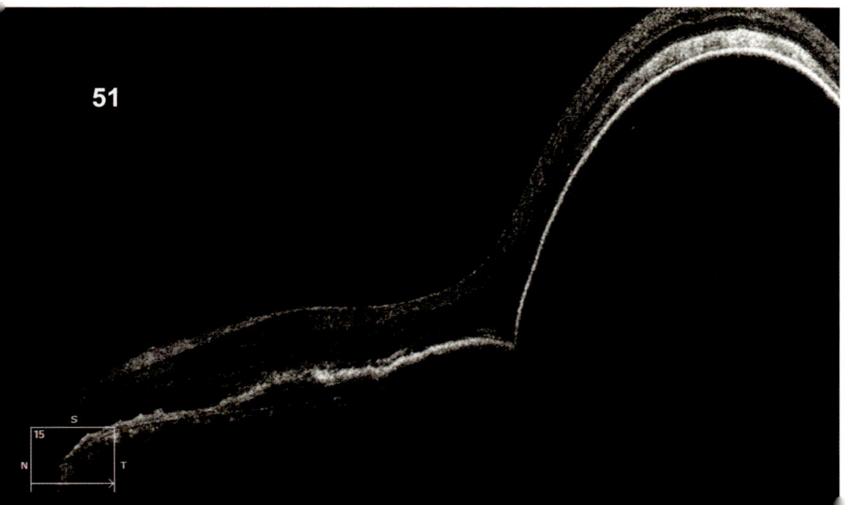


Figure 51 *Cross-sectional OCT scan passing through the fovea shows a dome-shaped large serous PED with presence of subretinal fluid suggesting it to be a vascularized PED.*

Figure 52 *Color fundus image at 3 months post anti -VEGF injection: Note the flattening of the pigment epithelial detachment following the treatment.*

Figure 53 *Cross-sectional OCT scan done at 3 months shows flattening of the PED with almost complete resolution of subretinal fluid.*

Figure 54 *Color fundus image at 5 months post anti-VEGF injection. The area of PED continues to flatten. There is significant reduction in the size and the height of the PED as compared to baseline.*

Figure 55 *Cross-sectional OCT scan done at 5 months shows further flattening down of the PED. No subretinal fluid is seen.*

Figure 56 *Color fundus image at 6 months post anti-VEGF injection. PED has completely flattened out.*

Figure 57 *Cross-sectional OCT scan done at 6 months shows straightening of the RPE layer at the site of PED.* □

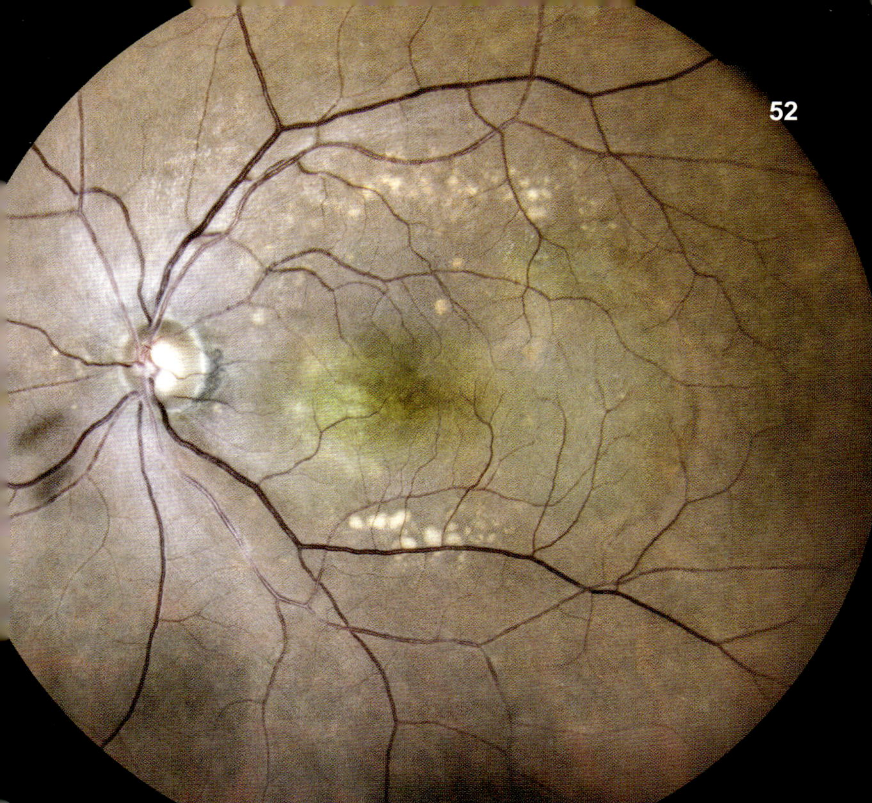

52

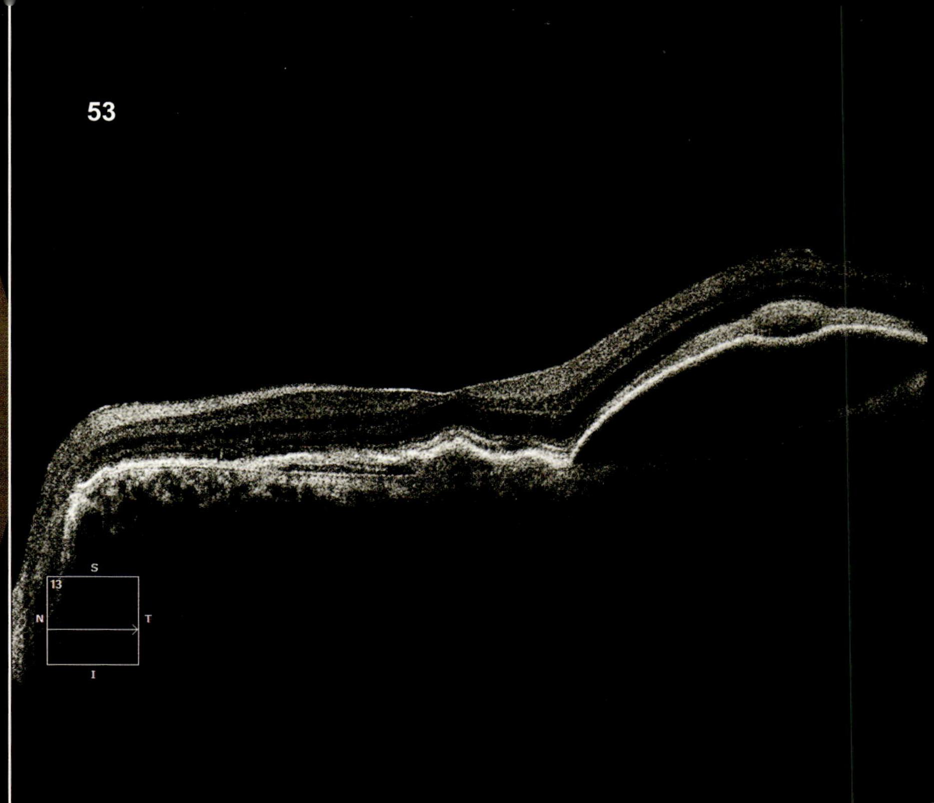

53

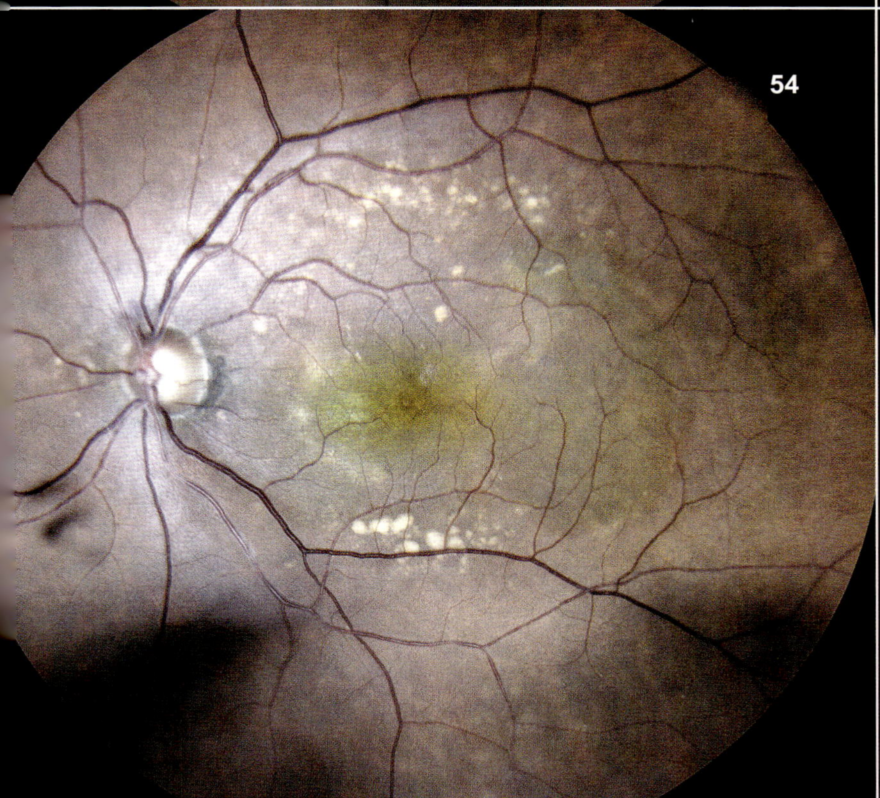

54

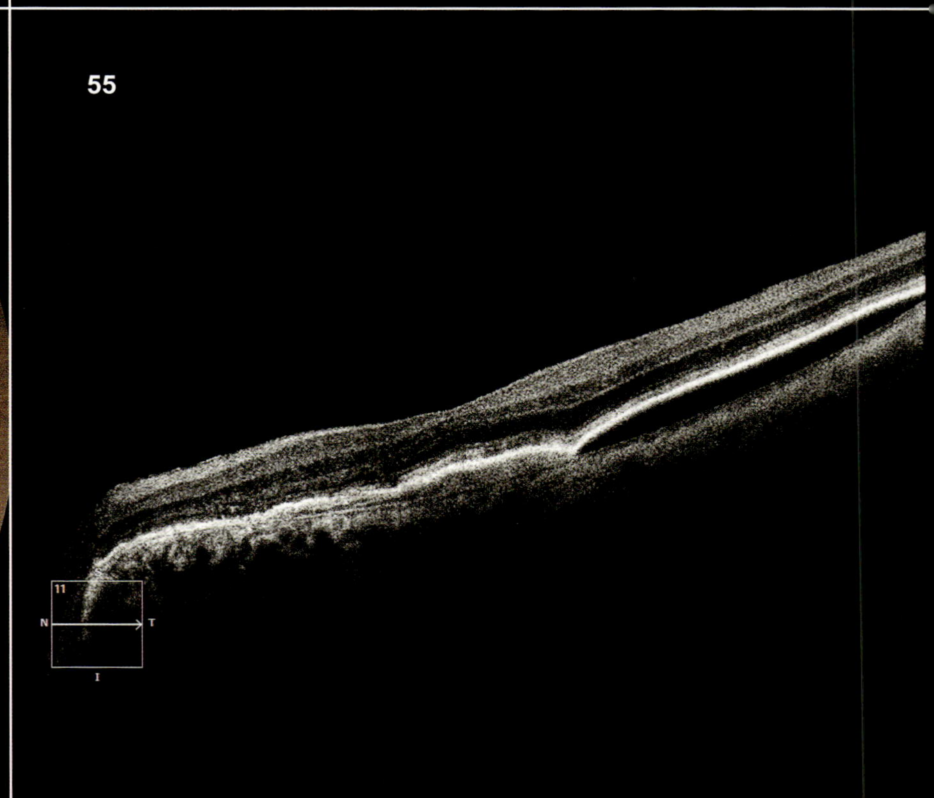

55

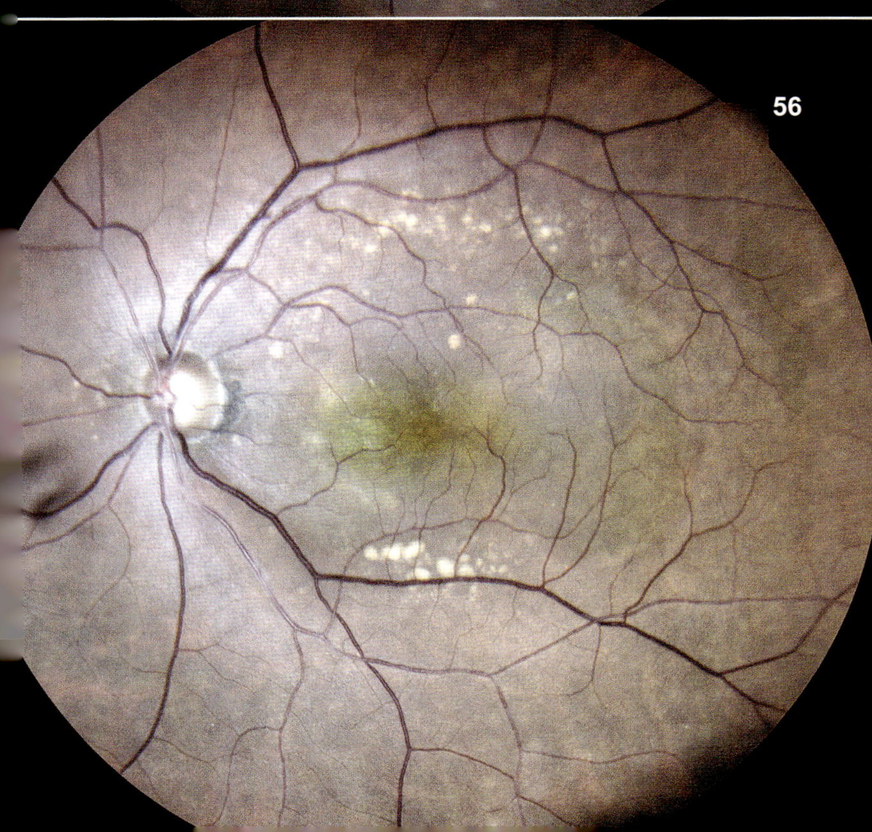

56

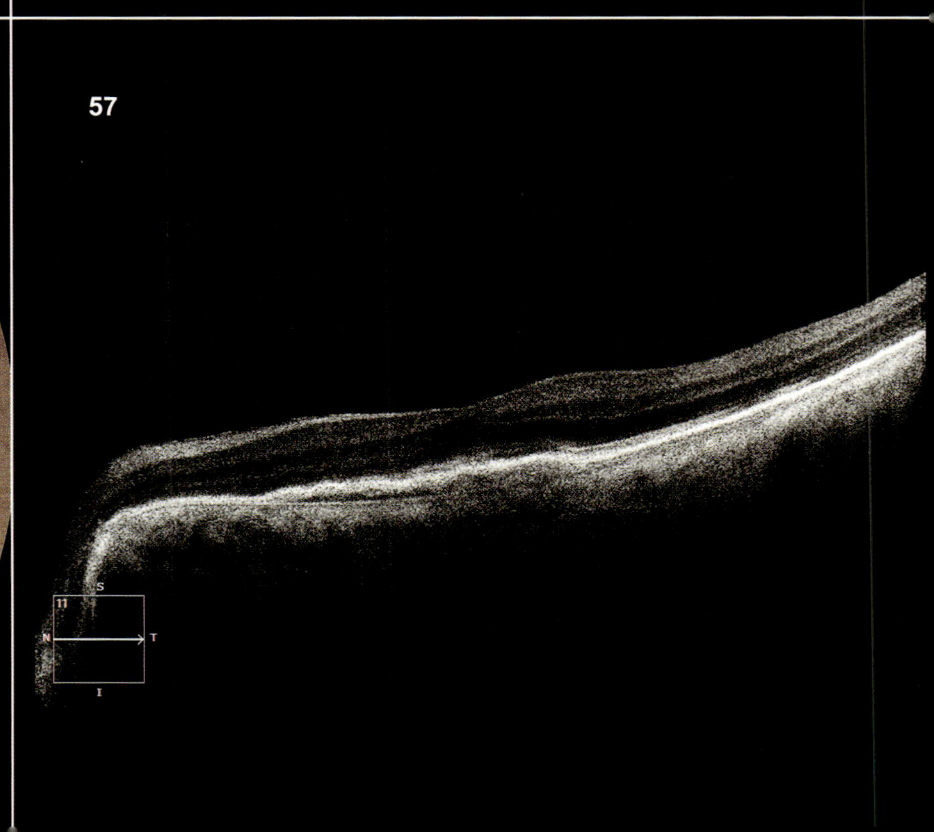

57

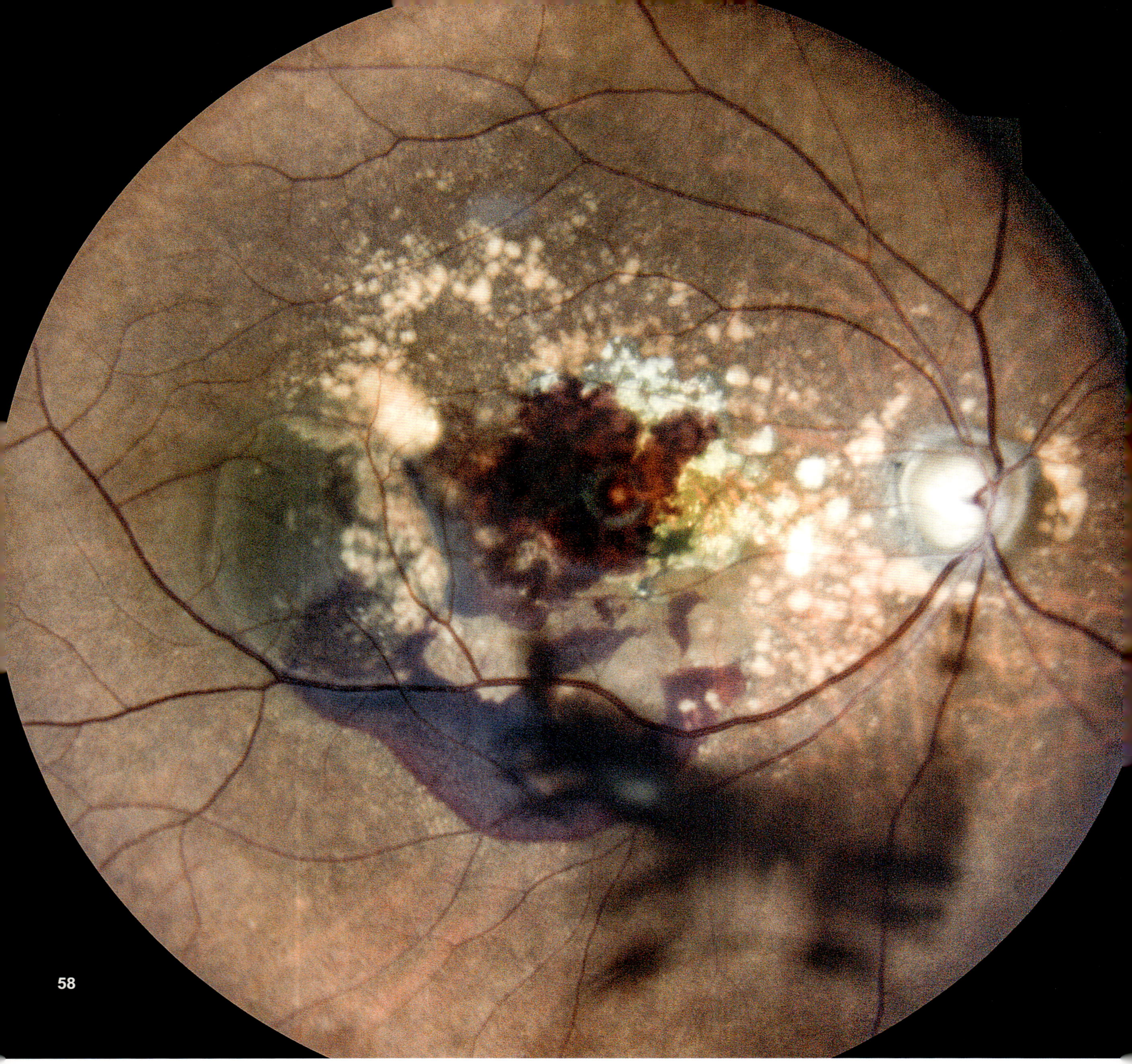


Figure 58 *Case of choroid neovascular membrane associated with geographic atrophy.*

Color fundus photograph shows multiple small to large drusen scattered all around the posterior pole with surrounding patches of atrophy.

*Note:* Large areas of subretinal hemorrhage seen along the inferotemporal arcade extending up to fovea suggestive of CNVM.

An 85-year-old male presented with sudden onset floaters and new onset scotoma. He had 5-year history of atrophic form of ARMD. Geographic atrophy and CNVM are usually considered as two distinct entities, former repressing advanced stage of nonexudative ARMD whereas latter results in exudative form of ARMD. However, at times geographical atrophy and CNVM can occur simultaneously in the same eye.

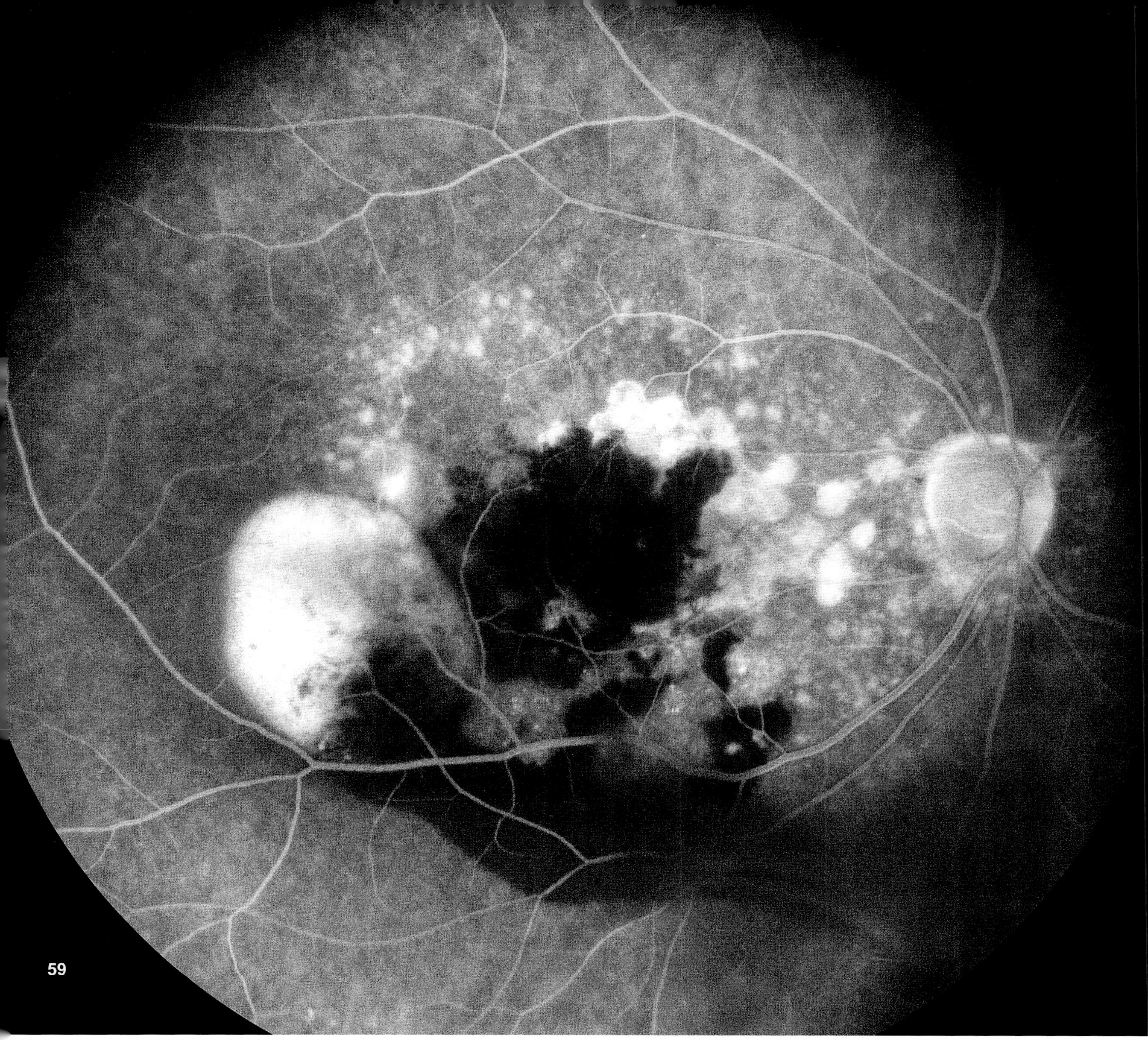

Figure 59 *FFA shows multiple small round hyperfluorescent lesions due to filling up of the dye within drusen, vascularized pigment epithelial detachment at inferotemporal macula and blocked fluorescence from the hemorrhage obscuring the underlying retina details.*

Figure 60 *Spectral domain OCT scan shows multiple drusen seen as small areas of RPE thickening with adjacent patches of RPE atrophy due to underlying geographic atrophy. Large pigment epithelial detachment (PED) with subretinal fluid is seen at temporal edge.*□

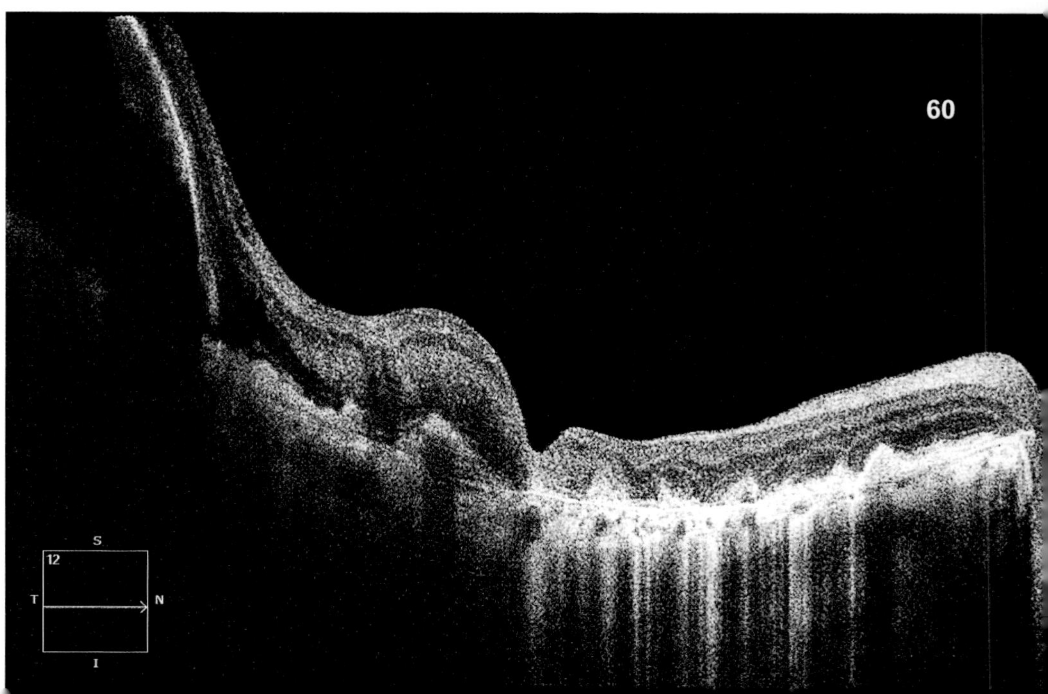

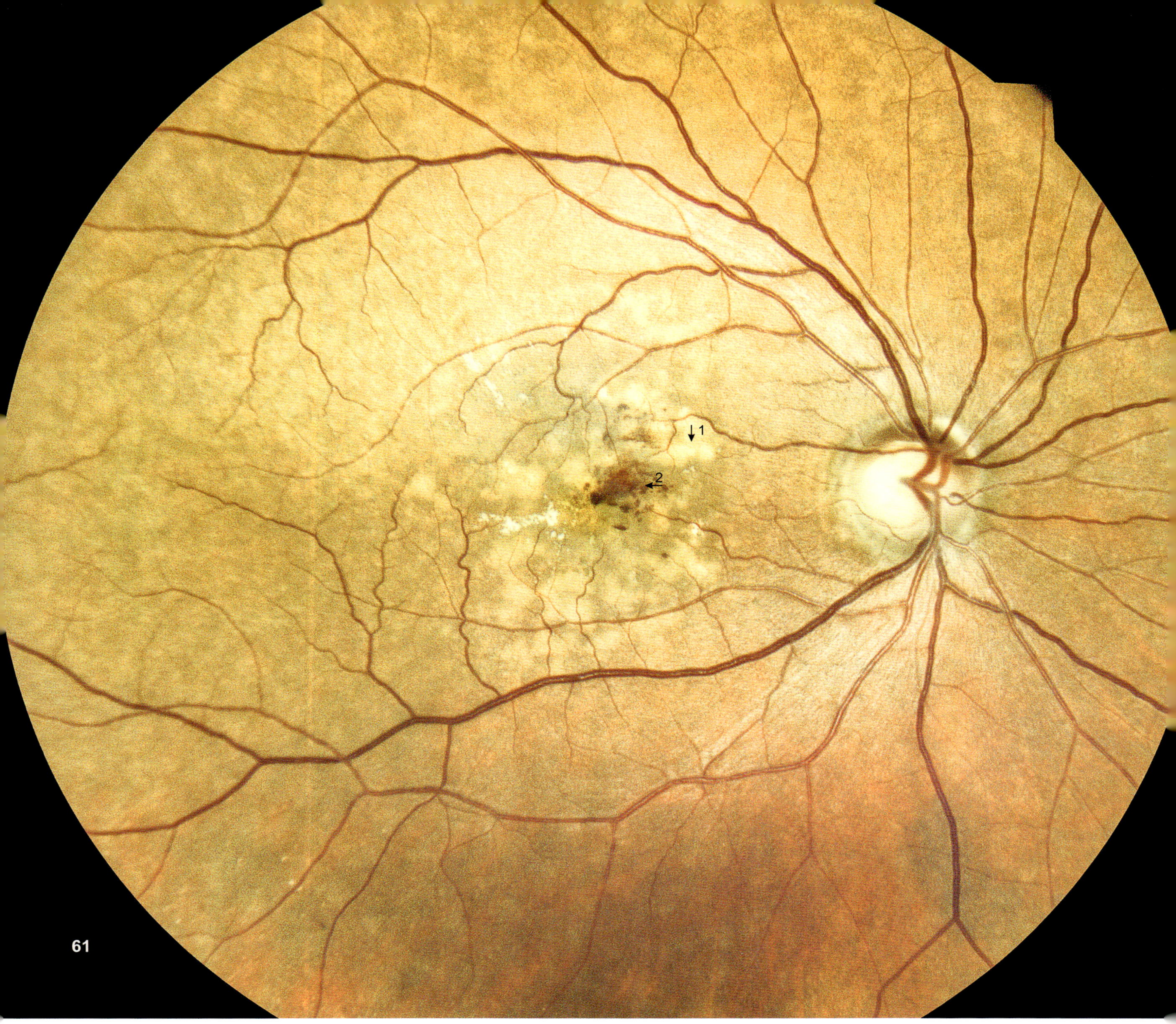


Figure 61 *Color fundus photograph of an 89-year-old female with retinal angiomatosis proliferans (RAP) type 3 choroid neovascular membrane. Note the presence of yellowish subretinal drusenoid deposits (1) at the macula and deep intraretinal dot hemorrhages (2) which are characteristic of RAP lesions.*

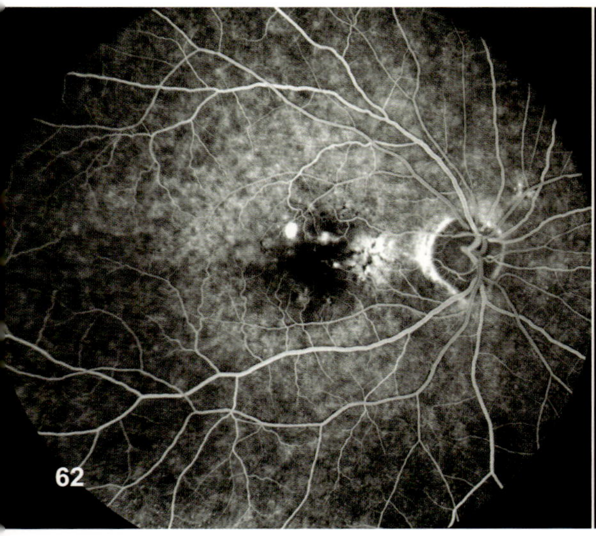


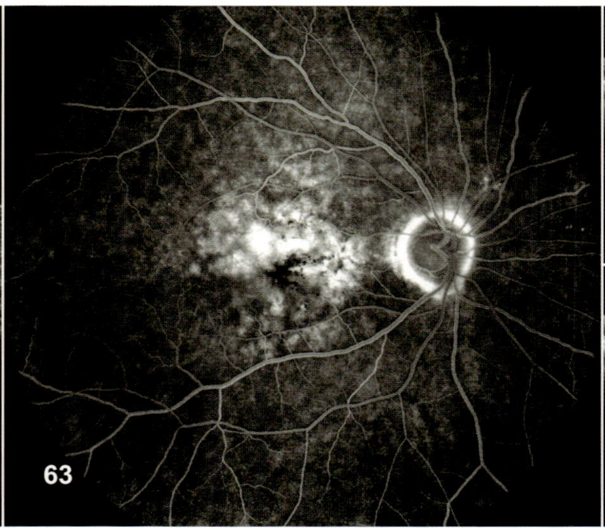


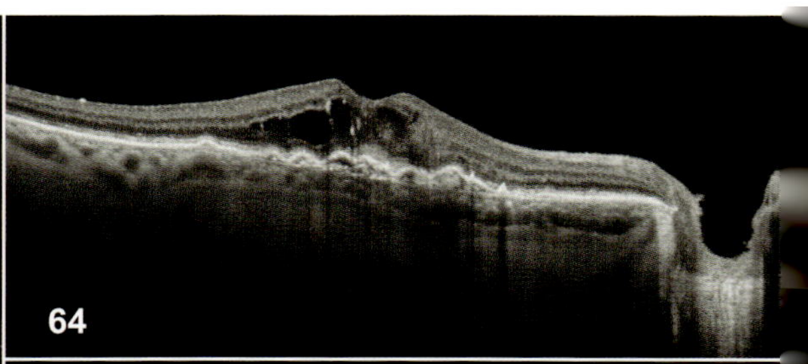


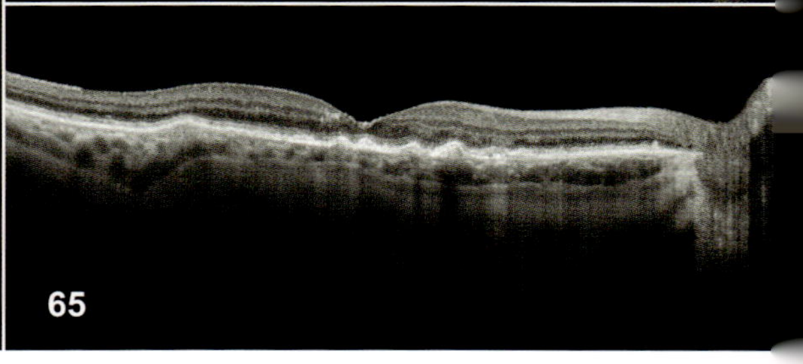


Figure 62 *Early frame of angiogram shows mixed pattern of hyperfluorescence from the soft drusens and drusenoid PED, tiny hypofluorescent dots from hemorrhages.*

Figure 63 *Late frame of angiogram demonstrates ill-defined late leakage.*

Figure 65 *OCT scan after intravitreal bevacizumab injection shows resolution of intraretinal fluid.*

Figure 64 *OCT scan shows RPE alterations and intraretinal cystic fluid. Intra-retinal hyperreflective patch extending in between the inner and outer retinal layers (RAP lesion).*□

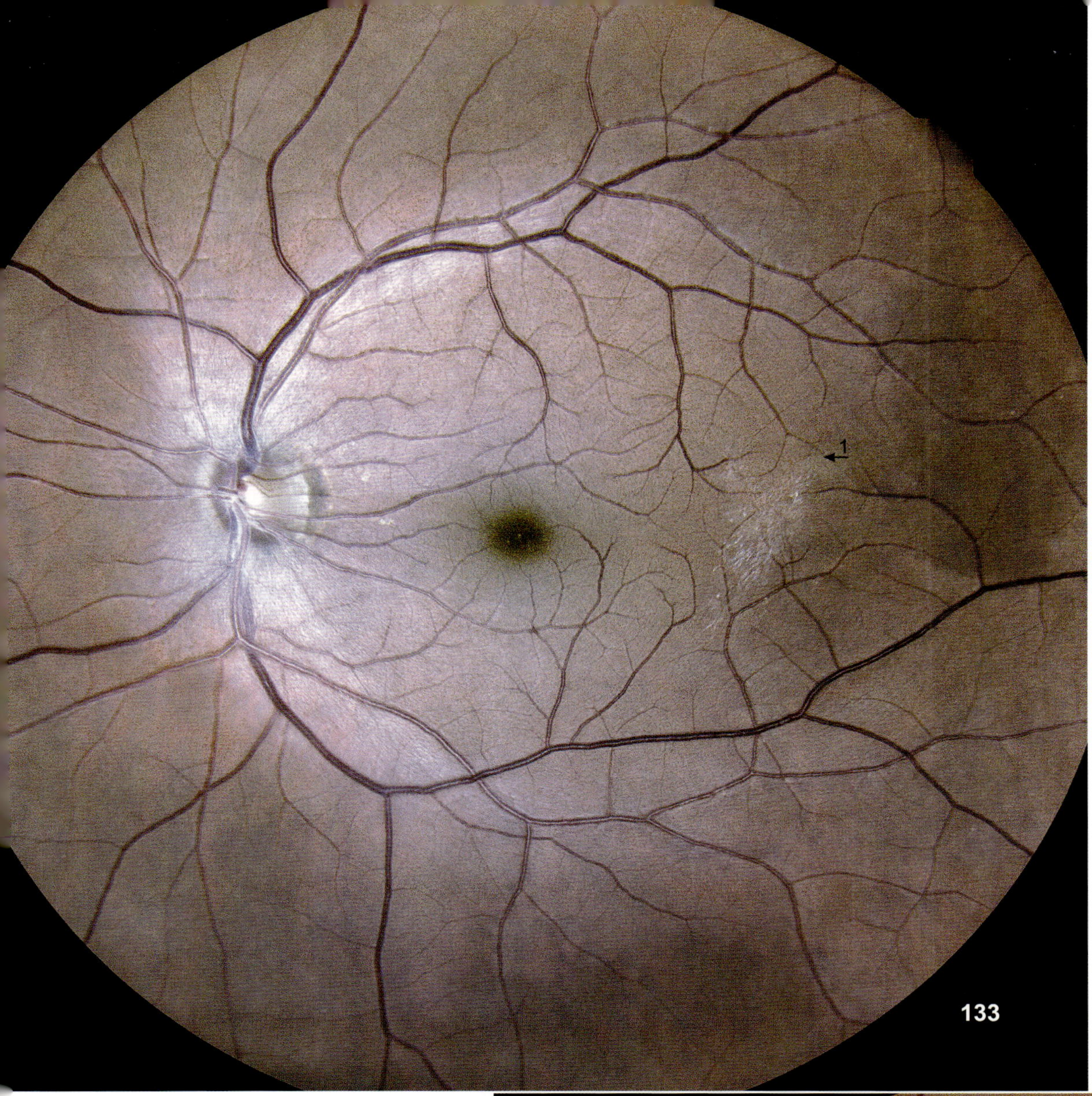


Figure 133

*Spontaneous resolution of epiretinal membrane.*

A 68-year-old male came for routine eye examination, BCVA was 6/6 in his left eye. Dilated fundus examination showed fine cellophane reflex temporal to the fovea at the macula suggestive of epiretinal membrane (ERM)(1). ERM was away from foveal center and not affecting visual acuity, was kept under monitoring.

Figure 134

*Follow-up after 6 months showed spontaneous regression of epiretinal membrane which is rare but has been reported in a few cases. Residual ERM is seen fragmented (1) and faint compared to previous visit.*

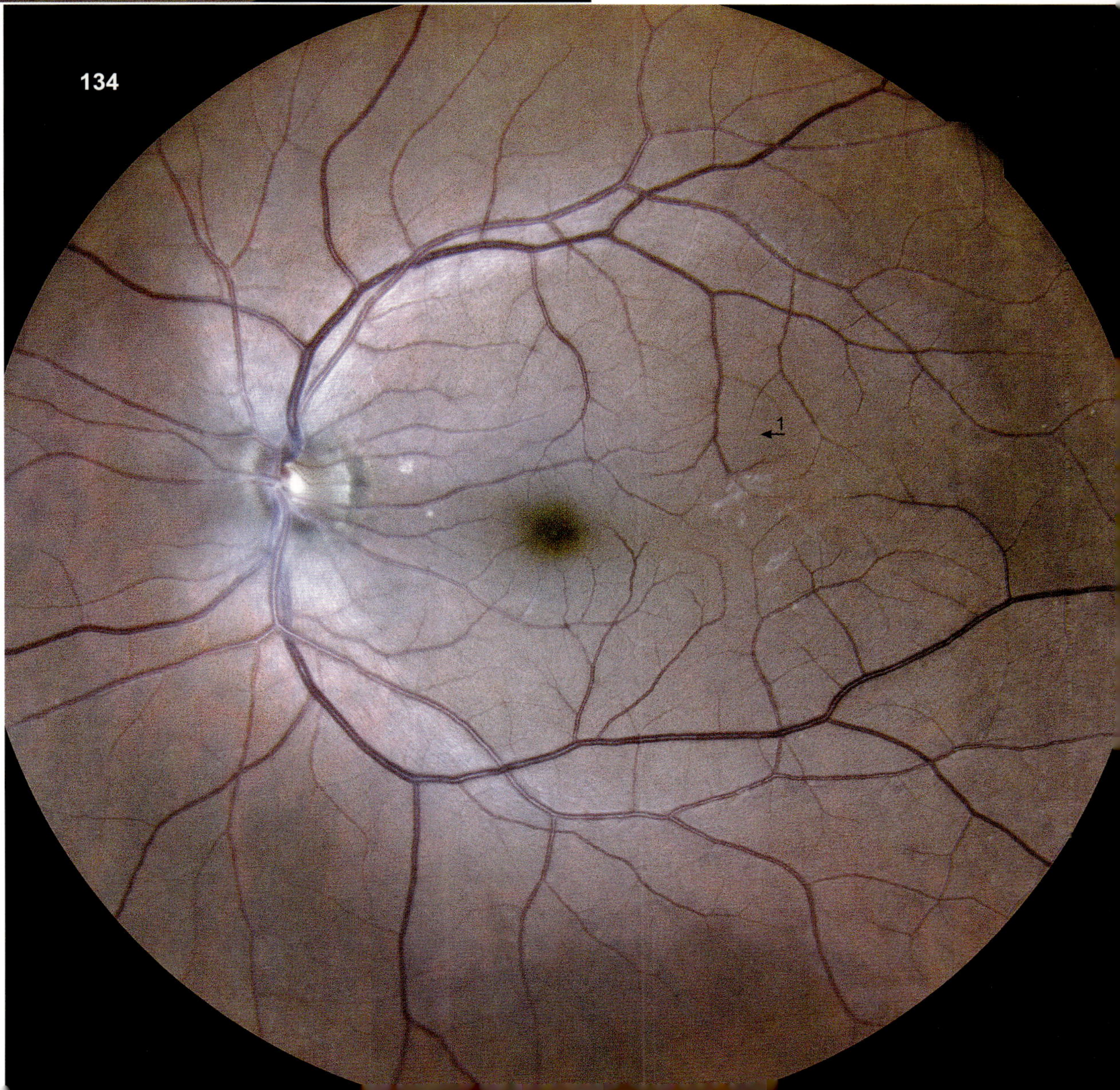

Figure 135

*A case of unilateral epiretinal membrane.*

A 70-year-old female came for routine follow-up after her cataract surgery in both eyes. She was known hypertensive on oral medication. BCVA was 6/6 in both eyes. Fundus photo of right eye shows changes in vessel wall and calliber suggestive of hypertensive retinopathy. Foveal reflex is bright.

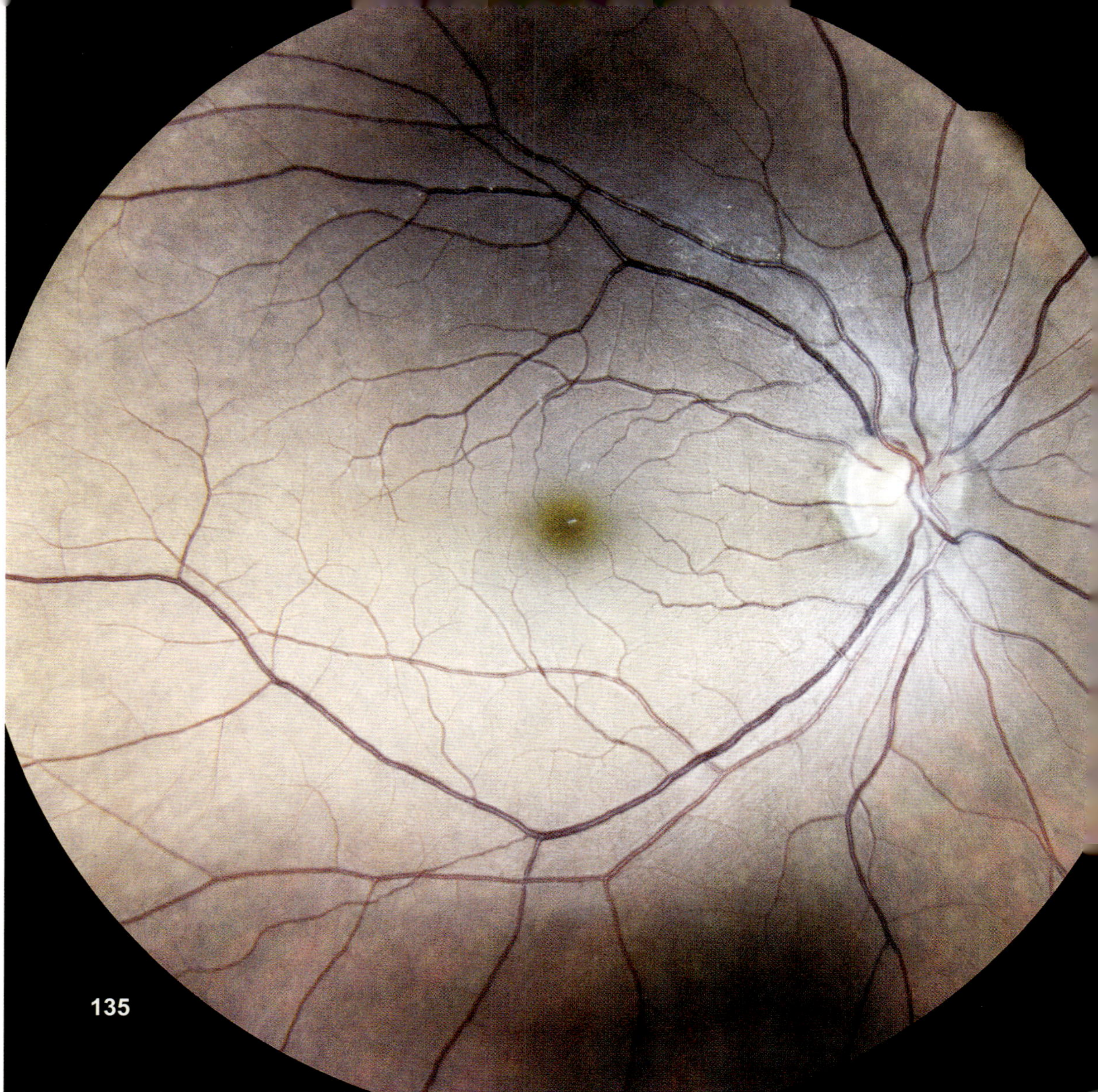


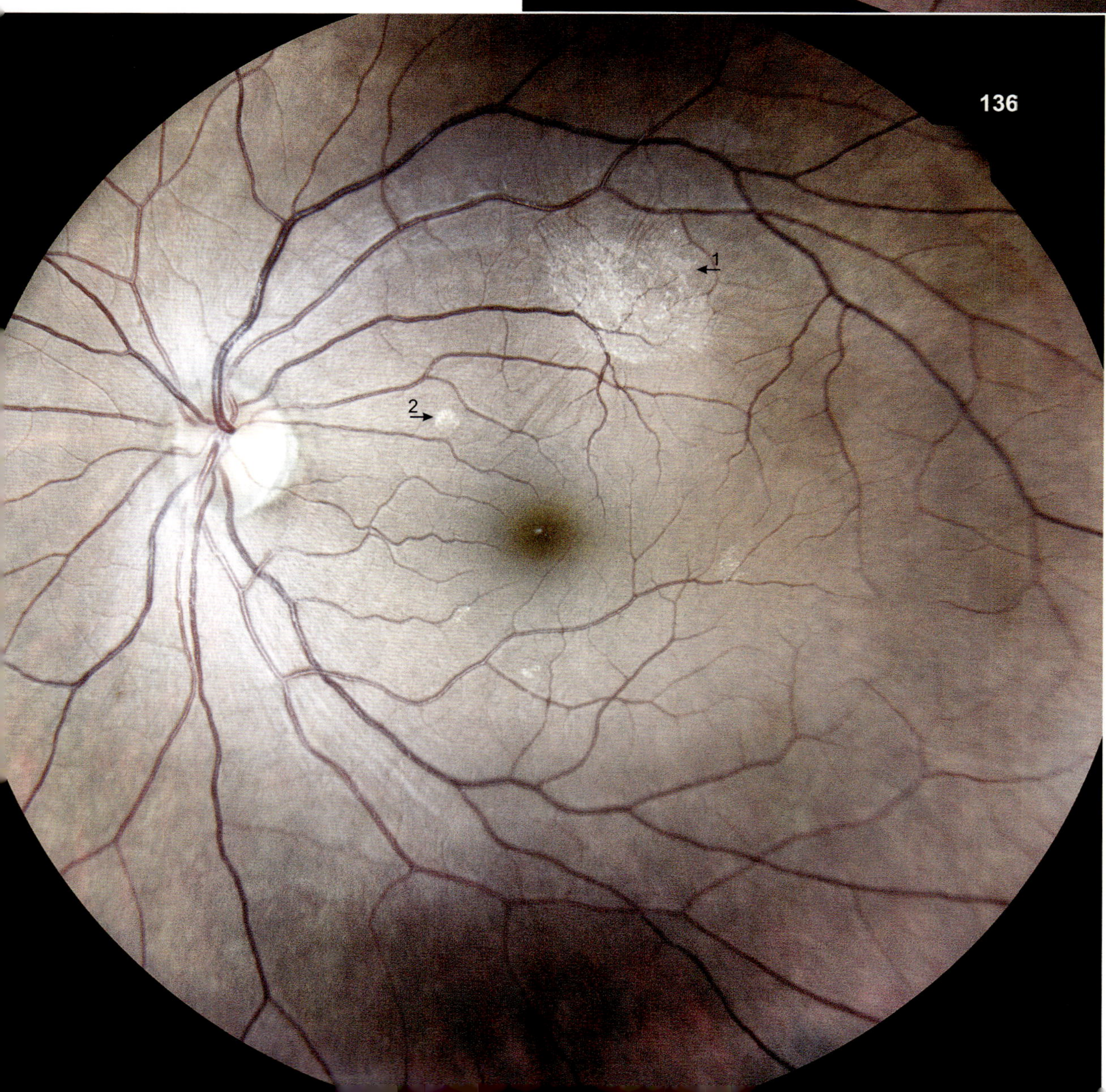


Figure 136

*The fellow left eye demonstrates a thin grayish translucent membrane like structure superotemporal to the fovea suggestive of epiretinal membrane (1). The tangential traction of epiretinal membrane is leading to formation of fine retinal striations which is however away from foveal center, hence no impact on visual acuity. Subtle retinal pigment epithelial changes were also visible over macula (2). Hypertensive retinopathy was evident in this eye as well.*

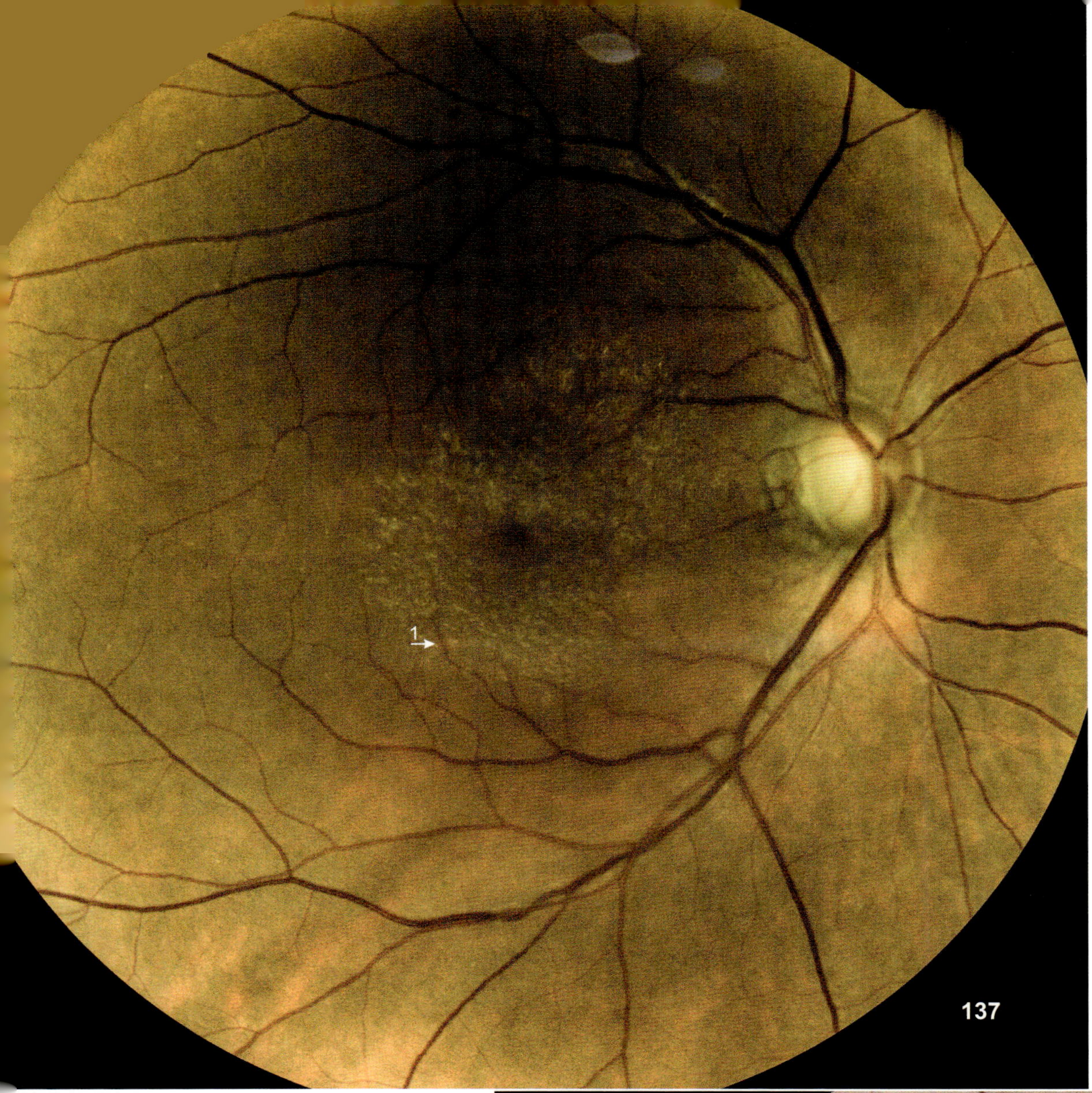


Figure 137

*A case of progression of epiretinal membrane.*

A 77-year-old male presented with complaints of blurred vision in his right eye since past four months, BCVA was 6/24. He had significant nuclear cataract grade 3 in his right eye. Color fundus photo demonstrates a thin sheet of fibrous tissue on the surface of macula causing surface wrinkling also known as cellophane maculopathy (1).

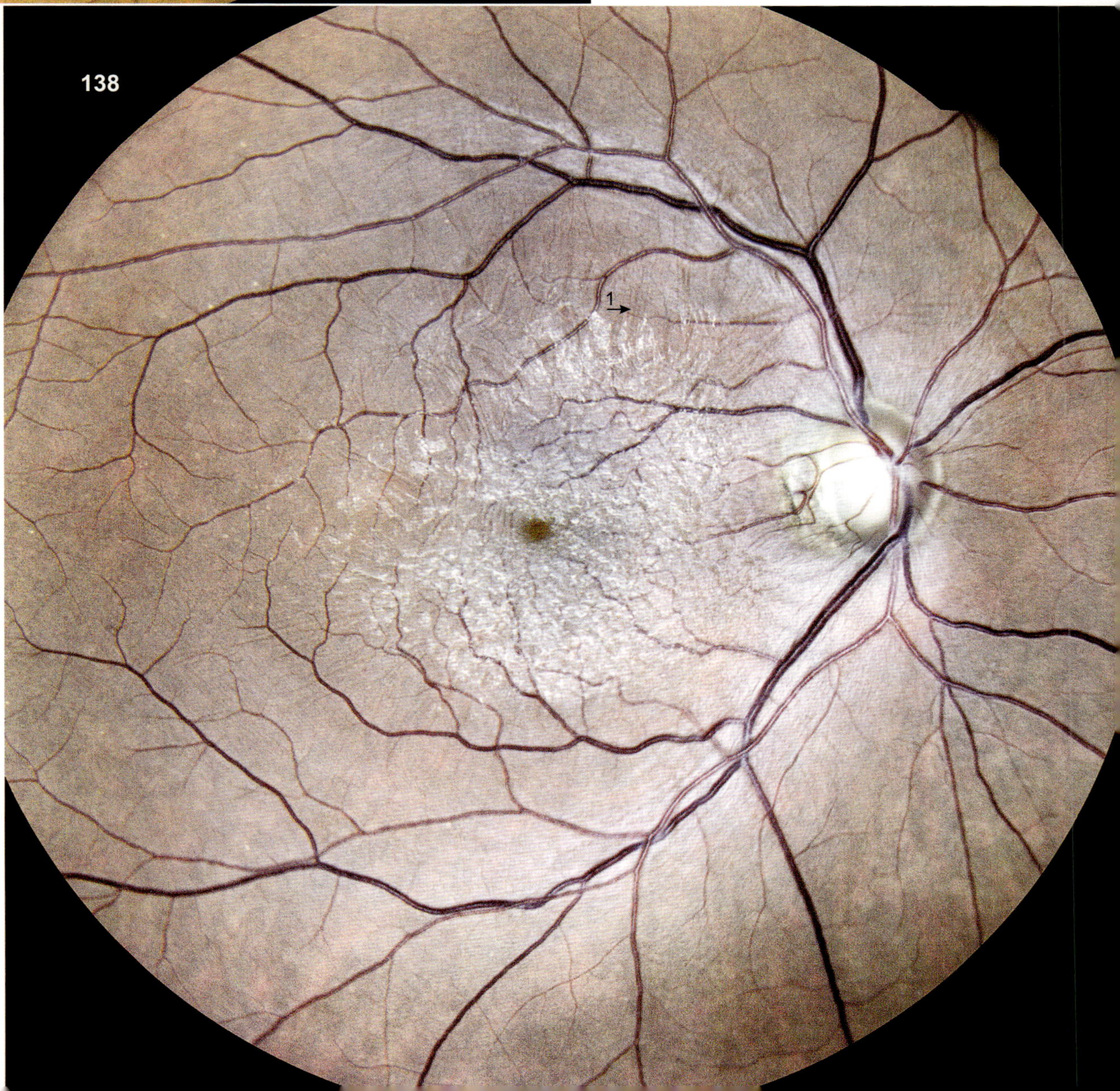


Figure 138

*He underwent cataract surgery with intraocular lens implant (note change in hue of color fundus photo). BCVA was 6/9. Four months postoperatively, one can see cellophane maculopathy at the macula which has increased in area to expand superiorly and temporally (1). However since it had minimal impact on his vision and he was able to carry on with routine activities for near as well as distance, no intervention was required.*

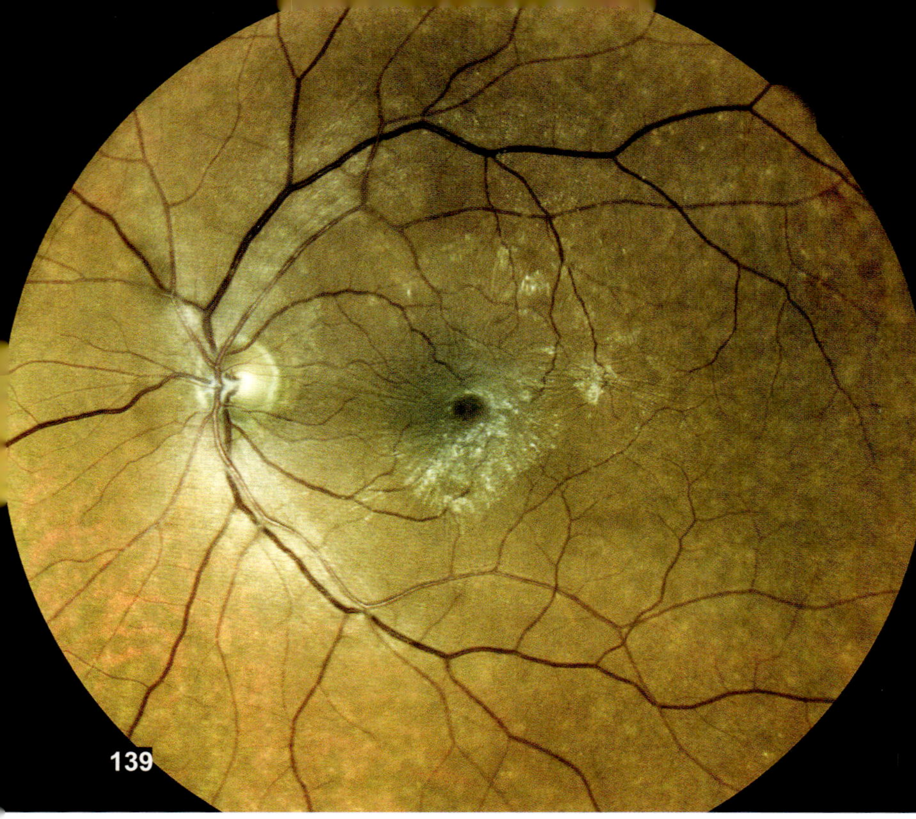


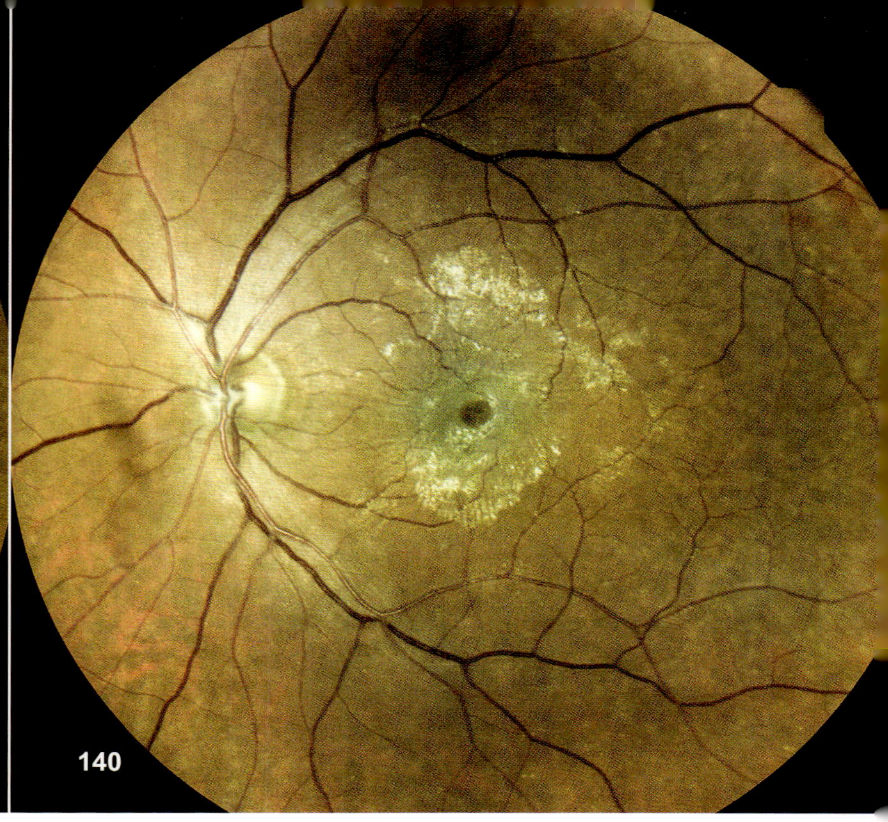


Figure 139 *Color fundus photograph of 77-year-old male with epiretinal membrane. Note the presence of a glistening reflex, more prominent at the inferior edge of the fovea accompanied by a dull foveal reflex, a pseudomacular hole appearance of the fovea and ILM folds.*

Figure 140 *Color fundus photograph of same patient done 3 months later demonstrating the progression of an epiretinal membrane. Note the region of abnormal cellophane reflex has grown and become prominent in the superior half of the macula.*

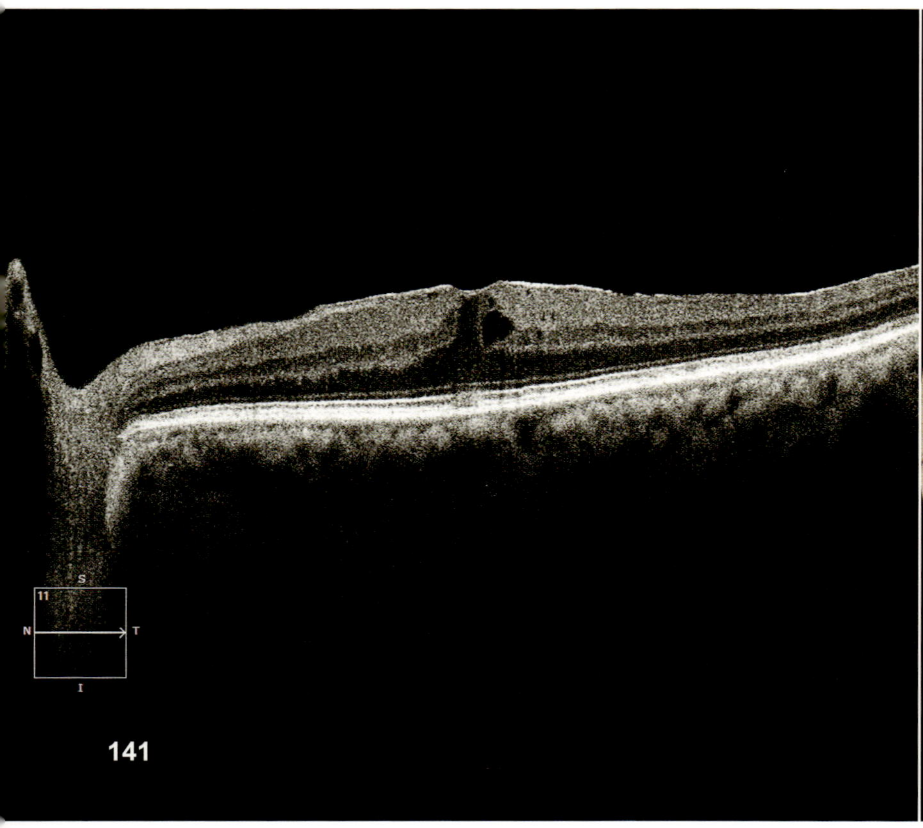


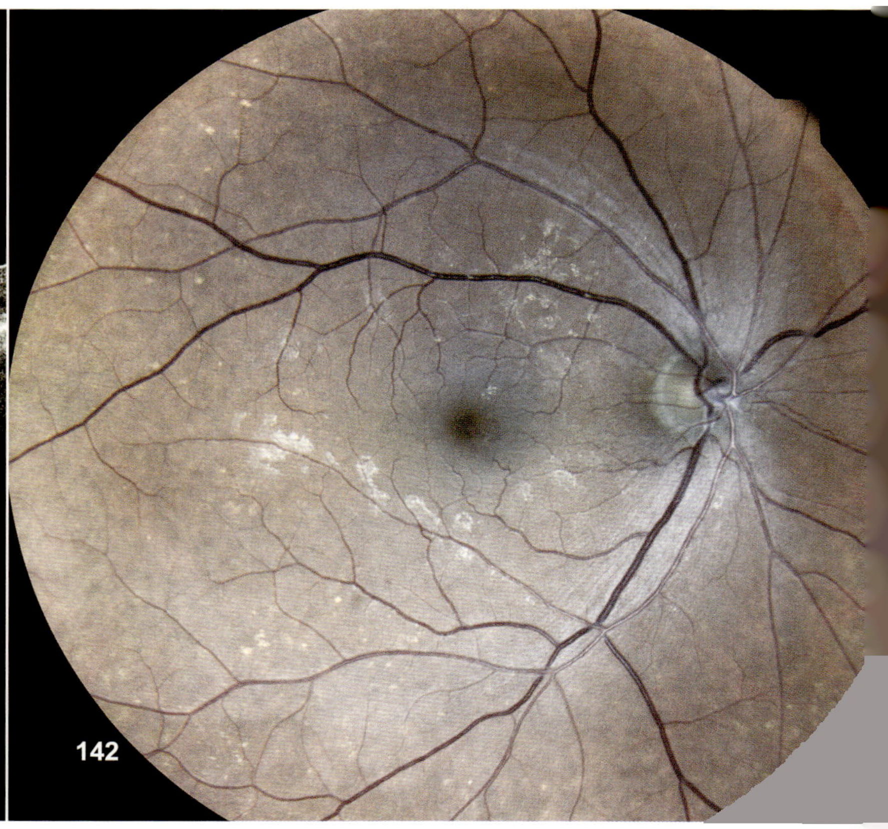


Figure 141 *OCT scan of the left eye demonstrating loss of foveal profile, hyper-reflective membrane at the surface of the retina and few cystic fluid pockets as a result of macular edema.*

Figure 142 *Color fundus photograph of the right eye demonstrates subclinical detection of cellophane reflex at the posterior pole. Patient is asymptomatic at this stage.*

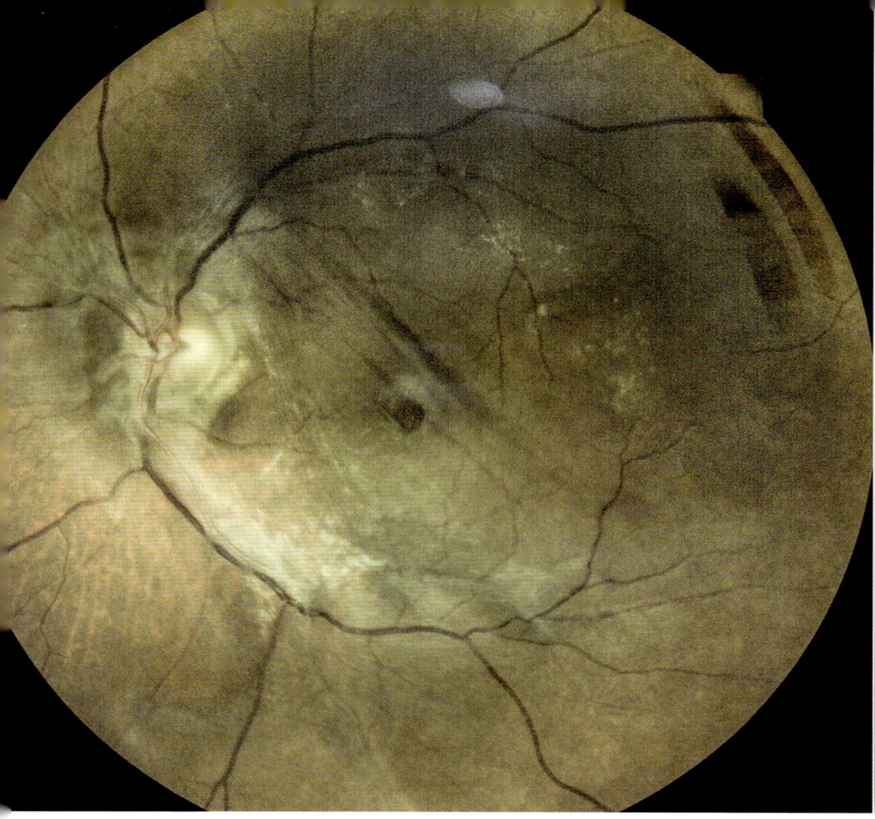

Figure 143 *A 74-year-old female presented with complaints of decrease in vision from her left eye for the past 2 months. She was known hypertensive. She also complained of metamorphopsia. BCVA was 6/36. Fundus photo of left eye shows a thick grayish membrane like structure extending from the disk inferotemporally to involve the macula, few oblique folds can be seen at the macula because of taut membrane. In some cases, epiretinal membranes may mimic the appearance of a macular hole, known as pseudohole. The same can be appreciated in the fundus photograph. Arteriosclerosis can also be seen in retinal blood vessels suggestive of hypertensive retinopathy. Media appears hazy due to nuclear sclerosis.*

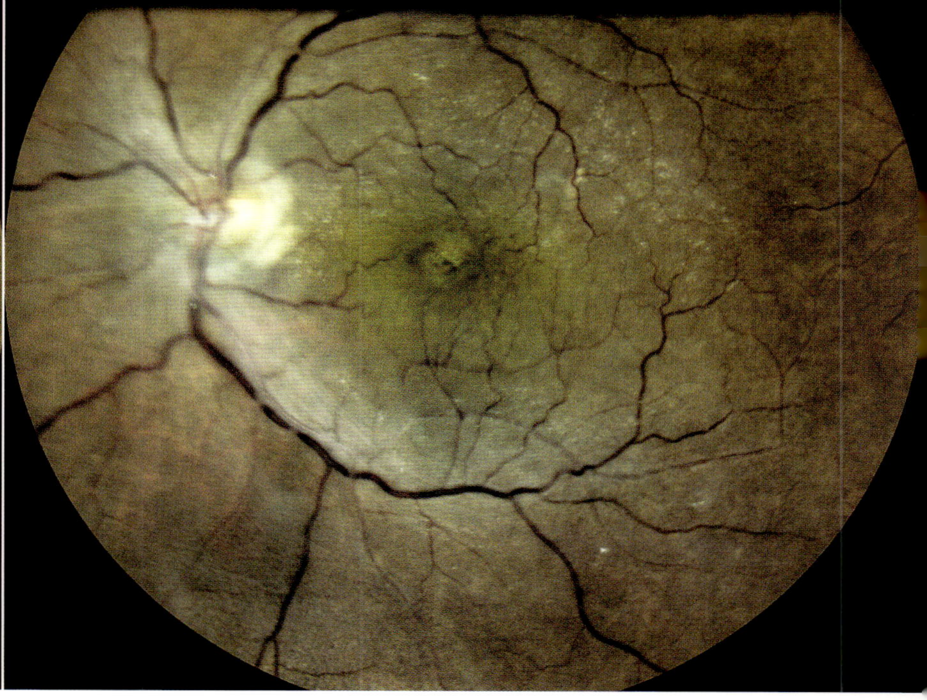

Figure 144 *Combined cataract surgery with intraocular lens implantation and 27-gauge pars plana vitrectomy to remove epiretinal membrane with intraocular tamponade using vital dyes (chromovitrectomy) which help visualizing intraocular tissues was done. At 3 weeks postoperative follow-up fundus photo shows complete removal of epiretinal membrane with residual intraocular gas bubble (around 20%), media clarity is also improved with implantation of intraocular lens.*

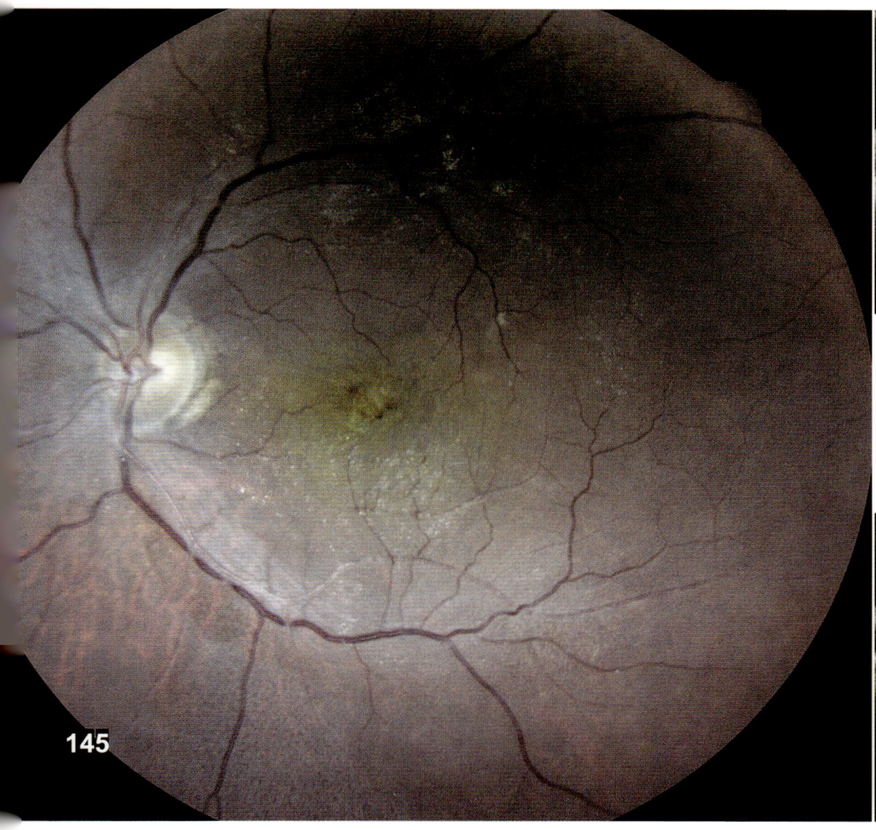


Figure 145 *At 6-week follow-up, the gas bubble diffused out completely, with BCVA of 6/24. Subtle retinal pigment epithelium alterations may persist in case of long standing chronic epiretinal membranes as can be seen in the foveal region, limiting visual acuity gain despite good anatomical outcome.*

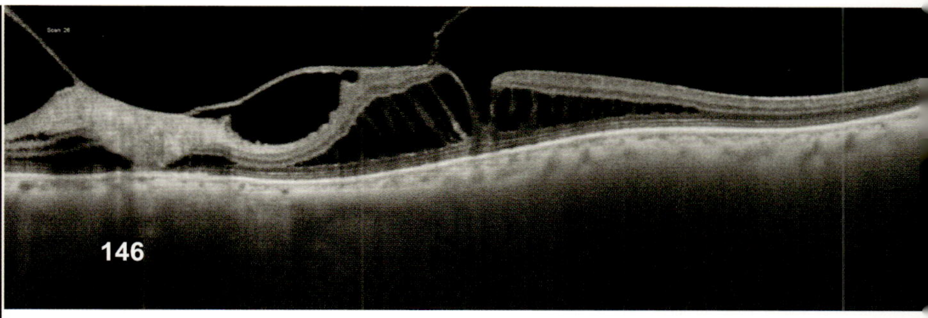


Figure 146 *OCT shows a thick hyperreflective membrane causing traction nasal to fovea and large vertical hyporeflective spaces suggestive of retinoschisis.*

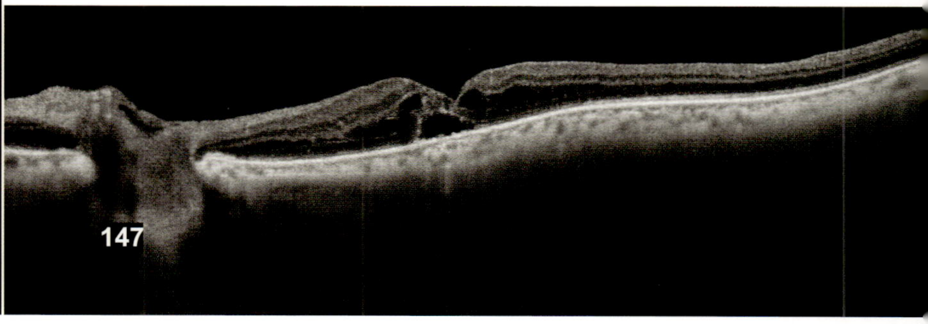


Figure 147 *Reduction in schitic spaces and total removal of epiretinal membrane can be seen on postoperative scan, shallow subfoveal fluid persists which may resolve with time.* □

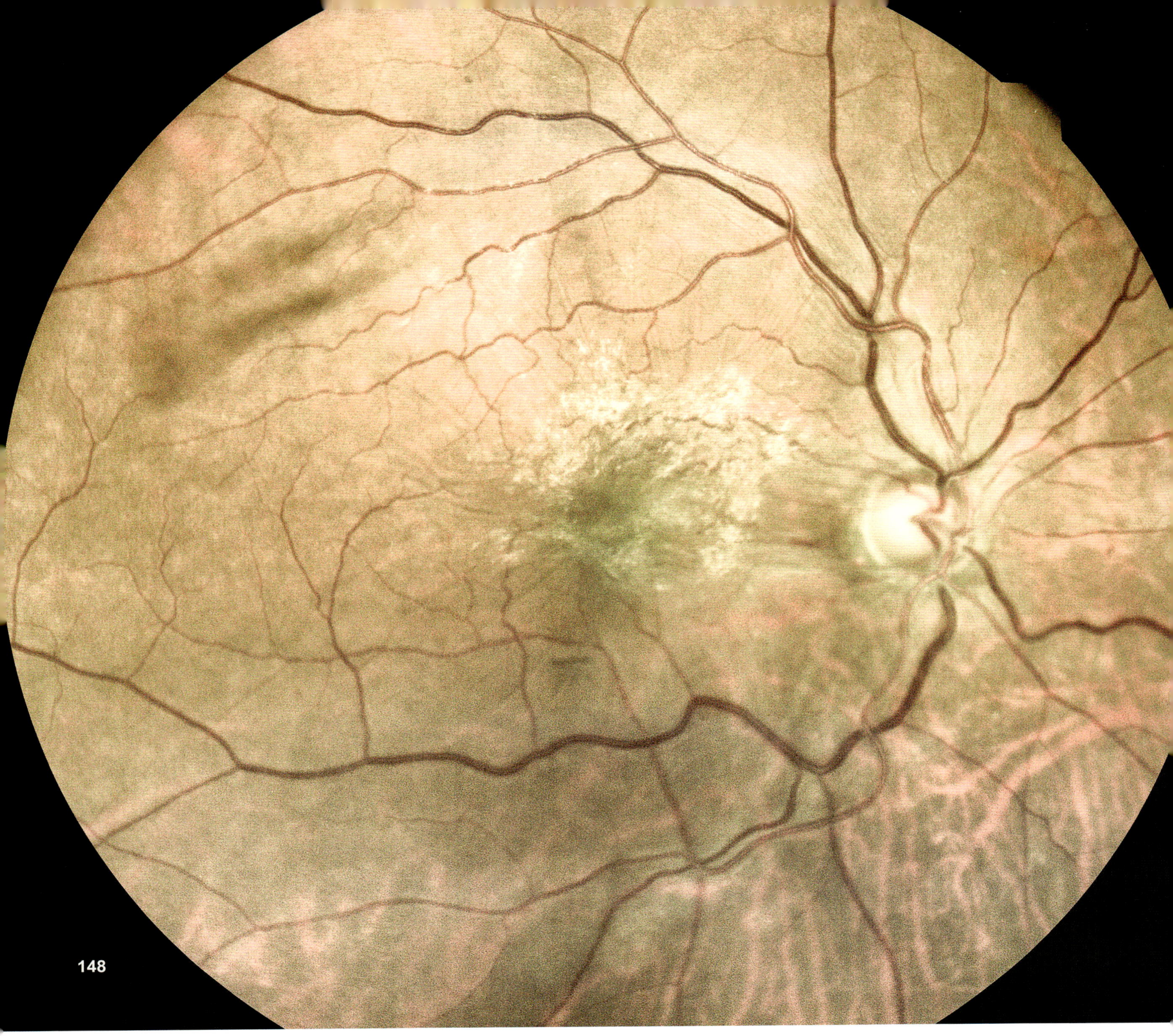


Figure 148 *A case of clinically significant epiretinal membrane managed with 25-gauge pars plana vitrectomy.*

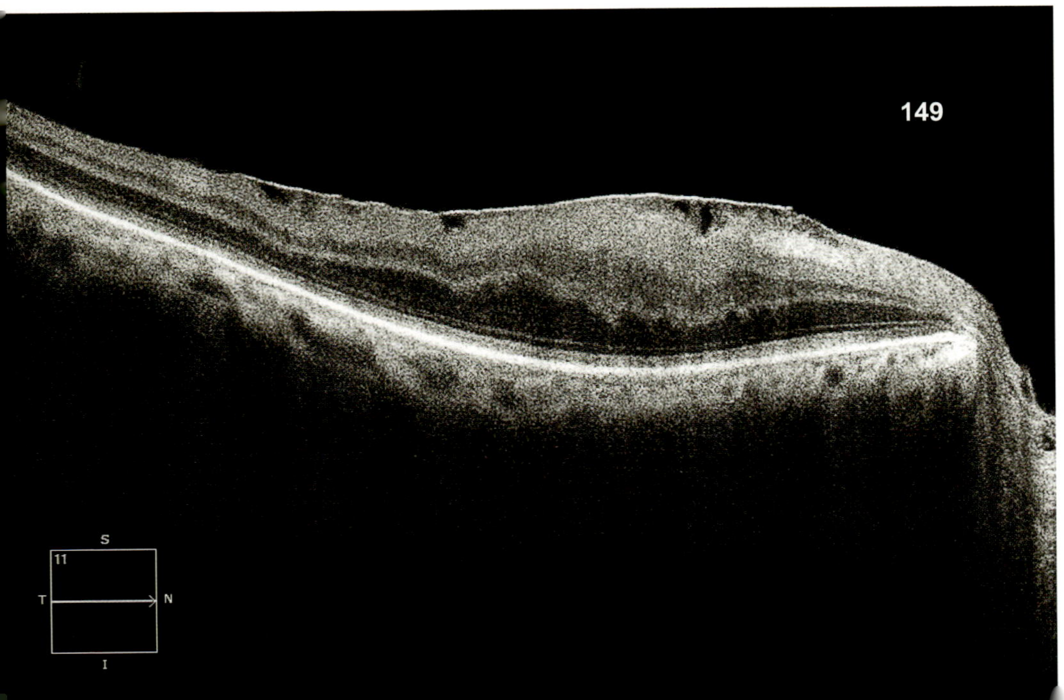


A 54-year-old male presented with complaints of decrease in vision and distortion from his right eye since 2 months. BCVA was 6/24.

Fundus photo of right eye shows a thick grayish white opaque fibrous membrane at the macula which is leading to retinal surface wrinkling also known as macular pucker. This epiretinal membrane is present at the fovea and in very dense leading to it being more clinically apparent as well as has a significant impact on vision and reading ability of the patient.

Figure 149 *OCT also shows thick hyper-reflective membrane on retinal surface involving fovea distorting foveal architecture and causing increase in central retinal thickness.*

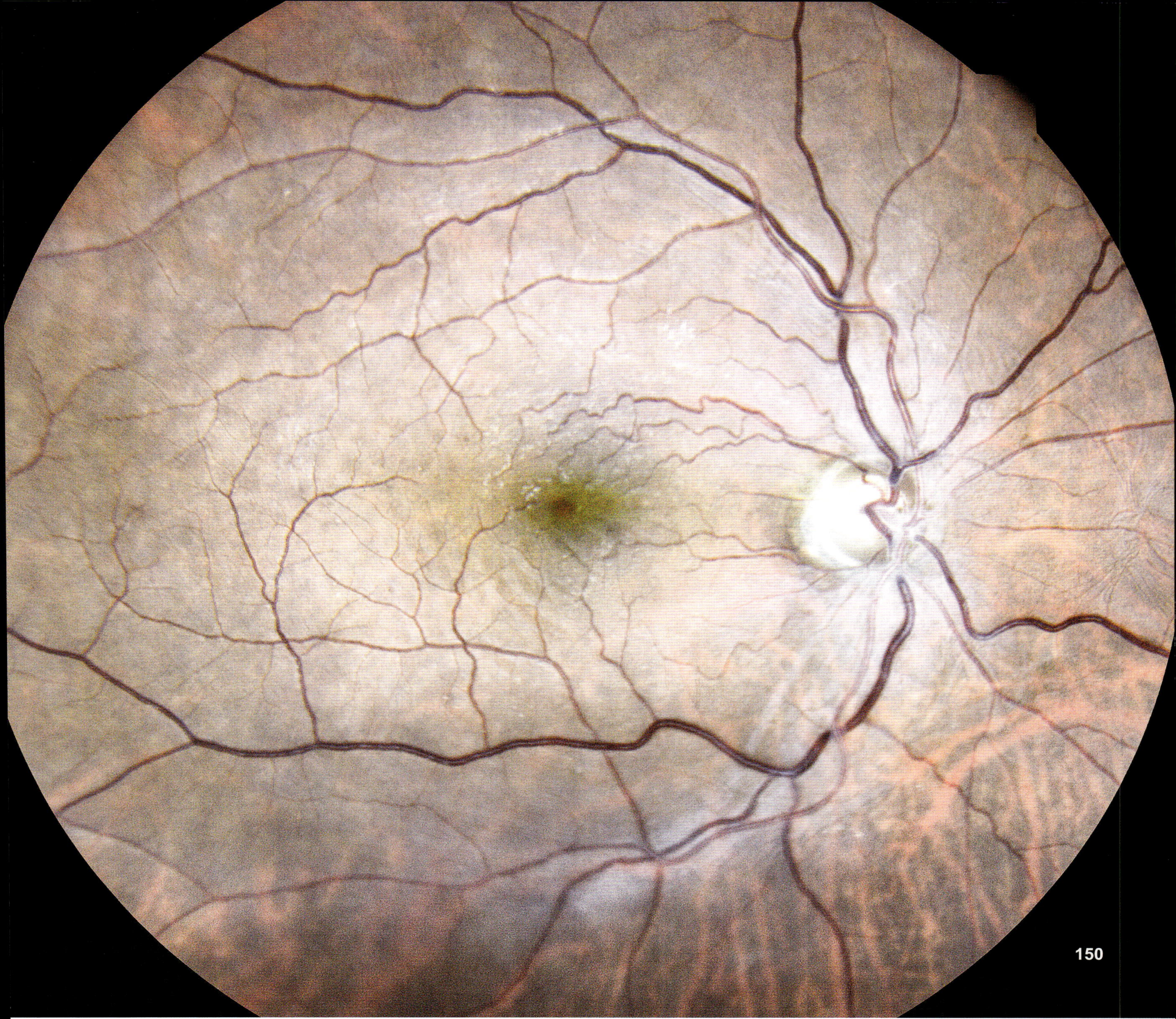


Figure 150 *He under went a 25G pars plana vitrectomy in view of visually significant metamorphopsia. Dyes like brilliant blue green to counter stain the internal limiting membrane may be used, which aids in highlighting the epiretinal membrane, helping ensure complete removal. Color fundus photo shows complete removal of the fibrous tissue presents at macula, foveal reflex can be appreciated and good anatomical contour of macula can be seen.*

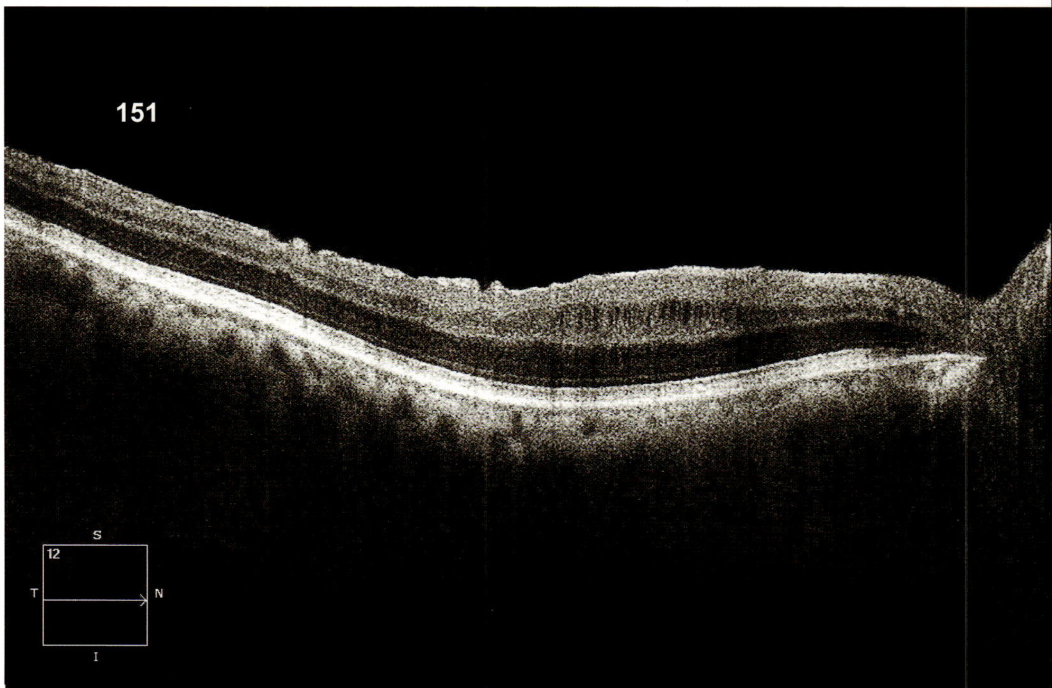


Figure 151 *Postoperative OCT shows complete removal of hyper-reflective membrane from the retinal surface, some residual retinal schitic spaces are seen which eventually may resolve with time and need no intervention.* □

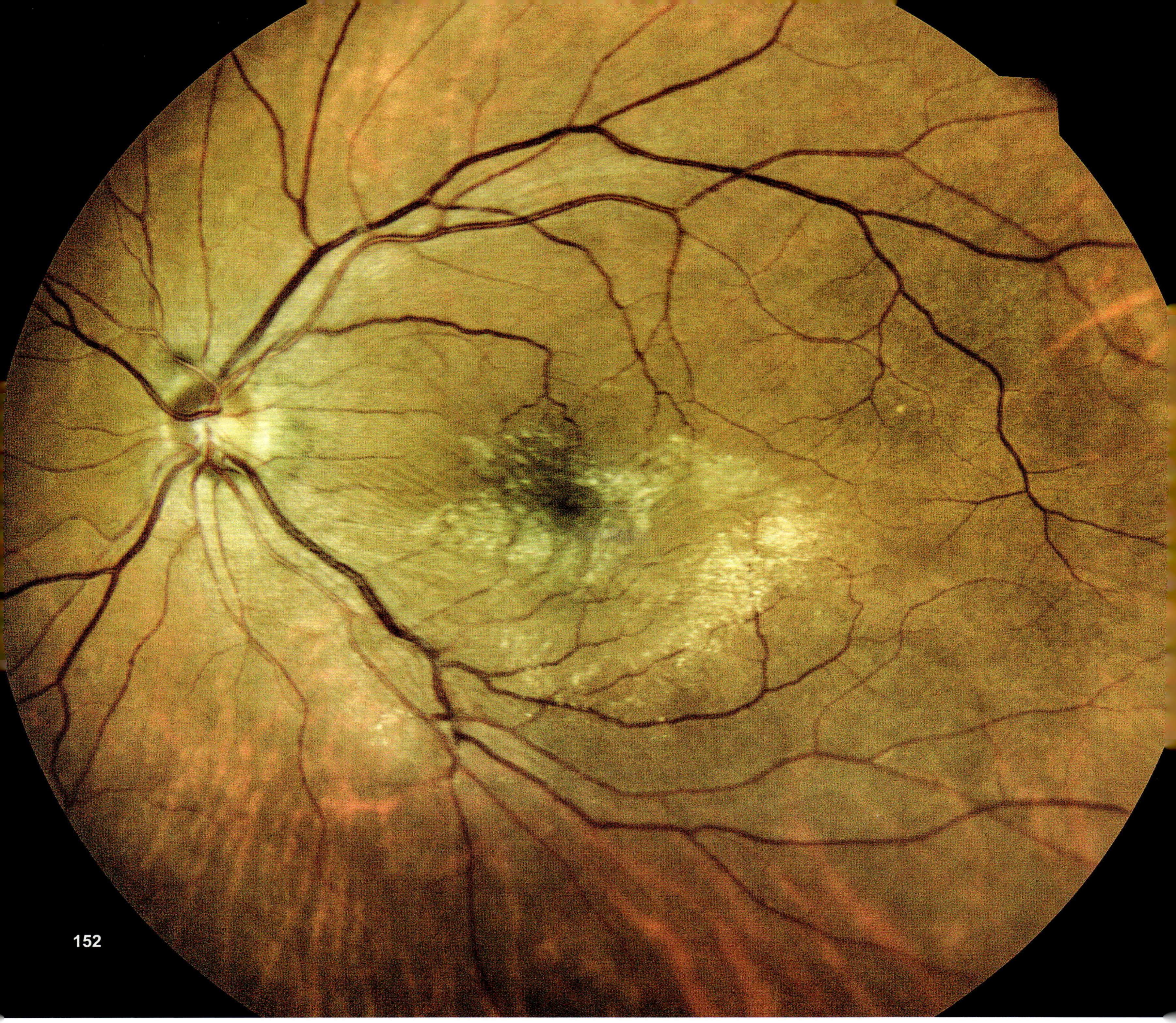

Figure 152 *A case of epiretinal membrane with cataract managed with combined cataract and pars plana vitrectomy. A 69-year-old female with BCVA of 6/9P, presented with complaints of distortion of vision from her left eye and difficulty in near vision since 2 months. Fundus photo of left eye shows grayish white cellophane reflex at the macula leading to retinal striations involving the fovea and a dull foveal reflex.*

Figure 153 *OCT of left eye demonstrates thick hyper-reflective membrane on top of the fovea, leading to distortion of underlying retina, increased central retinal thickness and loss of foveal pit. OCT of the right eye clearly demonstrates a bright hyper-reflective membrane like structure on top of the neurosensory retina temporally sparing the fovea. OCT is an excellent tool to monitor such cases.*

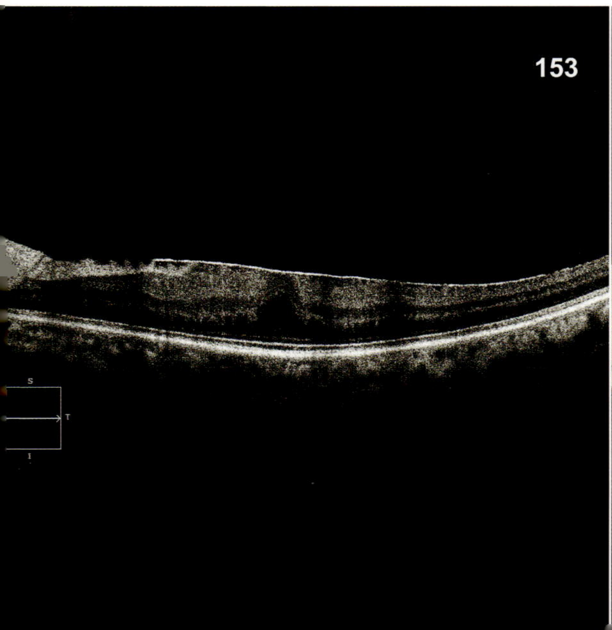

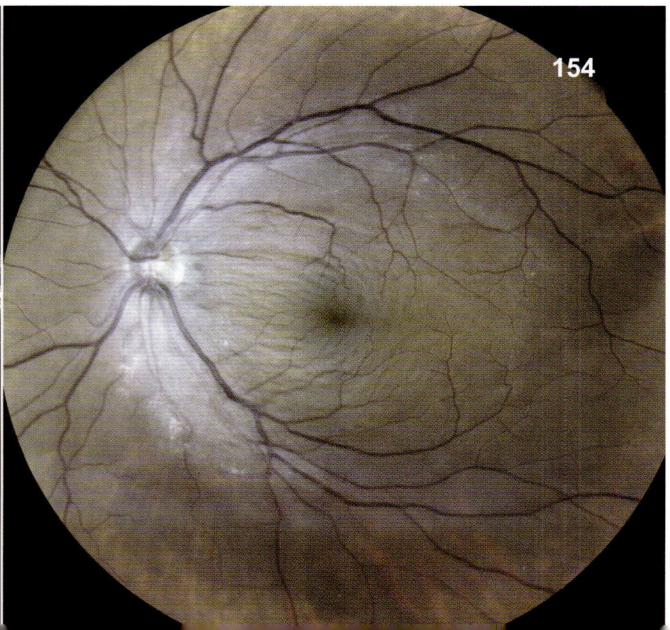

Figure 154

*25-gauge pars plana vitrectomy with epiretinal membrane peeling using adjuvants such as intravitreal dye was performed. Postoperatively complete removal of epiretinal membrane can be seen from the fovea. Some residual striations can be seen owing to long standing traction of the membrane which gradually may settle over few months.* □

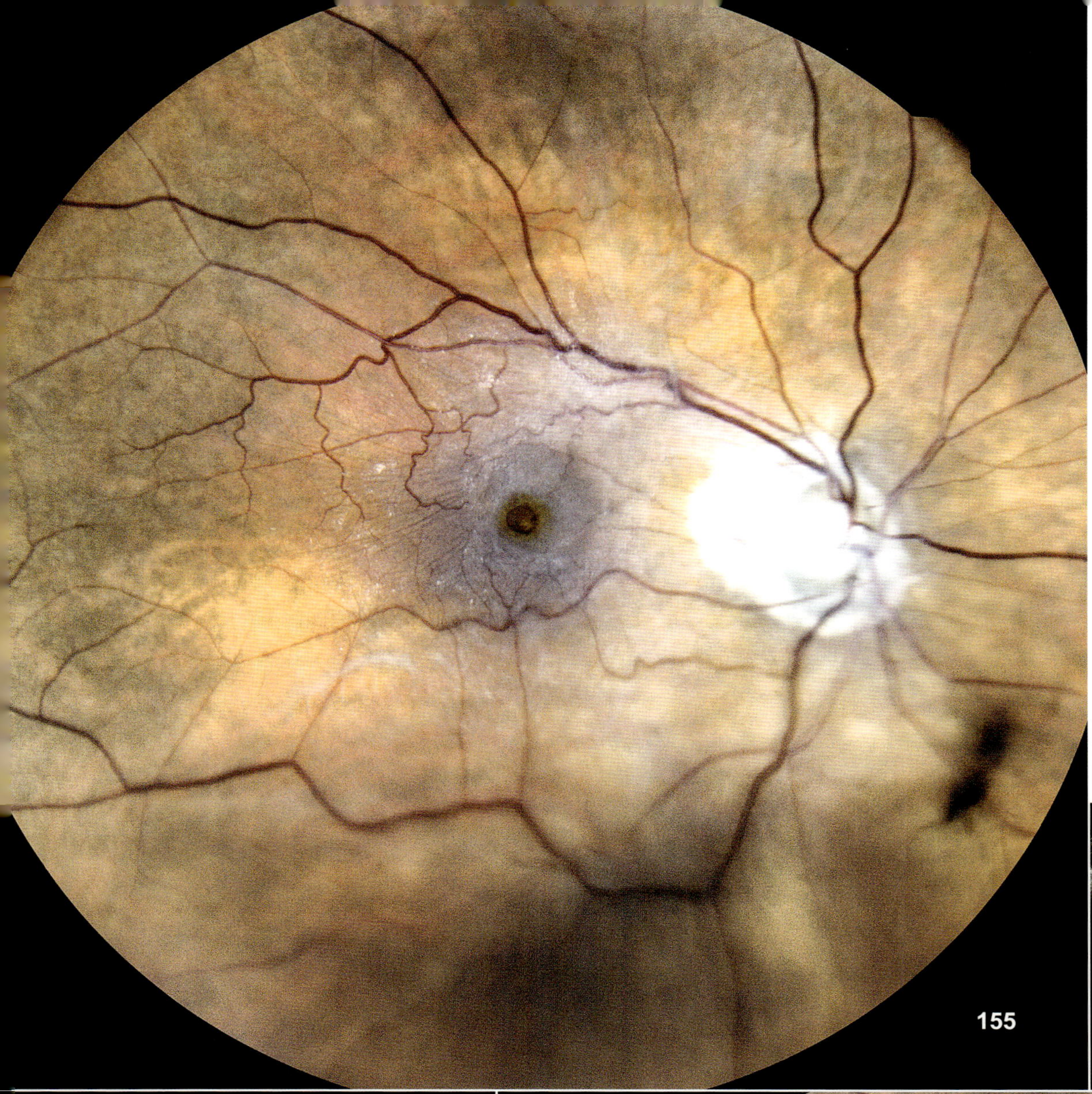

Figure 155

*An 88-year-old male presented with complaints of decrease in vision from his right eye since 2 months. BCVA was 6/9P in his right eye. Color fundus photo shows thick grayish white membrane at the macula involving the fovea causing folds on retinal surface suggestive of epiretinal membrane. At the fovea a bright reddish-orange circular defect is seen suggestive of pseudomacular hole.*

Figure 156

*Preoperative OCT demonstrates a fine linear hyper-reflective structure on top of retina distorting the fovea, increasing central retinal thickness, causing a vertically elongated hyporeflective cyst-like space at the fovea.*

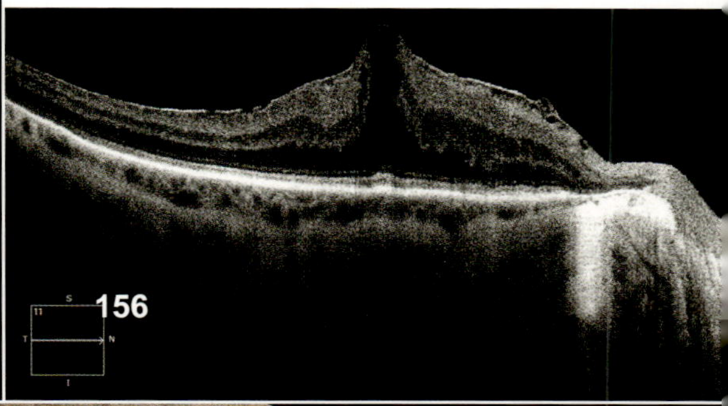

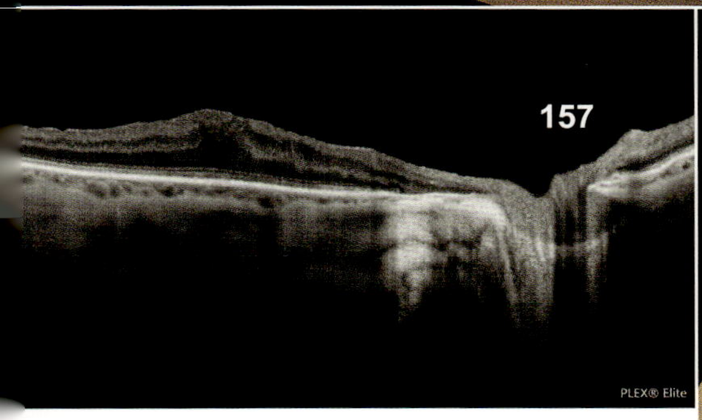


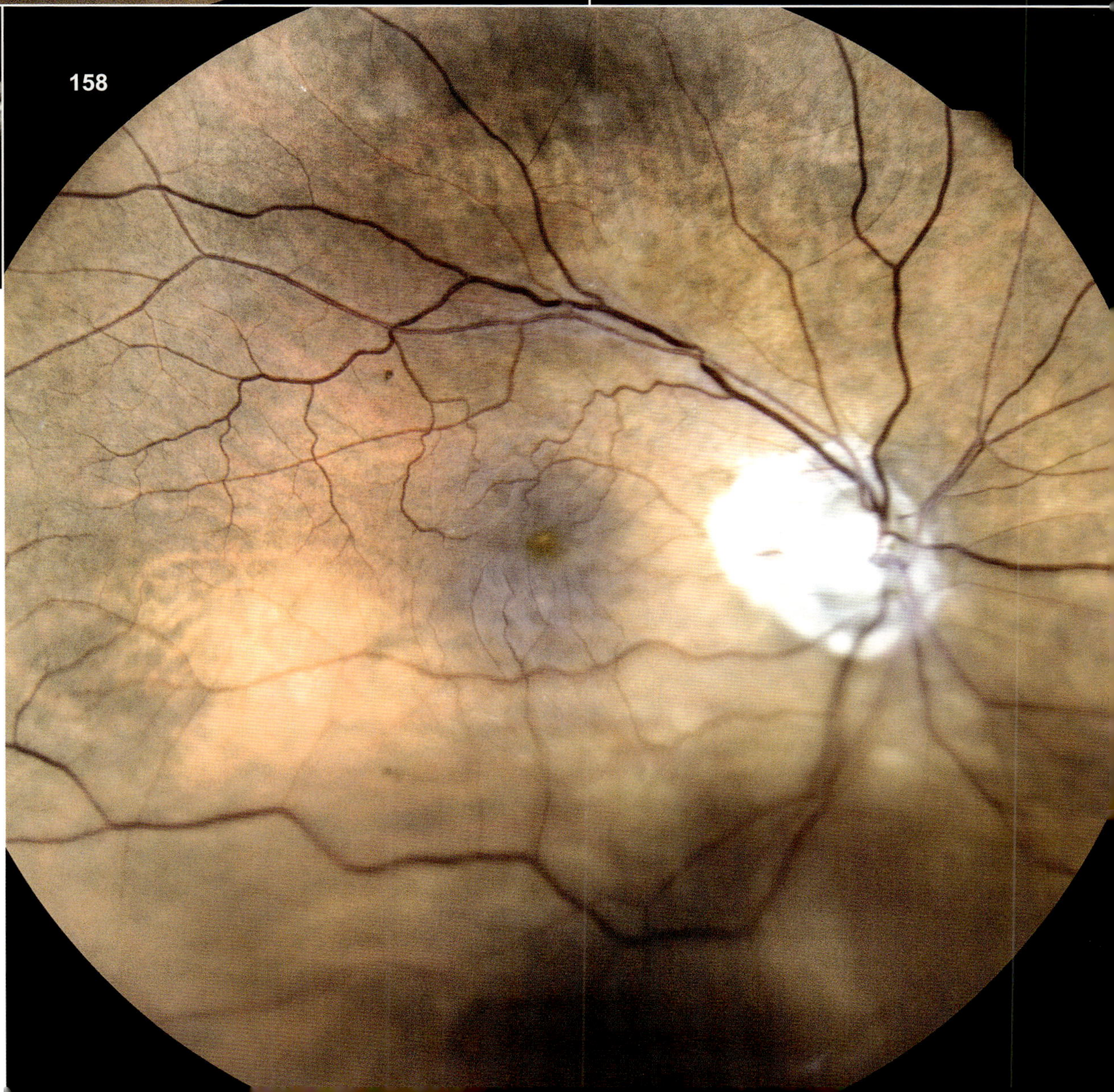

Figure 157

*Postoperatively there is complete removal of the hyper-reflective membrane, significant reduction in central retinal thickness, and also reduction in number of cystic spaces. Few hyporeflective spaces in nasal aspect of retina persist which may disappear over a few months of follow-up.*

Figure 158

*25G PPV with ERM peel with internal limiting membrane (ILM) peeling was done. Intraoperative use of dyes such as brilliant blue green assists in staining of internal limiting membrane in turn "negatively staining" the epiretinal membrane to help remove it entirely.* □

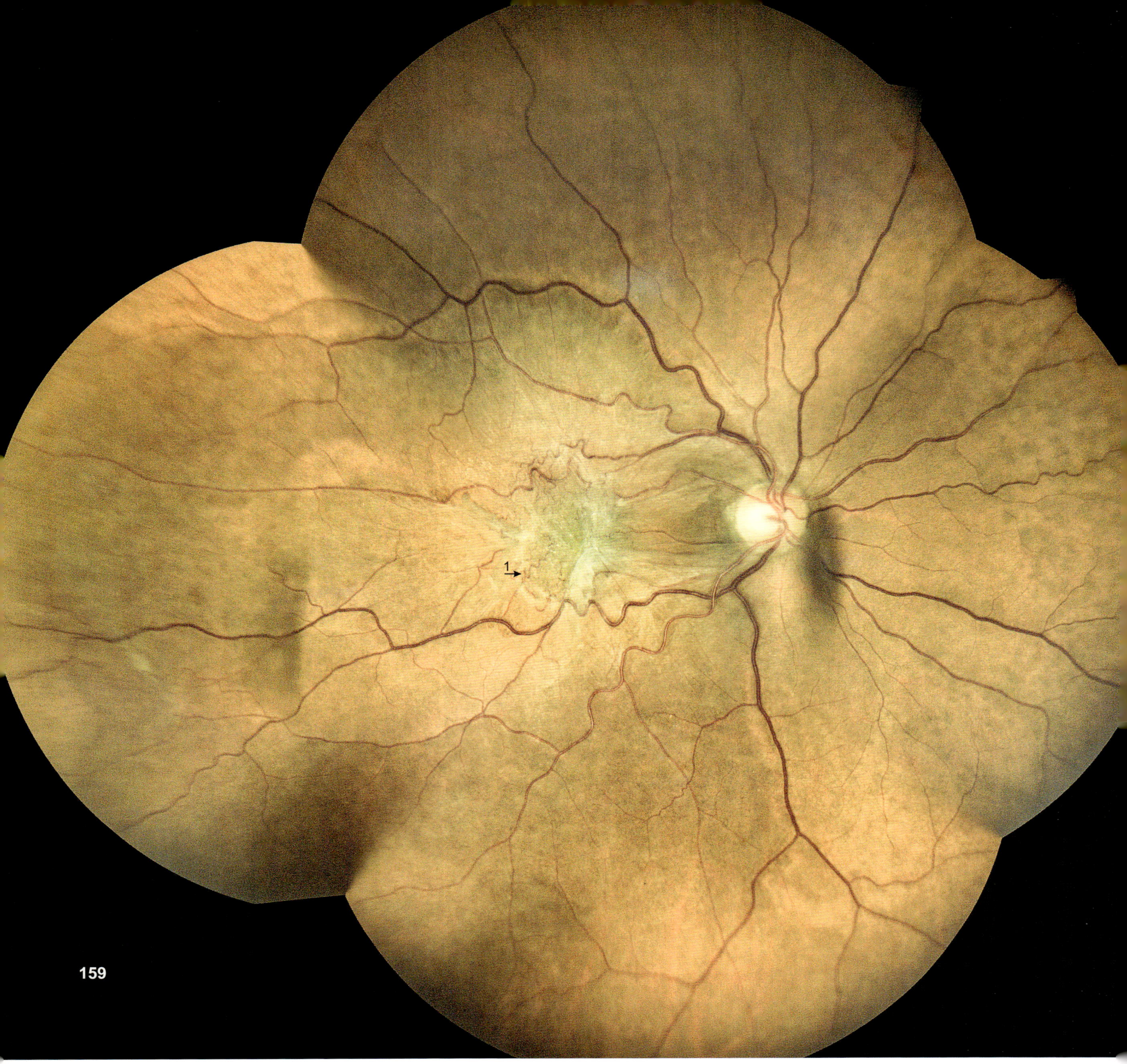


Figure 159 *A case of thick epiretinal membrane along with nuclear cataract managed with combined cataract and pars plana vitrectomy.*

A 68-year-old female presented with complaints of distortion of vision from her right eye since past 3 months. Fundus photo demonstrates thick grayish opaque membrane at the macula causing distortion of vascular architecture and macular puckering suggestive of pre-retinal macular fibrosis (1).

Most common etiology of macular pucker is age related, although it may be associated with several ocular conditions like previous retinal detachment surgery, diabetic retinopathy, venous occlusive disease or associated with intraocular inflammation.

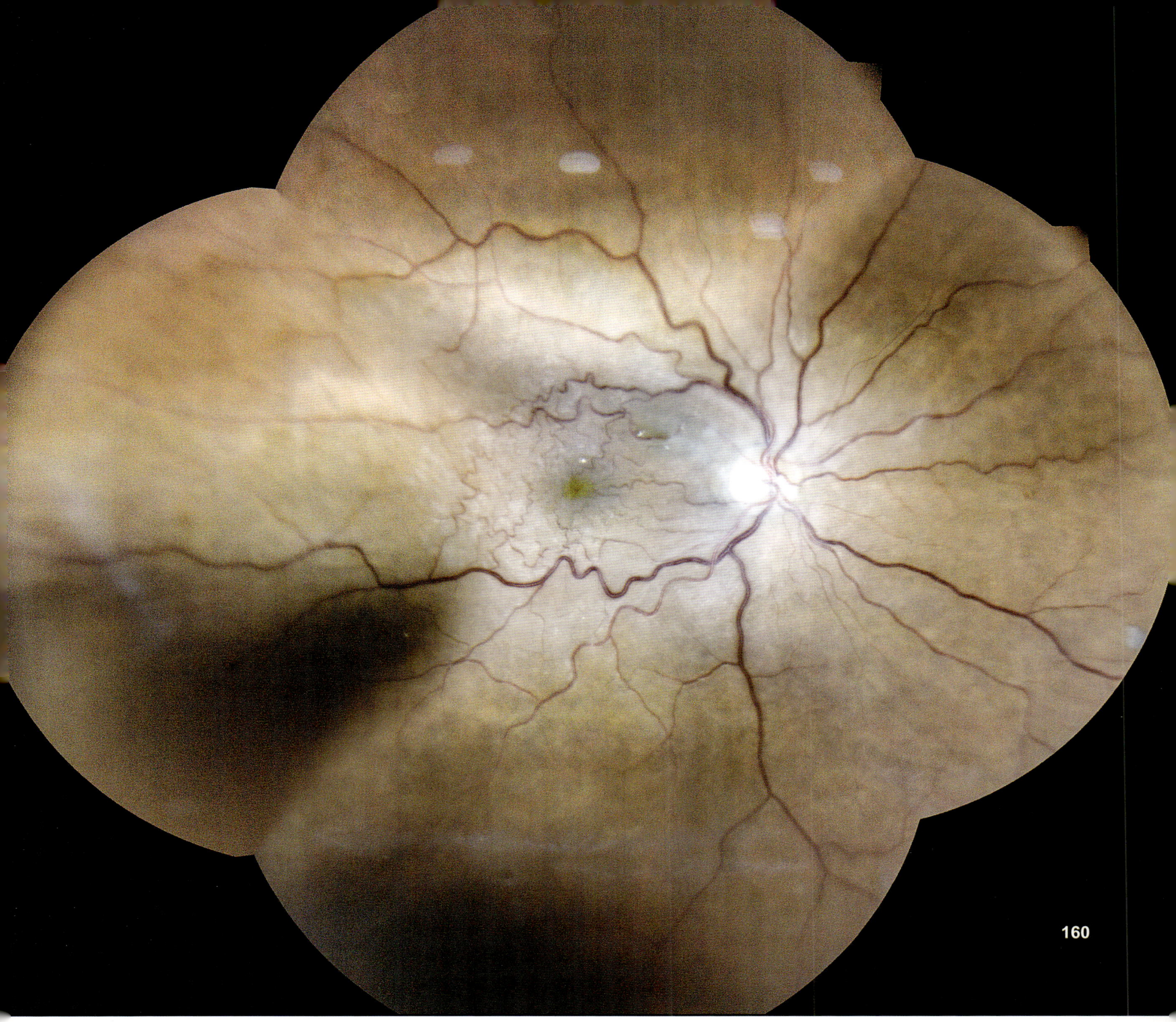

Figure 160 *25-gauge PPV was done, using intraocular dye to counter stain the epiretinal membrane against the highlighted internal limiting membrane. Postoperative photo shows complete removal of the grayish membrane like structure. Some amount of vascular network distortion persists at the macula.*

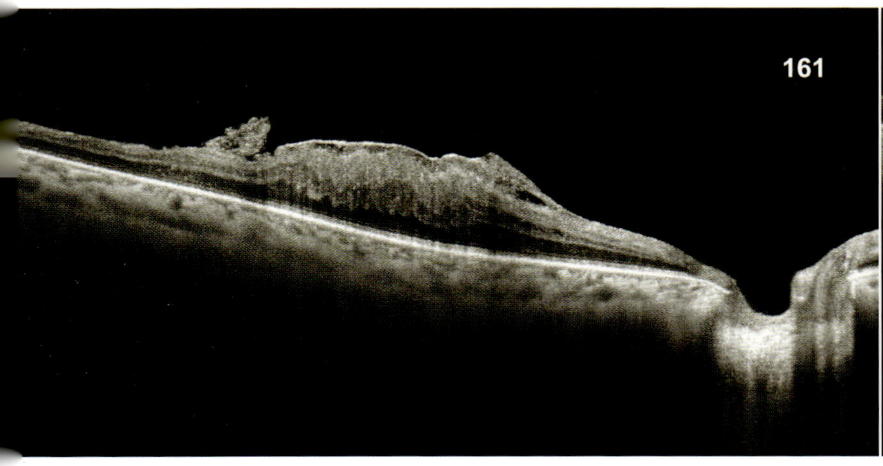

Figure 161 *SS-OCT demonstrated thick hyper-reflective membrane like linear structure at the macula causing gross increase in thickness of retina and significant distortion of inner retinal layers. Temporally thick fibrocellular tissue of epiretinal membrane has folded upon itself to form a globular elevated structure.*

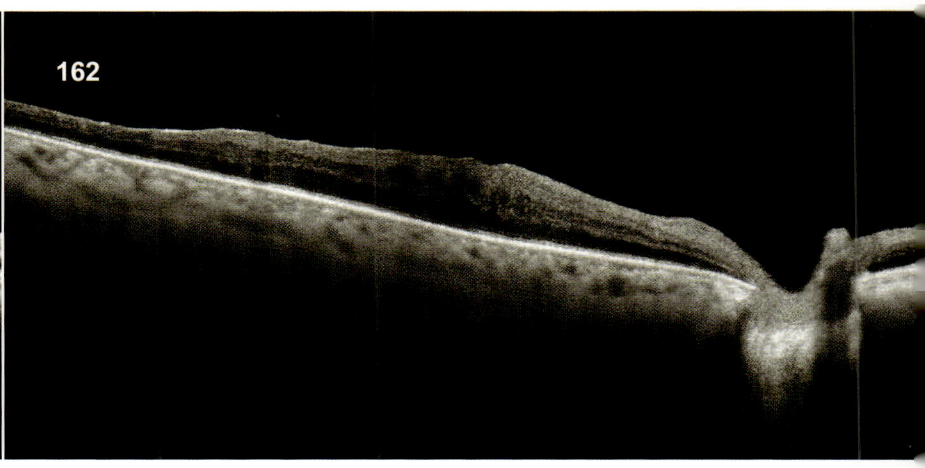

Figure 162 *OCT scan at 4 weeks postoperatively reveals complete removal of epiretinal membrane, reduction of central retinal thickness. However, some amount of residual retinal thickness persists which may decrease over a course of 3–6 months as the inciting traction is relieved and no additional intervention is required.* □

Figure 163

*A case of macular hole managed with 25-gauge pars plana vitrectomy.*

A 68-year-old female presented with complaints of recent drop in vision from her left eye. BCVA was 3/60 with near vision N60. Fundus examination of left eye shows well-defined circular defect at the fovea (1). Cuff of subretinal fluid can be seen all around it (2). Small yellowish precipitates can be seen at the base of hole. Age-related yellowish deposits can be seen at the macula (3).

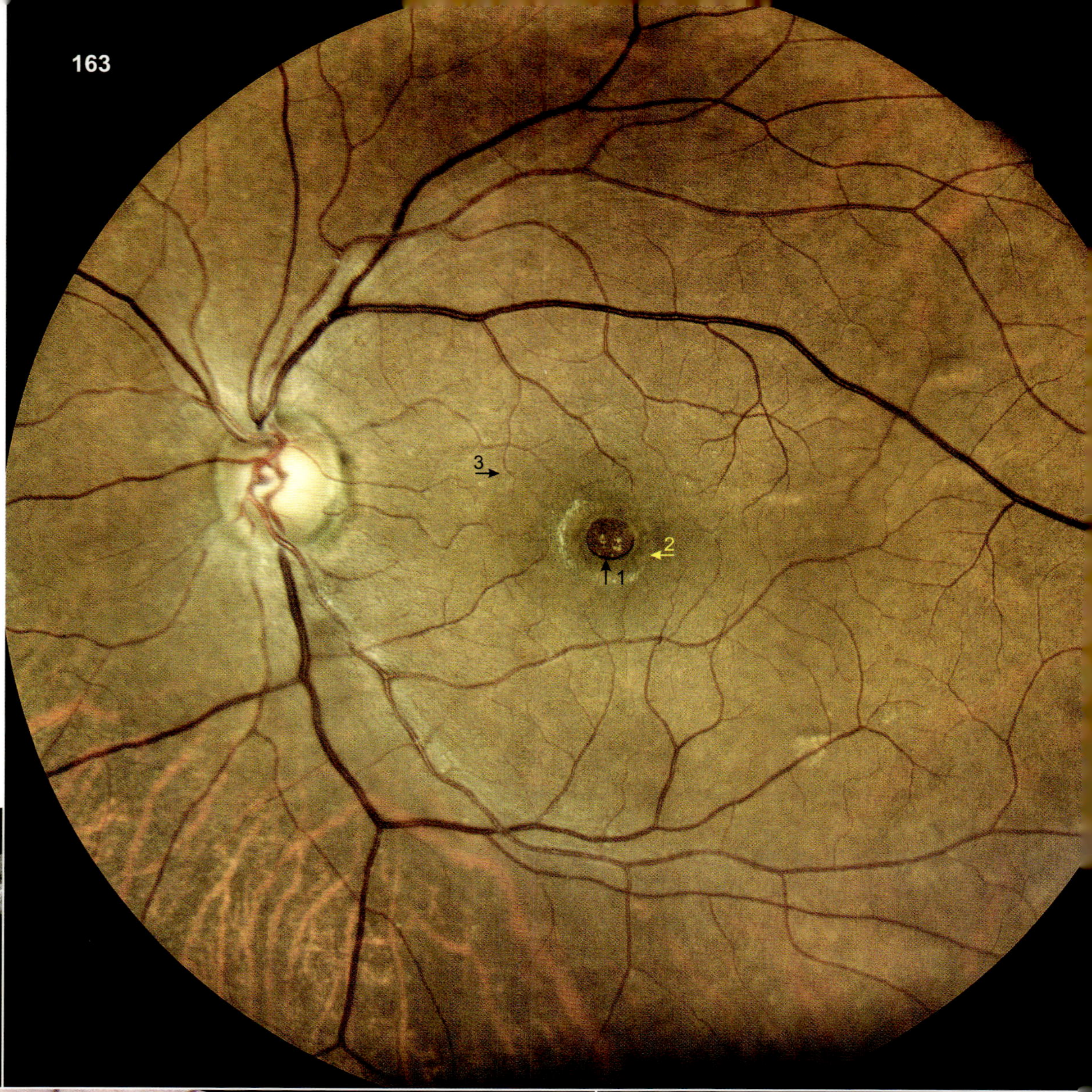


Figure 164

*OCT is gold standard for diagnosis, staging and management of macular holes. Here it shows a full thickness defect at the fovea along with few cystoid spaces in neurosensory retina at the edge of macular hole.*

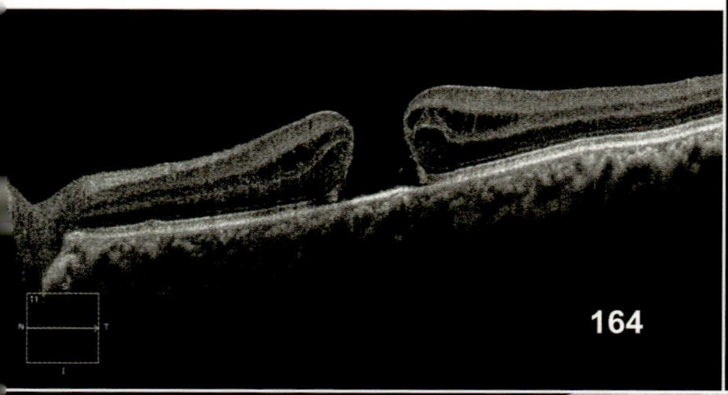


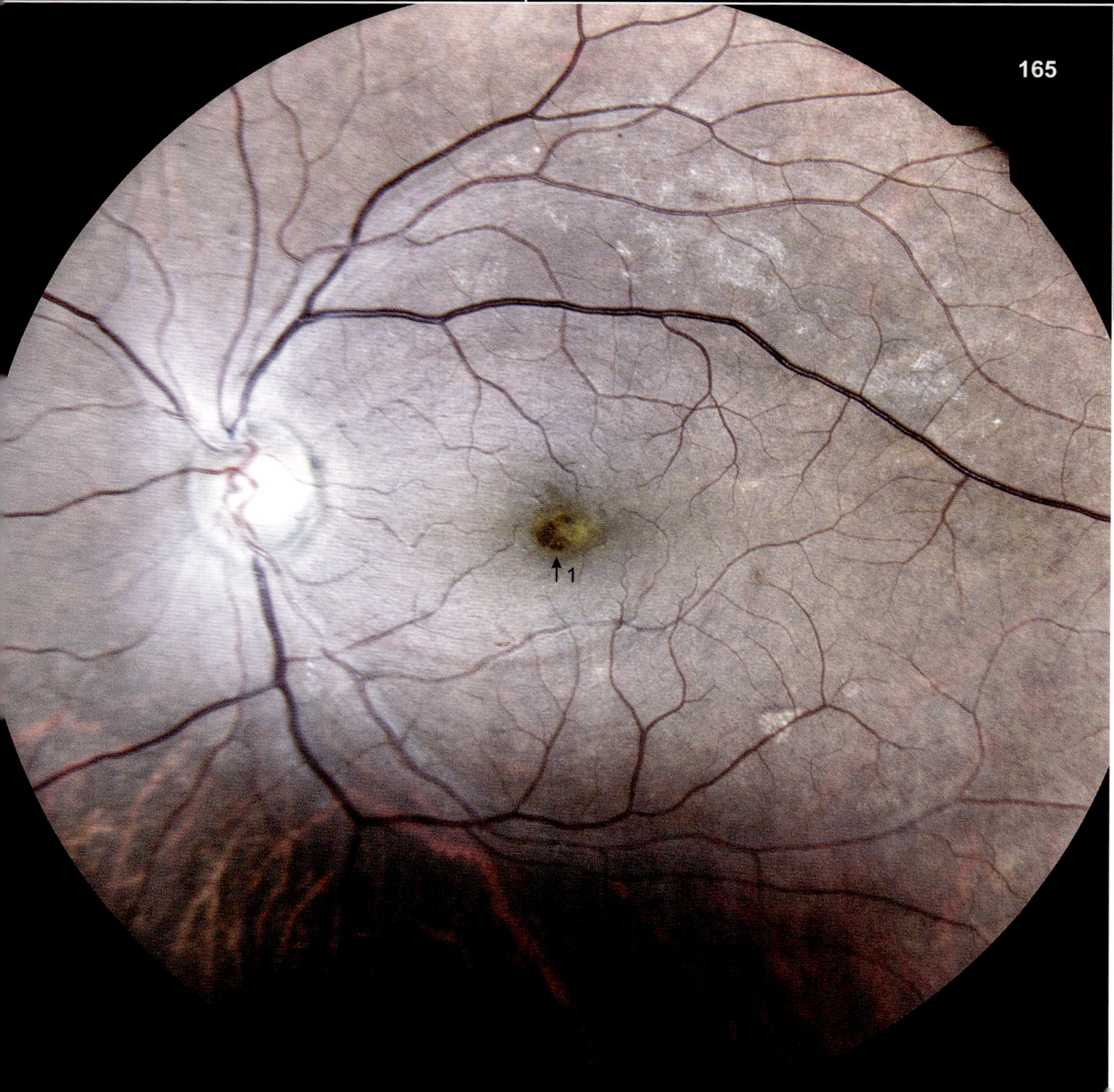


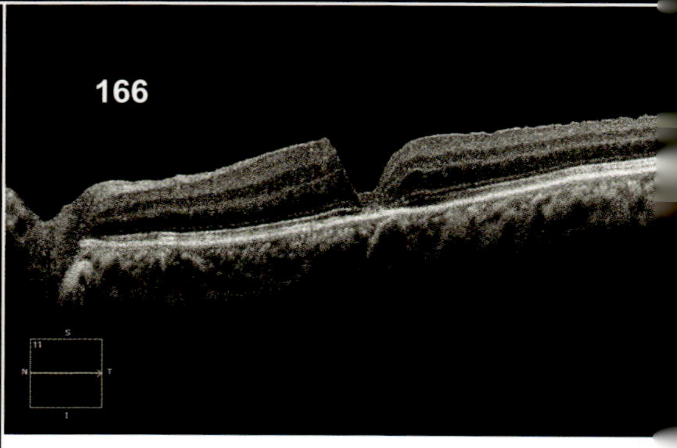


Figure 165

*A combined cataract surgery along with 25G pars plana vitrectomy with internal limiting membrane peel with internal tamponade (intraocular gas) was performed. Six weeks post-operatively intraocular gas resolved. Closed macular hole can be seen on fundus photo (1).*

Figure 166

*Postoperative OCT shows closed macular hole with type "V" closure. Subtle alterations of retinal pigment epithelium and IS-OS junction can be seen on OCT.* □

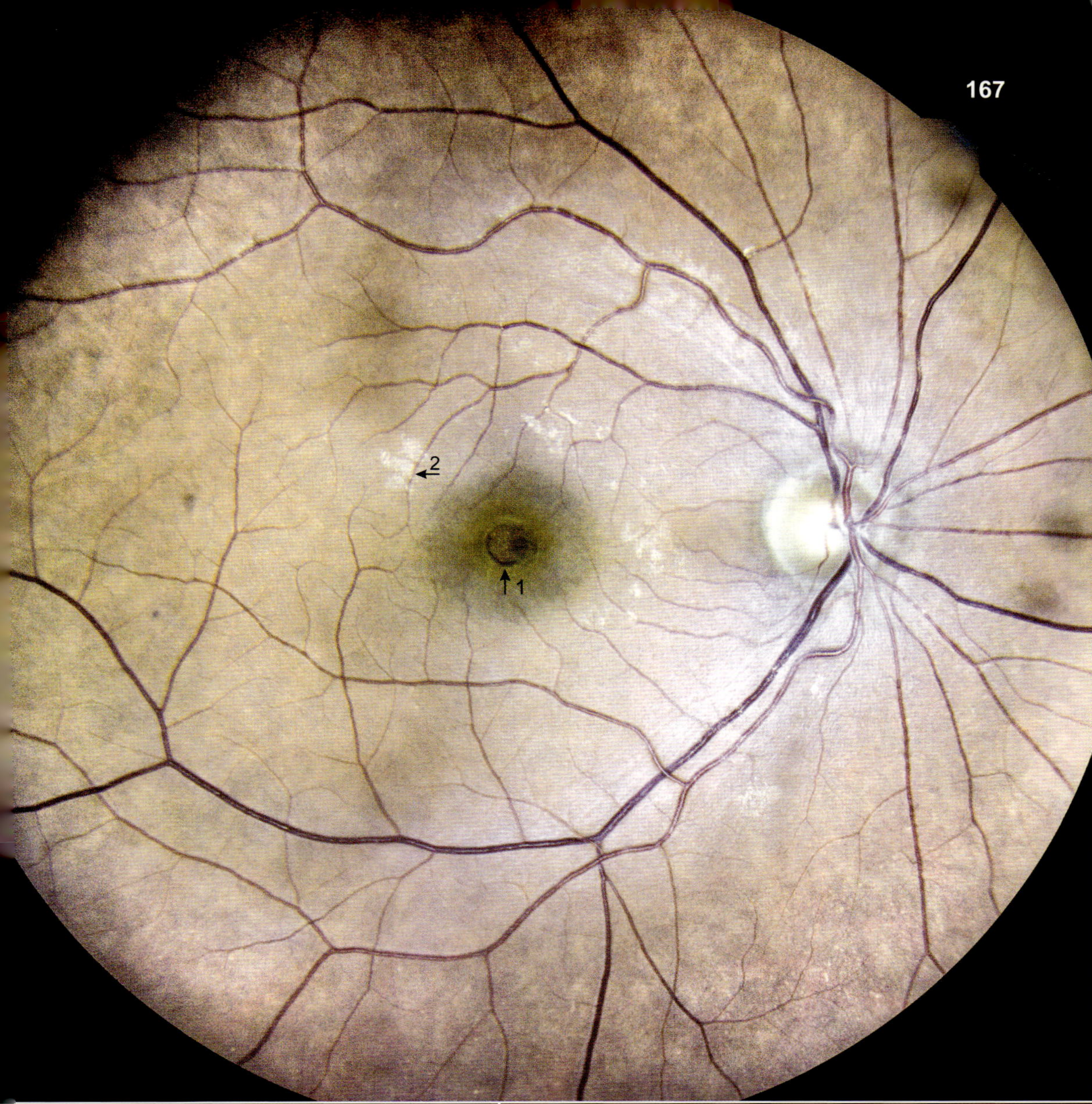


Figure 167

*A 75-year-old male presented with complaints of blurred vision for reading from his right eye since past 15 days. BCVA was 6/36. Fundus photo of right eye shows a full thickness circular defect at the fovea along with a rim of subretinal fluid all around it (1). Mild cellophane reflex can also be seen nasal and superior to the fovea suggestive of ERM (2).*

Figure 168

*OCT shows a full thickness macular hole visible as a complete defect in all retinal layers at the fovea with large cystoid spaces at the rim of the macular hole. Complete separation of vitreous from macula is seen as we can identify a linear undulating hyper-reflective membrane-like structure in vitreous cavity.*

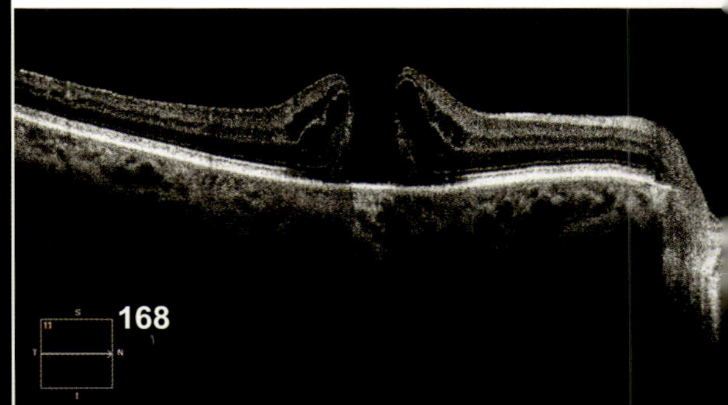


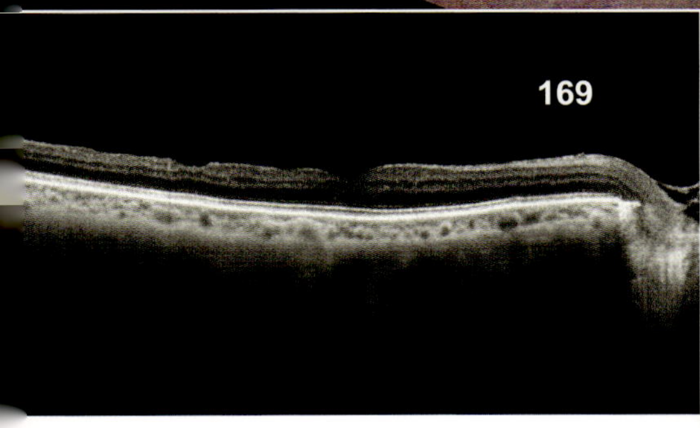


Figure 169

*Postoperative OCT demonstrates complete closure of macular hole with restoration of good foveal anatomy. IS-OS junction is intact accounting for good postoperative BCVA.*

Figure 170

*Postoperatively after 6 weeks, intraocular gas has escaped. Fundus photo shows macular hole is closed (1). BCVA was 6/9. No cellophane reflex is seen.* □

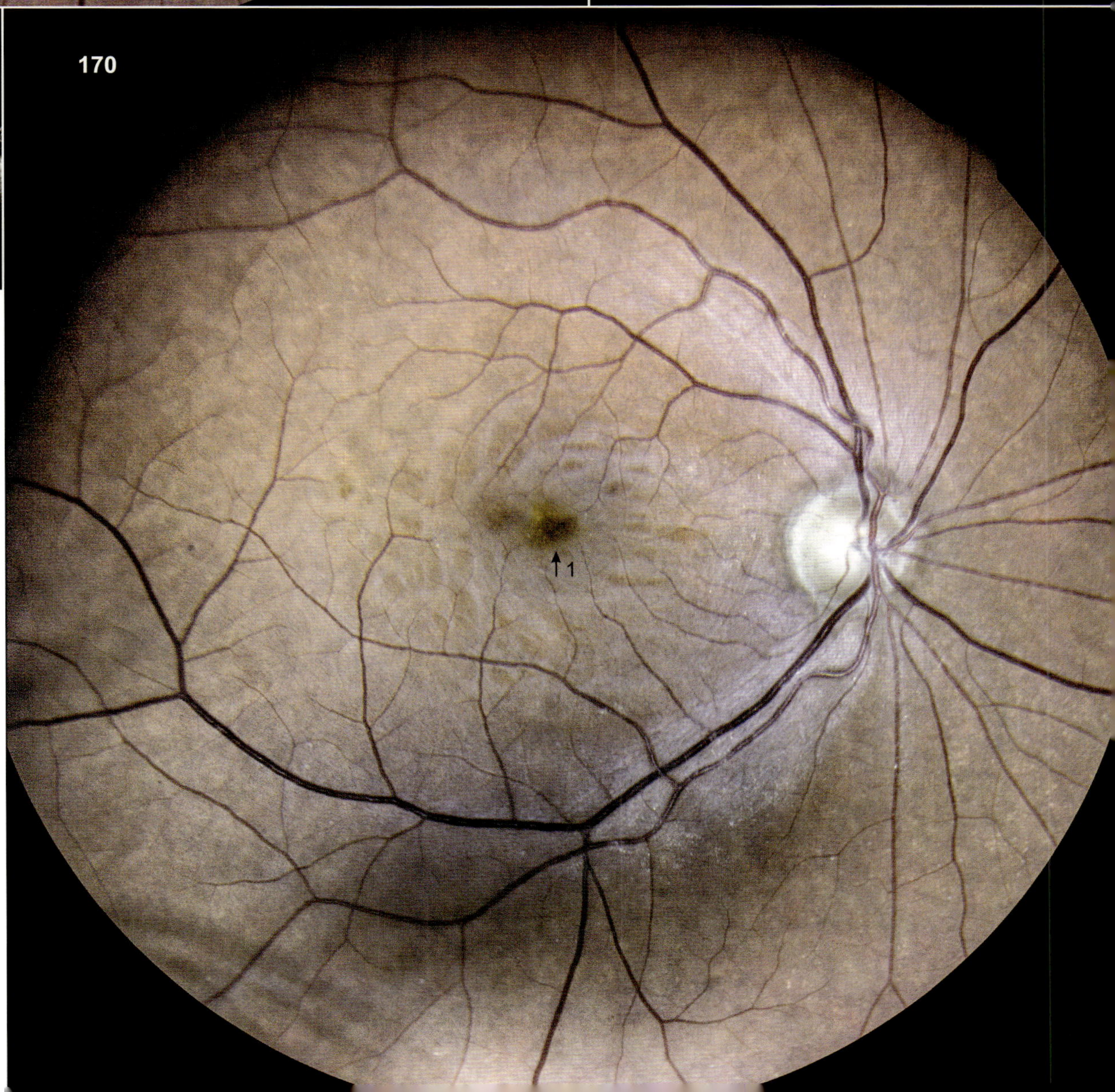

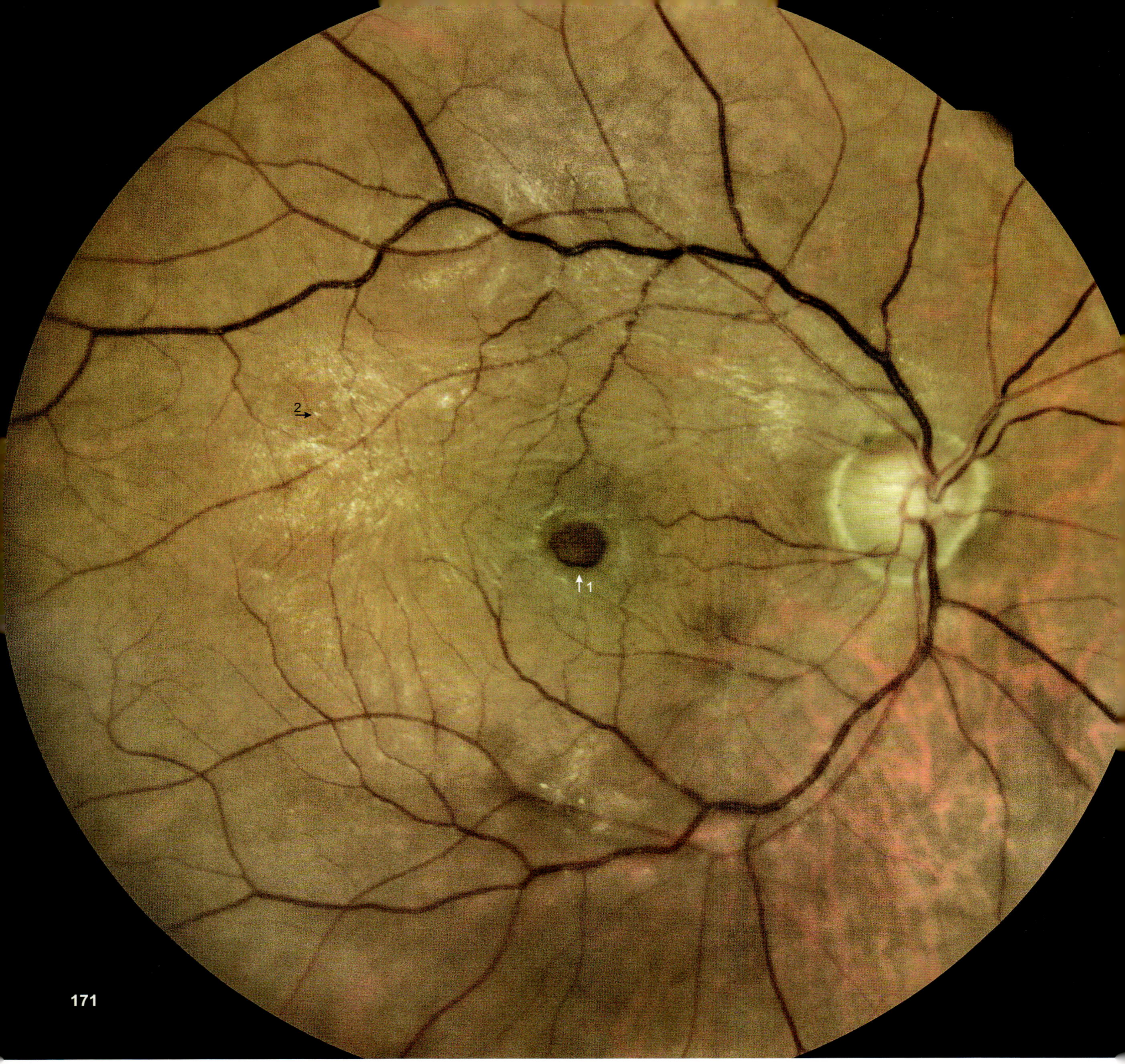


Figure 171 *A case of macular hole with epiretinal membrane managed with PPV with "double" membrane peeling.*

A 60-year-old male presented with complaints of decrease in vision from his right eye since 1 month. BCVA was CF 3 meters. Fundus photo shows a large reddish circular defect at the fovea, i.e. full thickness macular hole which is more than 400 microns (1). Cellophane reflex can be seen at macula encompassing the fovea suggestive of ERM (2).

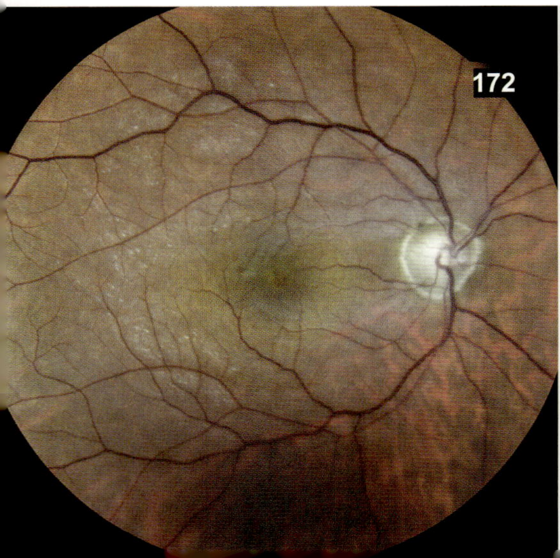


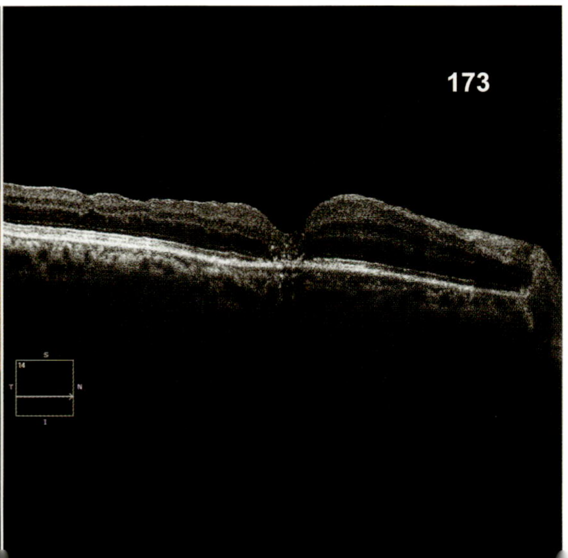


Figure 172 *He was planned for 25G PPV with epiretinal membrane removal with internal limiting membrane peeling using vital intraocular dyes. At 6 weeks postoperatively best corrected visual acuity is 6/60. Fundus photo shows media clarity grade 1 with closed macular hole and complete removal of epiretinal membrane.*

Figure 173 *OCT scan postoperatively shows complete closure of macular hole, however, there is disruption of outer retinal layers at fovea accounting for limited vision gain despite anatomical success of the procedure.* □

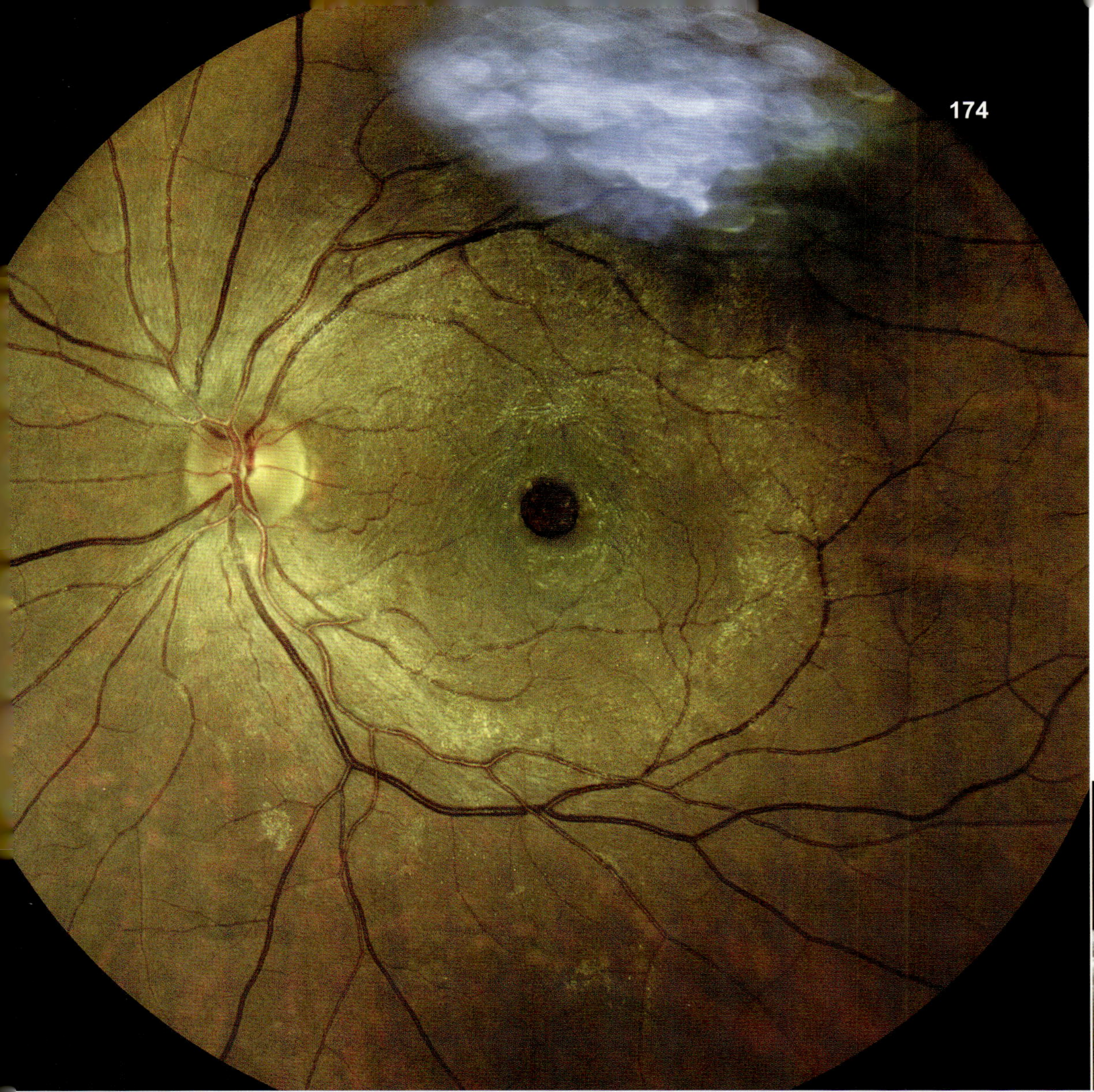

174

Figure 174

*Large macular hole managed with 25-gauge pars plana vitrectomy with internal limiting membrane (ILM) peel and ILM flap technique.*

A 63-year-old male presented with complaints of decrease in near vision from his left eye since past 8 months. Fundus photo shows a round reddish defect at the macula suggestive of macular hole, size of which was around 850 microns.

Figure 175

*SS–OCT shows large full thickness macular hole with inverted V-shaped configuration, with large basal diameter of around 2600 microns. Fine hyper-reflective membrane like structure anterior to neurosensory retina suggestive of complete PVD, hence a stage 4 macular hole.*

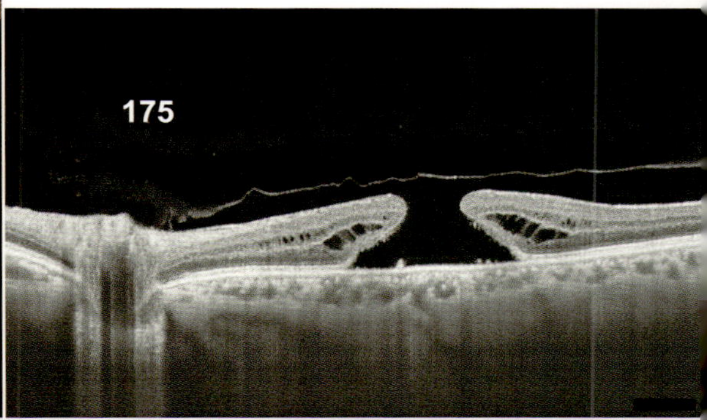

175

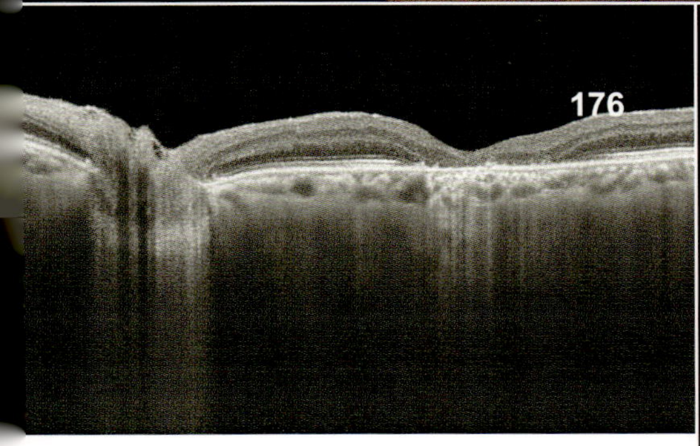

176

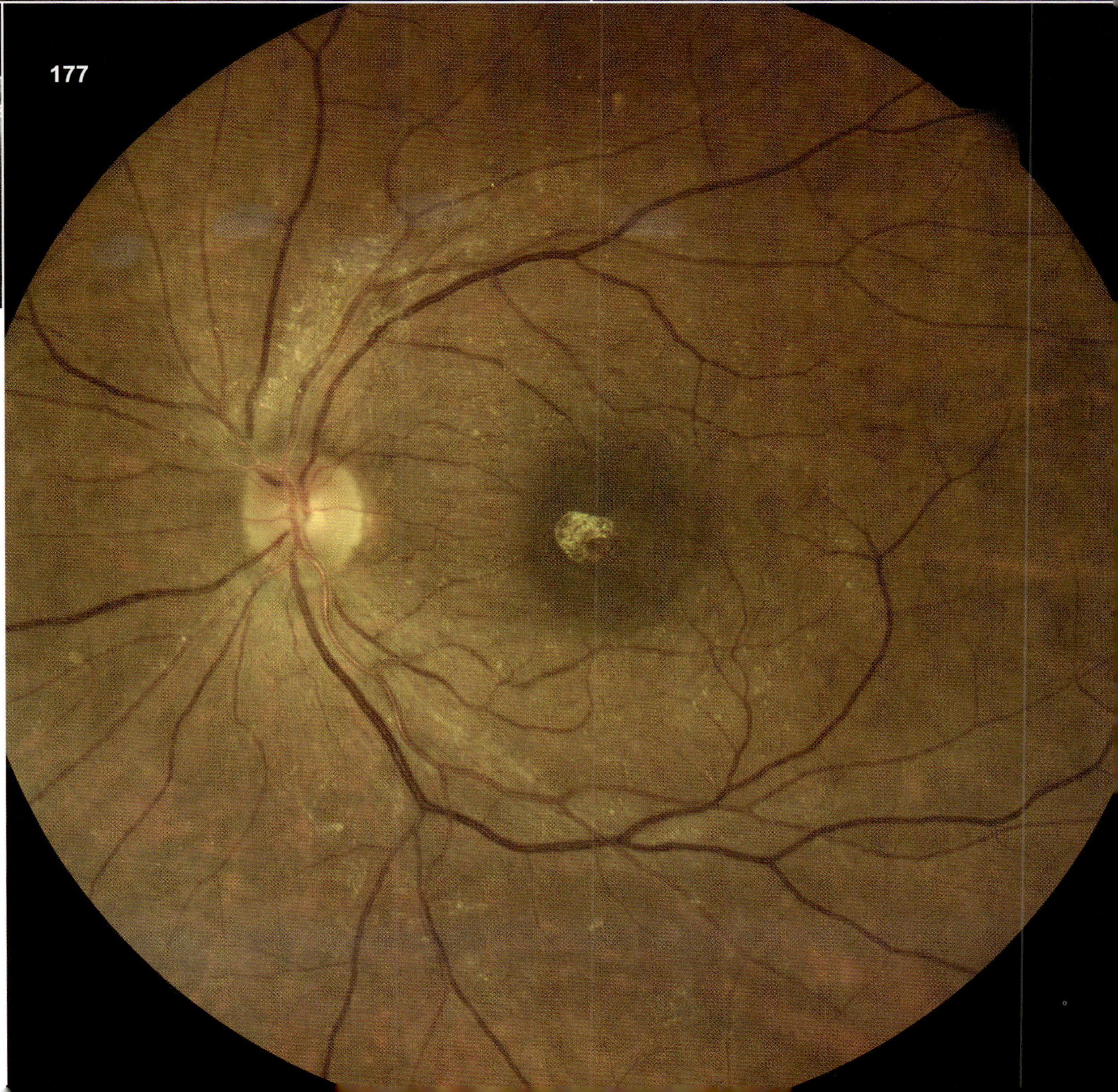

177

Figure 176

*SS-OCT postoperatively clearly shows complete closure of macular hole with significant retinal pigment epithelium atrophy at the fovea. There is also gross disintegration of inner retinal layers which is commonly seen in long standing and large macular holes.*

Figure 177

*At 2 months postsurgery there is complete resolution of intraocular gas. BCVA was 6/60. Macular hole is closed with significant retinal pigment epithelium atrophy at the macula, accounting for only modest gain in visual acuity.* □

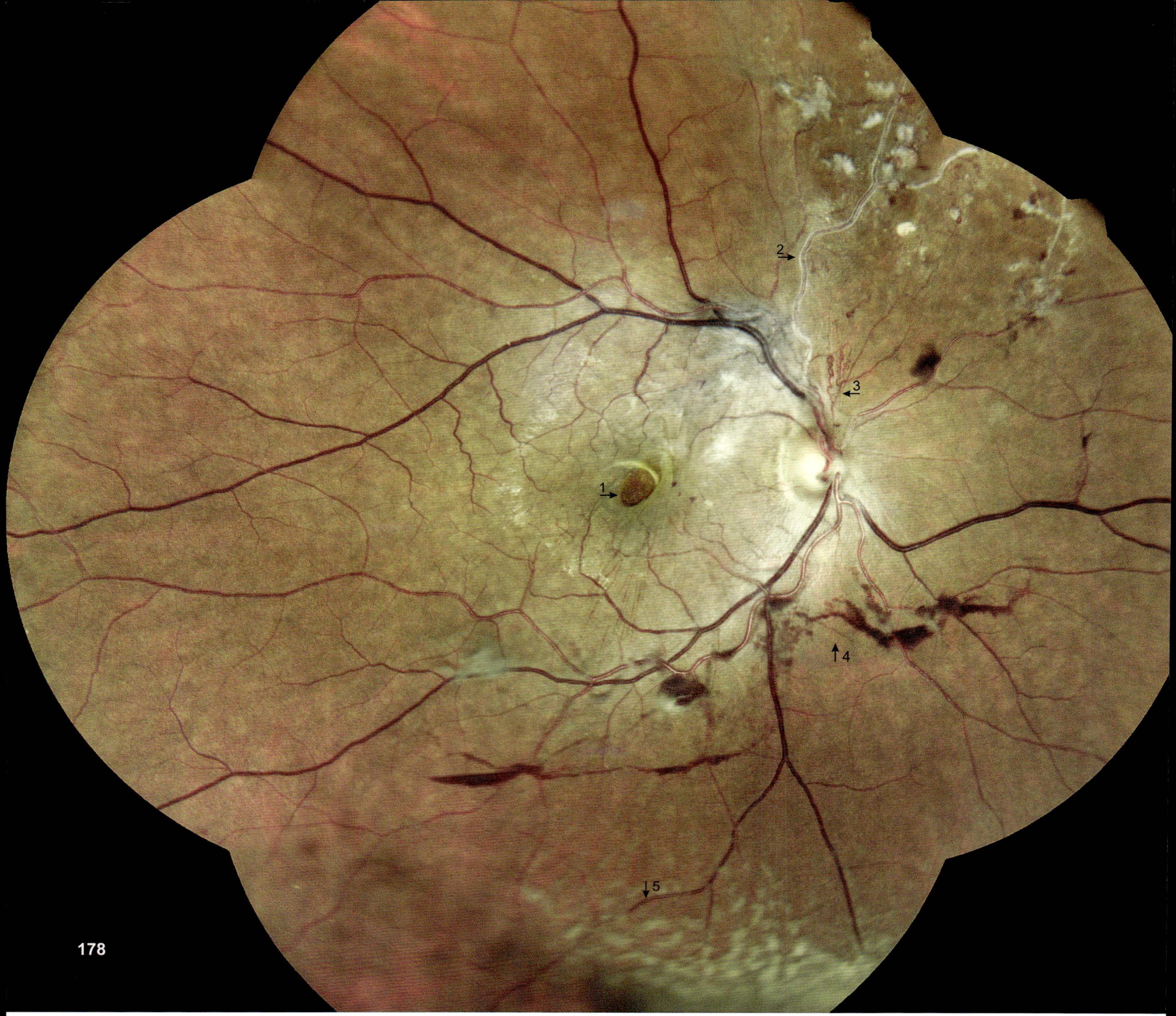


Figure 178 *A case of secondary macular hole secondary to epiretinal membrane traction following branch retinal vein occlusion.*

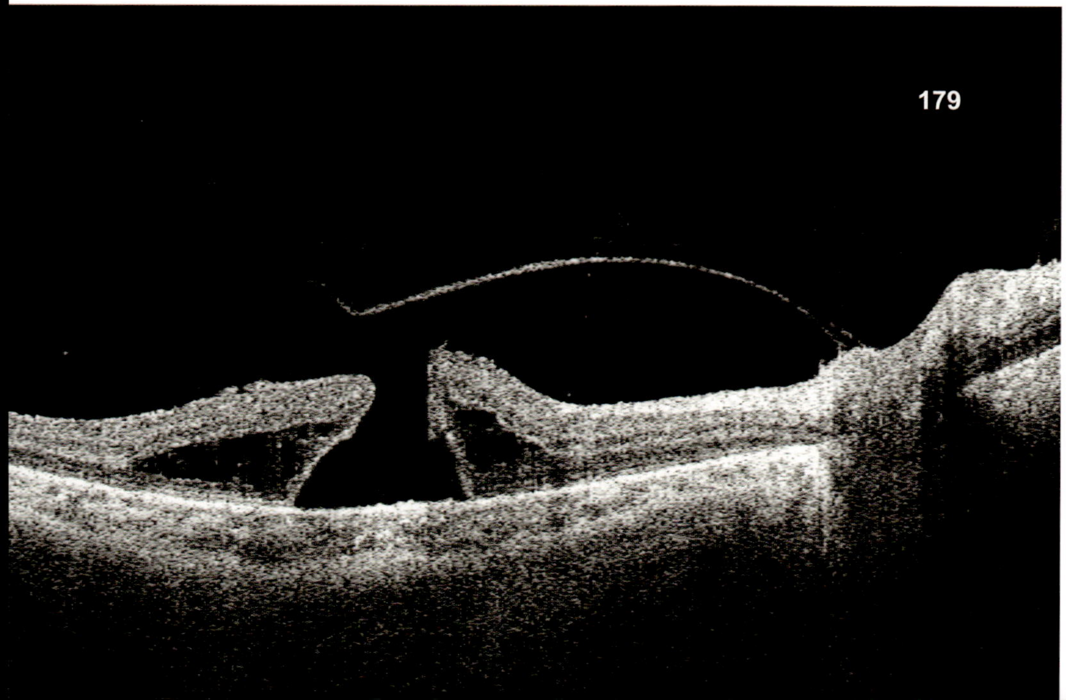


A 67-year-old male patient present with complaints of distortion of vision, metamorphopsia and decrease in vision from OD since 2 months.

Fundus photo of right eye shows thick grayish epiretinal membrane at the macula causing drag at the fovea and leading a circular vertically elongated defect at the macula "macular hole" (1) along with sclerosed vessel in superonasal quadrant suggestive of BRVO (2). Neovascularization can be seen superior to the disk (3). Preretinal hemorrhage can be seen inferior to the arcade (4), gray colored old vitreous hemorrhage can be seen (5).

Figure 179 *Preoperative OCT shows a full thickness defect at the fovea suggestive of macular hole with large maximum outer diameter owing to wide base which has been shown to be an important index predicting closure of macular hole.*

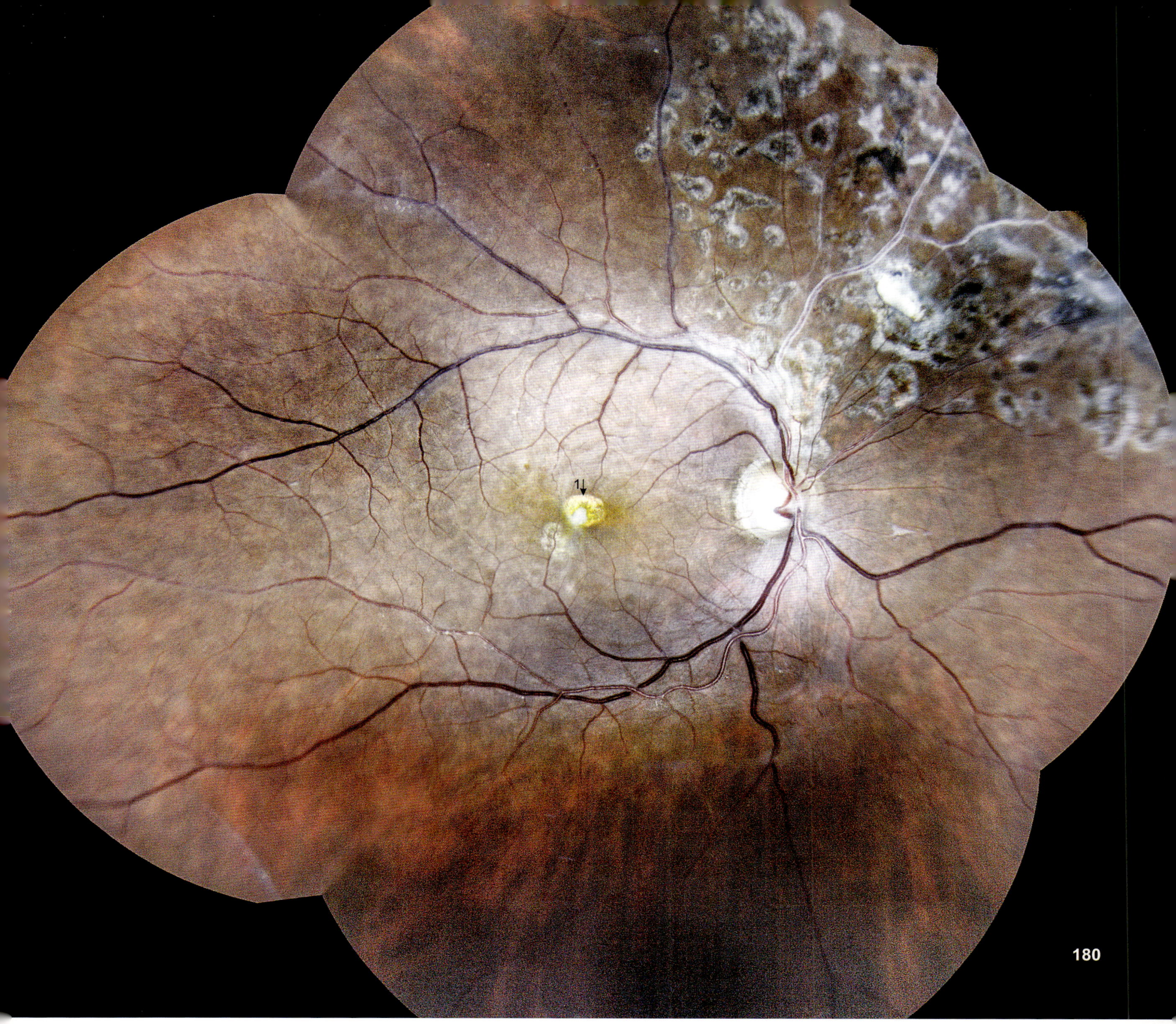


Figure 180 *25-gauge PPV was done, silicone oil tamponade was put 5 months after silicone oil removal was done fundus photo shows media clarity grade 1 with closure of macular hole, there is significant amount of retinal pigment atrophy at the fovea (1) accounting for low BCVA 6/36. Scatter marks can be seen superonasally with regression of neovascularization.*

Figure 181 *OCT scan after removal of silicone oil shows complete closure of macular hole with significant amount of retinal pigment epithelium atrophy and distortion of inner and outer layers of retina at the fovea. The epiretinal membrane causing traction was completely removed. There is resolution of cystoid spaces.* □

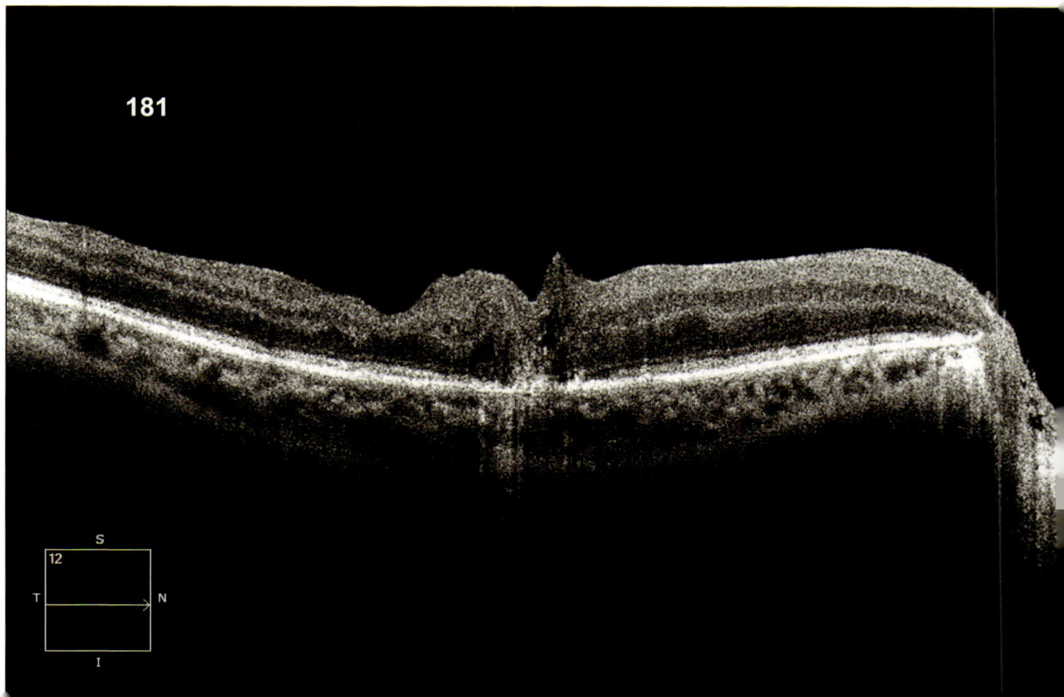

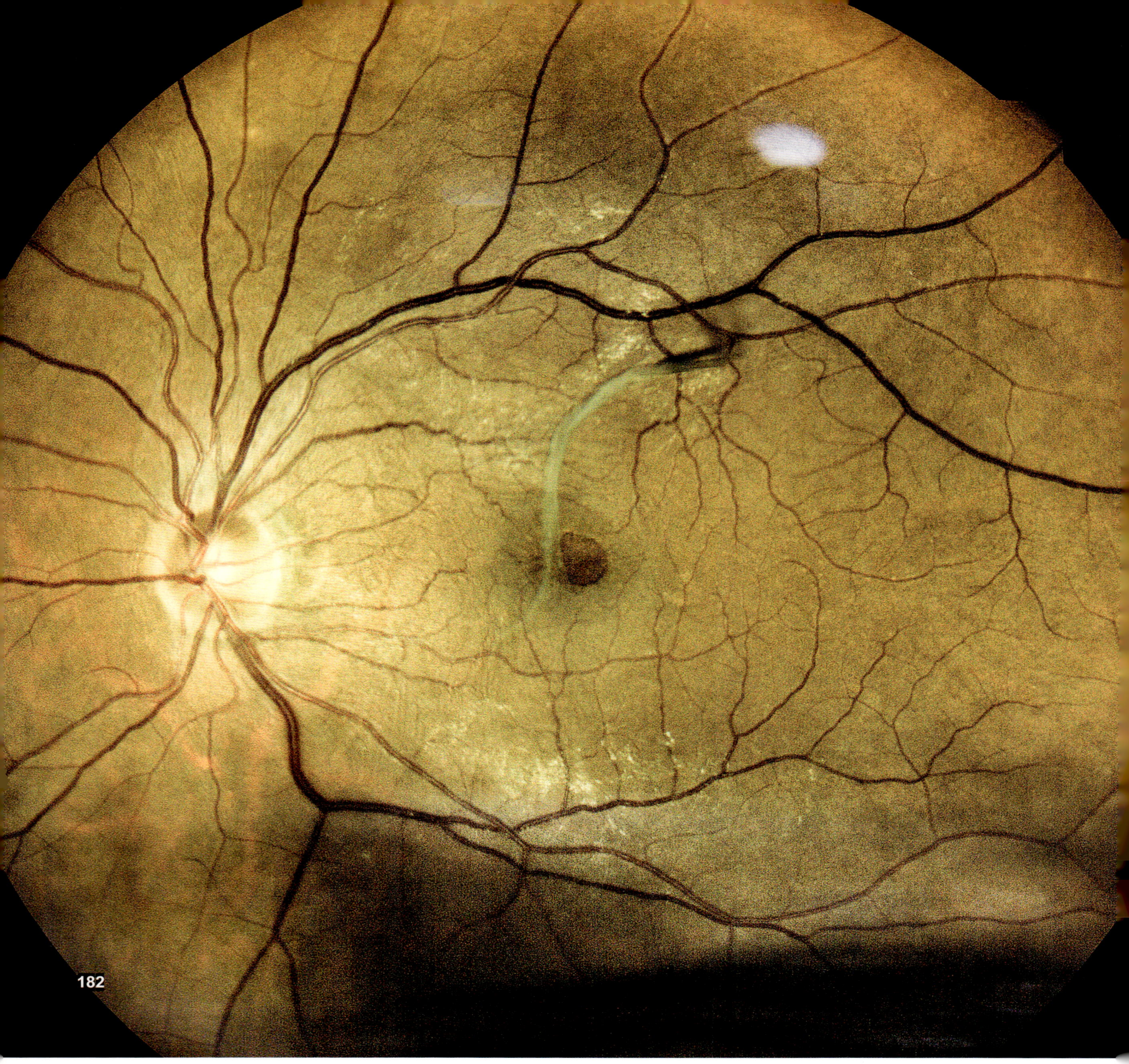


Figure 182 *A case of epiretinal membrane managed with 25G pars plana vitrectomy leading to secondary macular hole formation.*

A 64-year-old male presented with complaints of blurred distorted vision in his left eye since 3 months. BCVA was 6/24. Color fundus photo shows a thick grayish epiretinal membrane at macula along with a reddish circular defect at macula suggestive of pseudomacular hole as was confirmed on OCT.

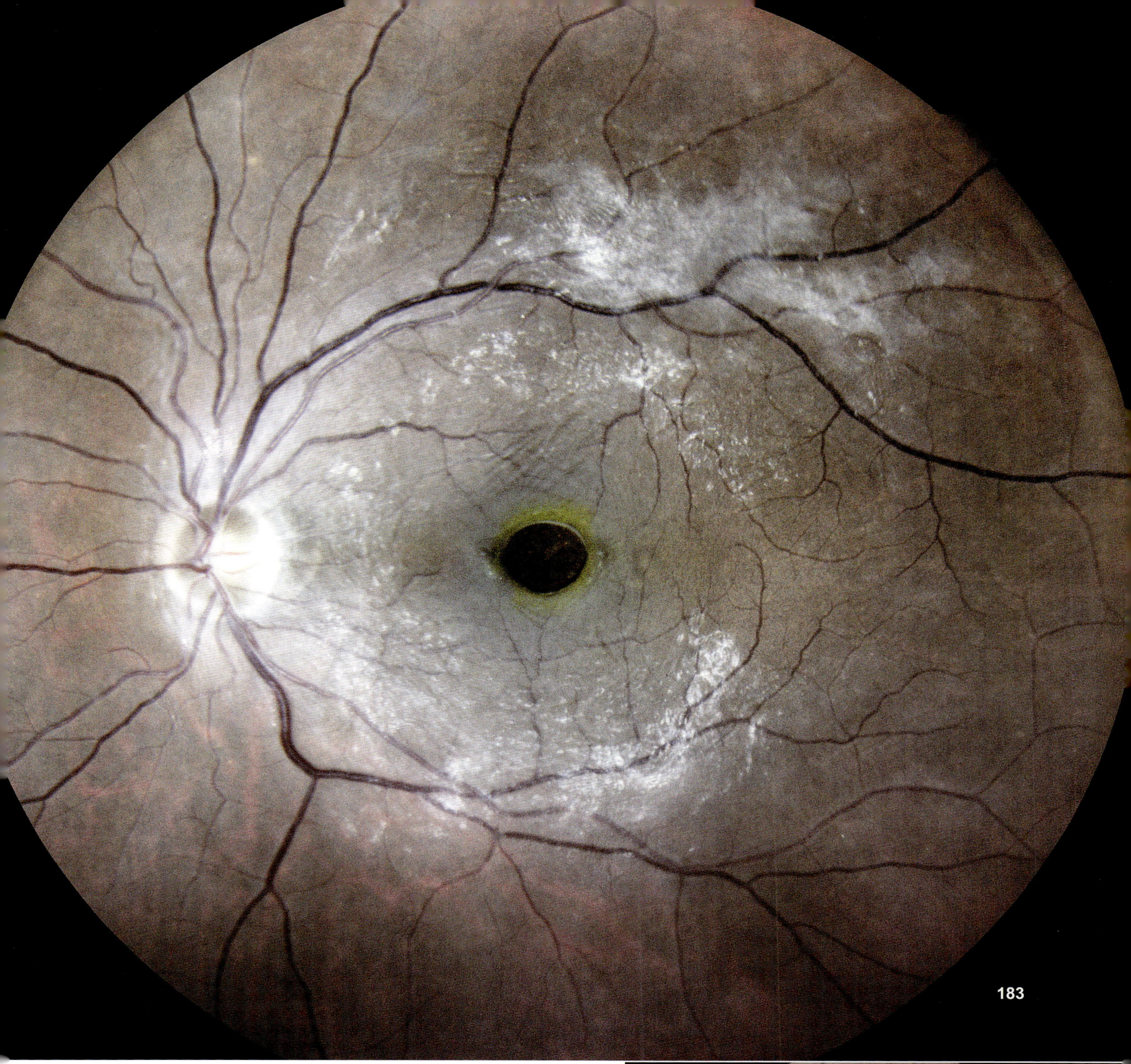

183

Figure 183 *Following PPV for epiretinal membrane a large full thickness hole can be seen at the fovea, BCVA was 6/60. He also complained of difficulty in near vision, rare but macular hole formation after PPV for epiretinal membrane peeling has been reported.*

Figure 184 *He underwent PPV again with removal of ILM using forceps and dye. 6 weeks after intraocular gas has resolved and macular hole is closed with best corrected visual acuity of 6/36.*

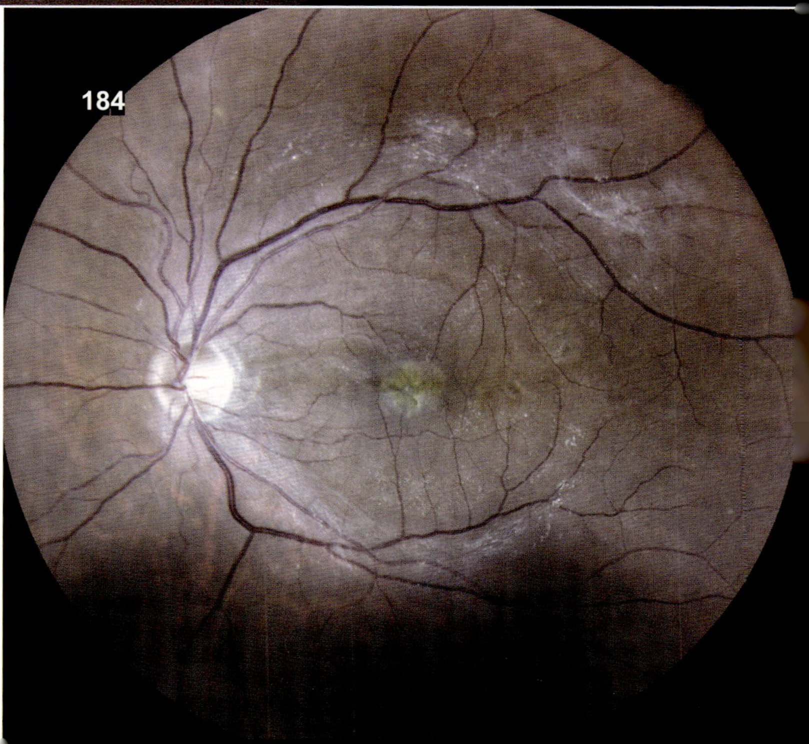

184

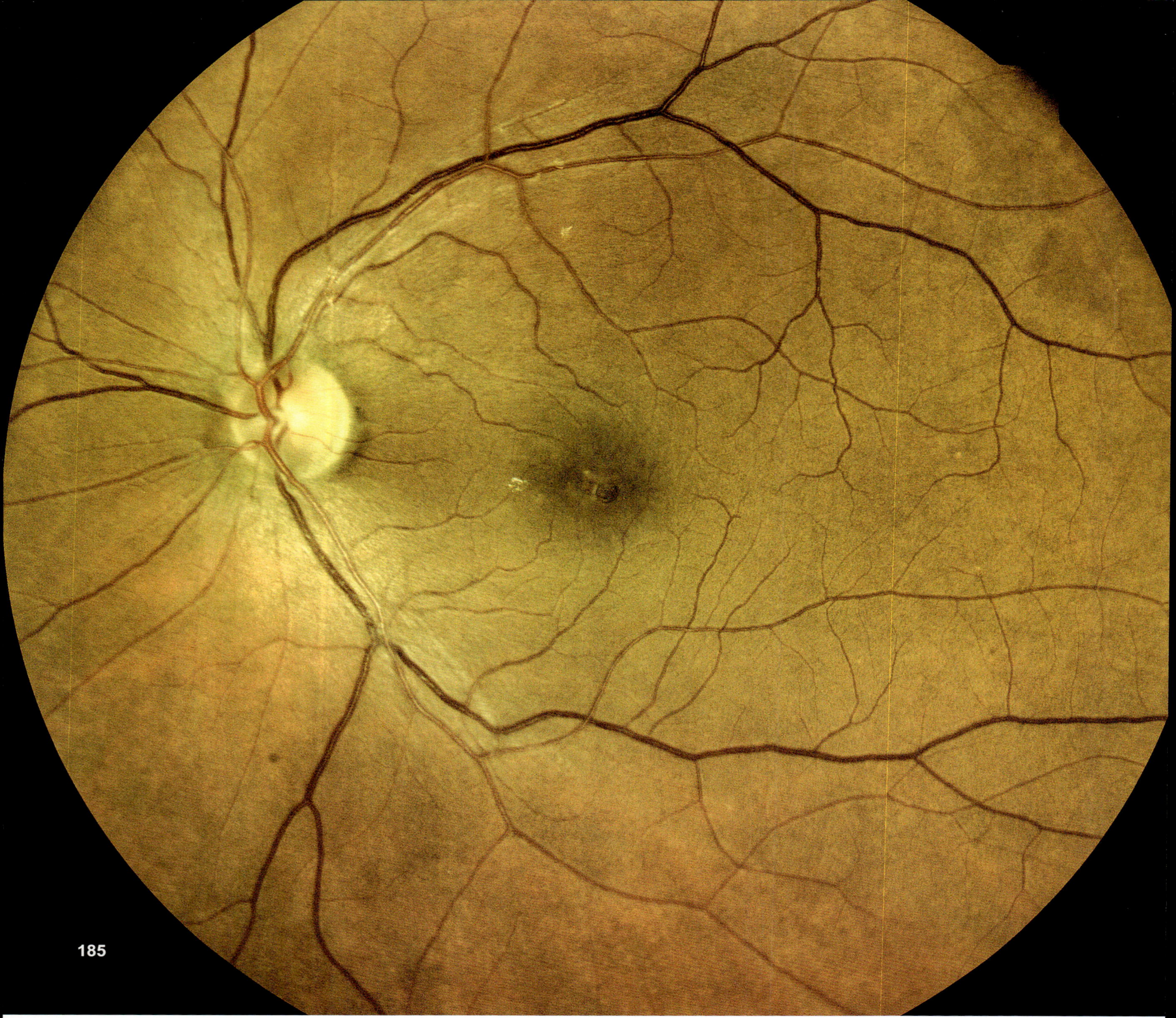


Figure 185 *A case of macular hole with juxtafoveal telangiectasia managed with 25G pars plana vitrectomy. A 60-year-old female presented with progressive blurring of central vision in her left eye. Color fundus photography demonstrated a gray sheen temporal to the fovea in both eyes, which is characteristic of juxtafoveal telangiectasia (JXT). In her fovea in left eye, there was a small circular reddish -yellow defect due to concurrent macular hole demonstrated by optical coherence tomography.*

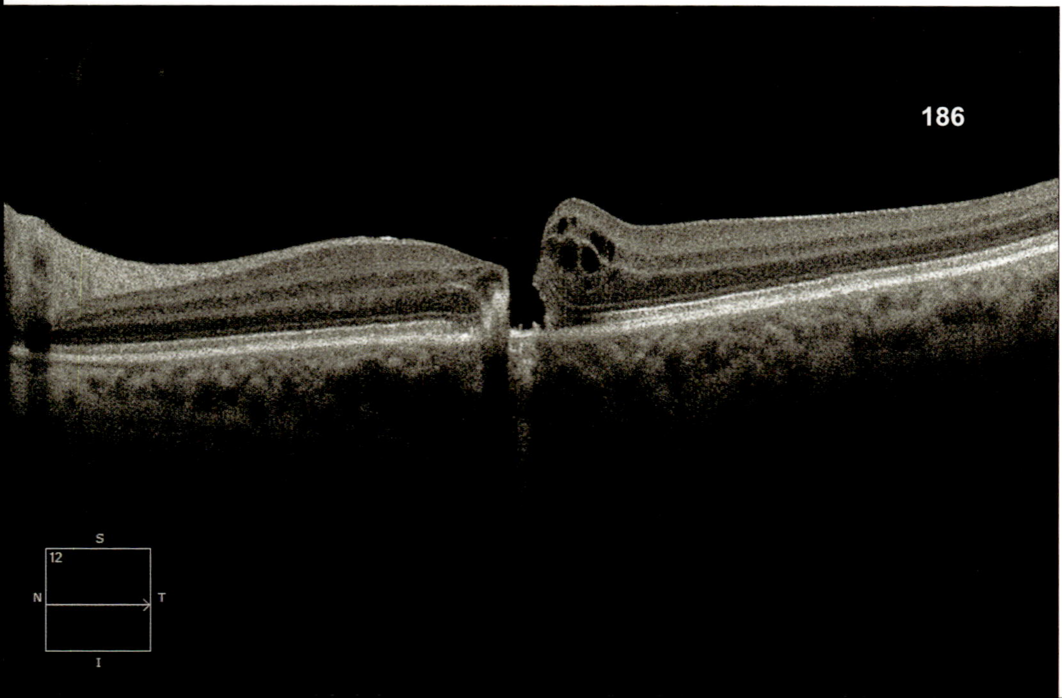


Figure 186 *Optical coherence tomography (OCT) shows small foveal defect, secondary to loss of outer nuclear layer and ellipsoid zone resulting in a full thickness macular hole that can encompass all retinal layers. Hyper-reflective areas on OCT correlate to areas of RPE hyperplasia and migration. Small hyporeflective cystoid spaces can be seen at the temporal edge of the defect.*

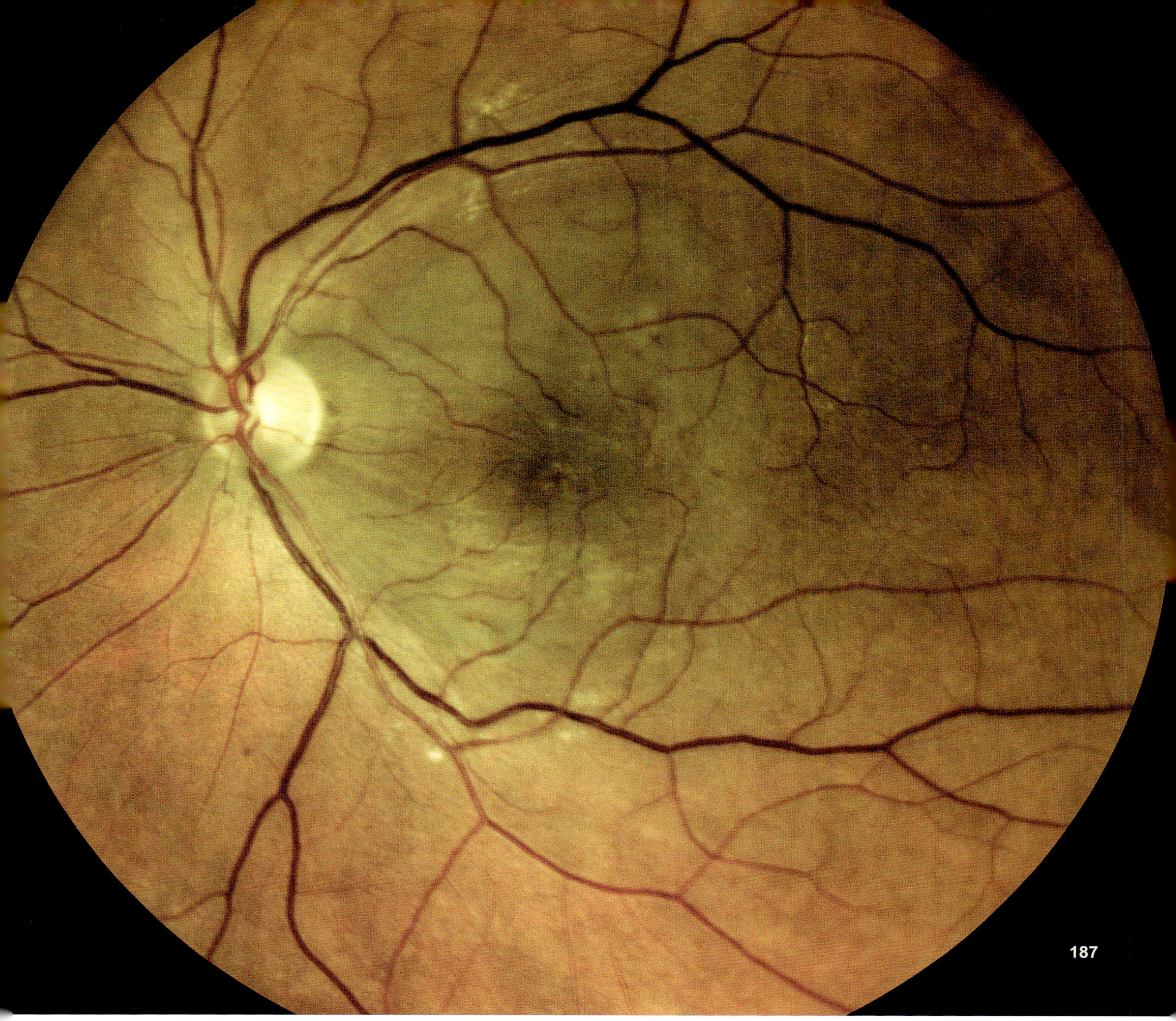


Figure 187 *Six weeks post-25-gauge pars plana vitrectomy with internal limiting membrane peeling with intraocular gas tamponade, fundus photo demonstrates complete closure of macular hole.*

Figure 188 *OCT postoperatively demonstrates complete closure of macular hole with persistent hyper-reflective areas on OCT correlate to areas of RPE hyperplasia and migration secondary to JXT.* □

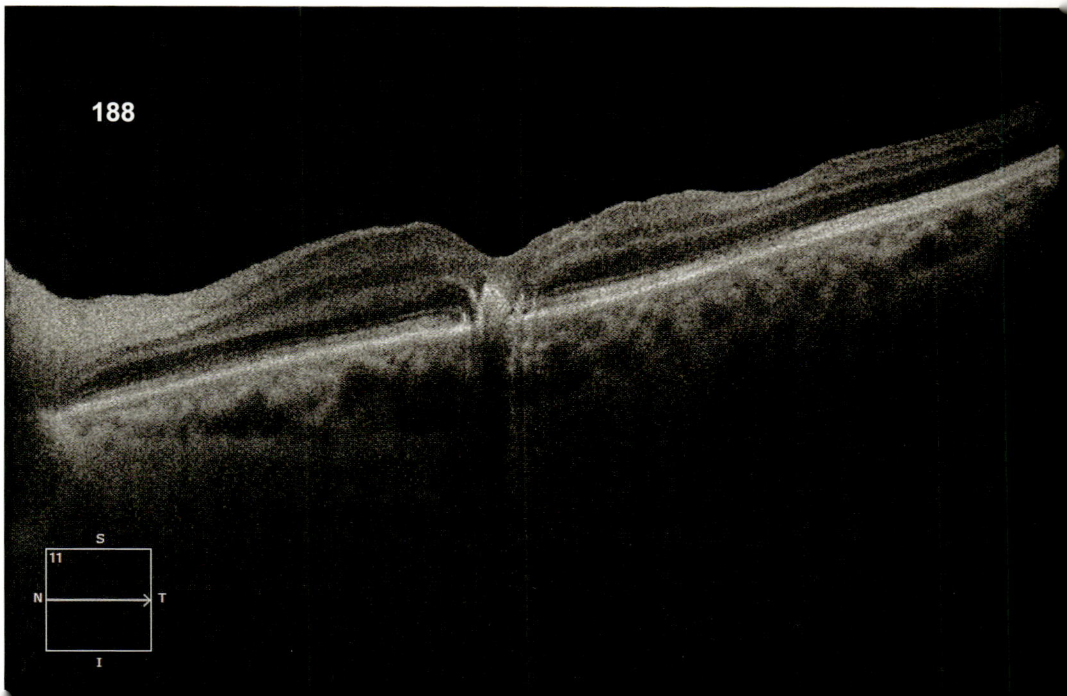

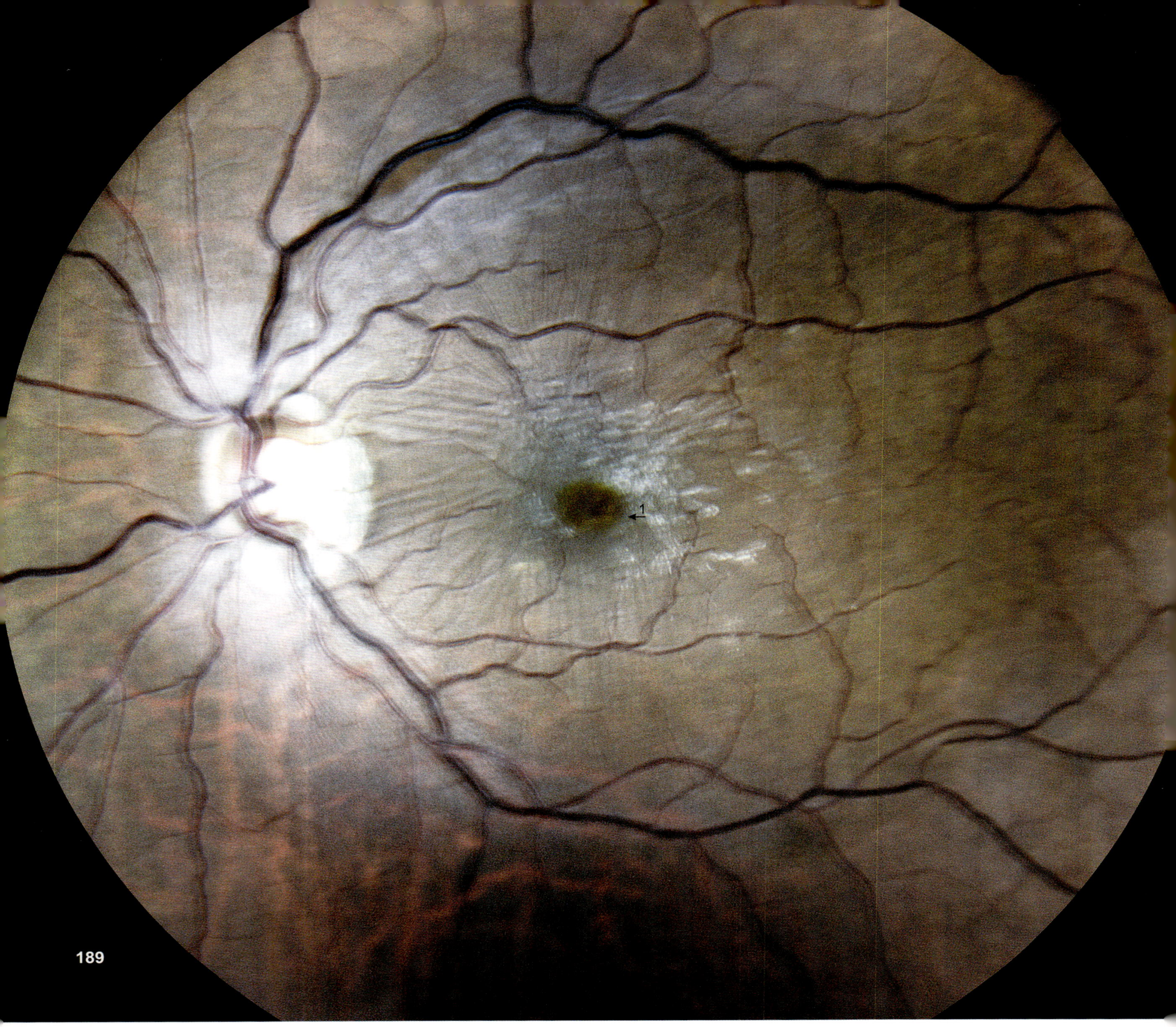


Figure 189 *A case of epiretinal membrane with, macular hole managed with 25-gauge PPV.*

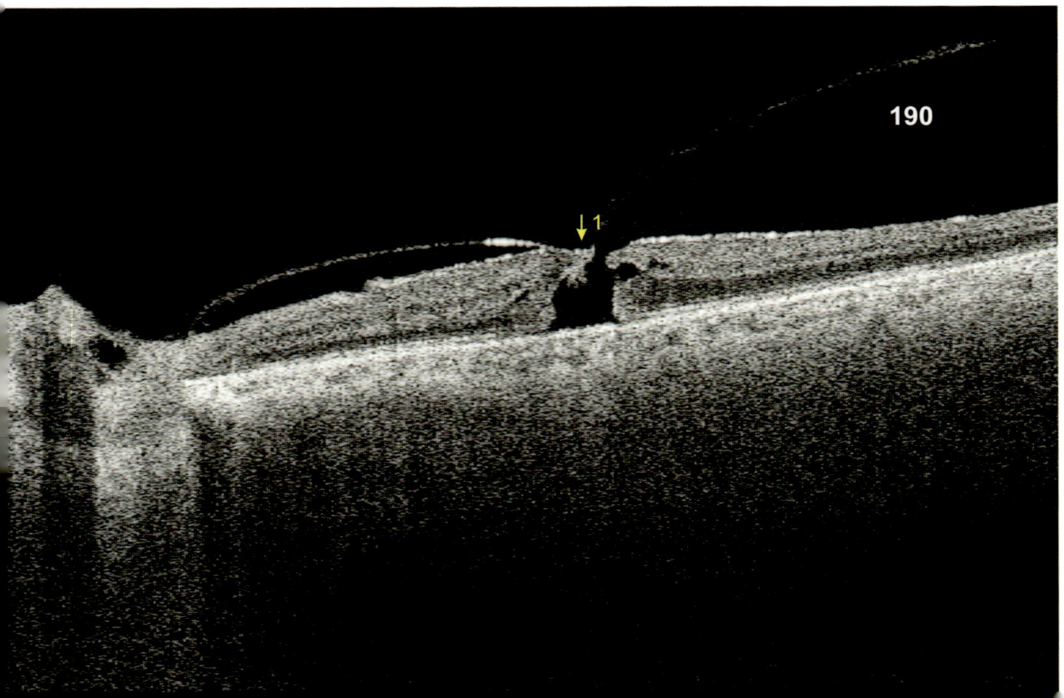


A 64-year-old female with complaint of decrease and distortion of vision since 4 months. BCVA was 6/60. Fundus photo shows epiretinal membrane with macular hole (1) which was managed with standard 25G vitrectomy with internal limiting membrane peeling with epiretinal membrane removal and intraocular tamponade sulphur hexafluoride.

Figure 190 *Preoperative SS-OCT shows densely adherent hyper-reflective epiretinal membrane attached to the edge of the macular hole (1) and resulting in traction and full thickness macular hole with ragged edges.*

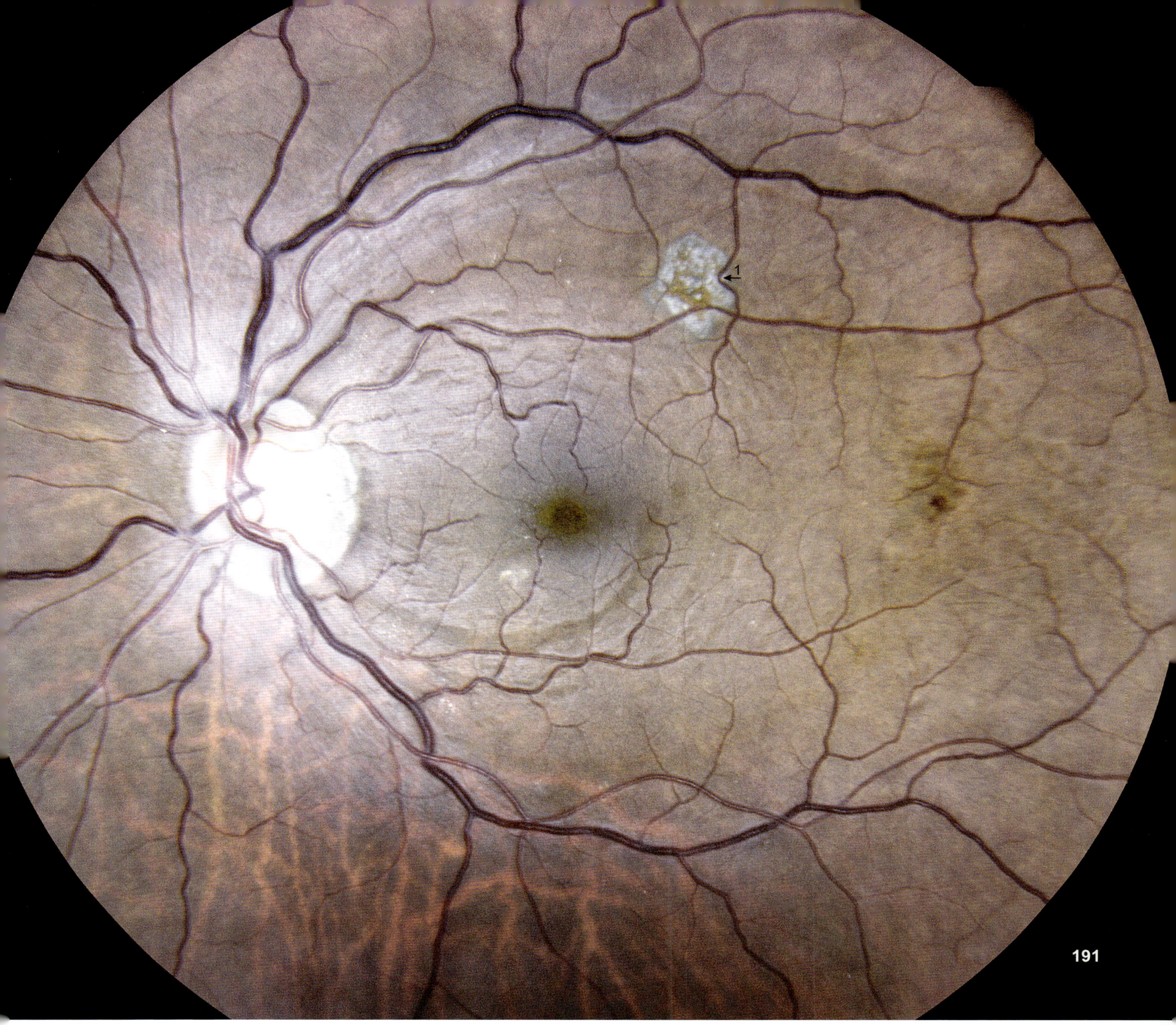


Figure 191 *Postoperatively macular hole is closed, one may get an iatrogenic break while trying to peel of the densely adherent membrane which is rare but should be managed with adequate laser barrage if away from center or ILM flap is close to center. Superotemporal iatrogenic break with laser marks around it can be seen (1).*

Figure 192 *Postoperative SS-OCT shows complete closure of the macular hole in "V" shaped closure. Epiretinal membrane is completely removed and there is disruption of outer retinal layers at fovea which was present preoperatively.* □

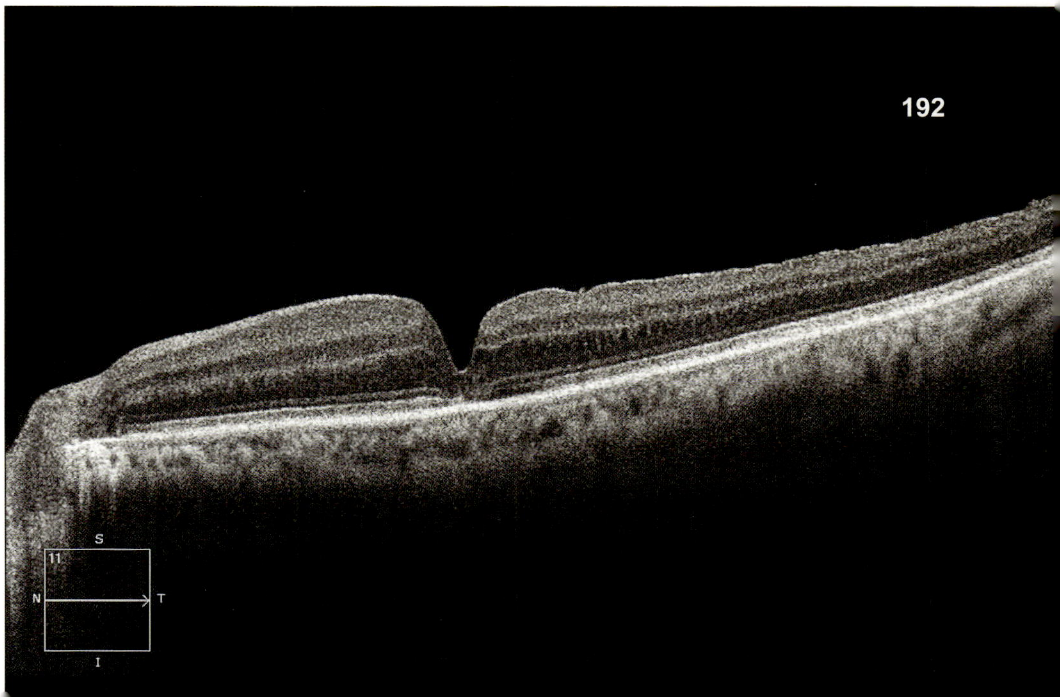

193

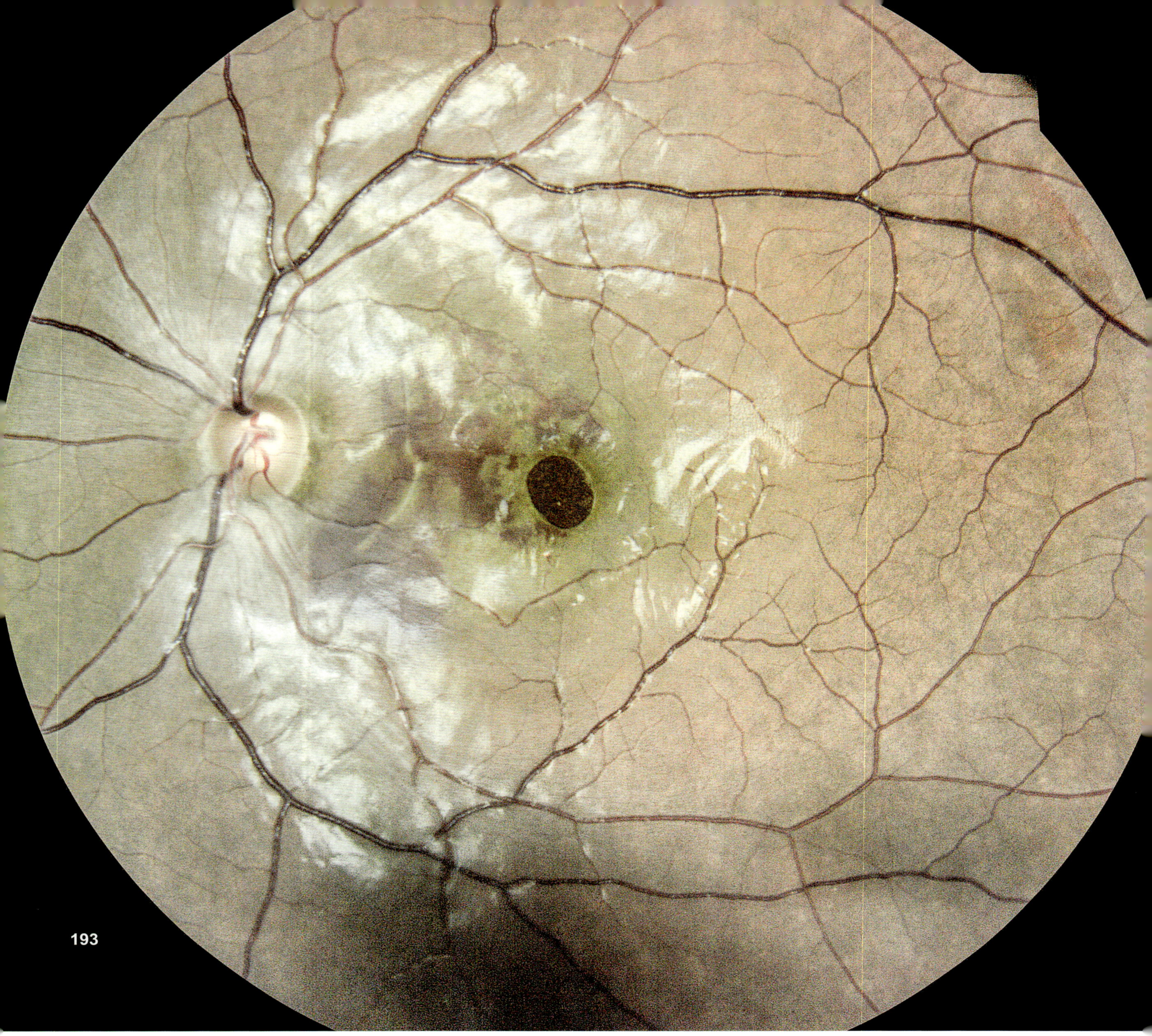

Figure 193 *Case of traumatic macular hole with choroidal rupture.*

Figure 194 *OCT demonstrating full thickness retinal defect at the fovea. There is presence of posteriorly concave area of disruption of RPE/choriocapillaris complex associated with loss of photoreceptors IS/OS and ELM reflectivity.*

194

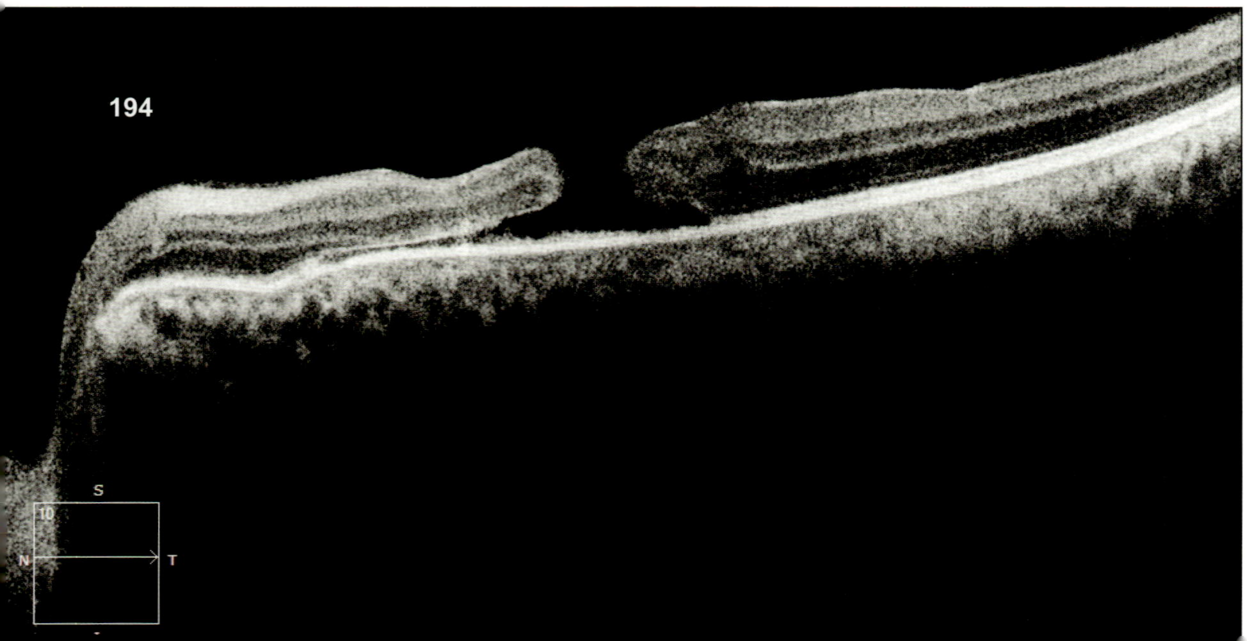


Note the presence of subretinal hemorrhage temporal to the disk, and a curvilinear white line concentric to the nasal margin of the disk, suggestive of a choroidal rupture. Also note a round reddish well-defined defect at the fovea as a result of traumatic macular hole.

Choroidal rupture are breaks in the choroid or Bruch's membrane as a result of direct or indirect trauma to the globe. Approximately 5–10% of the patients with blunt trauma to the globe may develop a choroidal rupture. □

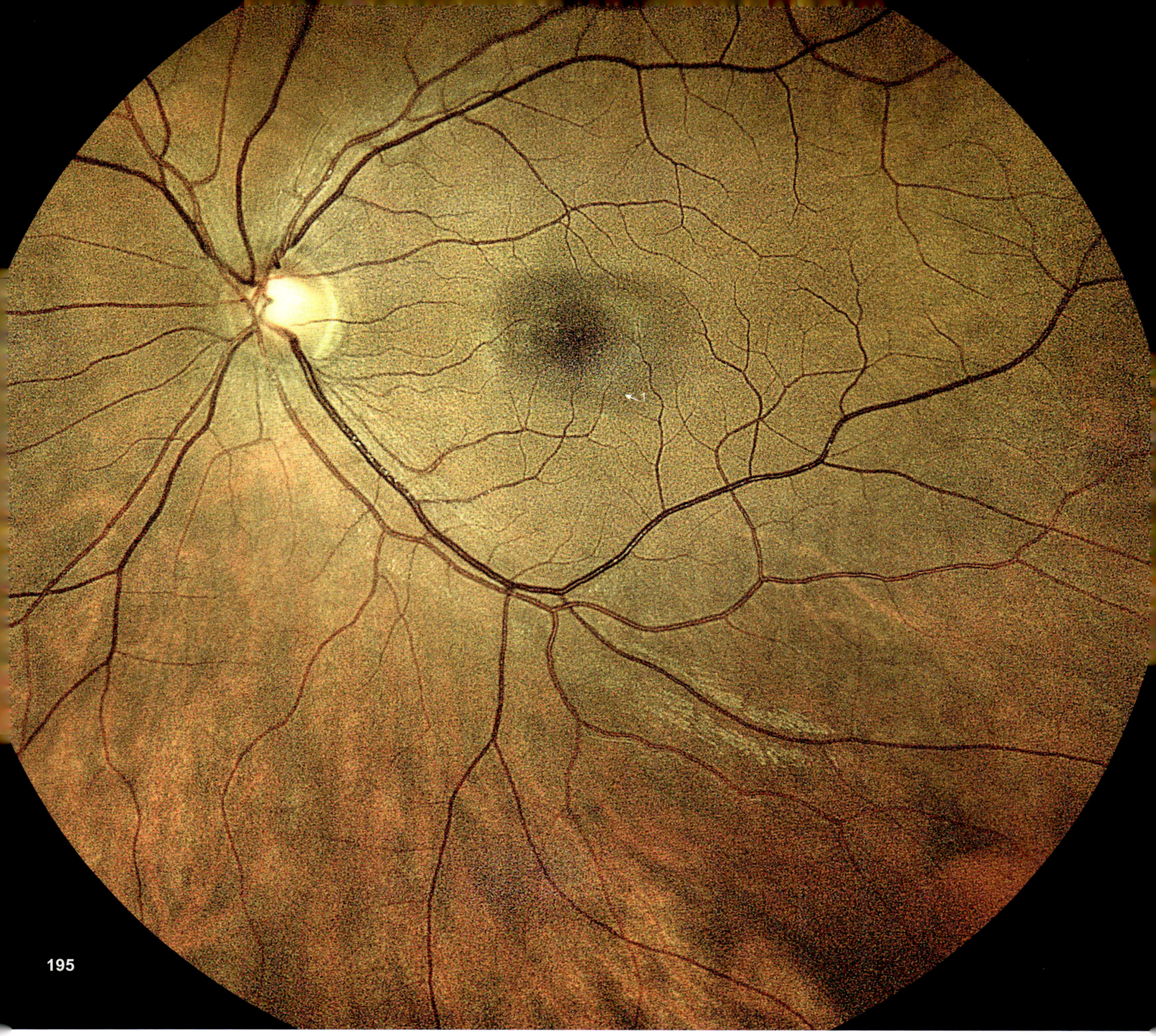


Figure 195 *Hydroxychloroquine (HCQ)-induced macular toxicity in a patient with long-term use of HCQ. There is a classic round area of central pigmentation, surrounded by annular zone of depigmentation of the retinal pigment epithelium (1) and loss of normal foveal reflex.*

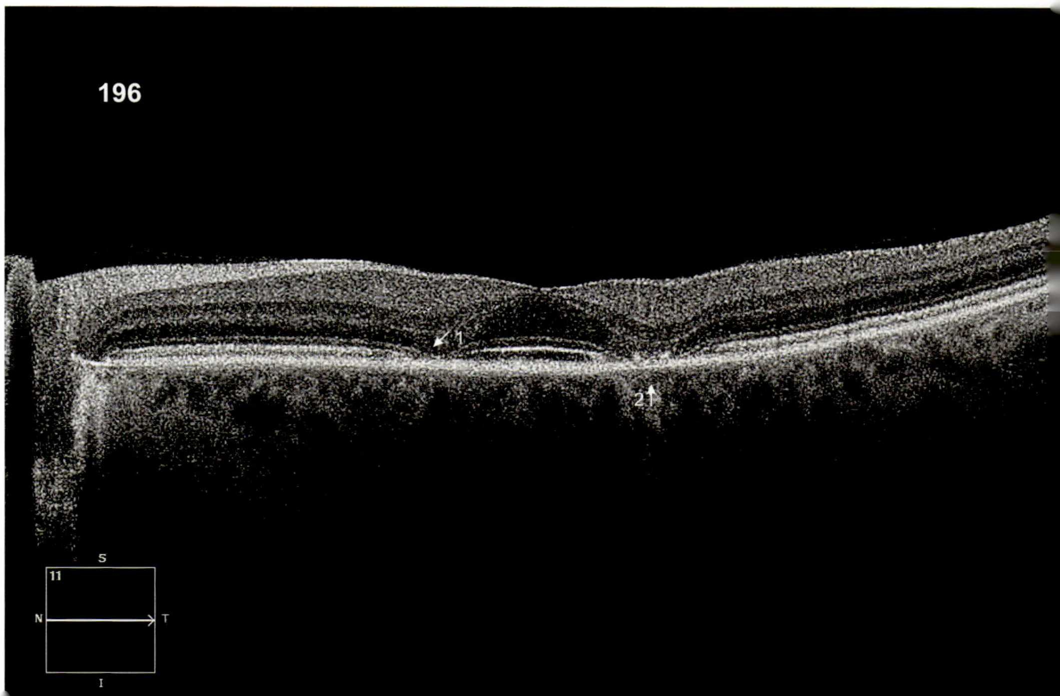


Figure 196 *SD-OCT demonstrating a classic presentation of HCQ associated "Bull's Eye Maculopathy." Note the presence of marked parafoveal thinning of retina, especially outer nuclear layer (1) and disruption of ellipsoid zone (2). Central foveal architecture is well preserved.*

HCQ is used for treatment of SLE, RA and other autoimmune disorder. Long-term use has been associated with irreversible maculopathy requiring discontinuation of therapy. Hence it is imperative that rheumatologist, medicine consultant and ophthalmologist are aware of this toxicity related to HCQ and regular eye screening should be advised as per the guidelines. □

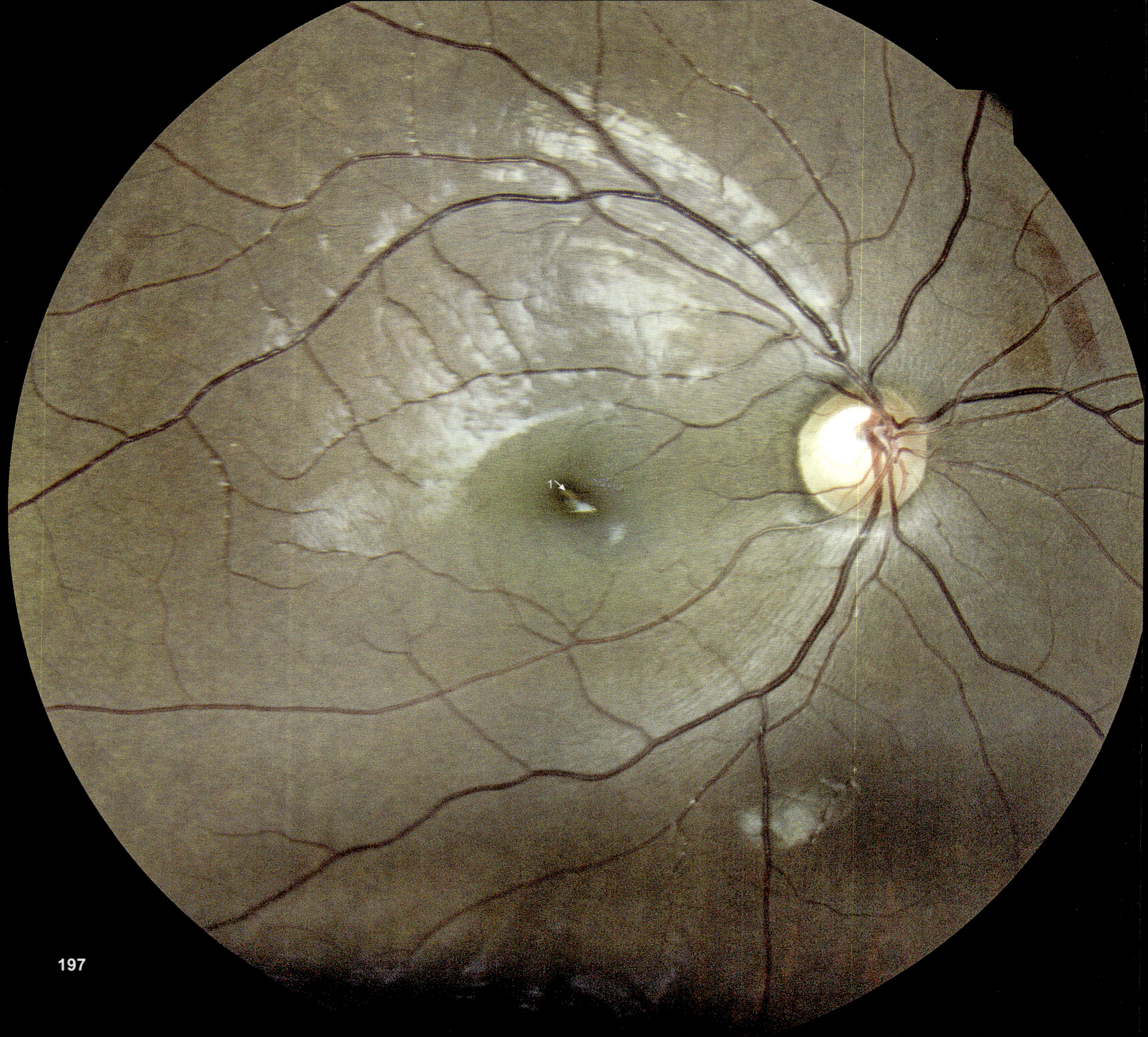


Figure 197 *A case of laser-induced retina phototoxicity. A young 30-year-old patient presented with sudden onset blurred vision after an accidental laser toy gun fired towards the eye. Note the presence of linear whitish lesion at foveal center (1). Rest of the retina appear normal.*

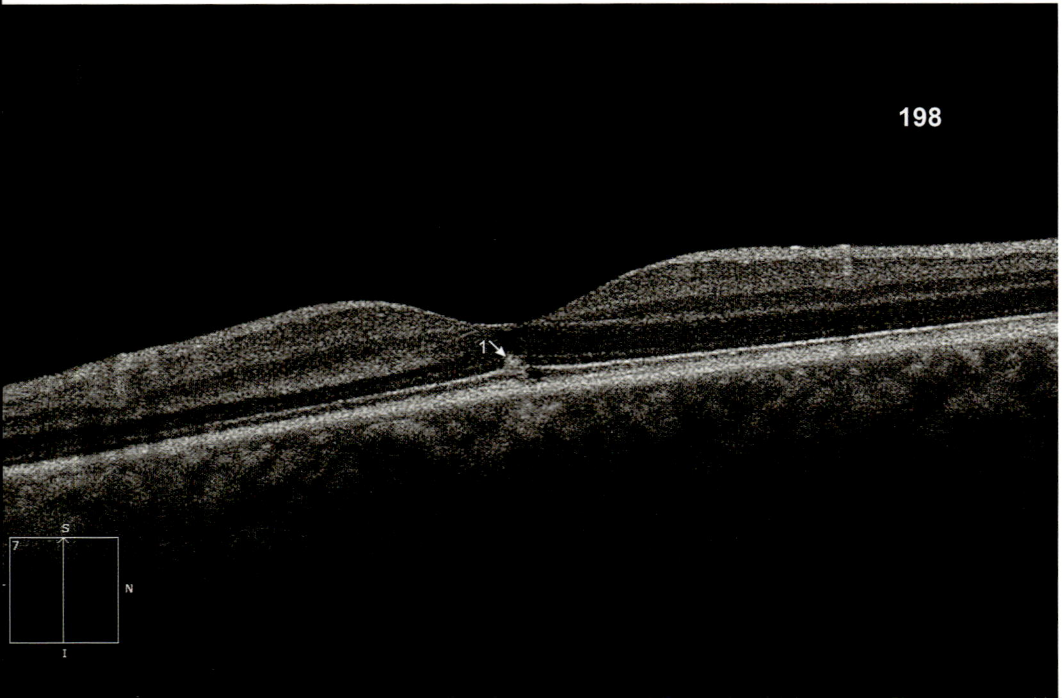


Figure 198 *Spectral Domain Optical Coherence Tomography (SD-OCT) scan in a case of laser-induced retinal phototoxicity. SD-OCT scan demonstrates disruption of ellipsoid zone and overlying external limiting membrane at the foveal center (1). Rest of inner retinal layers and RPE layers are normal and intact.* □

# CHAPTER 5

## RETINAL DETACHMENT

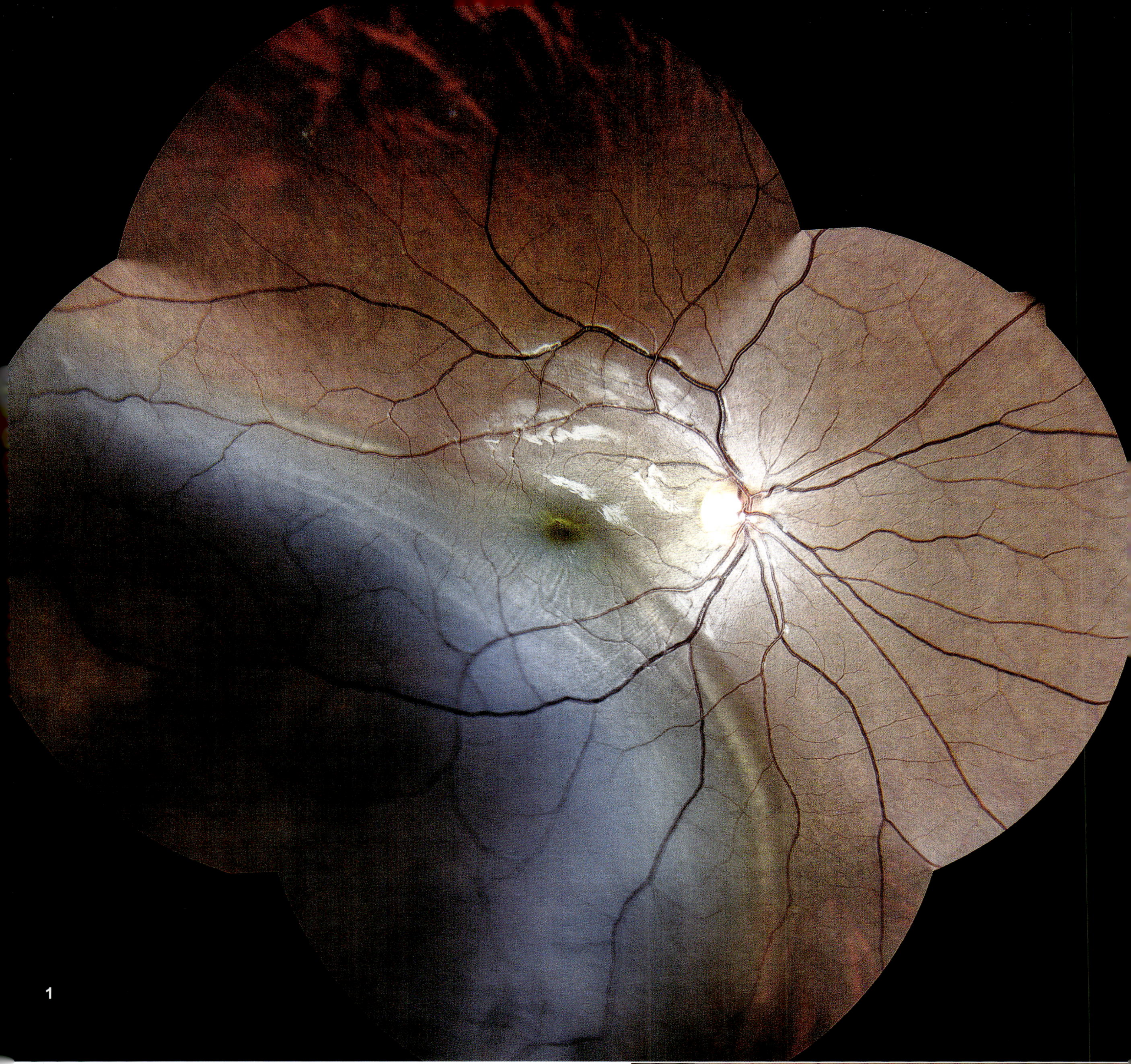

1

Figure 1 *Fundus photo shows grayish elevated retina in the inferotemporal quadrant, there was shallow detachment of macula. Indirect ophthalmoscopy localized a single break at 7 o'clock position.*

A 22-year-old female presented with blurring of vision from her right eye for past 7 days. BCVA was 6/6. She gave prior history of trauma. Fundus photo shows grayish elevated retina in the inferotemporal quadrant, there was shallow detachment of macula. Indirect ophthalmoscopy localized a single break at 7 o'clock position. She was advised a scleral buckling procedure with cryotherapy and subretinal fluid drainage. Scleral buckling employs episcleral implants to treat rhegmatogenous retinal detachment. One may lean in favor of scleral buckling in comparison to vitrectomy in case of phakic retinal detachments with clear lens and in younger patients where vitreous adhesions may be tenacious and complete dissection may be challenging.

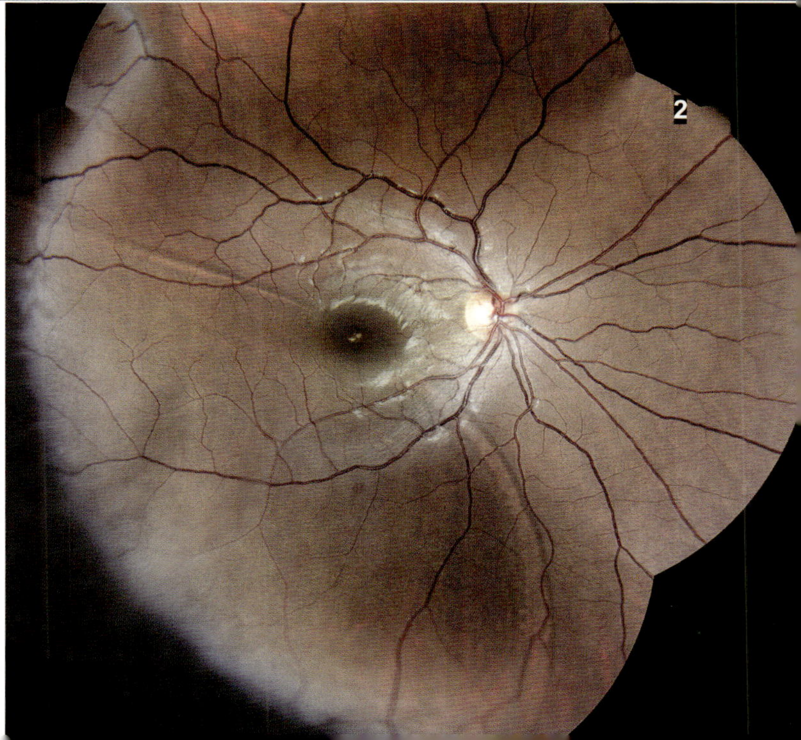

2

Figure 2 *Postoperatively retina was well-attached with indentation of the scleral buckling element visible from 6 o'clock hour to 9 o'clock hour. Prolonged accumulation of fluid can lead to subtle retinal pigment epithelium alterations, hence faint line demonstrating the extent of subretinal preoperatively can be seen.*□

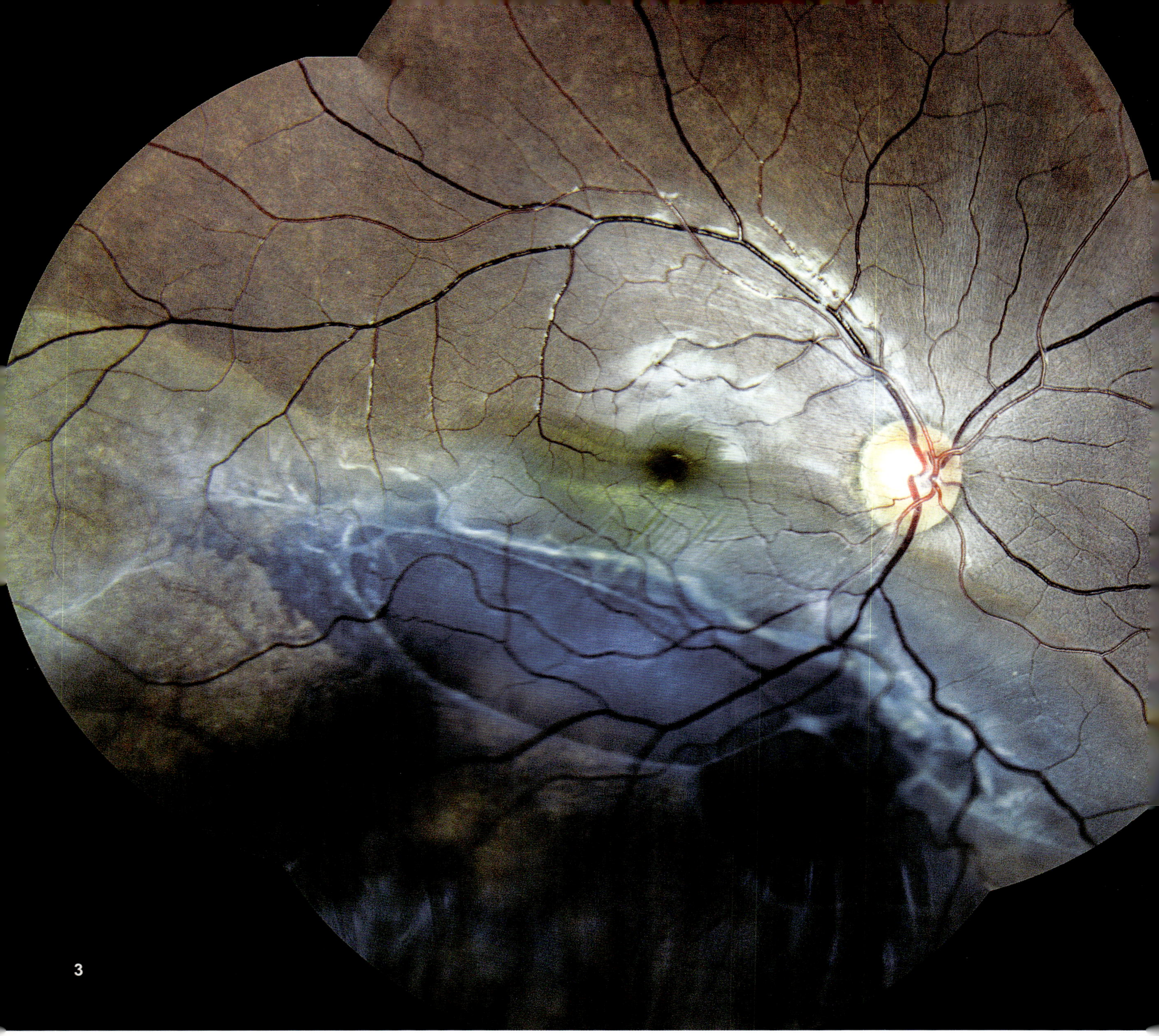


Figure 3 *A 21-year-old male presented with decrease in vision from his right eye since 10 days, BCVA was 6/12. Fundus photo demonstrates grayish detached retina in the inferior and temporal quadrant. Numerous whitish linear subretinal bands can be seen, retina appears to be thinned out and almost translucent, indicating this to be an old chronic retinal detachment. Dark purplish-red blood clot can be seen accumulated along the inferior arcade. Indirect ophthalmoscopy with indentation revealed a large break at 7 o'clock. Considering the younger age and phakic clear lens status of the patient, we planned a scleral buckling procedure with cryotherapy and subretinal fluid drainage.*

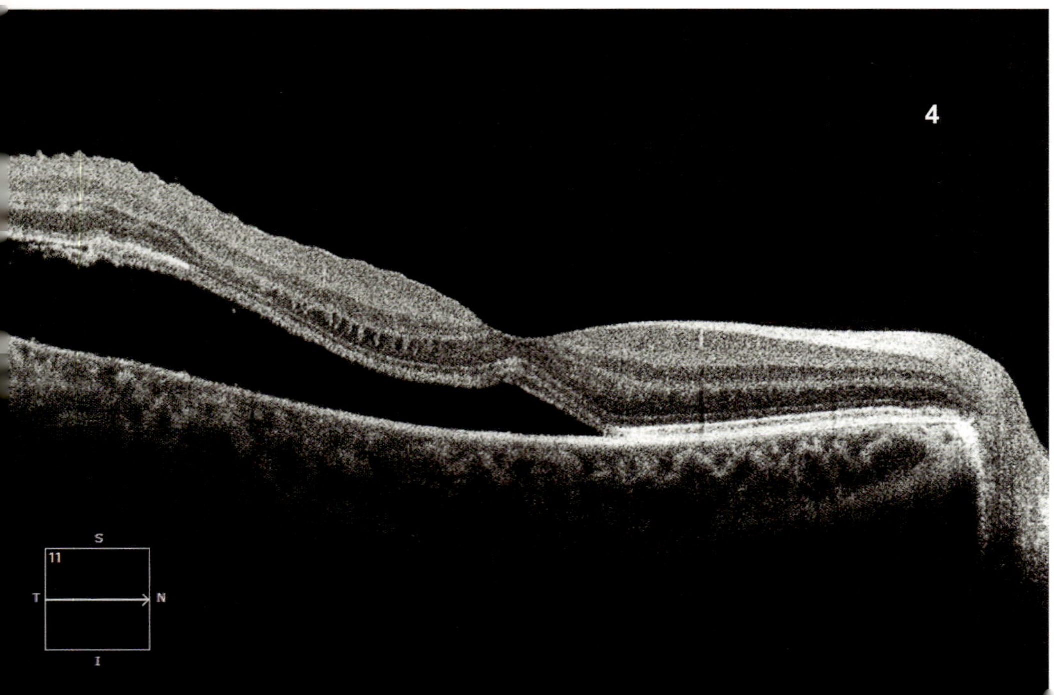


Figure 4 *OCT preoperatively demonstrates shallow hyporeflective fluid separating neurosensory retina from underlying retinal pigment epithelium involving the fovea which is an important prognostic indicator. Few hyporeflective cystic spaces can be seen in inner neurosensory retina which are common place in chronic long standing retinal detachment.*

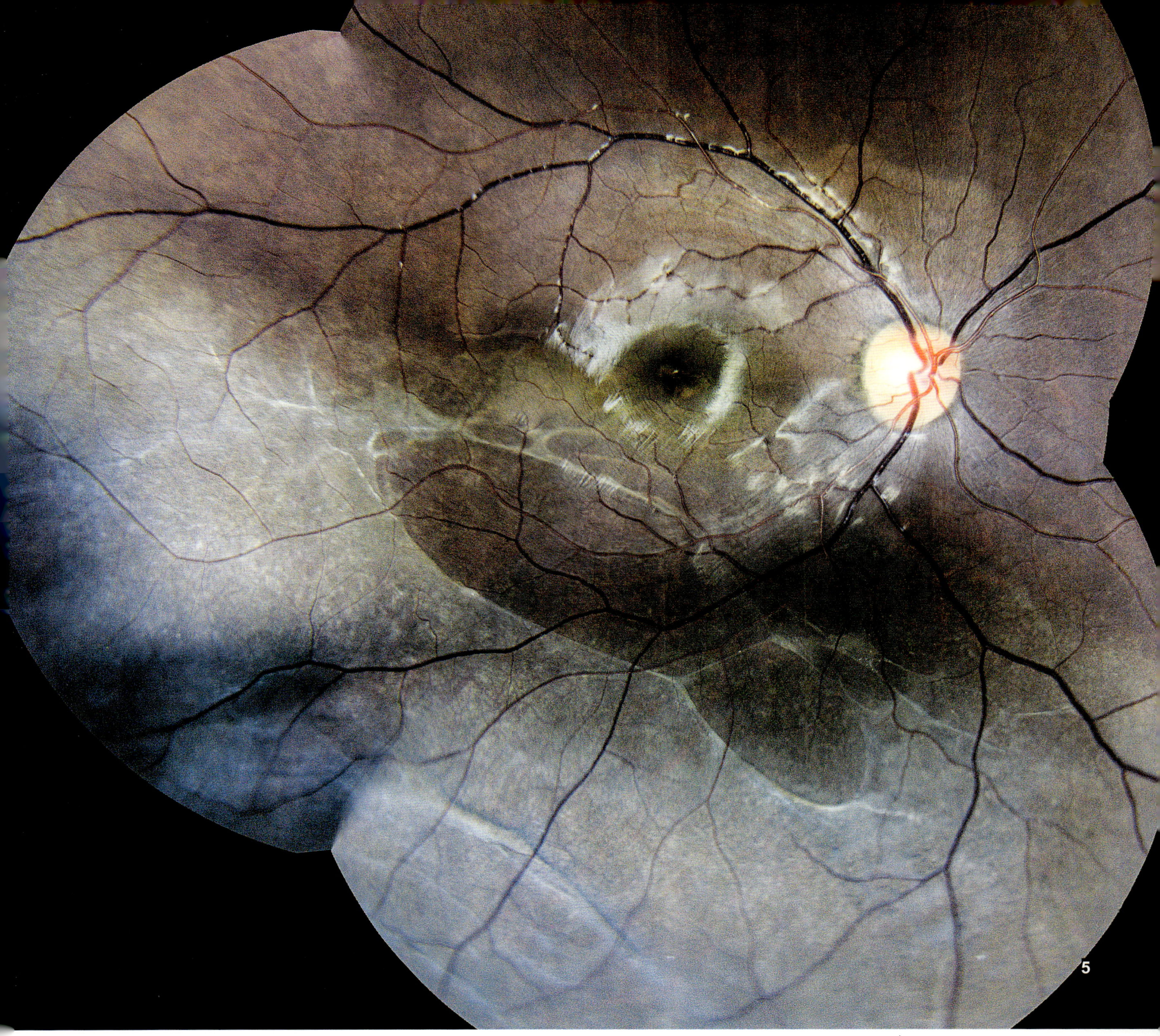


Figure 5 *Postoperatively, at 1 month, BCVA was 6/6, fundus photo demonstrates well-attached retina, bright foveal reflex, subretinal bleed has resolved, subretinal bands can be seen which are not hindering retinal reattachment. Reattached retina may appear mottled or depigmented compared to the normal retina in cases of long-standing retinal detachment, despite restoration of normal anatomy.*

Figure 6 *In quite a few cases managed with scleral buckling procedure, shallow pockets of subretinal fluid may persist, which resolve gradually over a course of a few months without need for any additional surgical intervention. Resorption of fluid can be monitored using serial OCT.* □

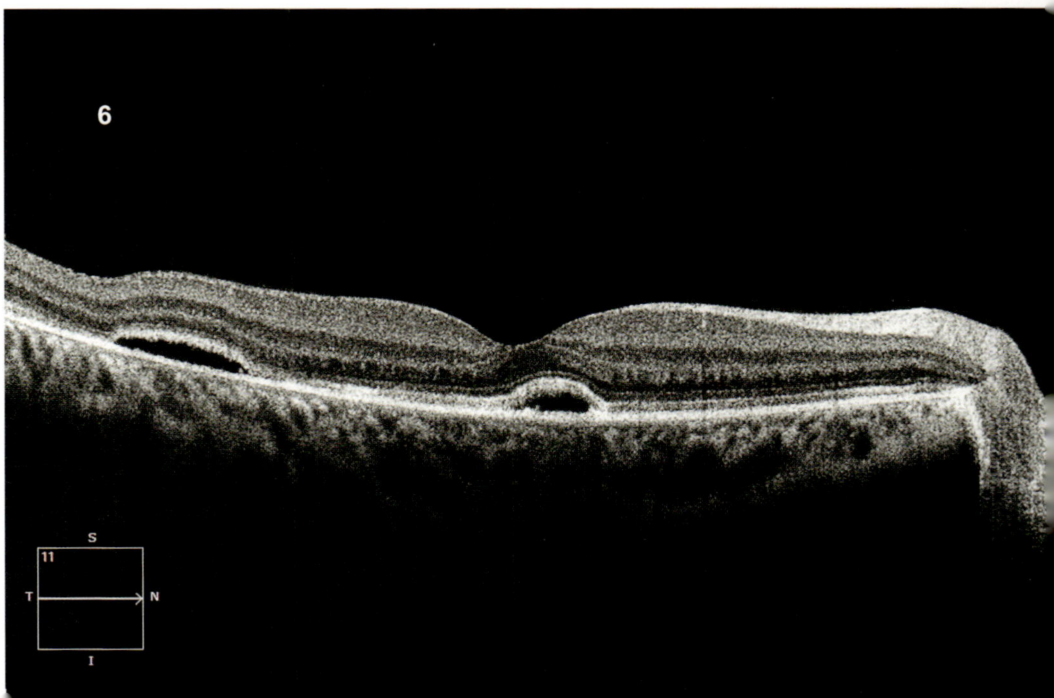

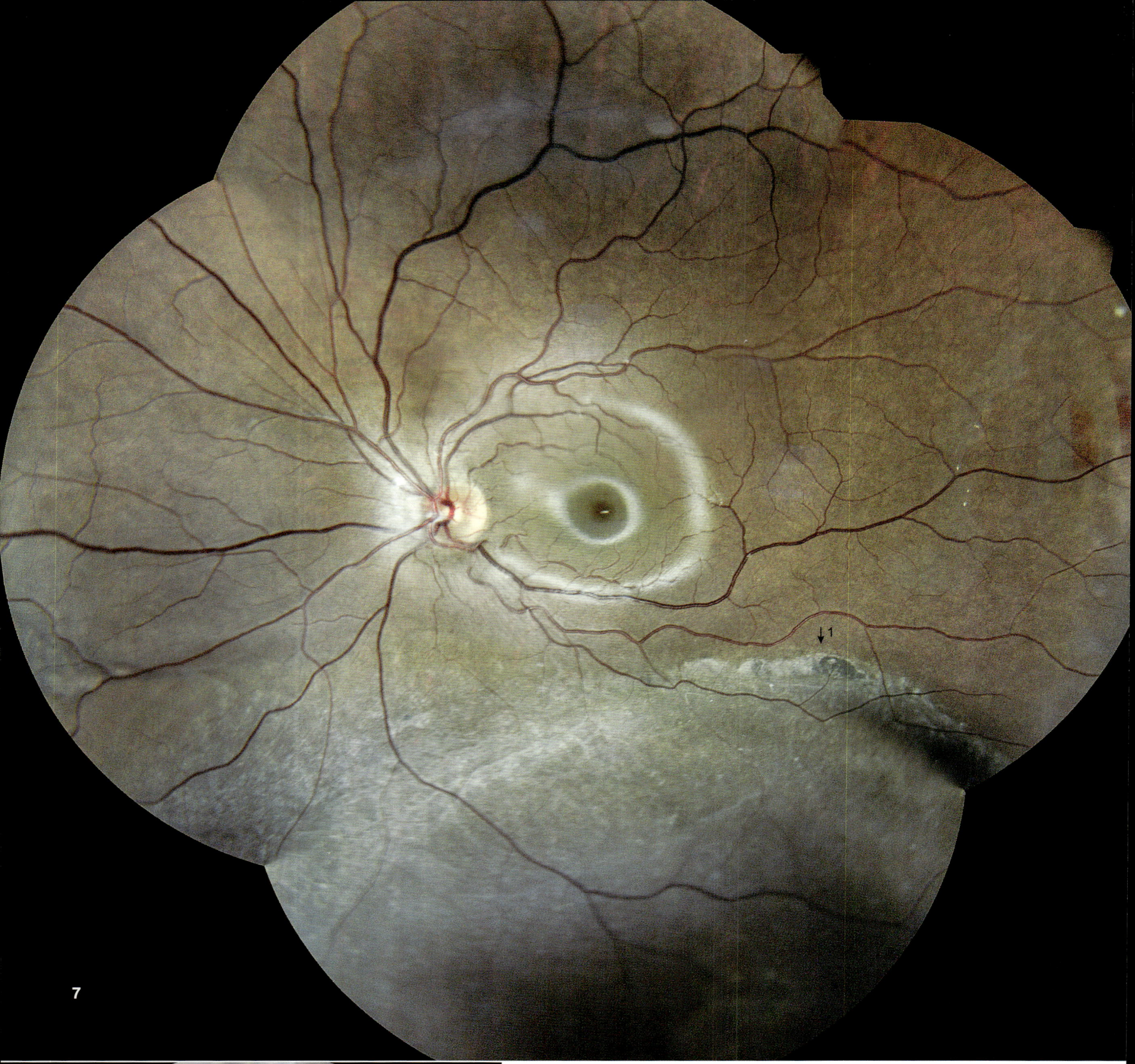


7

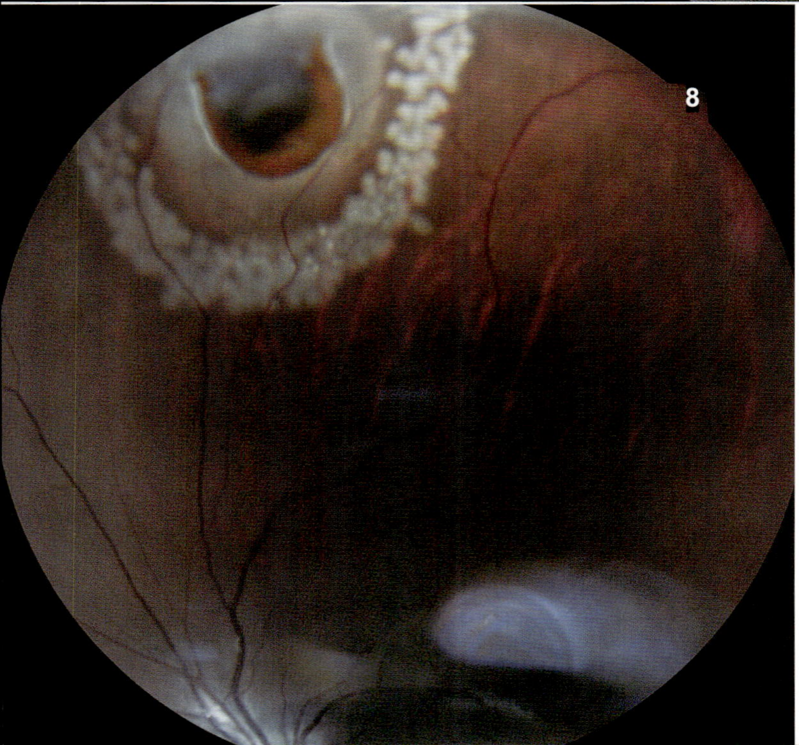

8

Figure 7 *A 26-year-old female came for routine eye check checkup and opinion for refractive surgery. Her BCVA was 6/6 in left eye. Fundus examination showed shallow inferior retinal detachment with significant retinal pigmentary epithelium changes suggestive of chronic nature of retinal detachment which may have gone unnoticed as it was not involving the macula. Demarcation line along the superior limit of fluid can also be seen (1). Foveal reflex is bright and optic nerve head appears healthy.*

Figure 8 *Immediate barrage laser photocoagulation to this horseshoe tear was done as they are associated with high risk of retinal detachment. Whitish fresh burns can be seen all around the horseshoe tear immediately after laser.*

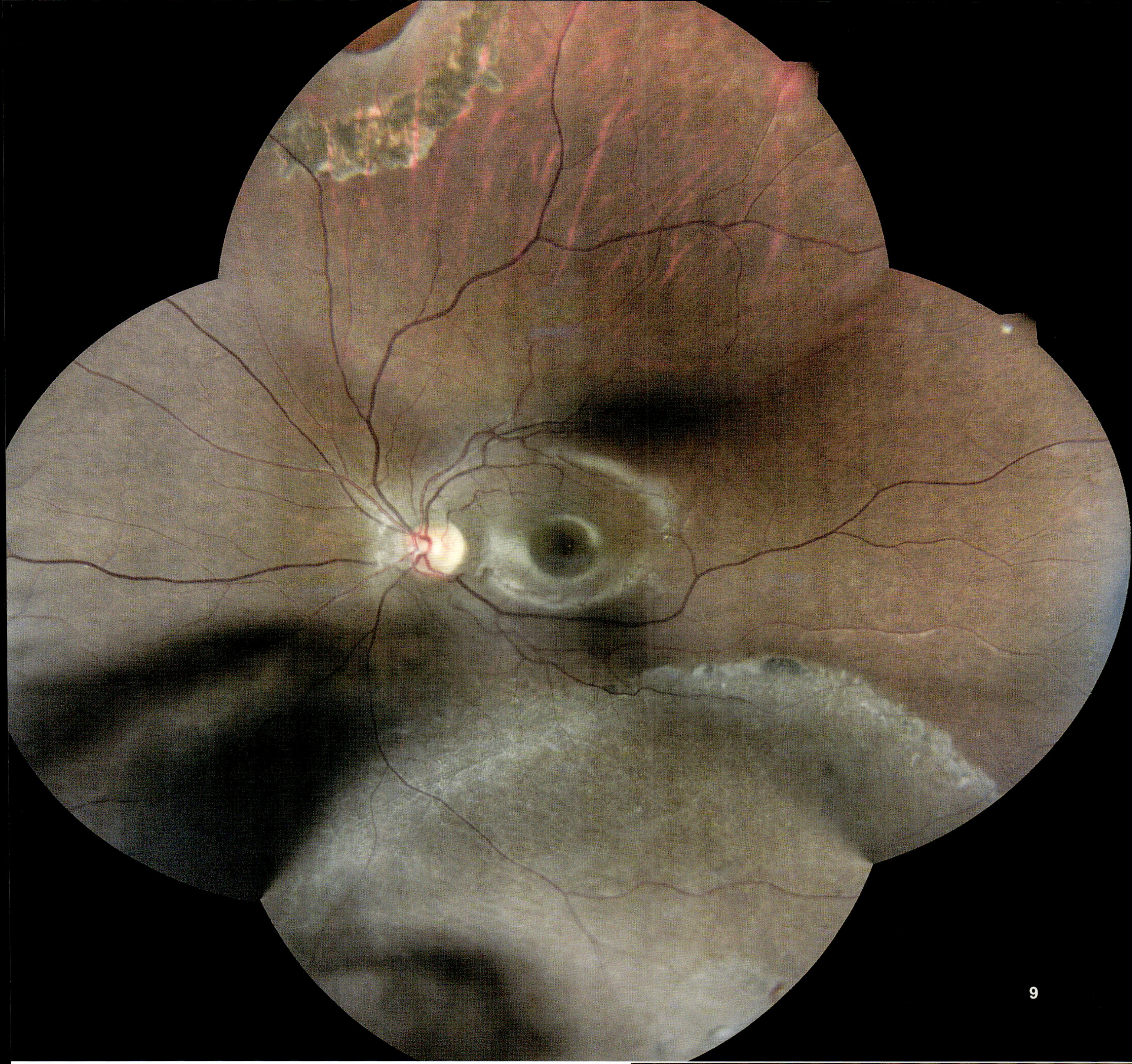

9

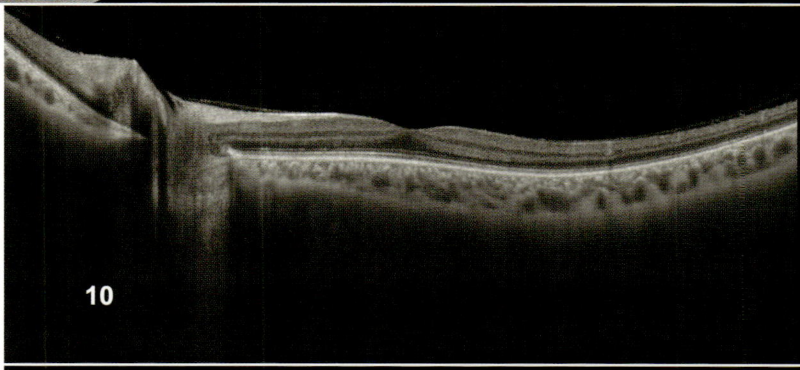

10

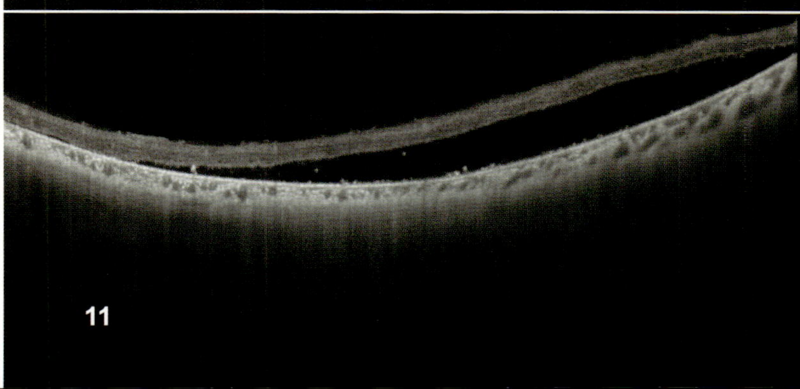

11

Figure 9 *At 3 months follow-up she maintained best corrected visual acuity of 6/6, retina was well-attached. Superiorly the laser marks at 11 o'clock have become more atrophic, pigmented and coalesced over a period of time.*

Figure 10 *SS-OCT through the macula shows well-attached retina with healthy retinal layers resulting in good visual acuity. Macula on retinal detachments usually have excellent visual prognosis and urgent surgical intervention to retain the same is must.*

Figure 11 *SS-OCT through inferior part of retina shows shallow fluid separating neurosensory retina from underlying retinal pigment epithelial layer. Disruption of outer retinal layers is evident due to long standing nature of pathology.* □

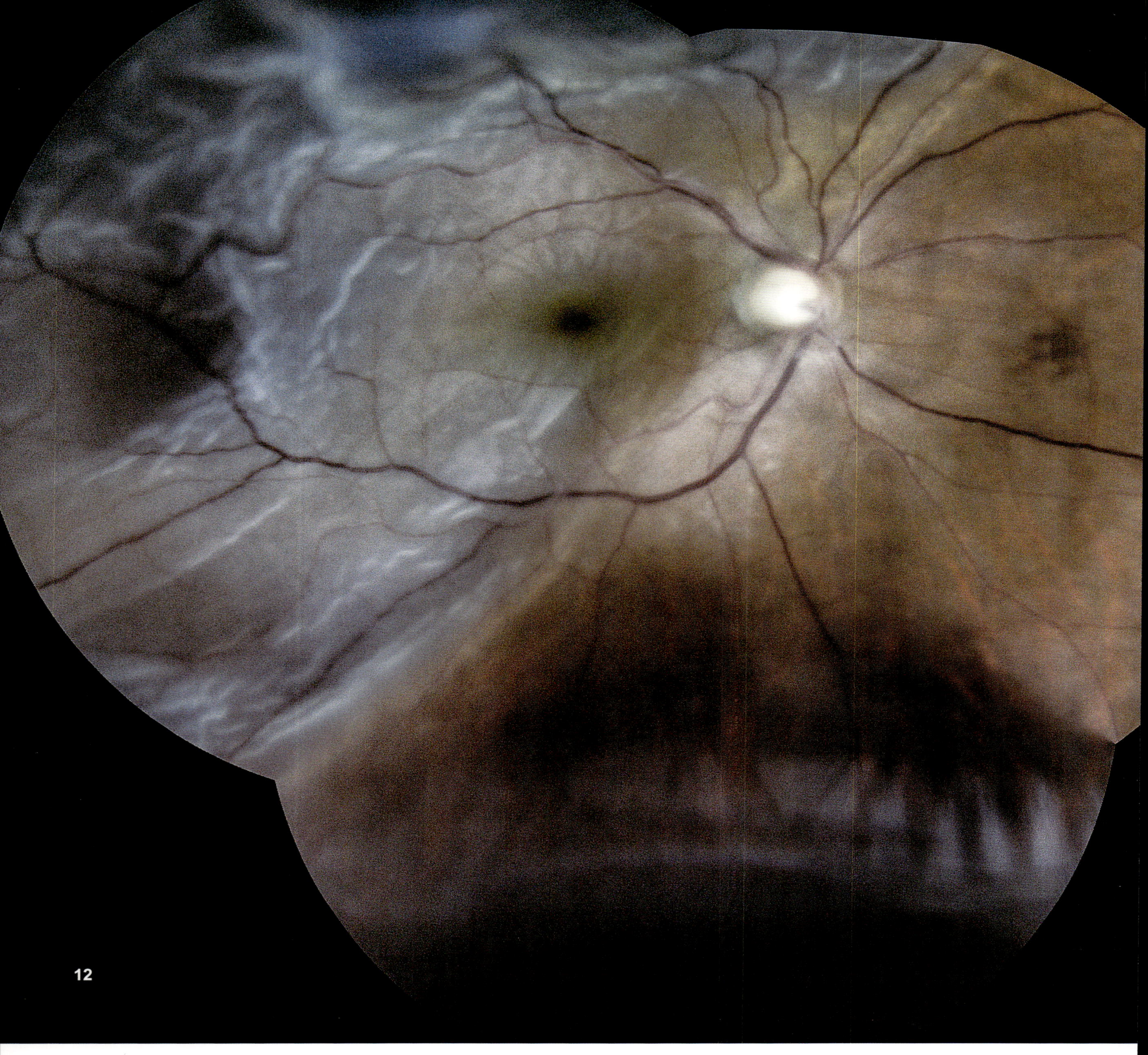


Figure 12 *Subtotal retinal detachment is a common presentation in routine vitreoretinal practice. These cases usually present early and have good prognosis. A 70-year-old male presented with complaints of sudden drop in vision from his right eye for 3 days, with BCVA CF1M. Fundus picture reveals grayish colored detached retina in superior-temporal quadrant with corrugated surface, the macula is detached (important prognostic indicator).*

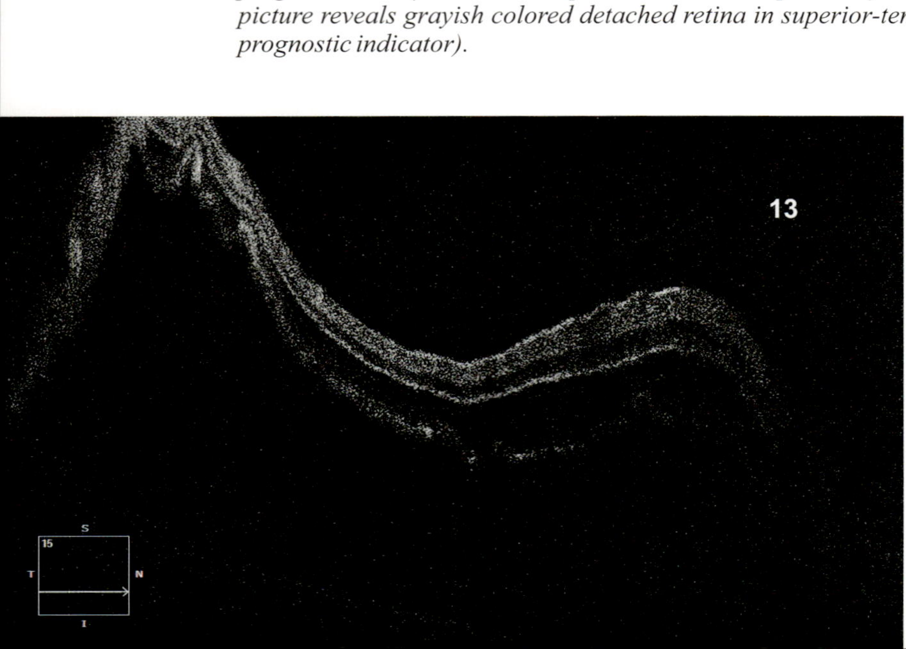


Figure 13 *OCT is an excellent tool and helps you in documenting and monitoring pathology. Subretinal fluid accumulation between neurosensory retina and underlying retinal pigment epithelium is visible on OCT scan.*

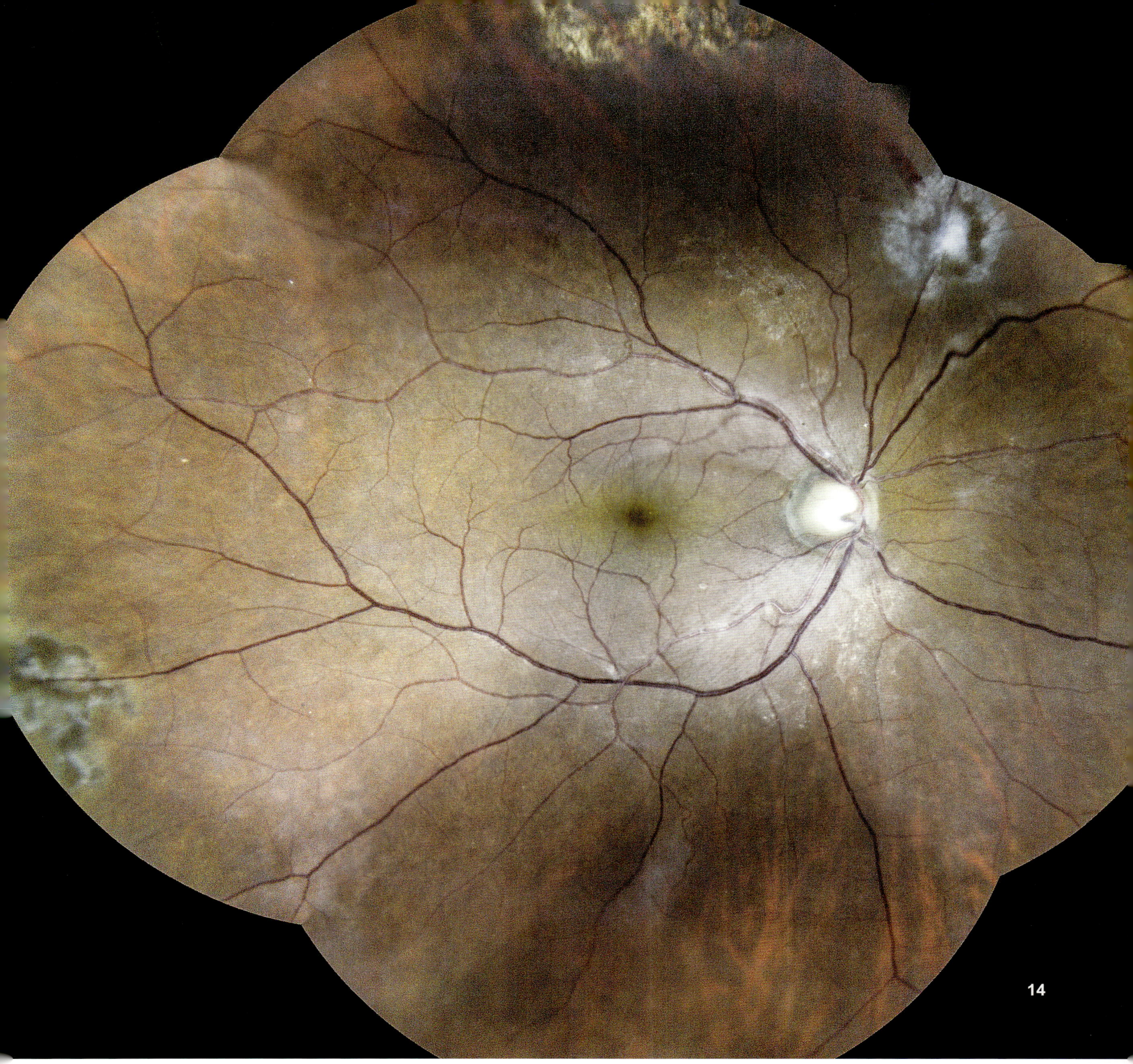

14

Figure 14 *Eventually gas escapes 4–6 weeks after procedure and normal anatomy of retina is restored as is seen in the fundus picture above. Laser marks are clearly visible around the retinotomy site and around pathological breaks which are well sealed now.*

He was advised pars plana vitrectomy (25G) with internal gas tamponade (C3F8 gas 14%), as it was relatively recent onset detachment and no significant proliferative vitreoretinopathy changes in retina. Post-operative prone positioning is critical to ensure success of the procedure.

Figure 15 *Postoperatively OCT demonstrates total restoration of retinal anatomy, with no fluid in between neurosensory retina and underlying retinal pigment epithelium. IS-OS junctions seems intact, accounting for good visual recovery of 6/9.* □

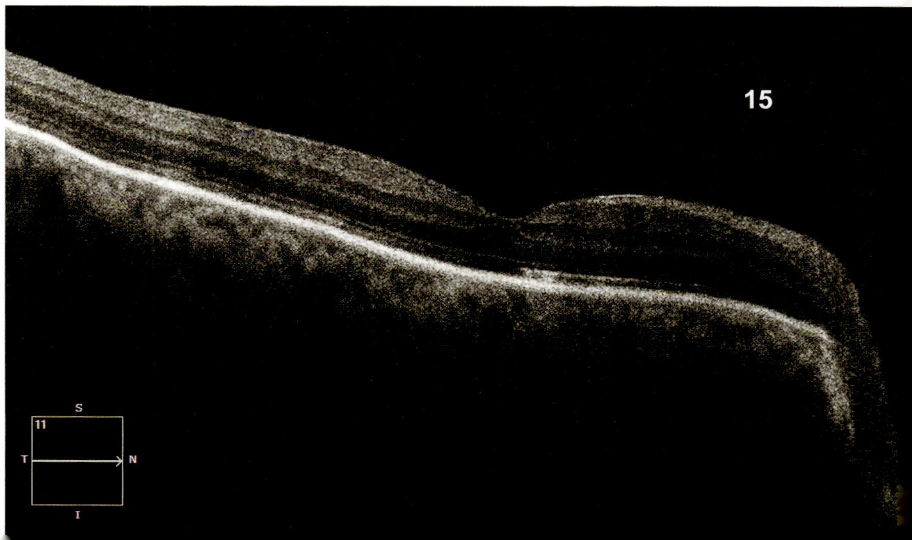


15

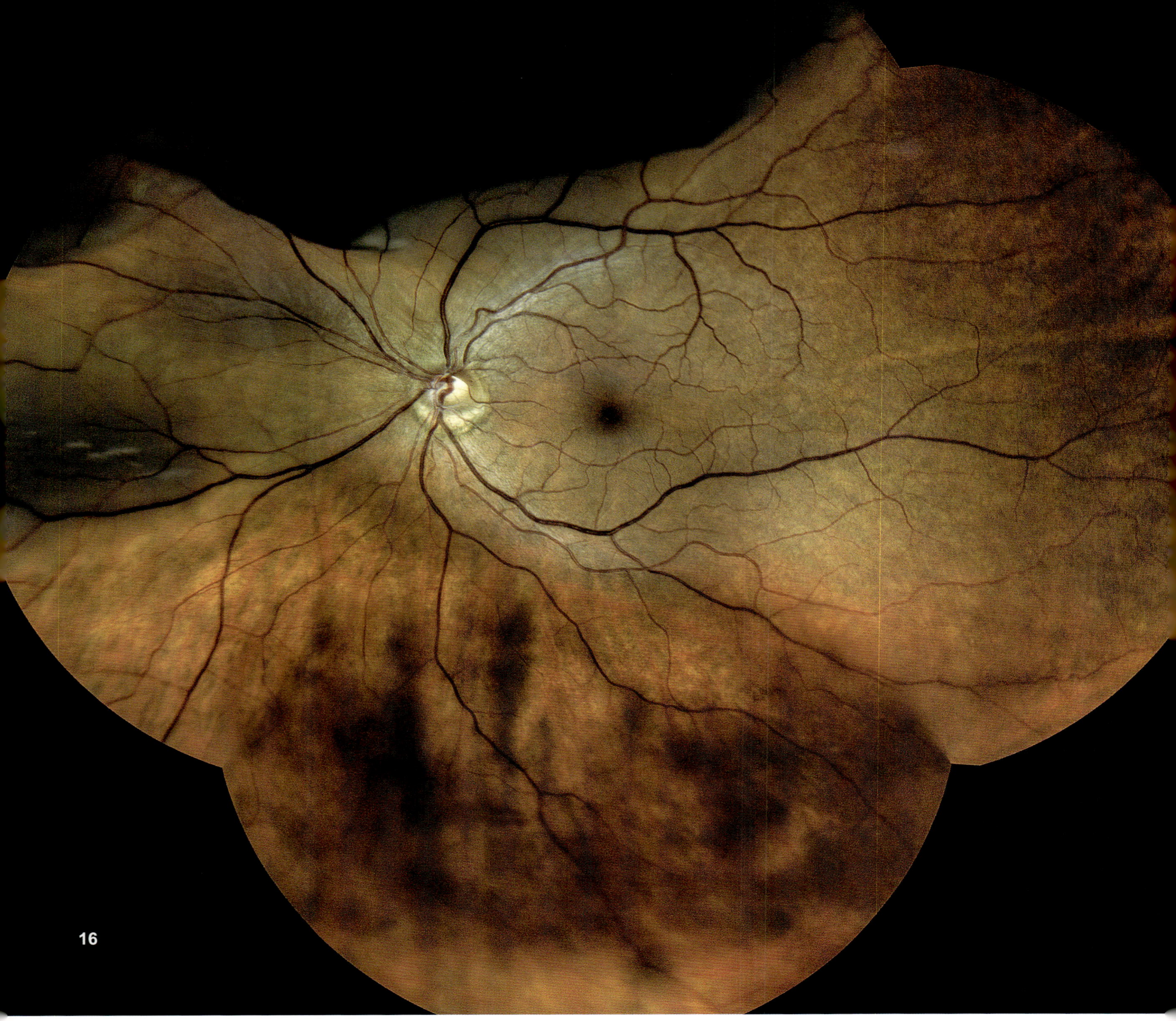

Figure 16 *Rhegmatogenous retinal detachment is caused by liquified vitreous passing through a retinal break into potential space between neurosensory retina and retinal pigment epithelium.*

Macula sparing retinal detachment yield best outcomes, if surgical intervention is done prior to involvement of macula. Hence, in routine practice it is ideal to proceed with emergent surgical intervention.

A 51-year-old male presented with complaints of black curtain like appearance in his left eye, BCVA 6/6. Fundus photo demonstrates detached grayish retina in superonasal half of the retina. Indirect ophthalmoscopy revealed a break at 11 o'clock position. The detachment however spared the macula.

He was pseudophakic and advised emergency pars plana vitrectomy (25G) with internal tamponade (c3f8) in view of superior break and macula sparing retinal detachment. While choosing intraocular gas as tamponade it is important to ensure patients compliance for post-operative positioning.

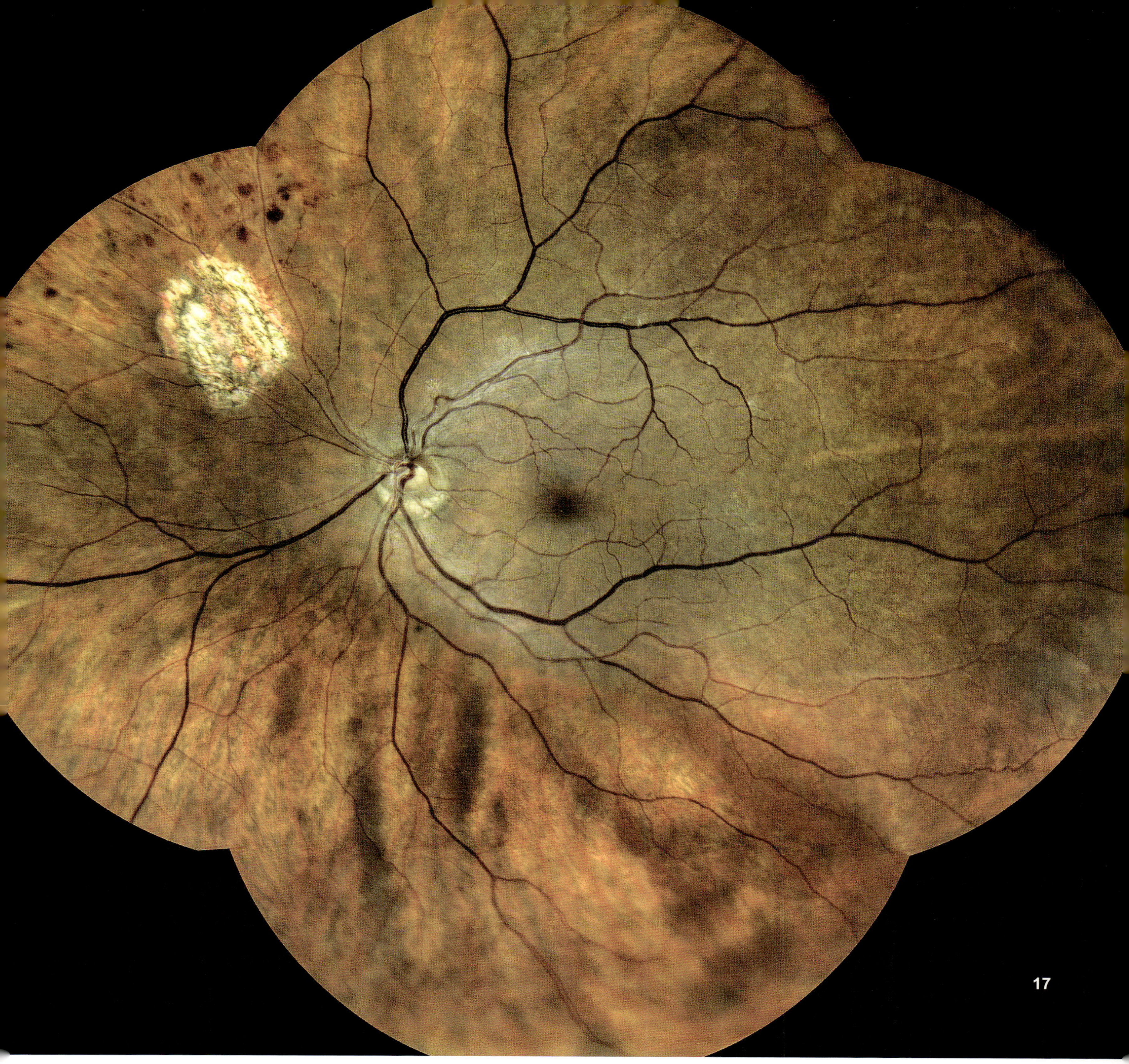


Figure 17 *Intraocular gas tamponade can last for 4–6 weeks, well-attached retina with restoration of normal anatomy can be see postoperatively, BCVA 6/9P laser marks around internal drainage retinotomy site can be seen. Superficial hemorrhages in superonasal quadrant were visible which resolved over 3 months of follow-up.*□

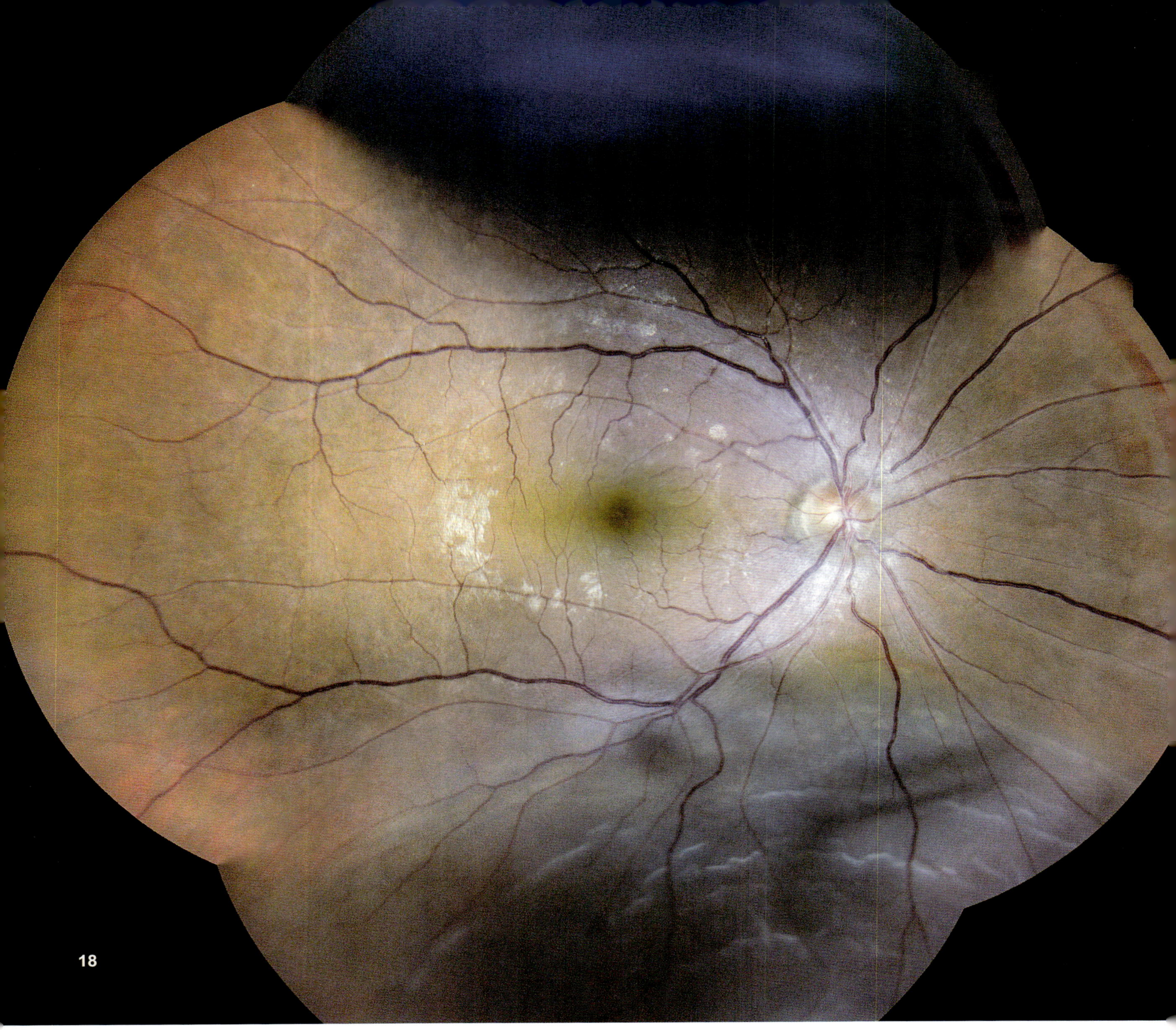


Figure 18 *A 68-year-old male presented with complaints of seeing a black shadow in front of his right eye in superior half for past 10 days. BCVA was 6/9 fundus photo shows a shallow grayish inferior detached retina extending up to the inferior arcade however sparing the macula, a large break can be seen inferiorly at 6 o'clock hour. Being a macula sparing retinal detachment it is best to ensure an emergent surgical procedure to ensure best prognosis.*

Figure 19 *At 3 months follow-up, he complains of decrease in vision, BCVA was 6/60, he also complained of distortion and difficulty in reading, fundus photo shows grayish membrane-like structure at the macula under silicone oil causing retinal folds indicative of epiretinal membrane leading to macular puckering.*

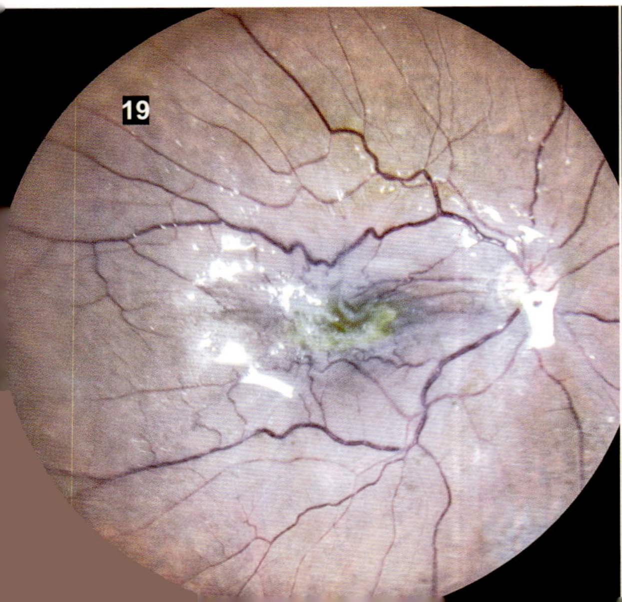


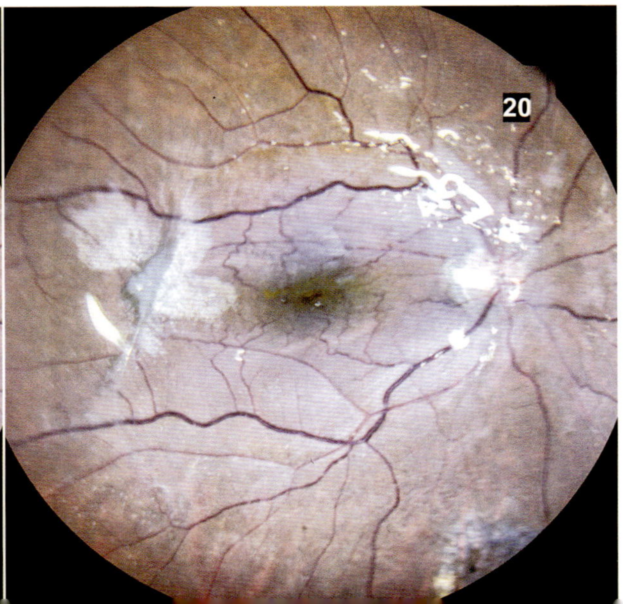


Figure 20 *At 4-month follow-up, he reported back with BCVA 6/18p, his visual acuity had improved and fundus shows grayish rolled up membrane lying temporal to macula and sparing the fovea. There was a spontaneous separation of epiretinal membrane under silicone oil. It is rare for epiretinal membrane to spontaneously separate, however if same is observed clinically or on optical coherence tomography is it ideal to wait and observe for release of traction on fovea and surgical intervention can be deferred.* □

Figure 21 *In yet another similar case, 2 months post-25G pars plana vitrectomy with silicone oil tamponade in situ, there was drop in visual acuity from 6/60 to 6/36 with complaints of metamorphopsia, fundus photo shows grayish membrane-like structure at the macula, indicating formation of epiretinal membrane.*

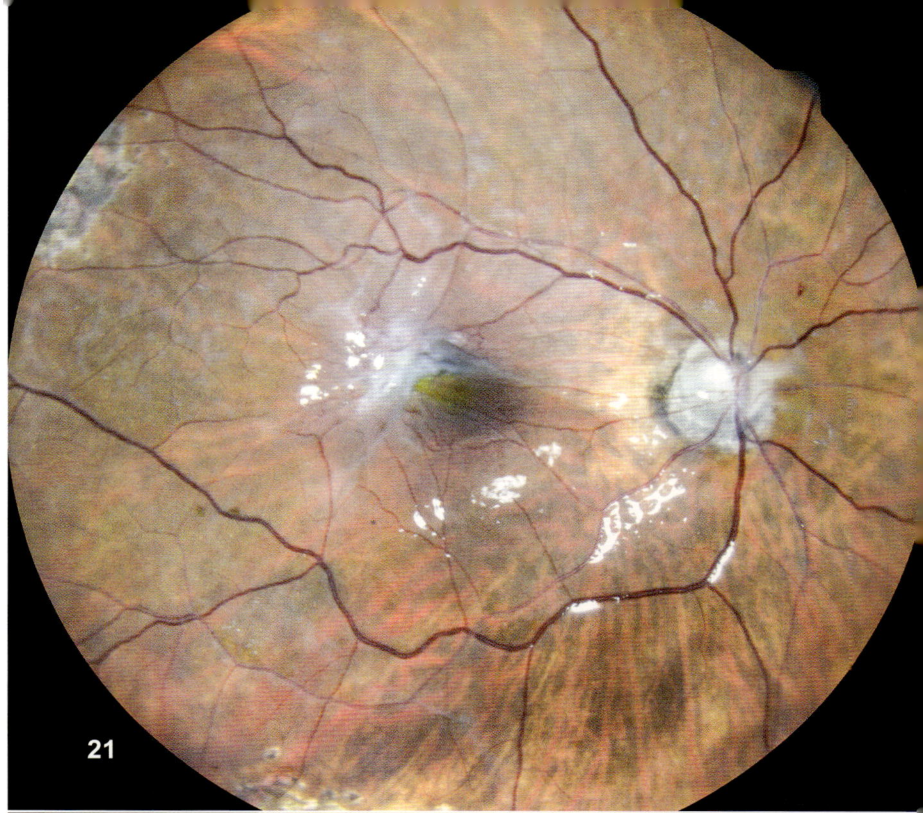


Figure 22 *At 3 months postoperative BCVA improved to 6/12p and fundus photo reveals spontaneous separation of epiretinal membrane under oil folding temporal to fovea relieving the traction at fovea. It is best to observe for more separation to occur spontaneously at this stage to relieve traction at the fovea.*

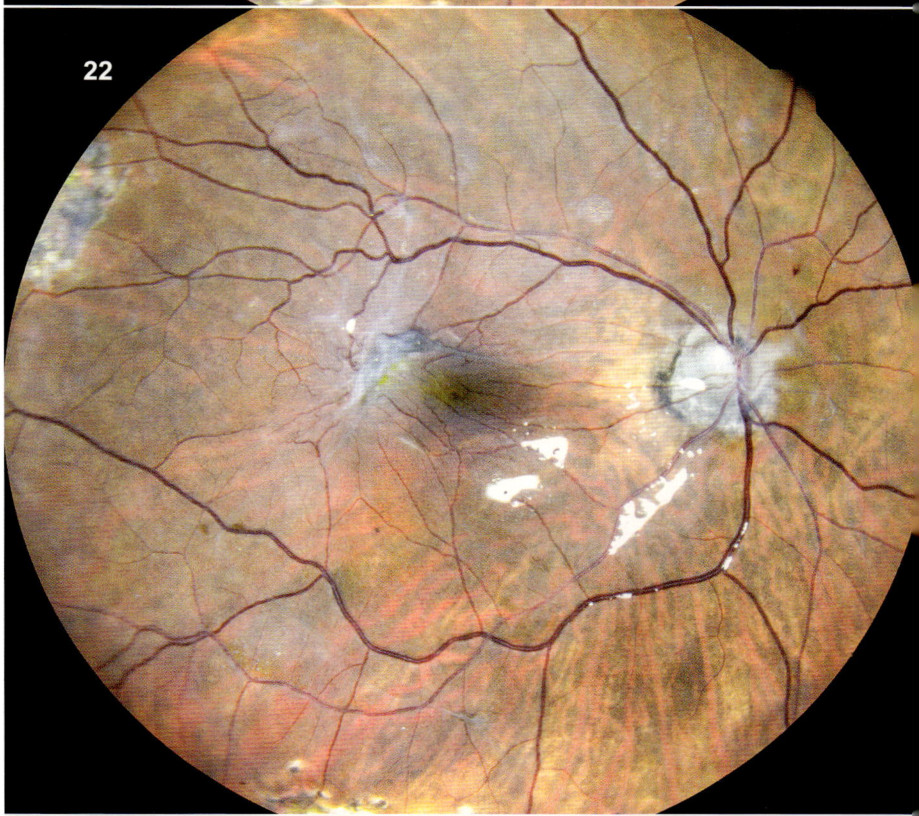


Figure 23 *At 7 months postsilicone oil removal and epiretinal membrane removal BCVA improved to 6/9 with restoration of normal contour of macula.* □

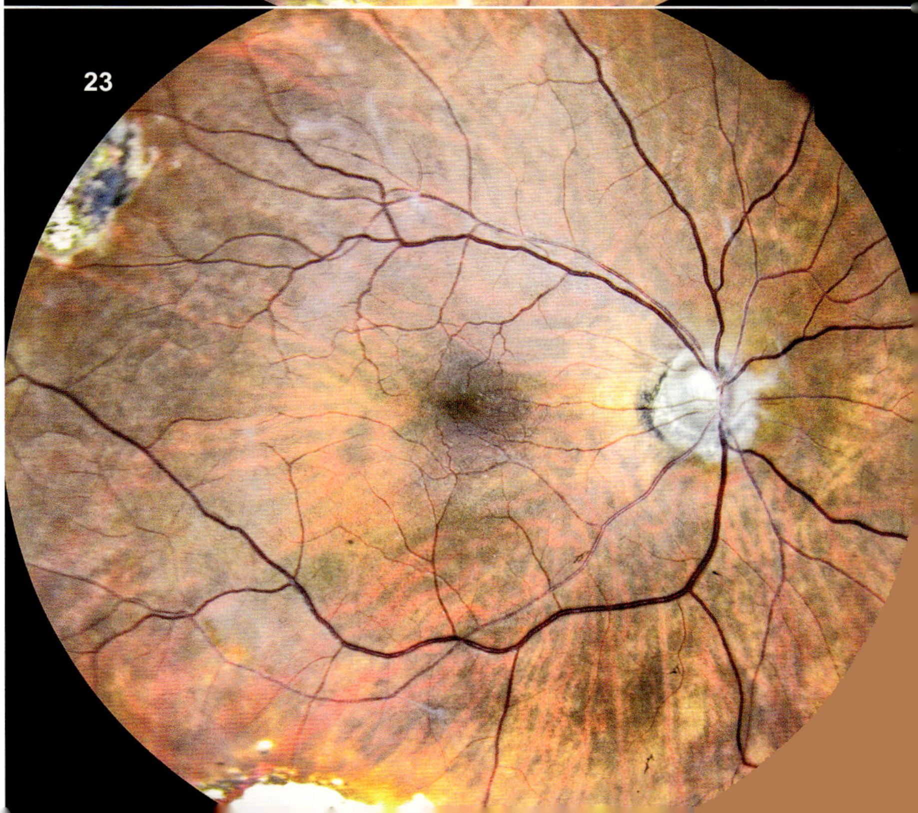

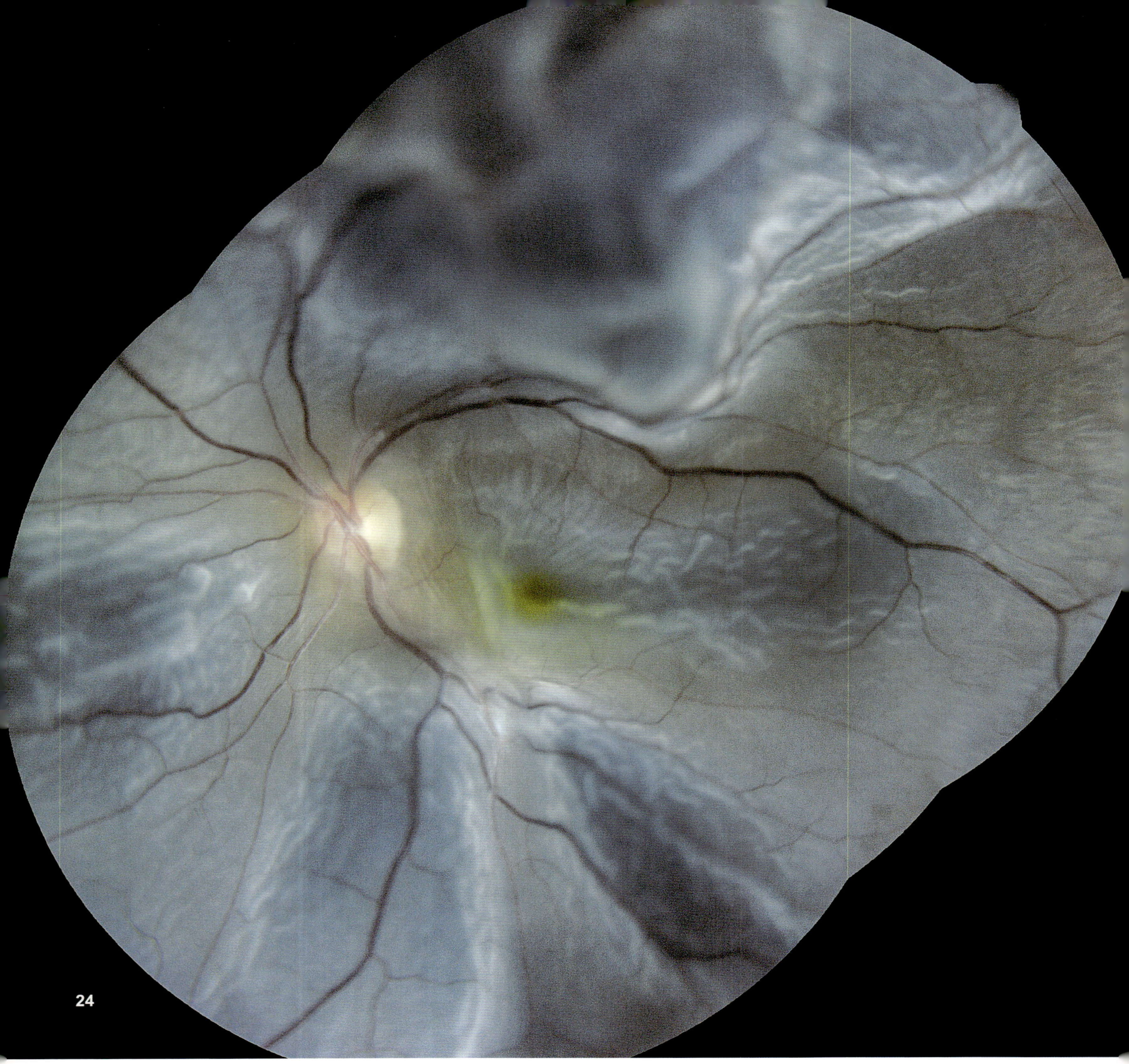

Figure 24 *Epiretinal membrane proliferation under silicone oil, in a case of long-standing rhegmatogenous retinal detachment managed with pars plana vitrectomy with silicone oil tamponade.*

A 66-year-old female presented with complaints of total loss of vision in her left eye for 2 months. She gave history of cataract surgery in the same eye. Fundus photo shows grayish detached retina with corrugated folds suggestive of total retinal detachment involving the macula.

Early proliferative vitreoretinopathy can be seen as slight puckering along the inferotemporal arcade with dragging of retina with folds visible extending up to temporal aspect of optic disk.

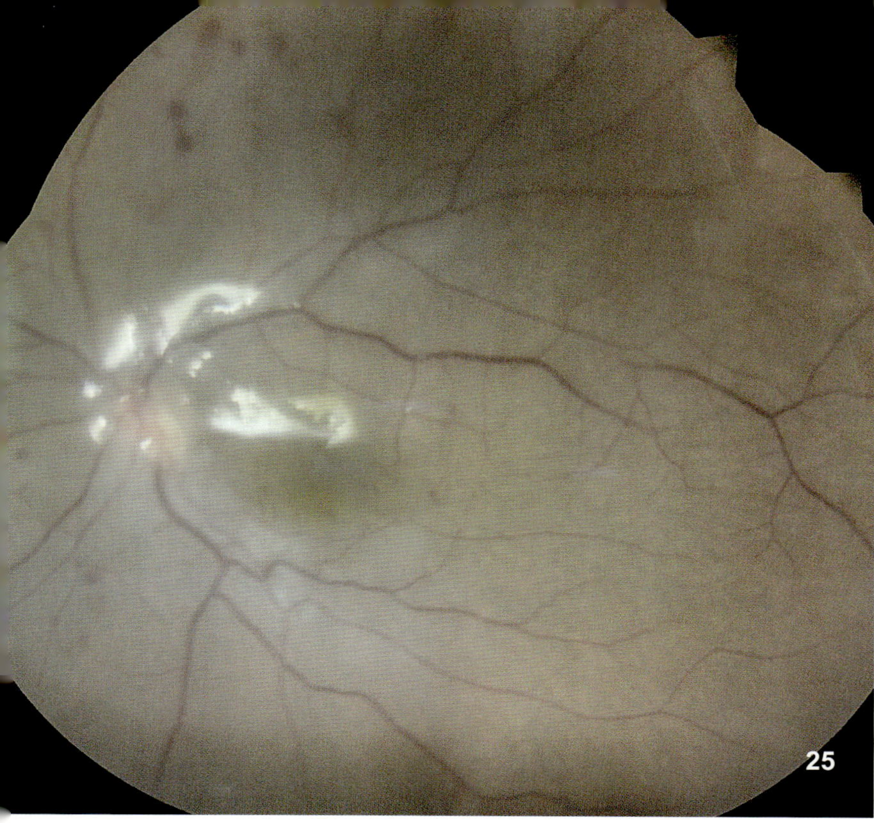

Figure 25 *25-gauge pars plana vitrectomy was performed in the left eye with silicone oil in situ. Long-acting tamponade-like silicone oil may be preferred in such cases as retinal detachment is long-standing, and also inability of patient to maintain prone position postoperatively. Fundus photo shows attached retina with silicone oil in situ. Laser marks can be seen nasally around drainage retinotomy site. Few superficial hemorrhages are present nasally.*

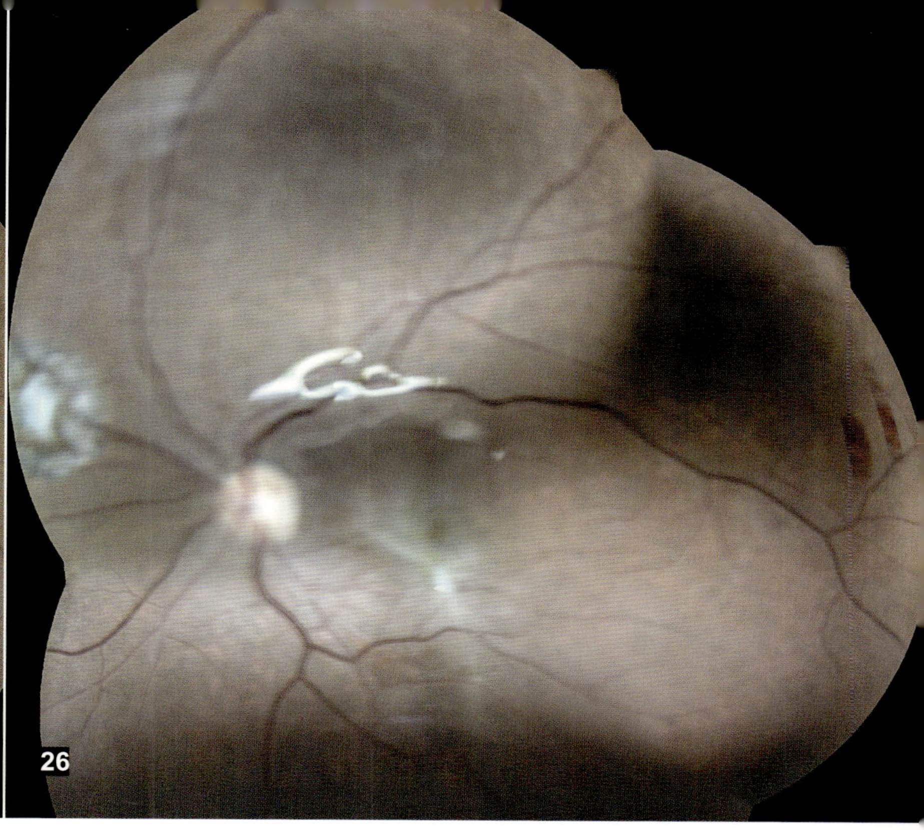

Figure 26 *Epiretinal membranes may develop in eyes filled with silicone oil, especially after it was used in cases with rhegmatogenous retinal detachment with pre-existing proliferative vitreoretinopathy. At 3-month follow-up BCVA was 6/60 and she complained of distortion of vision. Fundus photo shows well-attached retina with silicone oil in situ. However, one can appreciate a grayish white membrane-like structure over the surface of retina extending from the temporal end of the disc to inferiorly involving the fovea.*

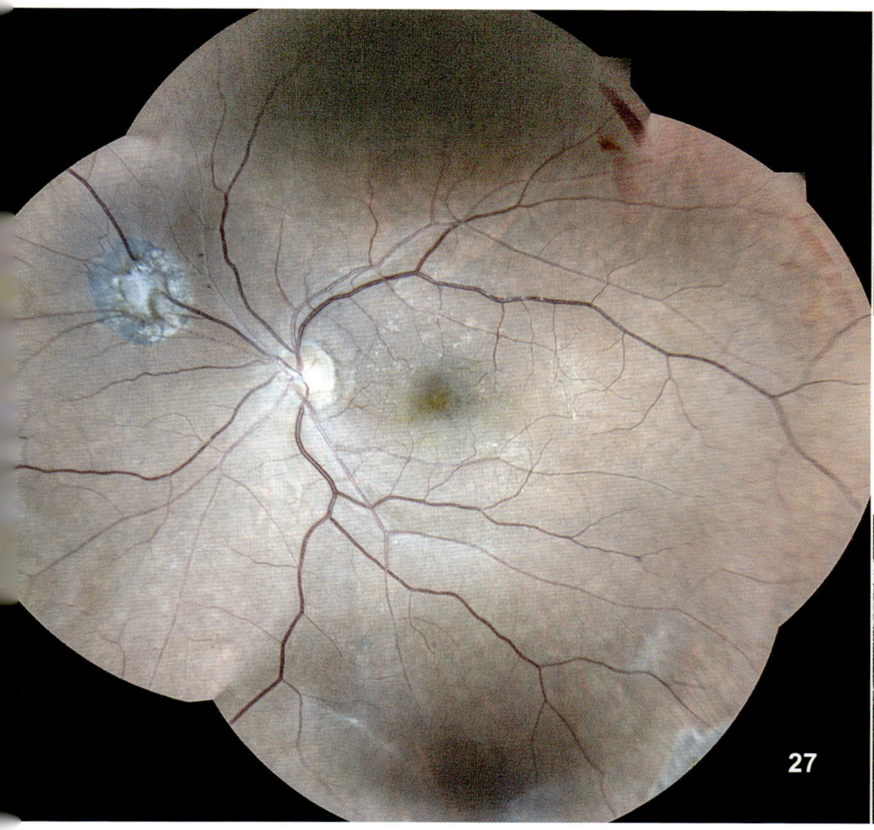

Figure 27 *She was planned for silicone oil removal along with epiretinal membrane removal. Epiretinal membrane removal using membrane forceps can be done with ease under silicone oil which provides for a counter traction force. Surgery with intraocular silicone oil in situ is called as "interface vitrectomy". This was followed by complete removal of silicone oil with multiple fluid air exchange to remove all emulsified oil. Postoperatively retina is well-attached and epiretinal membrane is removed completely removing any drag on macula. BCVA was 6/24.*

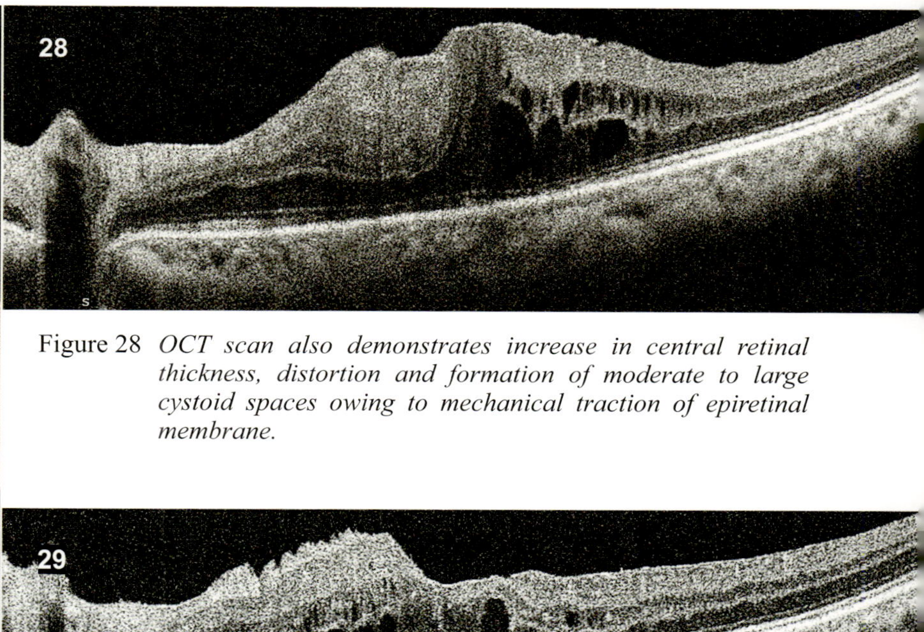

Figure 28 *OCT scan also demonstrates increase in central retinal thickness, distortion and formation of moderate to large cystoid spaces owing to mechanical traction of epiretinal membrane.*

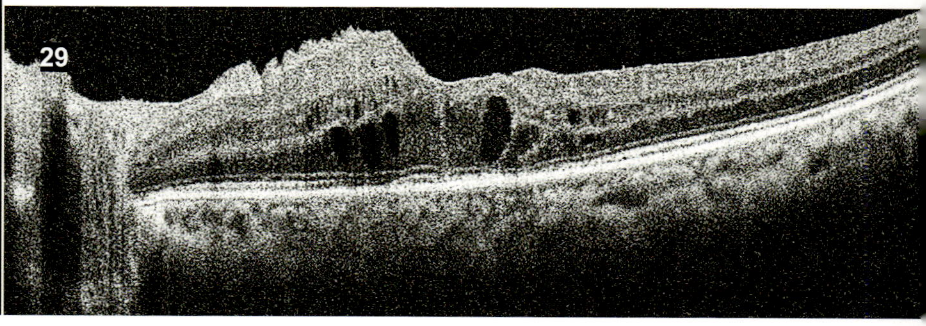

Figure 29 *OCT postoperatively at 2 weeks shows reduction in number of cystoid spaces and retinal thickening which eventually keep on decreasing with passage of time.* □

A 58-year-old male presented with complaints of sudden appearance of black spots in front of his left eye and decrease in vision for past 1 day. Best corrected visual acuity was counting fingers close to face. He gave history of retinal barrage laser in his fellow right eye one year ago.

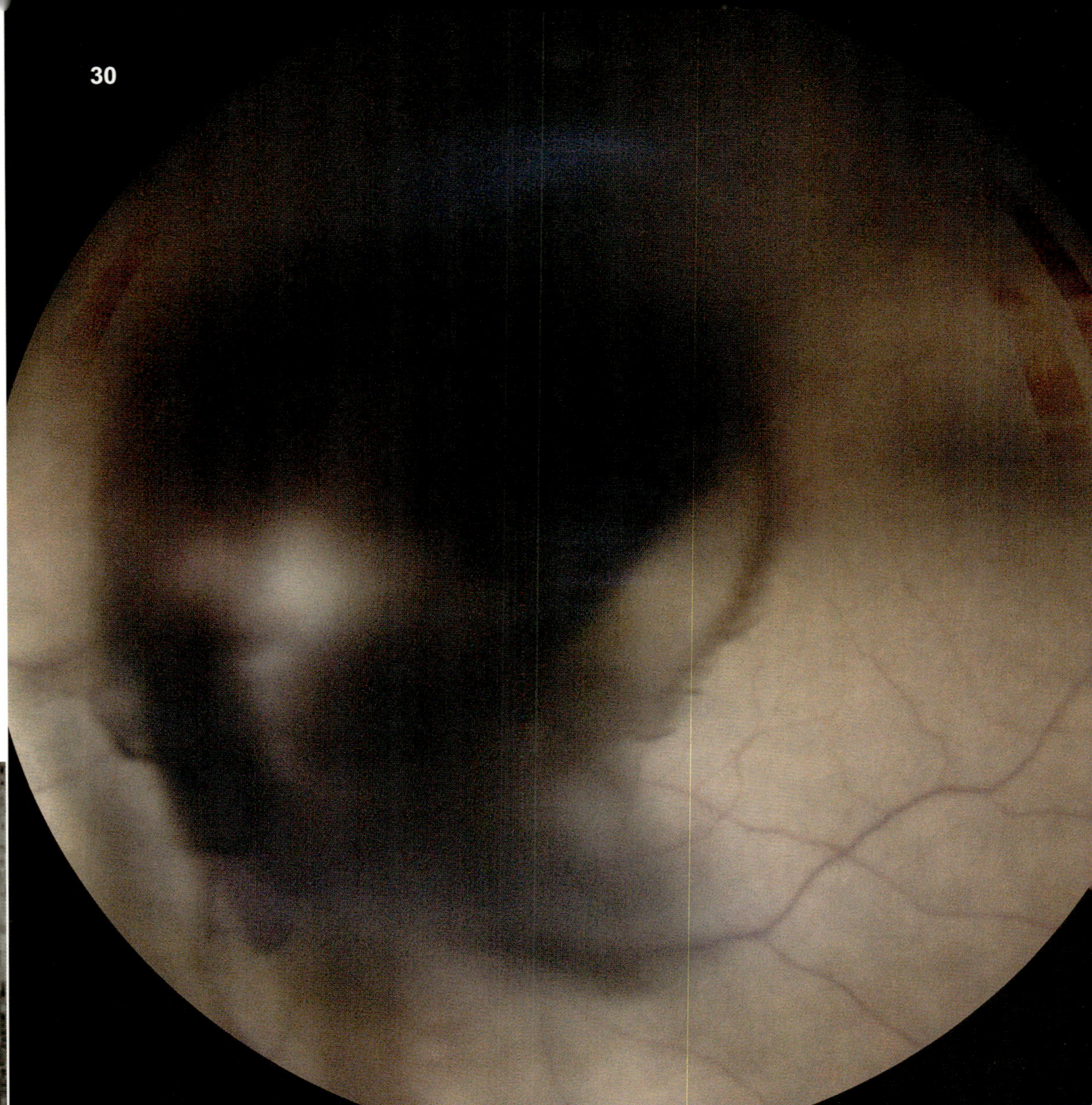

Figure 30

*Fundus photo shows dense vitreous hemorrhage obscuring most of the view of fundus at disc and macula. Media clarity was grade 2. A horse-shoe tear was seen on indirect ophthalmoscopy at 1 o'clock position however margins were obscured with hemorrhage and there was cuff of serous fluid around it.*

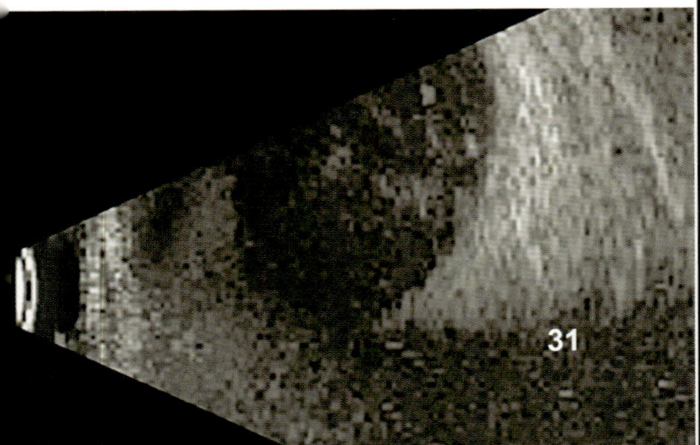

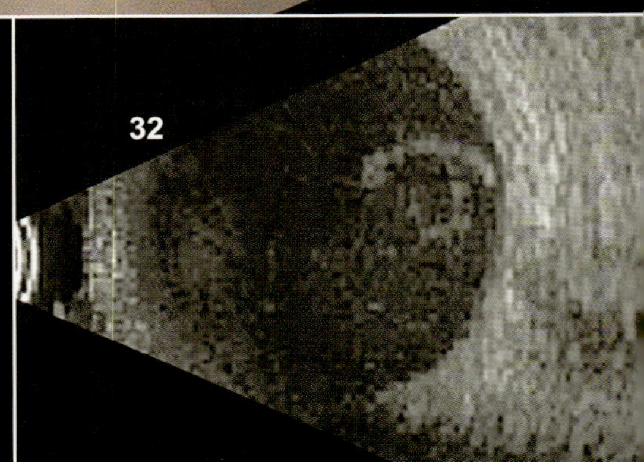

Figures 31 and 32

*It is essential to perform ultrasonography in such cases wherein it may not be possible to view the retina owing to media opacity. Ultrasound of left eye shows moderate amplitude echoes in vitreous cavity suggestive of vitreous hemorrhage. The retina was attached.*

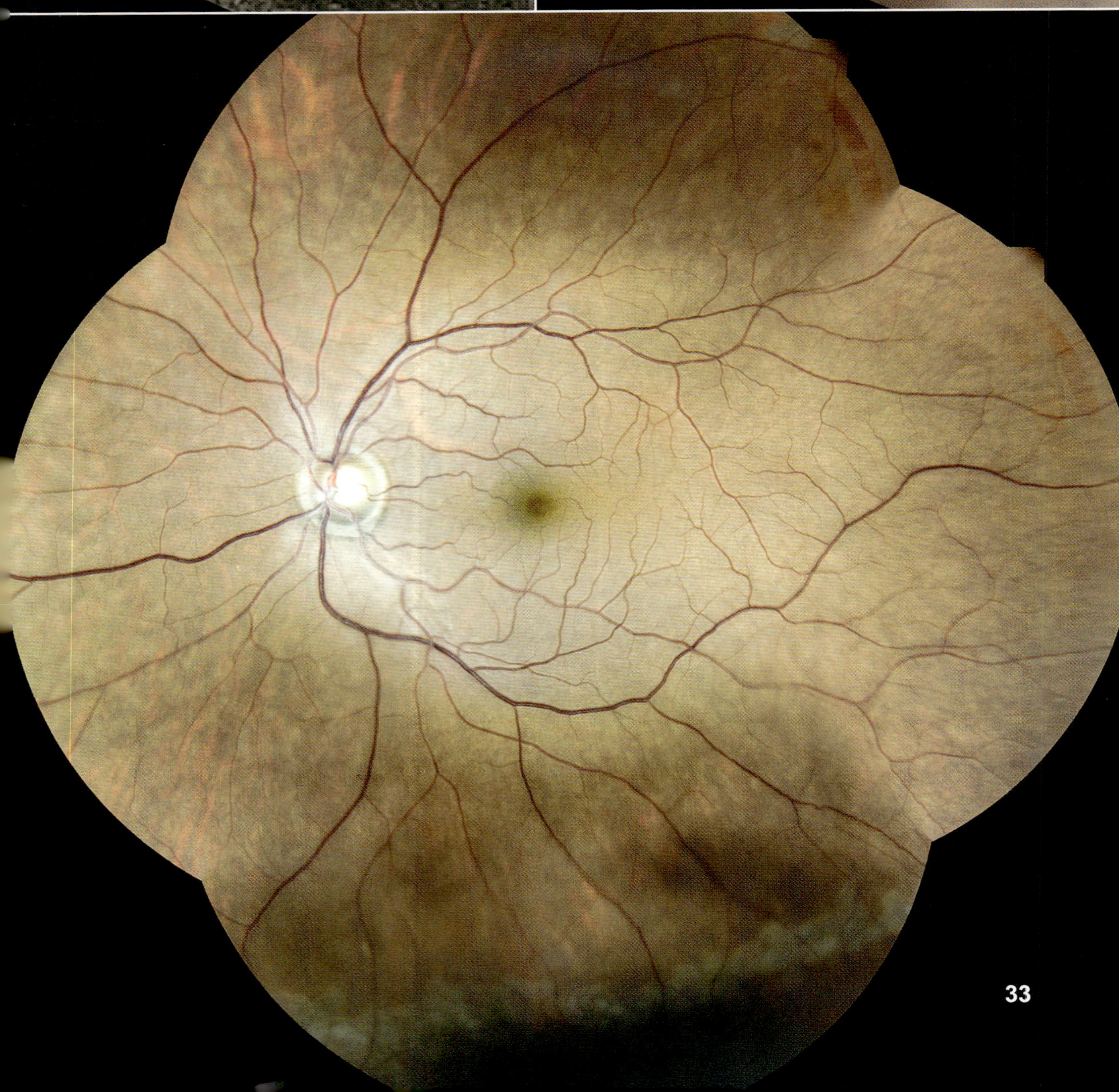

Figure 33

*Urgent 25-gauge pars plana vitrectomy was done in to prevent detachment of retina, as it was not possible to laser the tear through the dense hemorrhage. Postoperatively at one week BCVA is 6/6 media clarity is grade 1, optic disc and macula are seen clearly.* □

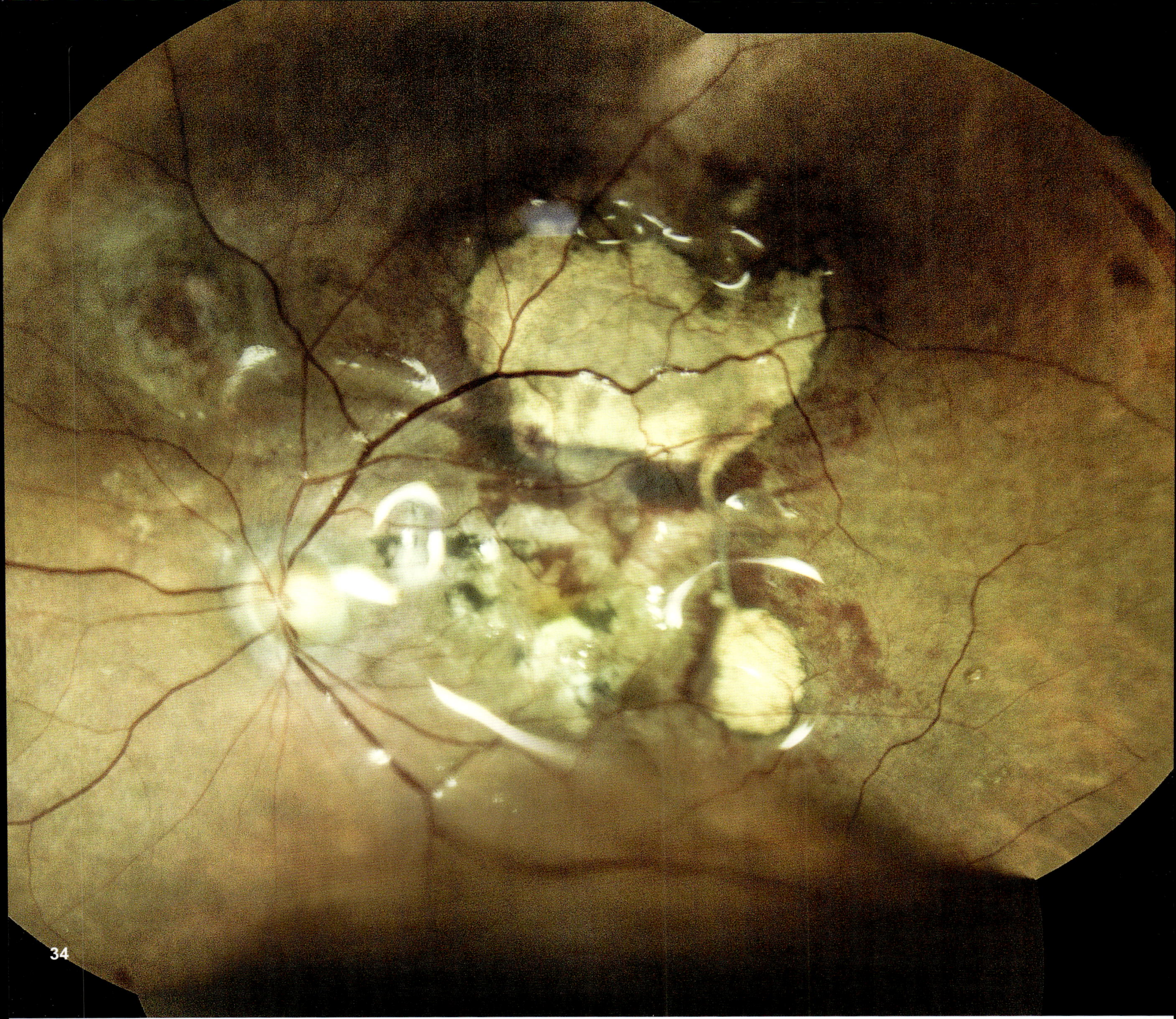

Figure 34 *An urgent 25-gauge pars plana vitrectomy was performed, vitreous hemorrhage was cleared using vitreous cutter, following that posterior vitreous was removed after staining with triamcinolone acetonide and vitreous base dissection was complete, fluid air exchange was done followed by silicone oil tamponade. Silicone oil is preferred in uniocular patients in view of faster visual rehabilitation, also the patient was unable to maintain prone positioning for prolonged period of time. Postoperatively retina is well-attached with media clarity grade 1, nasal retinotomy site can be seen superonasally with laser marks all around. Fresh red colored subretinal hemorrhage and old partially dehemoglobinized bleed can be seen at the macula. Diffuse retinal pigment epithelium atrophy is also present at the macula suggestive of age-related macular degeneration.*

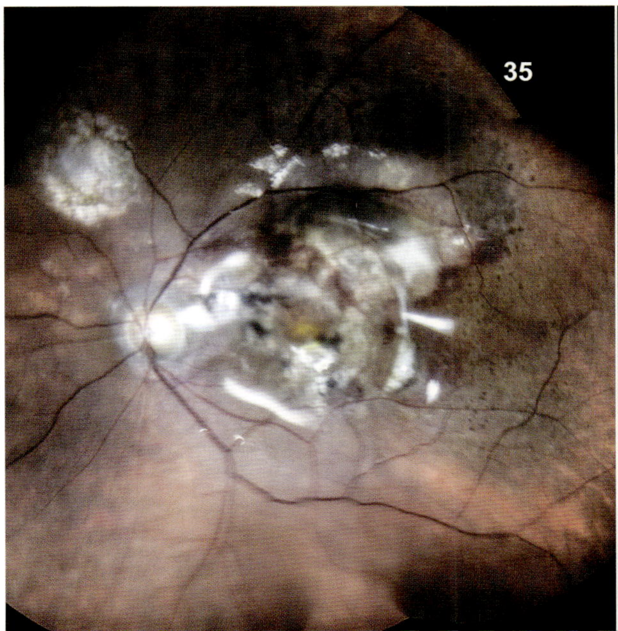

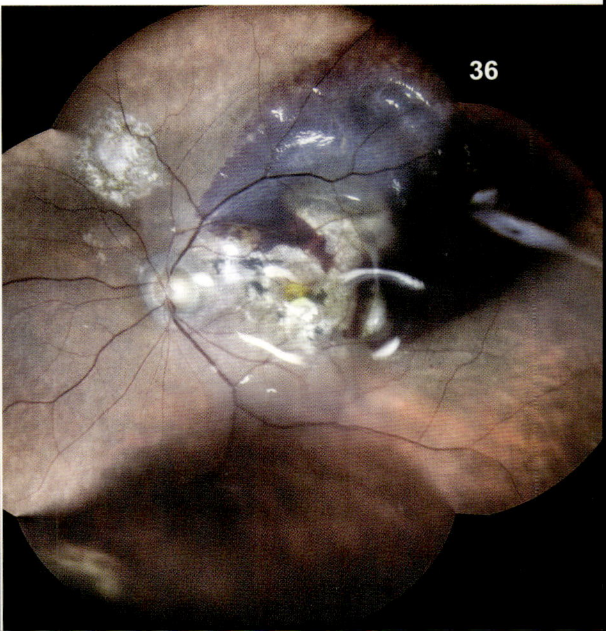

Figure 35 *He was advised for intravitreal injection of anti-VEGF in his left eye as he was uniocular patient. BCVA of 6/60 on fundus photo postinjection there was significant reduction in preretinal bleed however some of it still persisted which need further injections.*

Figure 36 *At 6 weeks follow-up retina was well-attached with silicone oil in situ however there was significant increase in subretinal bleed suggestive of active exudative age-related macular degeneration.* □

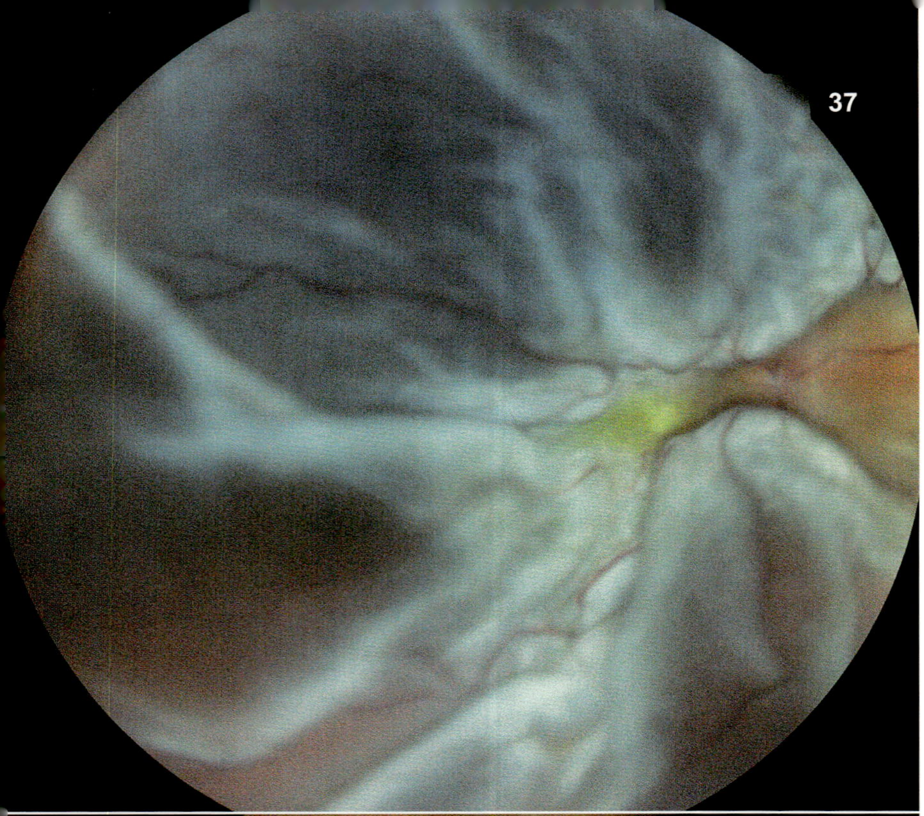


Figure 37 *A 62-year-old male presented with complaints of diminution of vision from his right eye for 4 months. BCVA was counting finger close to face. Fundus photo shows rhegmatogenous retinal detachment with multiple surface wrinkles and folds in all quadrants extending up to the macula, suggestive of proliferative vitreoretinopathy (PVR), which is associated with retinal stiffness and decreased mobility on eye movement. It was classified to be PVR D-1, having fixed folds in all quadrants with wide funnel-shaped configuration.*

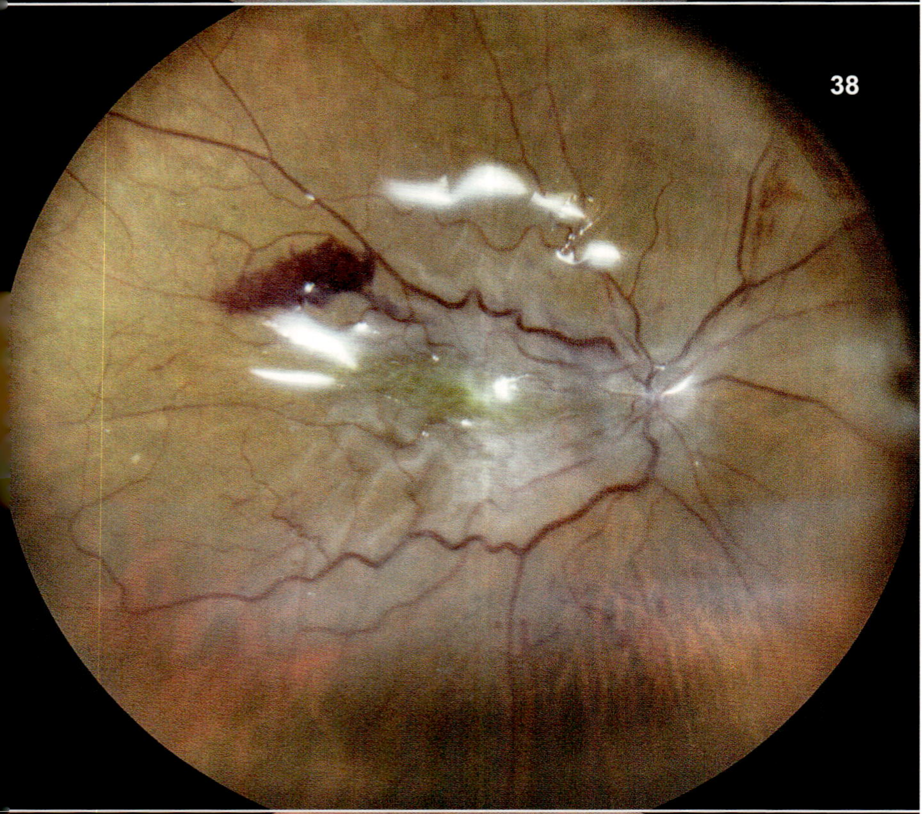


Figure 38 *At 3-month follow-up membranes progressed to cause further PVR with puckering of macula, narrowing of arcade and deep subretinal hemorrhages at superotemporal aspect owing to traction. These membranes can usually be peeled off from retinal surface at the time of planned silicone oil removal, while silicone oil is in-situ to provide for counter traction.*

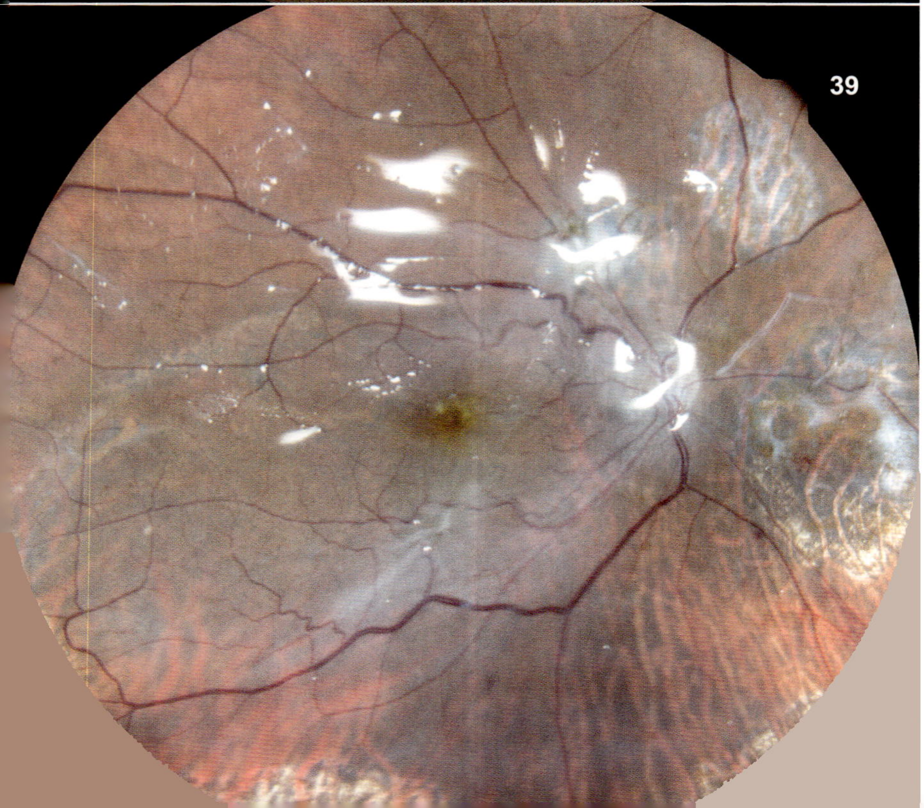


Figure 39 *25-gauge pars plana vitrectomy was done with silicone oil tamponade. Such cases usually carry poor prognosis and are at high risk for reproliferation following retinal detachment surgery and must be kept under close follow-up. At 2-month follow-up early PVR as a gray membrane causing pucker can be seen developing along the inferior arcade.* □

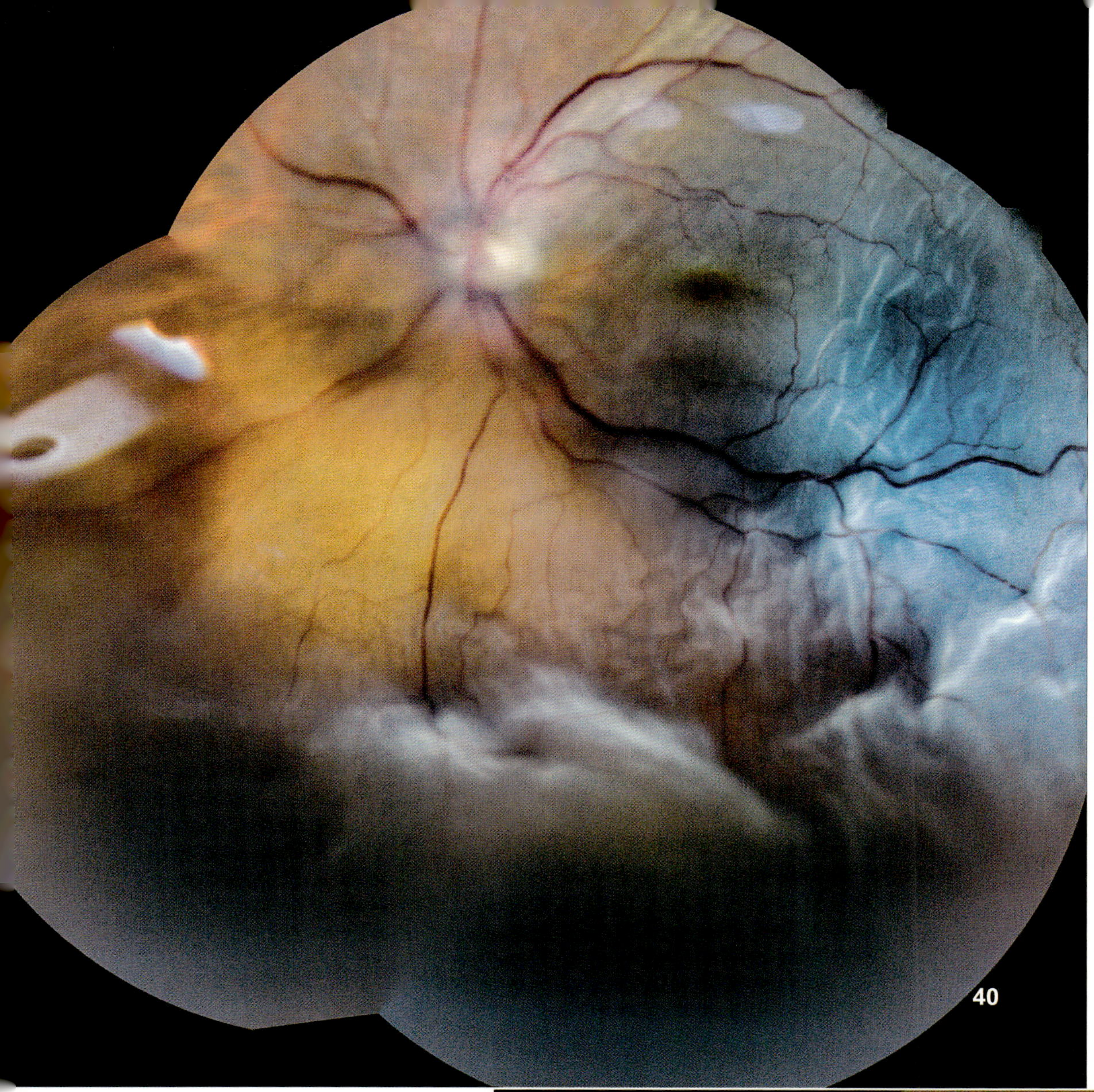


Figure 40

*A 72-year-old male presented with complaints of decrease vision in left eye for 6 months. Fundus examination showed gray elevated detached retina with corrugated surface. It was involving inferior and temporal retina. Superior and nasal retina was still on, indicating a subtotal retinal detachment. There was a retinal hole at 5 o'clock hour.*

Figure 41

*He underwent a 25-gauge pars plana vitrectomy with internal tamponade. Fundus photo shows reattached retina with silicone oil tamponade in situ. In cases of inferior retinal detachment silicone oil as tamponade may be preferred over intraocular gas. Internal drainage retinotomy site can be seen inferonasally. Position of drainage retinotomy can be chosen according to the configuration of retinal detachment.*□

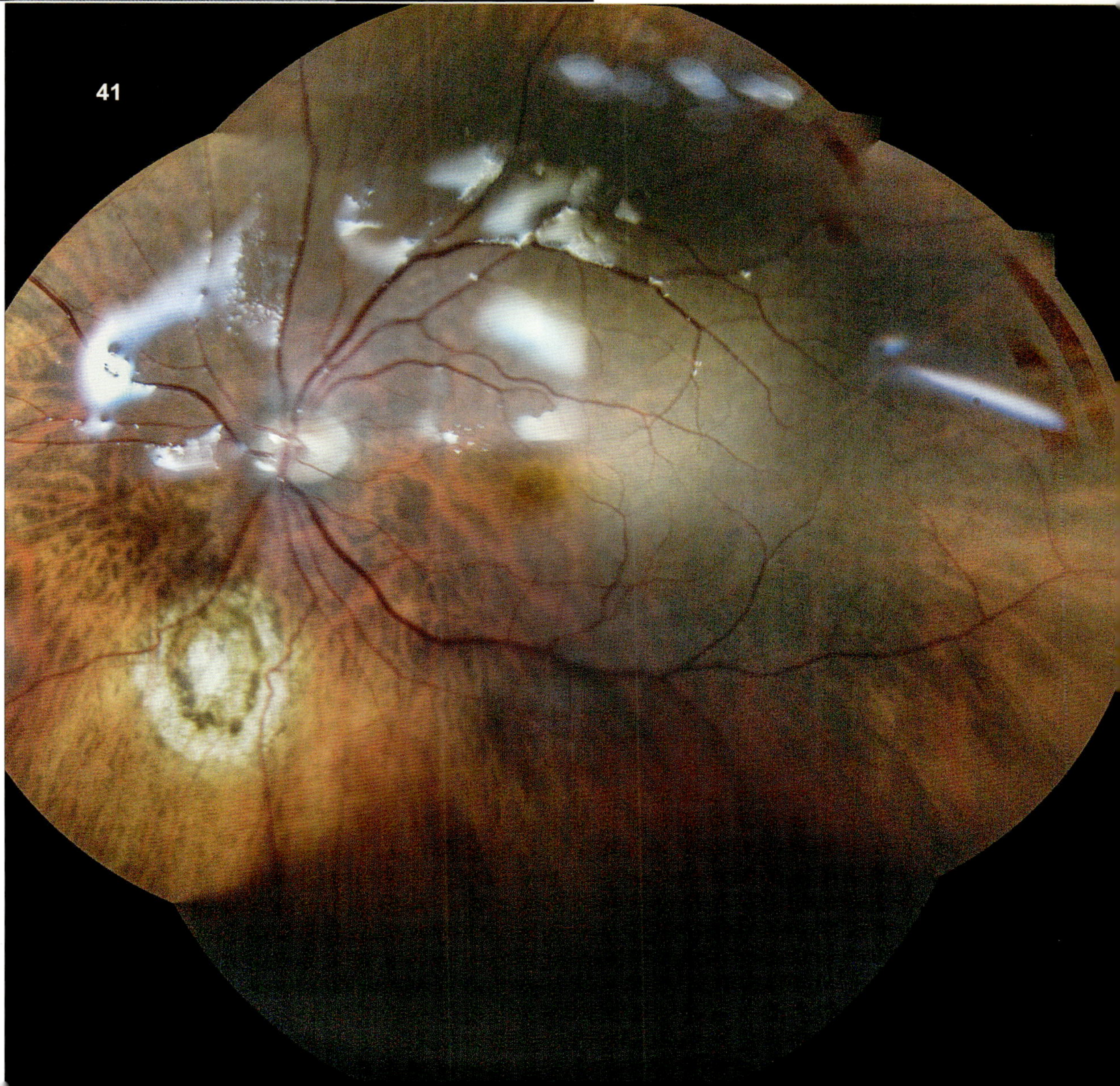

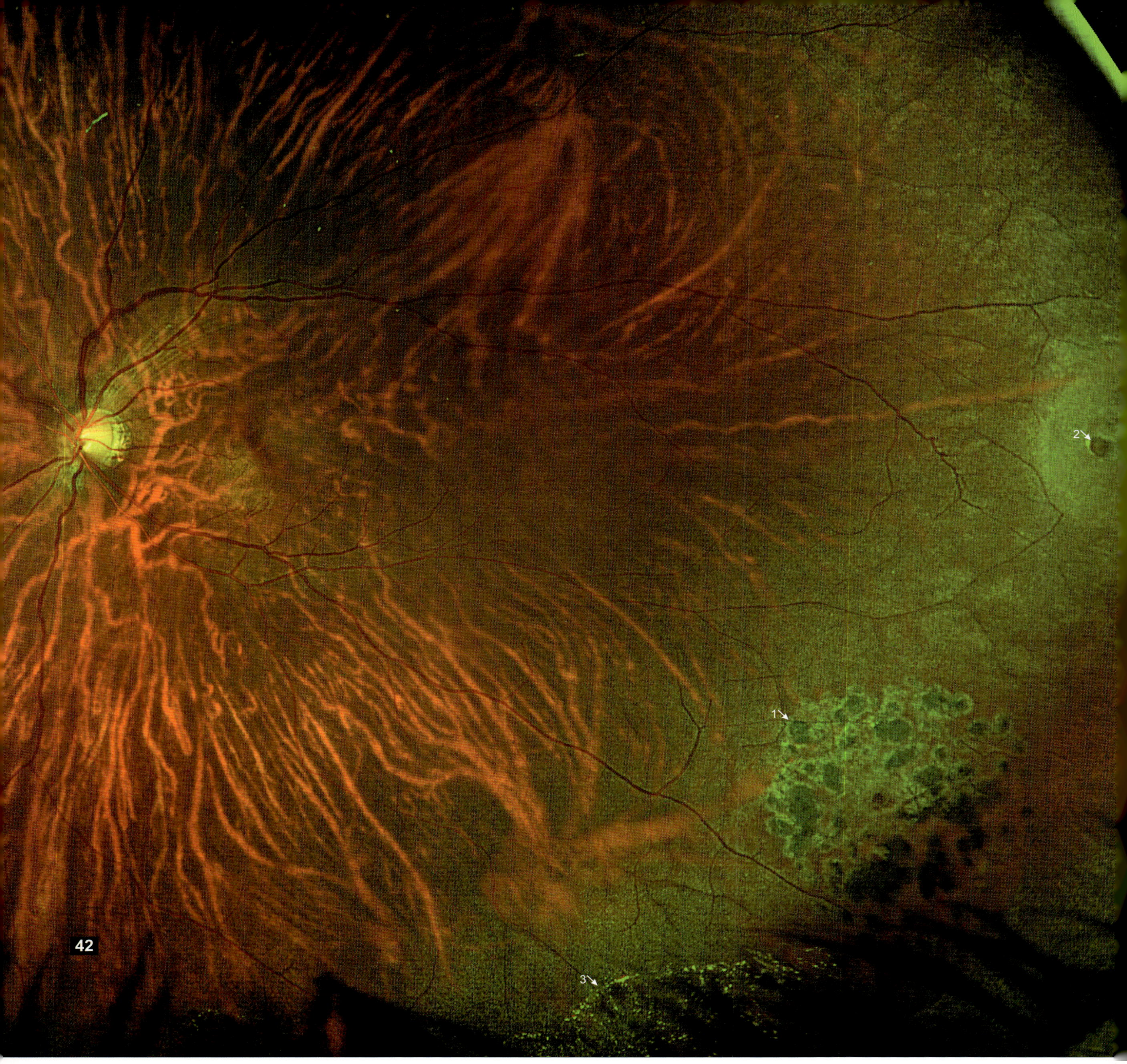


Figure 42 *Wide field color fundus montage image demonstrating lasered retinal holes (1), unlasered retinal holes (2) and unlasered retinal holes associated with lattice degeneration (3) in a young 30-year-old myope.*

Retinal holes are commonly encountered in retinal periphery during dilated fundus examination in an asymptomatic and symptomatic patients. Retinal holes are sometimes contained within lattice degeneration and may be partial or full thickness. There is no clear consensus of management of atrophic retinal hole. So many ophthalmologist elect to monitor. However, full thickness retinal hole can allow transmission of fluid from vitreous cavity and subretinal space and may result in retinal detachment. Laser prophylaxis may reduce risk of retinal detachment as done in this particular case. Usually, retinal holes do not immediately result in serious vision problems. □

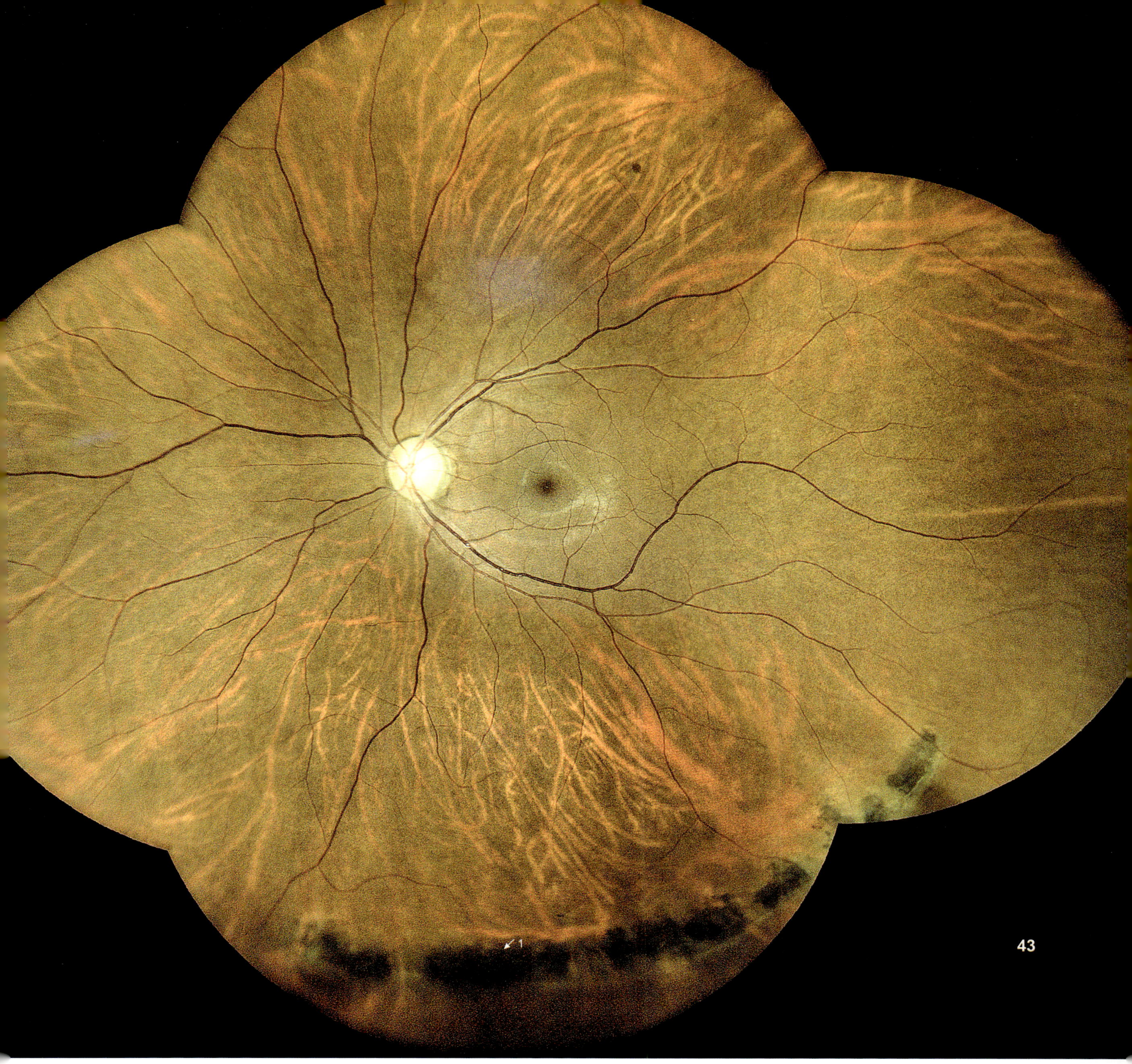


Figure 43 *Ultrawide fields montage image of a patient with incidental finding of pigmented lattice degeneration. Note the presence of horizontally placed black oval patches of RPE pigmentation all along the inferotemporal quadrant in the equatorial region of retina (1).*

Lattice degeneration affects vitreous are inner retinal layers with secondary changes of RPE clumping and pigmentation and are variably located within equatoriale region of fundus, typically inferotemporal patients with lattice degeneration are typically asymptomatic and lesions are usually detected during routine indirect ophthalmoscopic examination, acute onset of floaters and flashes of light may indicate presence of retinal break, i.e., complication of lattice.

RD is a relatively rare complication of lattice degeneration (<1% of patients with lattice degeneration), but lattice degeneration is associated with as many as 40% of all rhegmatogenous retinal detachments.□

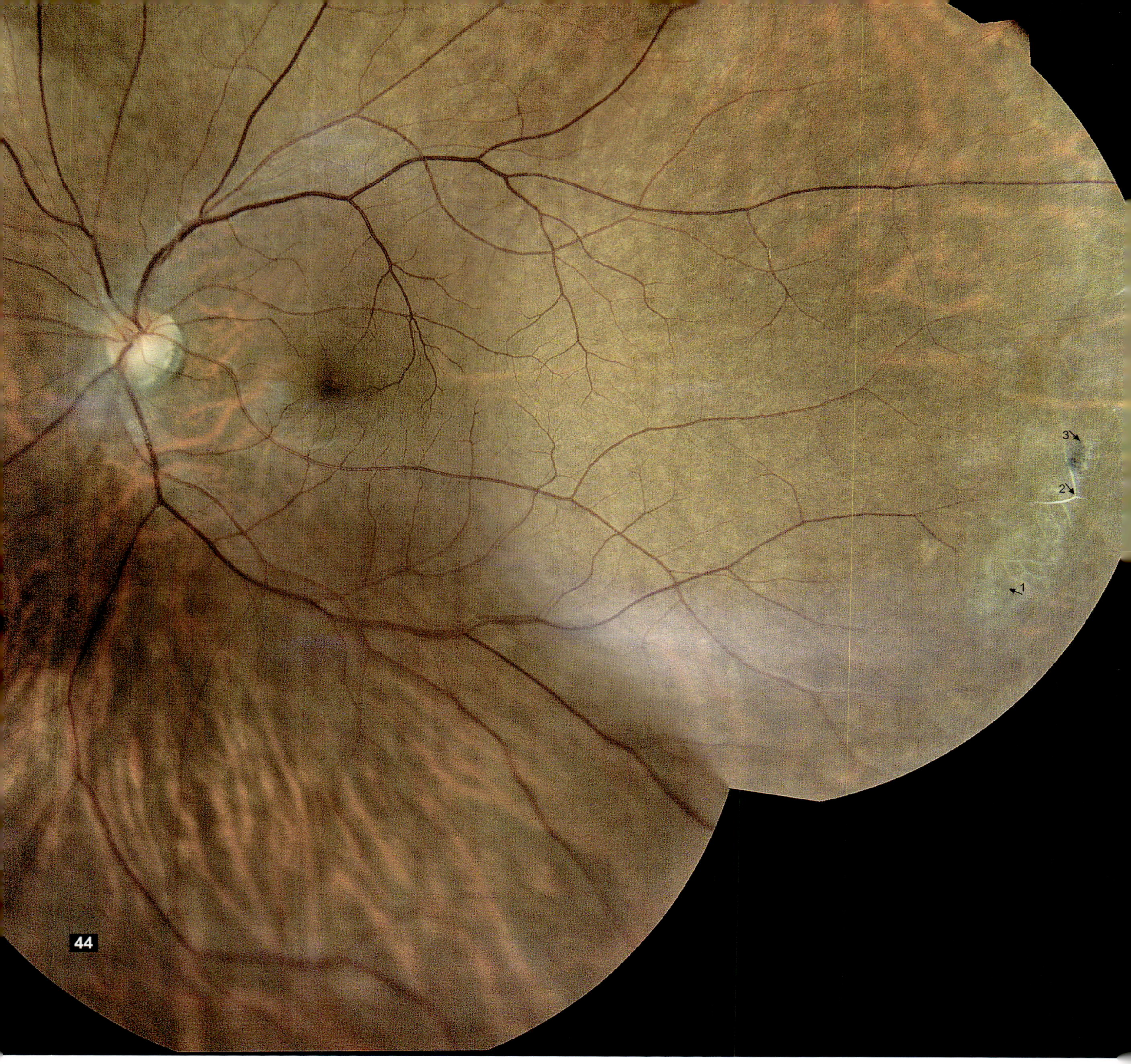


Figure 44 *Color fundus montage image of lattice degeneration. Note the presence of whitish patch of thinned retina (1) in the extreme periphery of temporal retina accompanied by cross hatching pattern formed by sclerotia vessels (2) and a few pigment clumps (3).*

Lattice degeneration is a type of peripheral retinal degeneration that is prevalent in 6–10% of general population, although myopes are mostly affected. Patient with lattice degeneration carries a low risk of development of rhegmatogenous retinal detachment later. But, it has been observed that patients who develop retinal detachment, 40% have associated lattice degeneration. There has been no consensus or randomized controlled trail regarding the benefit of laser or cryopexy for such lesions.□

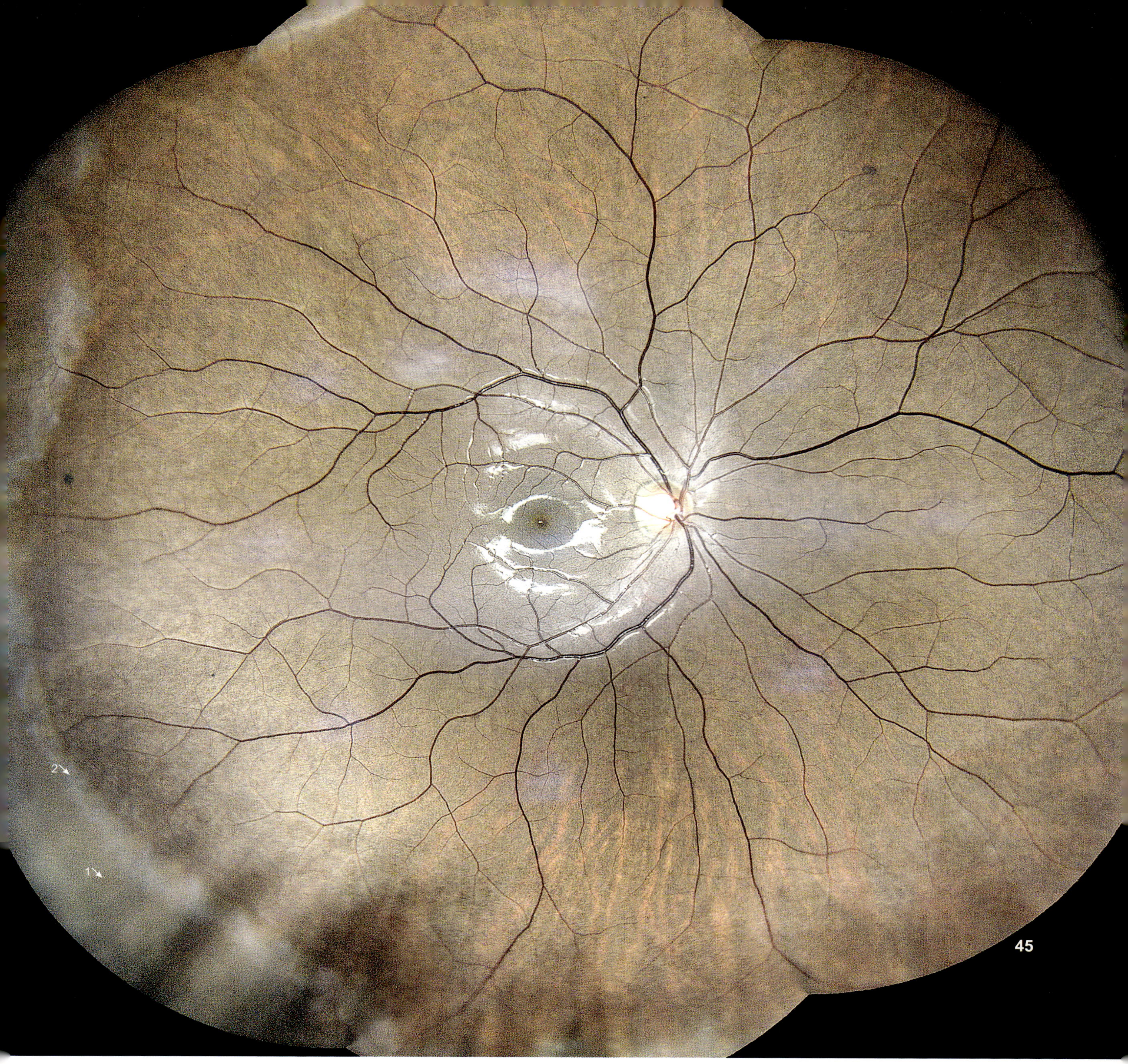


Figure 45 *A case of peripheral retinal degeneration: Ultra-wide field color fundus montage image demonstrating "white without pressure" (WWOP) type of peripheral retinal degeneration WWOP is an area of the retina that is translucent white to gray in color (1) in the periphery region of lesion and is sharply demarcated from normal retina (2).*

White without pressure (WWOP) has been described as a form of retinal degeneration, where a certain whitening of peripheral retina is apparent even without scleral indentation.

Retina breaks usually do not develop in patients with WWOP and hence prophylactic laser is not recommended. □

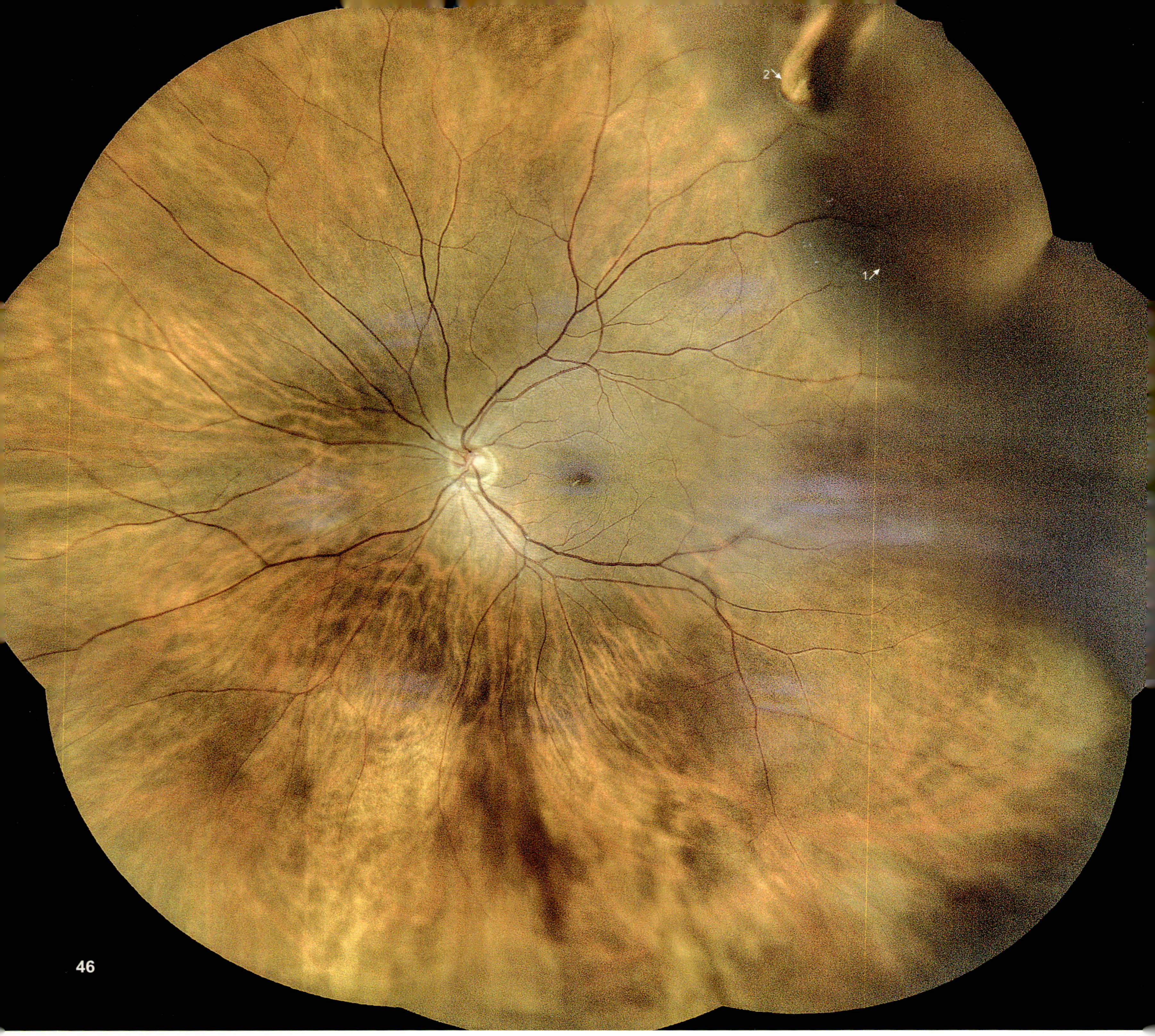


Figure 46 *Ultra-wide field montage image in a case of recent onset superotemporal retinal detachment. Note the dome-shaped area of retina elevation with elevated retinal vessels representing localized retinal detachment (1). Horseshoe tear can be seen superotemporally (2). Rest of the retinal architecture is well preserved and macular is normal.*

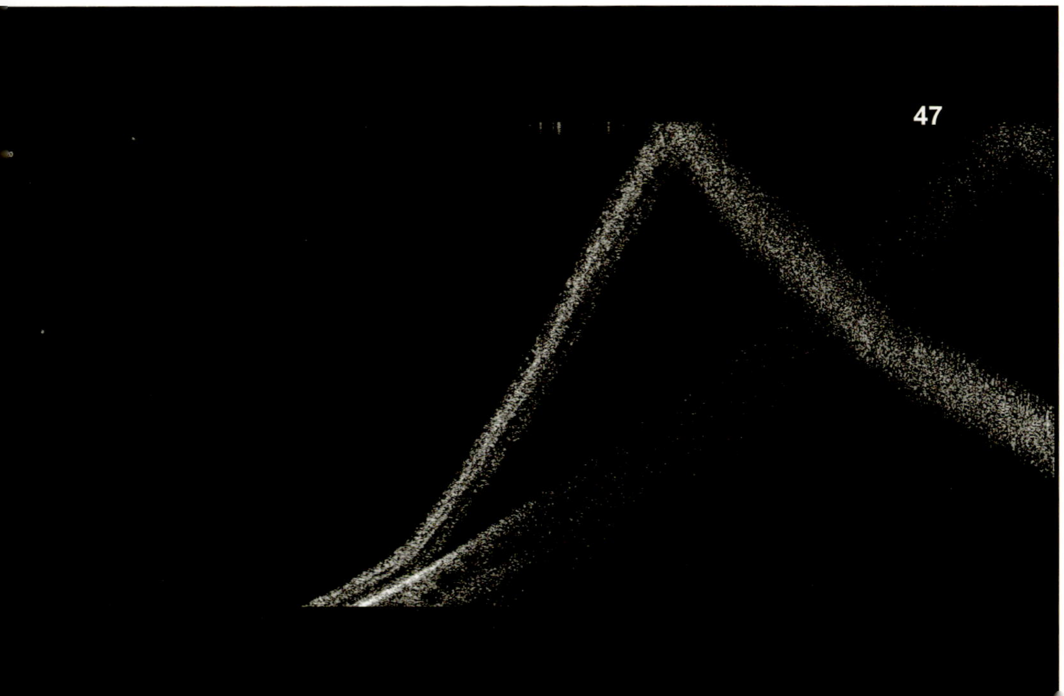


Figure 47 *Swept source optical coherence tomography demonstrating retinal detachment. Horizontal line scan passing through the area of abnormal elevation of retina superotemporal shows clear splitting of neurosensory retina from outer retinal layers.*

Ultra-wide field OCT has the ability to capture the details of the peripheral retina and that has allowed for its new and expanded clinical application. Retinal detachment is one such disease entity where utility of ultra-wide field OCTs has been well demonstrated as shown in our case. OCT image helps to differentiate retinal detachment from retinoschisis where in the former case splitting is seen between neurosensory and outer retina and in the latter splitting of outer plexiform and outer nuclear layer is present.□

# CHAPTER 6

## INFLAMMATORY

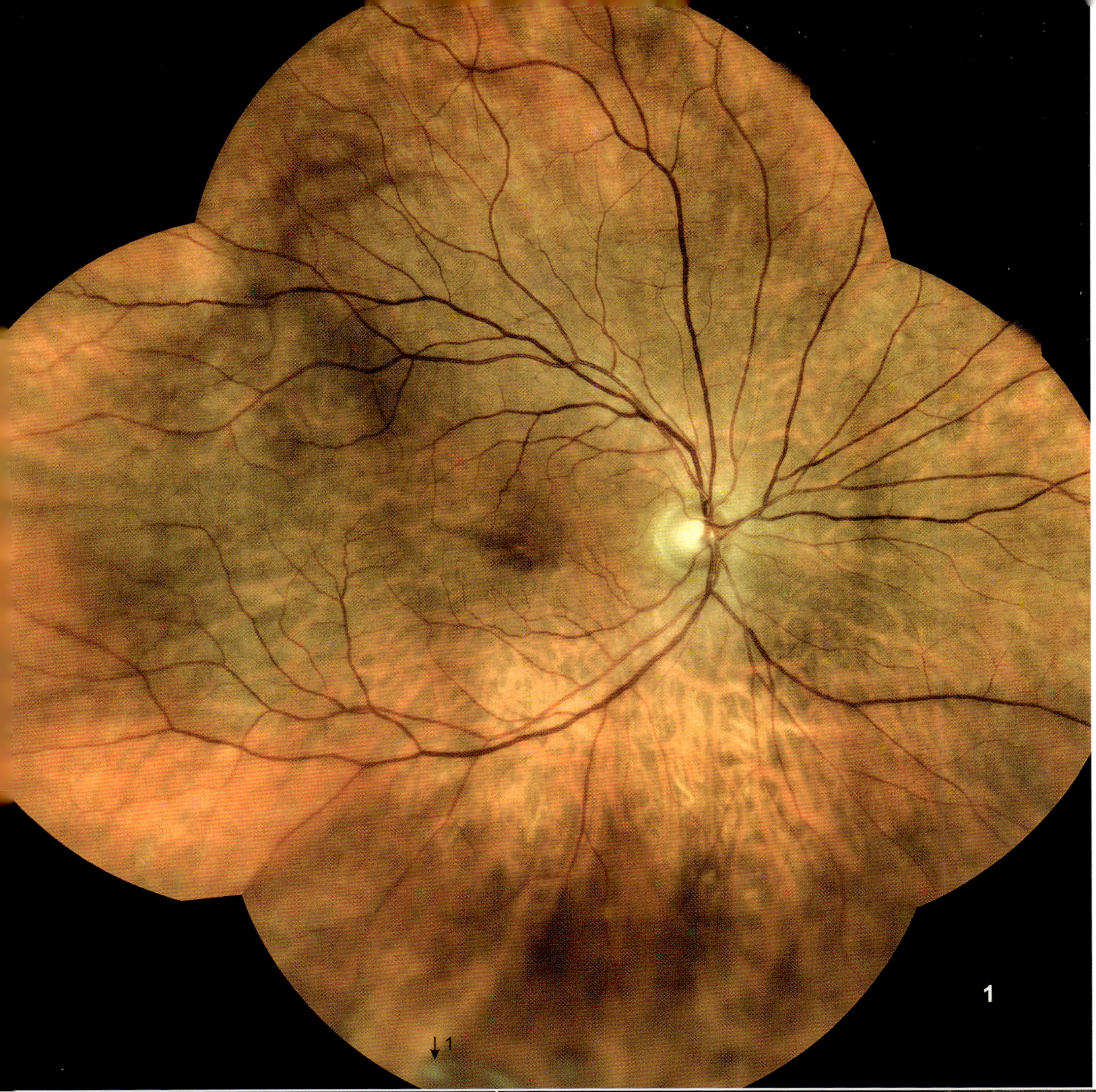


Figure 1

*Case of intermediate uveitis demonstrating vitreous snowballs (1).*

Color fundus montage photograph shows normal looking retina with fluffy whitish deposits in the inferior vitreous—snowballs. Vitreous infiltration with inflammatory cells commonly occur in intermediate uveitis. However, when this vitreous debris collects and coalesce in the inferior vitreous cavity it is then called vitreous snowballs.

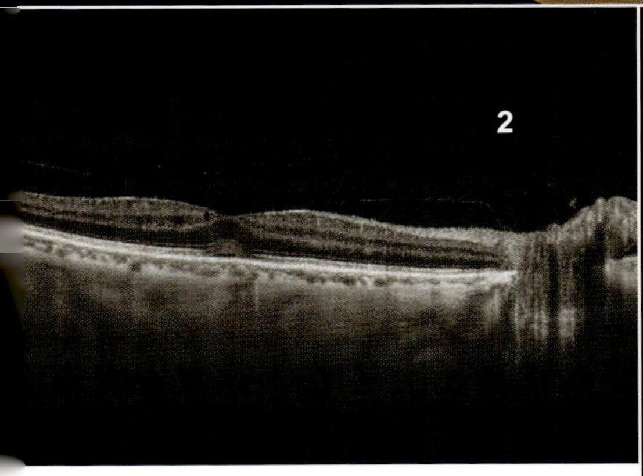


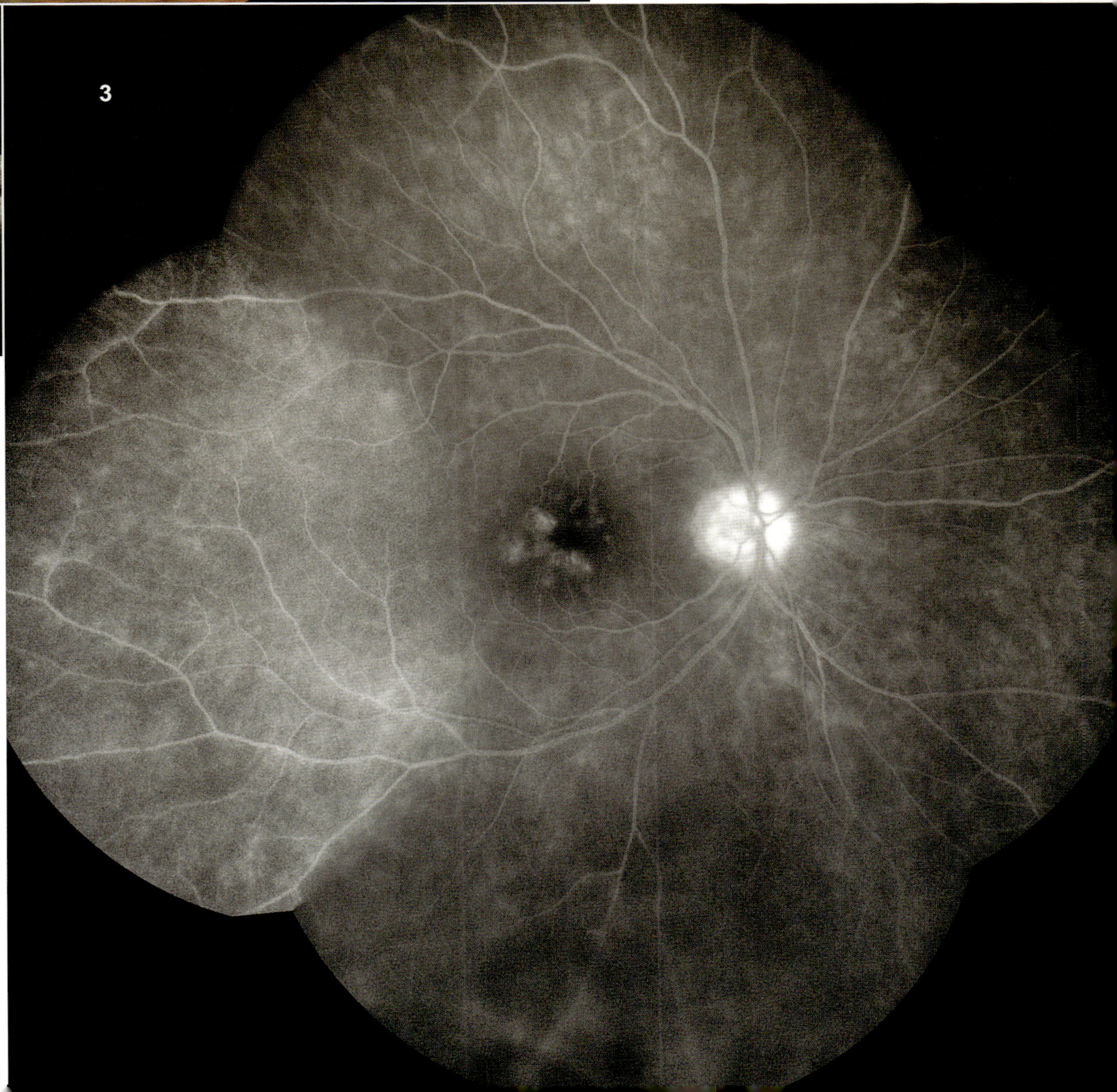


Figure 2

*Swept source OCT scan in a case of cystoid macular edema secondary to intermediate uveitis.*

Figure 3

*Fundus fluorescein angiogram montage detects vascular hyperpermeability that appears as hyperfluorescent perivascular leakage along the peripheral retinal veins. There is late accumulation of dye in the parafoveal cystic spaces giving the characteristic petaled pattern of macular edema. Optic disk is hyperfluorescent.* □

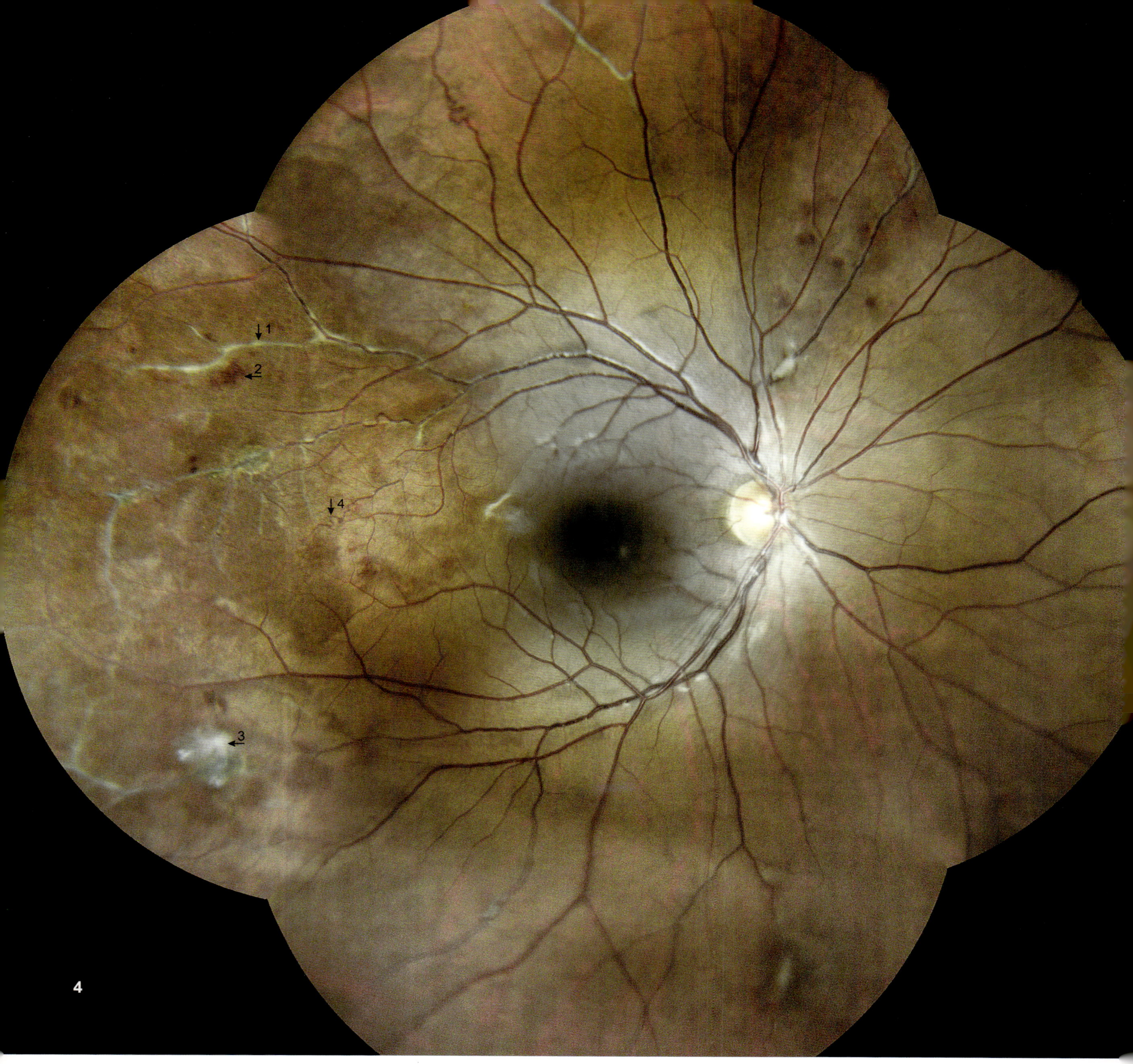


Figure 4 *Case of tubercular occlusive retinal vasculitis: Fundus montage shows prominent perivascular sheathing (1) associated with retinal hemorrhages (2), fibrosed retinal neovascular frond (3) and venous remodeling (4) at the junction of perfused and nonperfused retina.*

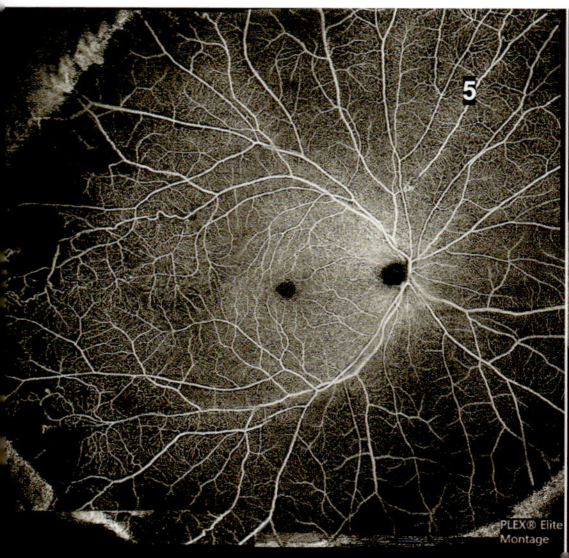


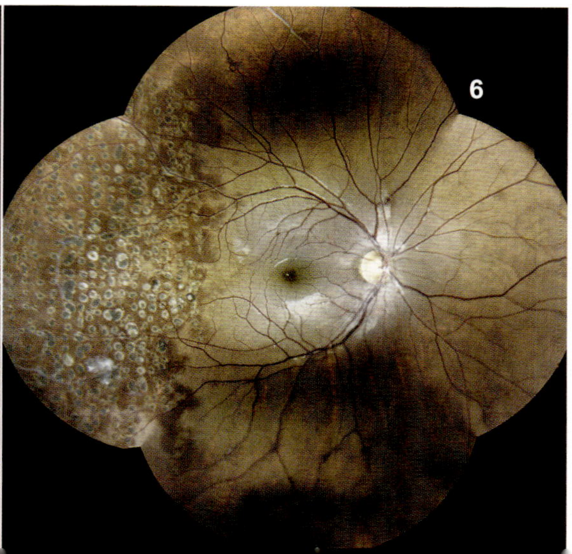


Figure 5 *OCTA montage image demonstrating nonperfused temporal quadrant and well-perfused retinal vasculature in other quadrants.*

Figure 6 *A case of tubercular occlusive retinal vasculitis—1 year after treatment, laser photocoagulation scars are visible. No NVE was seen and no new patch of retinal periphlebitis has developed.*

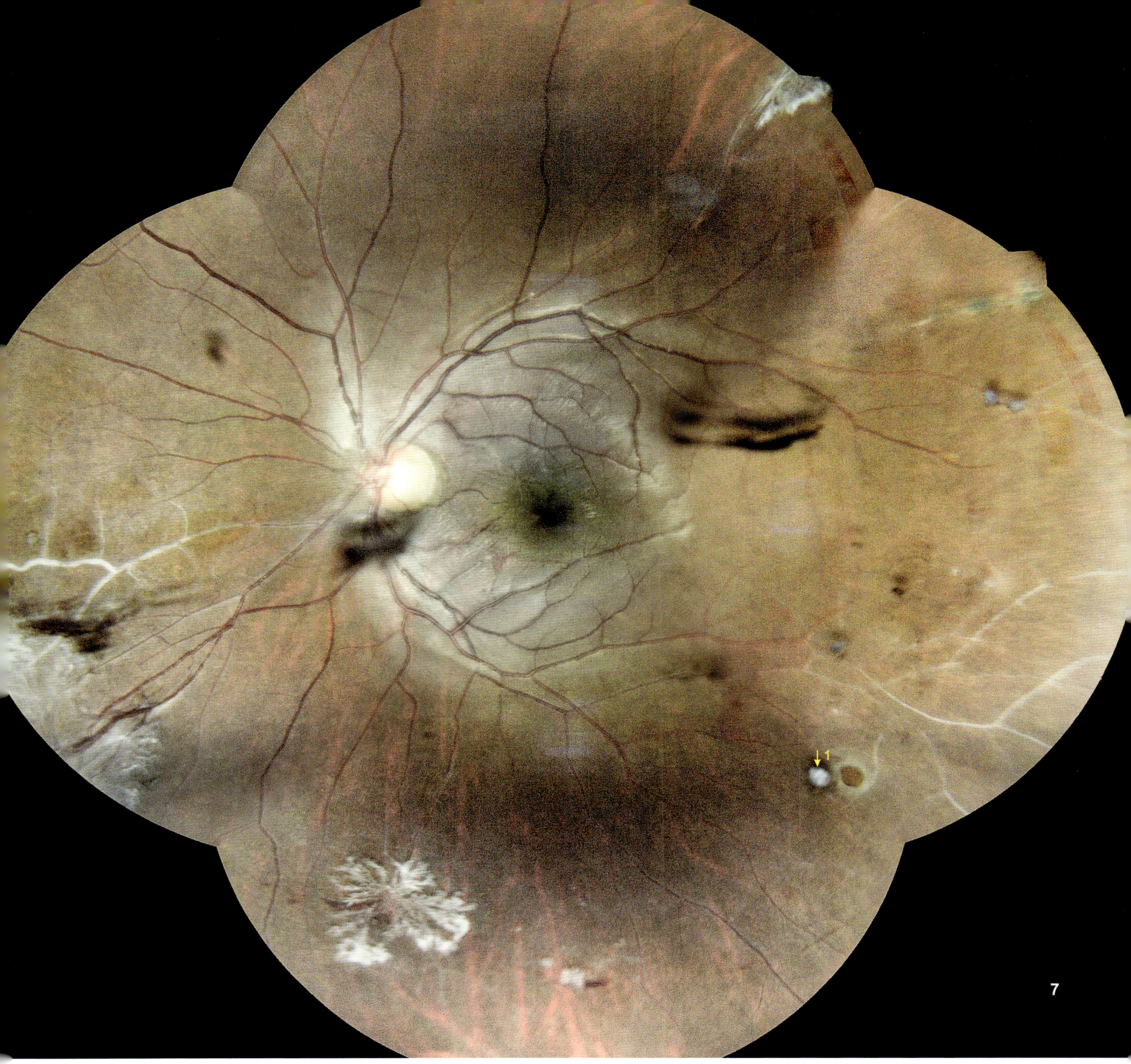


Figure 7 *Left eye fundus montage of the same patient shows unusual retinal hole (1) in the setting of the other classic signs of retinal vasculitis.*

Figure 8 *Case of tubercular occlusive retinal vasculitis—post-treatment photographs. Note the disease is in its quiescent stage with no recurrences at 1 year.*

Figure 9 *OCTA montage demonstrates retinal non-perfusion in nasal half and large non-perfusion area in inferotemporal retina.* □

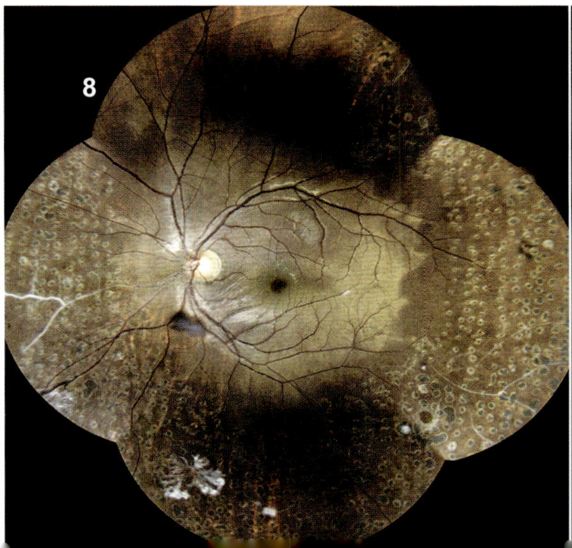


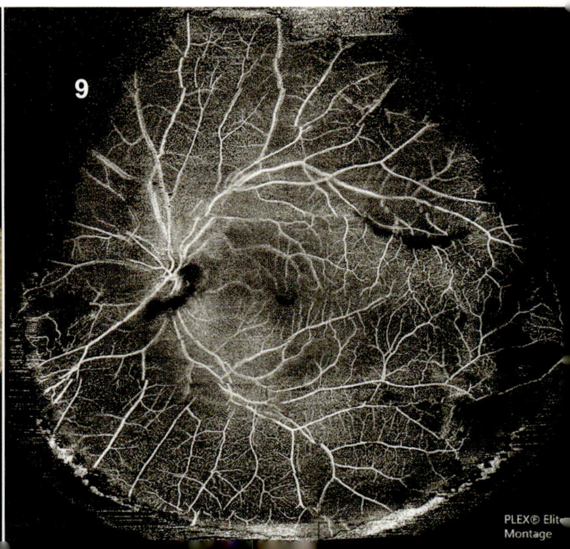

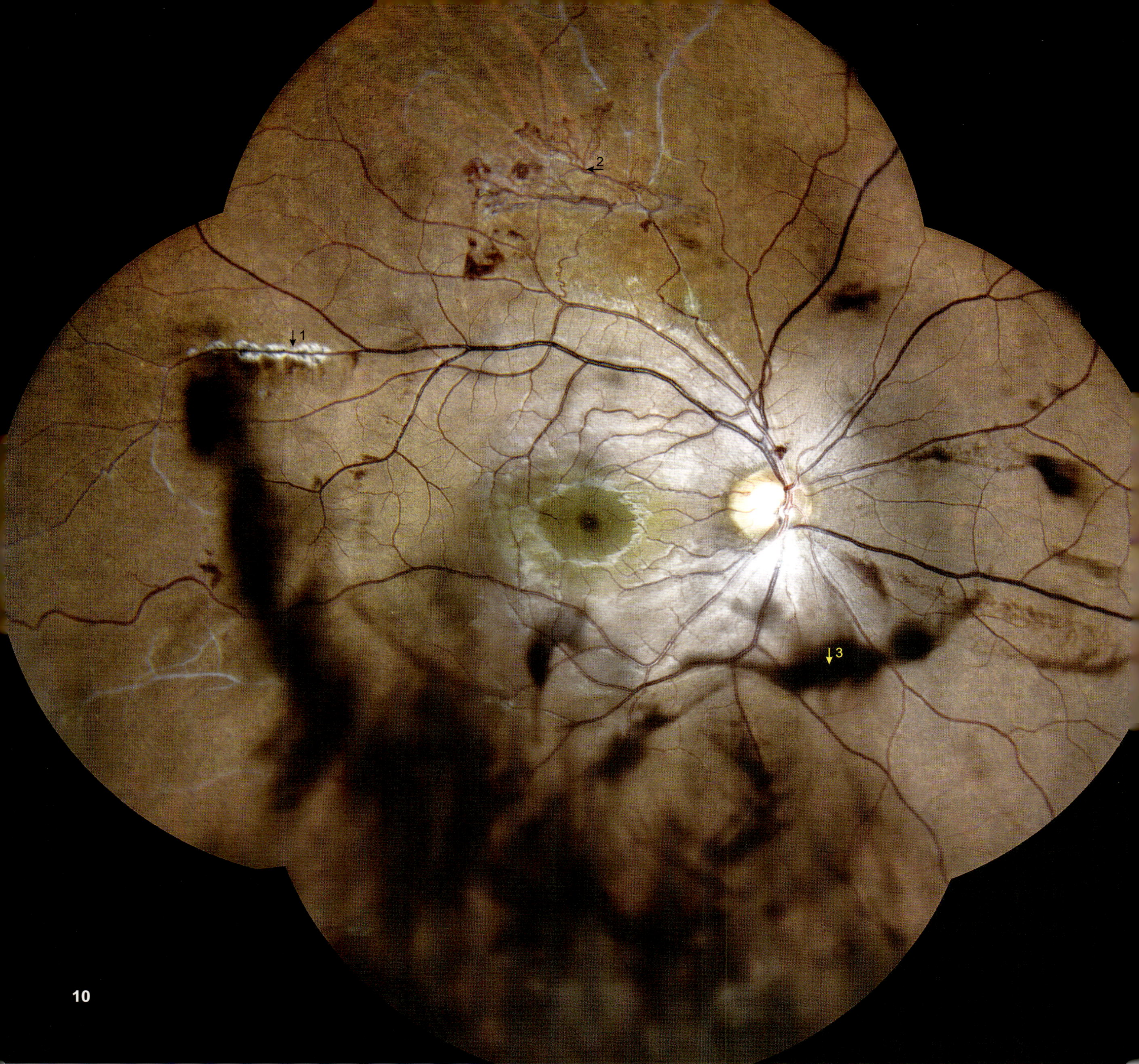


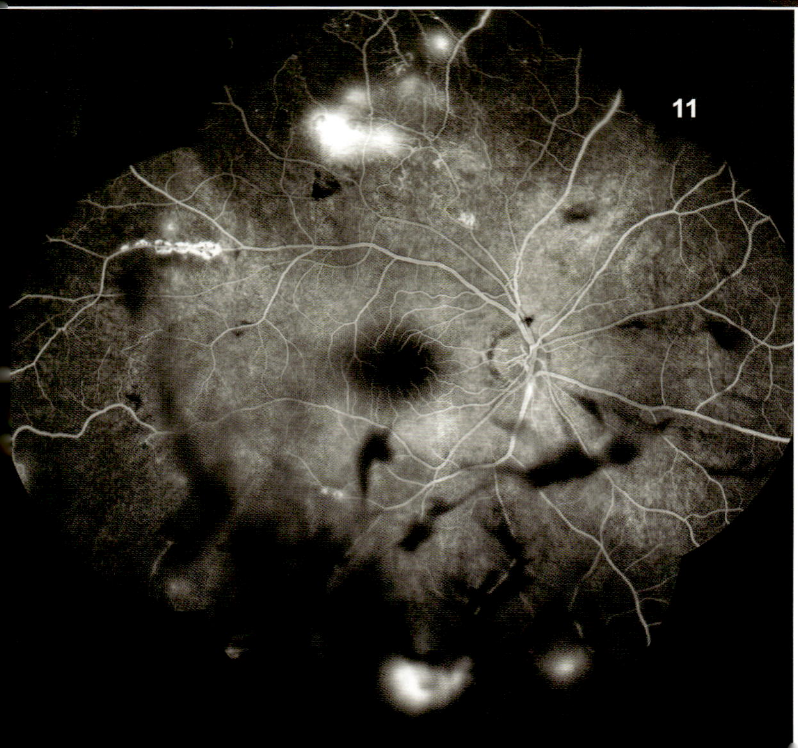


Figure 10 *Unilateral occlusive retinal vasculitis with vitreous hemorrhage.*

Young 35-year-old male presented with sudden onset floaters in his right eye. Color montage photograph demonstrating retinal periphlebitis (whitish retinal exudates along the retinal veins) (1) neovascularization (2) and vitreous hemorrhage (3).

Retinal vasculitis is a sight threatening inflammatory disorder of retinal vessels that may occur as an isolated idiopathic condition as in our case or as a part of spectrum of systemic inflammatory disease, (autoimmune vasculitis, neoplastic, sarcoidosis) or infective pathologies.

Figure 11 *Fundus fluorescein angiogram demonstrating multiple areas of retinal neovascular leakage's and fluorescein perivascular leakage from the affected vessel (large temporal vein).*

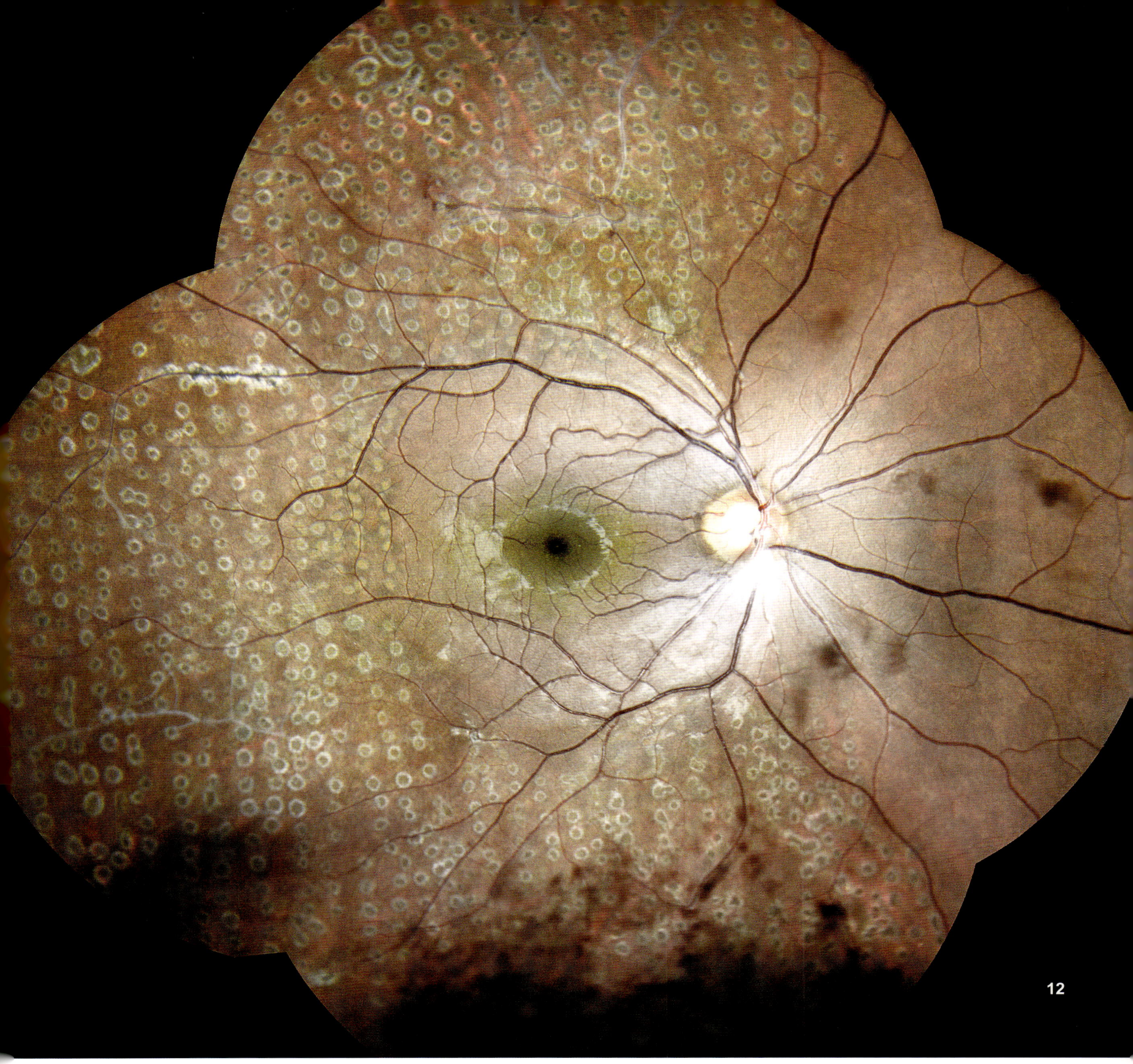

Figure 12 *Unilateral occlusive retinal vasculitis with vitreous hemorrhage—2 months after treatment.*

Patient underwent laboratory investigations to rule out any associated infective disease (negative for TB/ syphilis/lyme) or systemic autoimmune pathology. He was given a single intravitreal anti-VEGF injection, oral steroids were started at the dose of 1 mg/kg body weight.

A sector PRP laser was done to areas of nonperfusion. Such patients need a regular 3–6 months follow-ups as chances of recurrence are high, long-term immunosuppression is also required in most of the cases to prevent recurrences. □

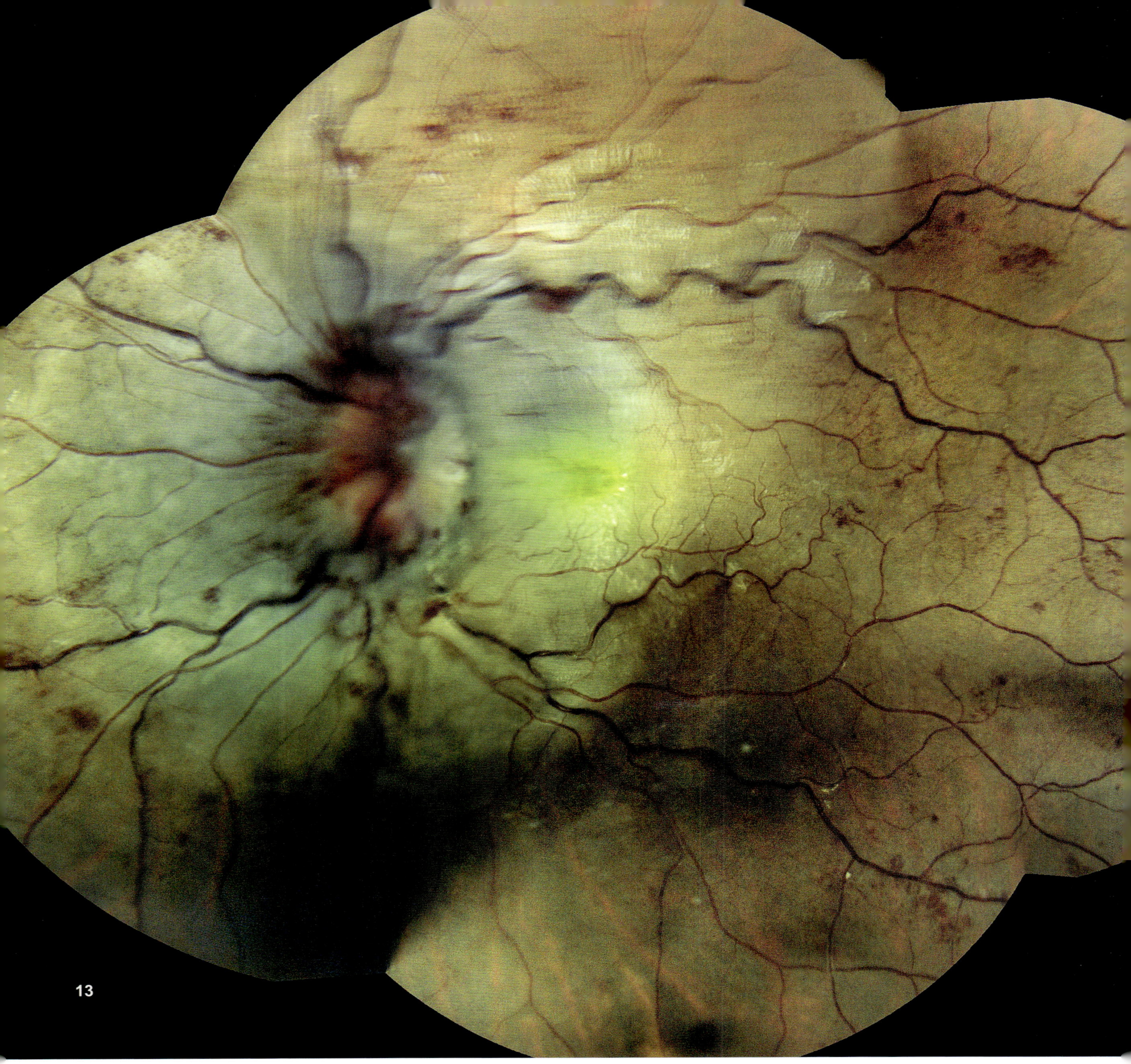


Figure 13 *Case of tubercular neuroretinitis.*

A 25-year-old young female presented with complaints of blurred vision, progressively worsening over the past few days. At presentation her visual acuity was perception of light (PL +) only in her left eye. Fundus photograph shows massive edema involving the optic disk with splinter hemorrhages seen at the level of optic disk. Macular area is also elevated as a result of associated neurosensory detachment. Tortuous retinal vessels, intraretinal hemorrhages are present, suggestive of an associated retinal vein occlusion due to pressure effect on the retinal vein at the level of optic disk. Her clinical picture was suggestive of neuroretinitis.

Neuroretinitis is an inflammation of the neural retina and optic nerve. It was originally described by Leber in 1916 as a stellate maculopathy, but later Don Gass in 1977 challenged that and renamed it as neuroretinitis citing that disk edema precedes macular edema.

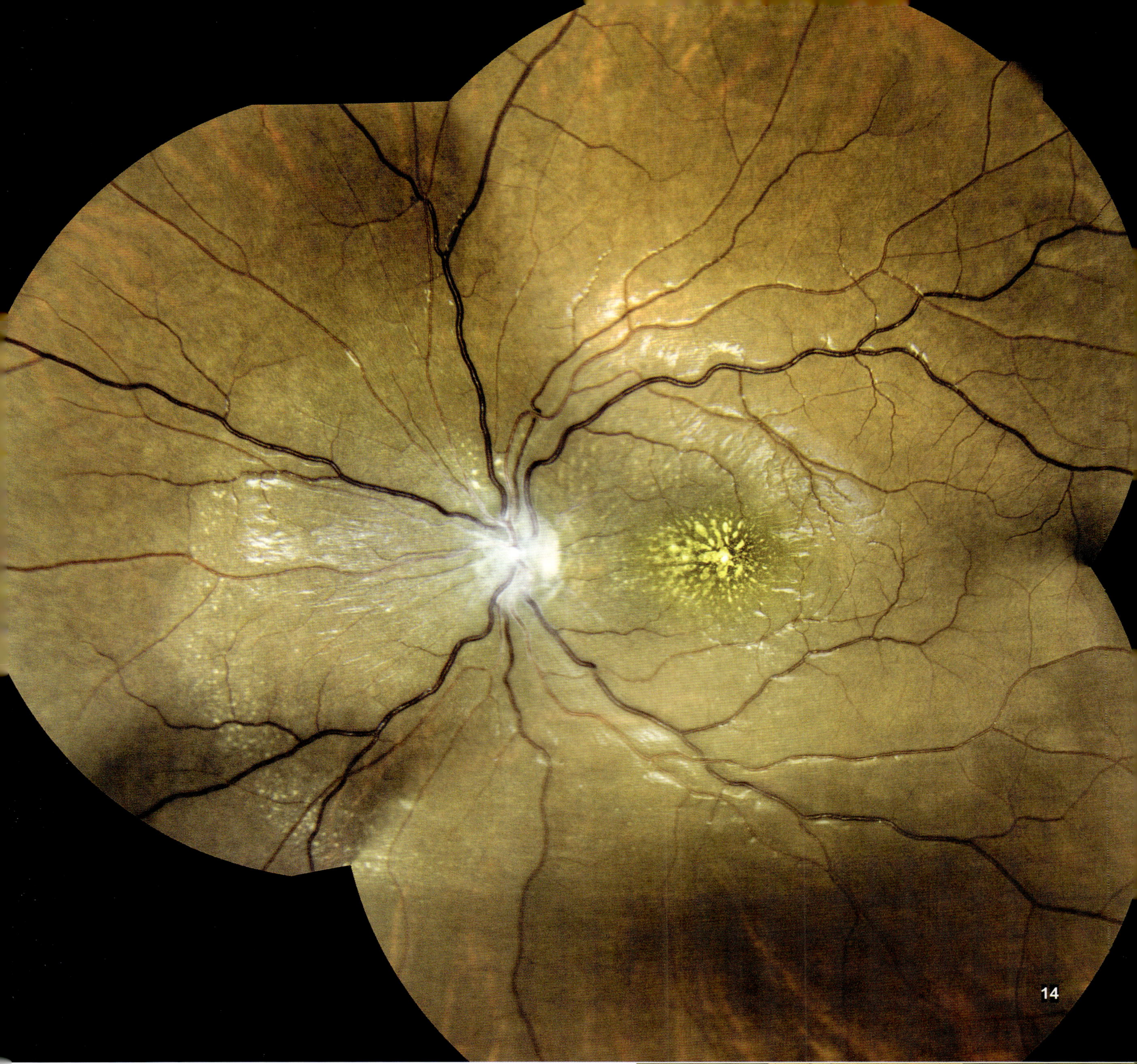


Figure 14 *Case of tubercular neuroretinitis—1 month post-treatment.*

She was subsequently managed on systemic immunosuppressives and antitubercular treatment. Color image a month later, shows resolution of disk edema, but there is pallor of the optic nerve and hence visual acuity was counting fingers close to face. Macular edema has resolved. There is an accumulation of hard lipid exudates at the fovea giving the appearance of typical stellate retinopathy.

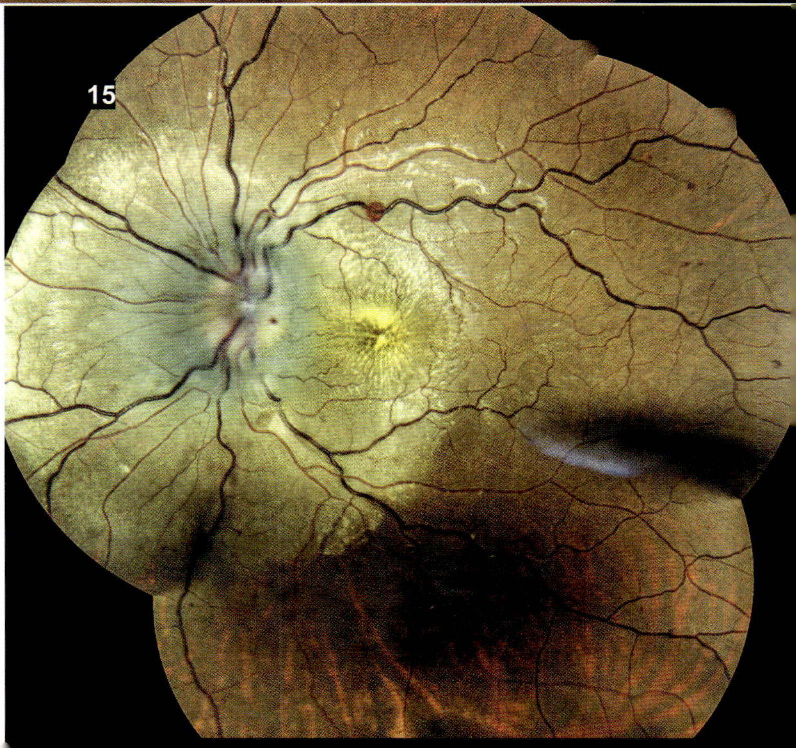


Figure 15 *Case of tubercular neuroretinitis—color fundus montage 3 days after IV methylprednisolone and initiation of antitubercular treatment.*

She underwent complete laboratory investigations to rule out infective/autoimmune diseases. Her Mantoux skin test was positive with an induration of 25 mm × 25 mm, Quantiferon gold test for tuberculosis was also found to be positive. She was treated as a presumed case of tubercular neuroretinitis. She was given a course of pulse IV methylprednisolone 1 g/day for 3 days followed by oral steroids and antitubercular treatment was initiated. Color fundus montage image three days after initiation of treatment shows reduction in macular thickening, optic nerve edema has resolved drastically, vessels appear less tortuous and retinal hemorrhages from the retinal periphery have resolved. □

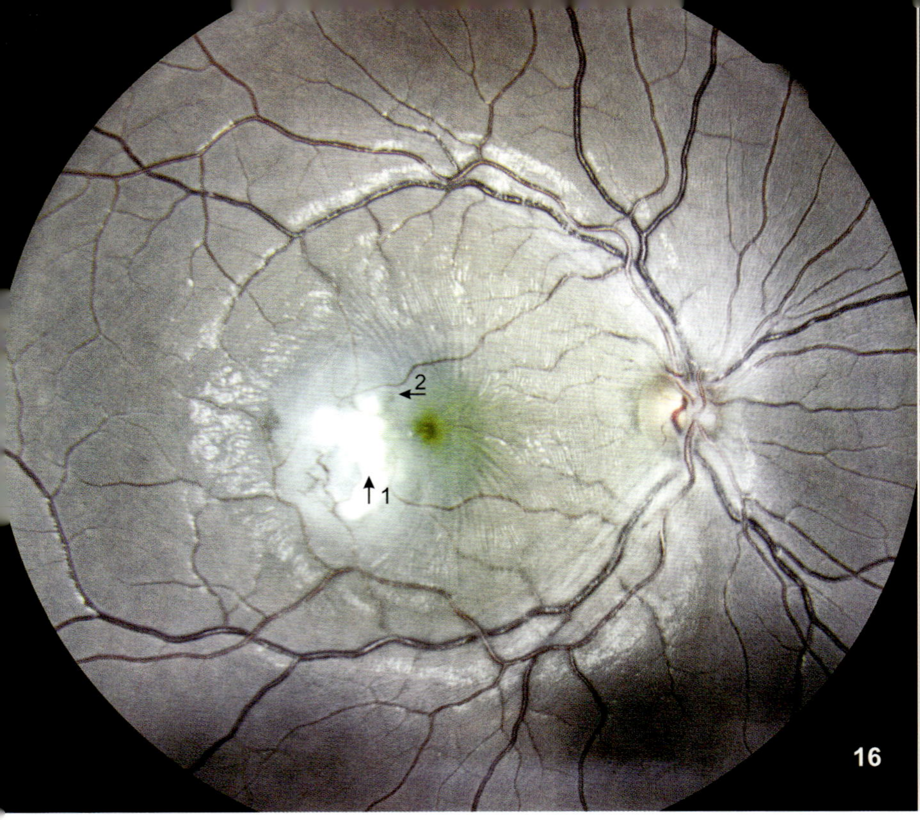


Figure 16 *Case of idiopathic acute necrotizing retinitis.*

A 17-year-old boy presented with sudden onset painless blurred vision in his right eye. At presentation his visual acuity was counting fingers 2 meters in the right eye. Anterior segment examination was unremarkable. On fundus examination, note the presence of crescent-shaped whitish patch of necrotizing retinitis (1), with underlying hemorrhages and serous macular detachment (2) as a result of inflammation.

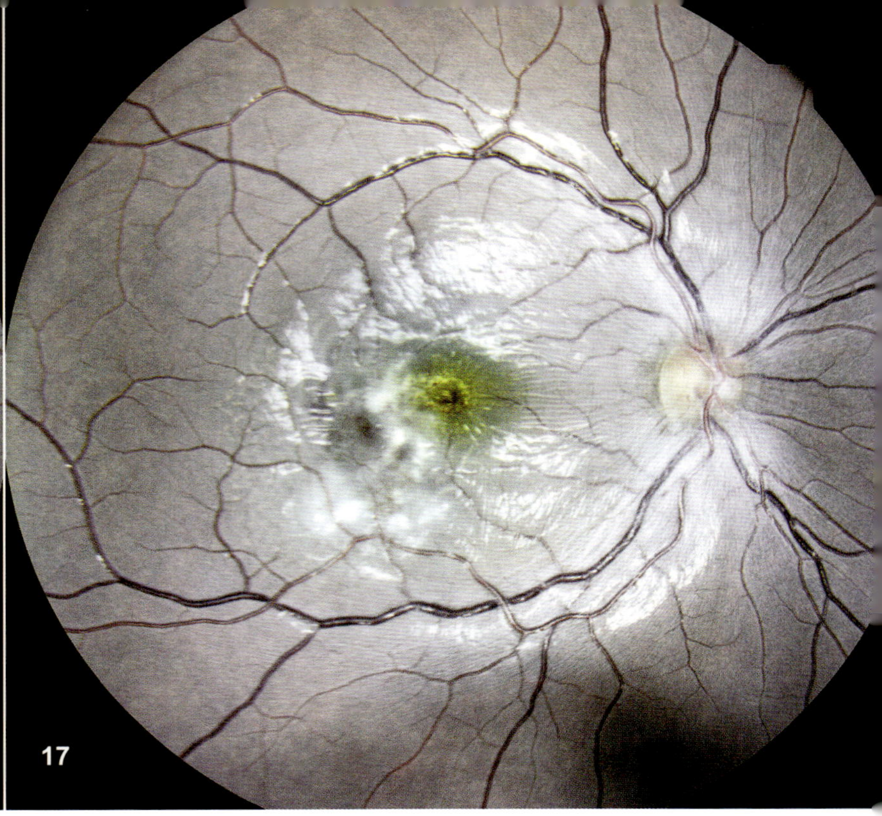


Figure 17 *Color image 3 days after pulse dose of IV methylprednisolone treatment.*

Aqueous sampling and laboratory test did not show any viral/bacterial pathology. IV methylprednisolone pulse dose was given (1 g/day for 3 days). Color photo shows reduction in the lesion activity as suggested by the reduction in fluffy white patch, SRF has reduced. Lipid exudates were now seen near the fovea as a result of rapid resolution of SRF.

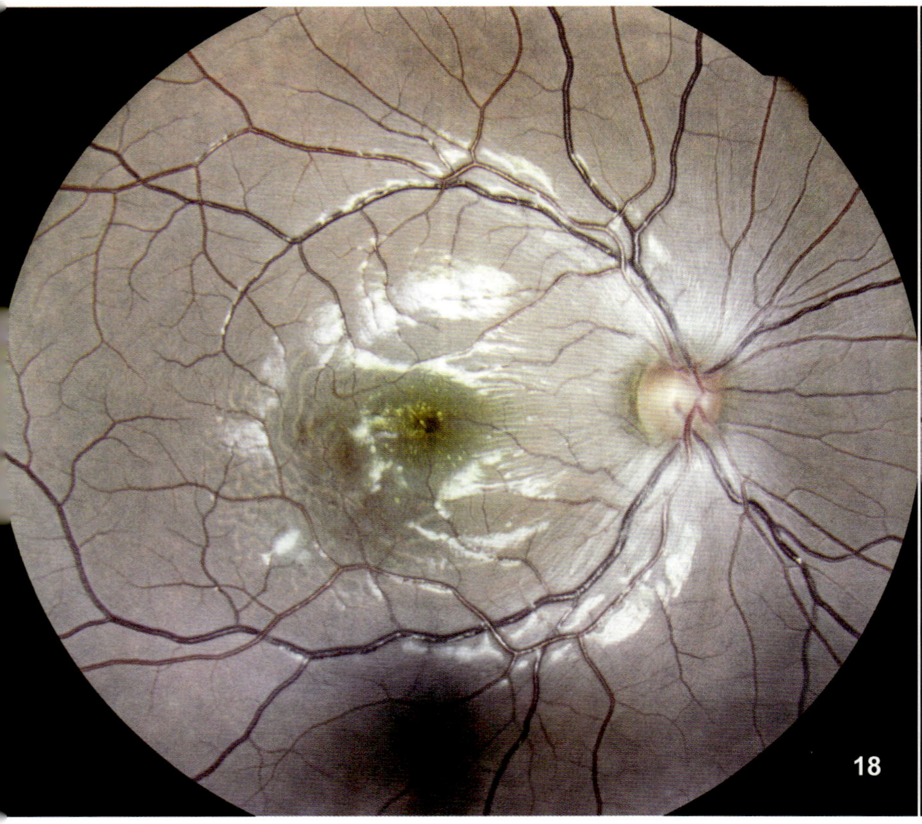


Figure 18 *Color image done 1 month post-treatment.*

Note the complete resolution of active retinitis patch with underlying choroidal folds seen. Choroidal folds are formed due to undue stretching of the retina and choroid as a result of inflammatory activity.

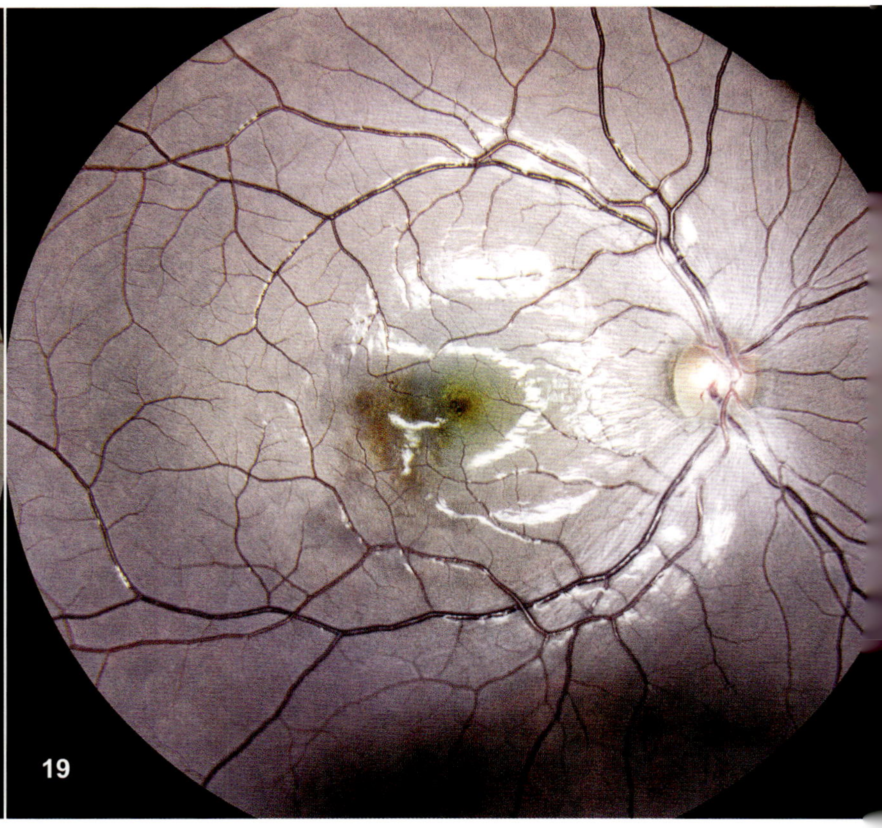


Figure 19 *Color image done 1 year postinitial event.*

Macula appears normal except slight discoloration in the temporal fovea and disappearance of choroidal folds. His visual acuity was 6/6 at 1 year.

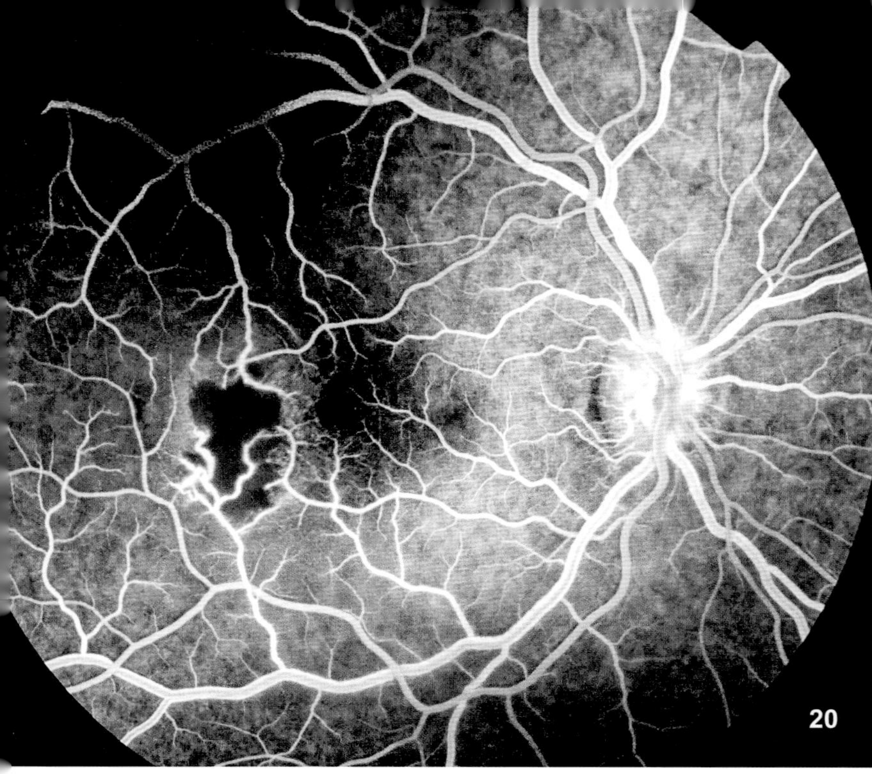


Figure 20 *Early frames of angiogram demonstrating hypofluorescence at the site of active patch of retinitis.*

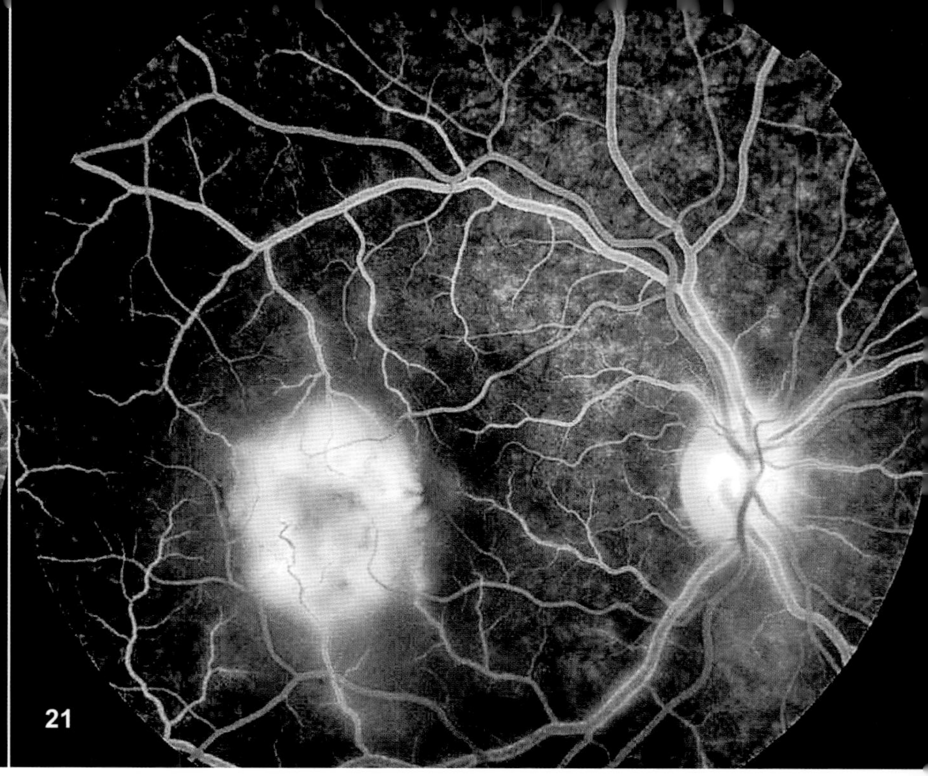


Figure 21 *Late frame of angiogram shows increasing hyperfluorescent inflammatory leakage.*

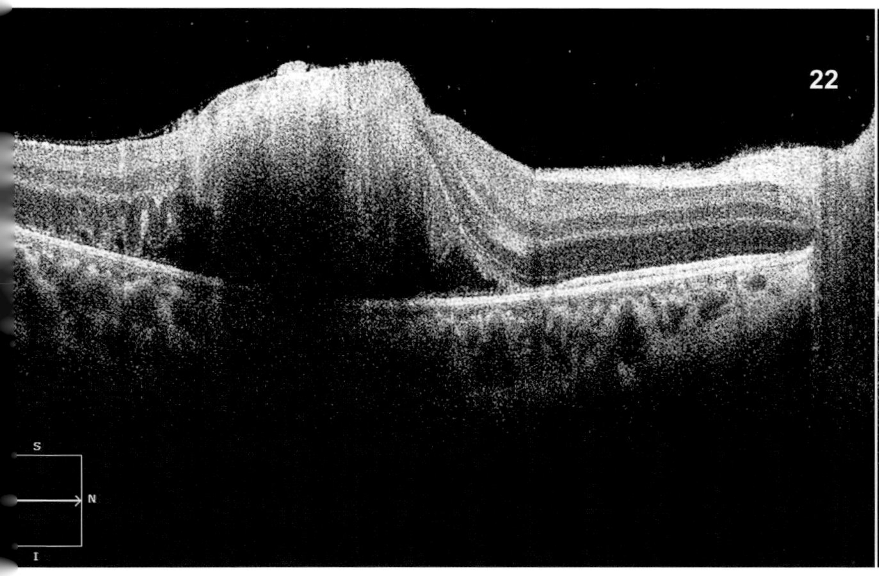


Figure 22 *Spectral domain OCT scan passing through the lesion demonstrates hyper-reflectivity in the inner retina with adjacent retinal thickening and presence of retinal fluid.*

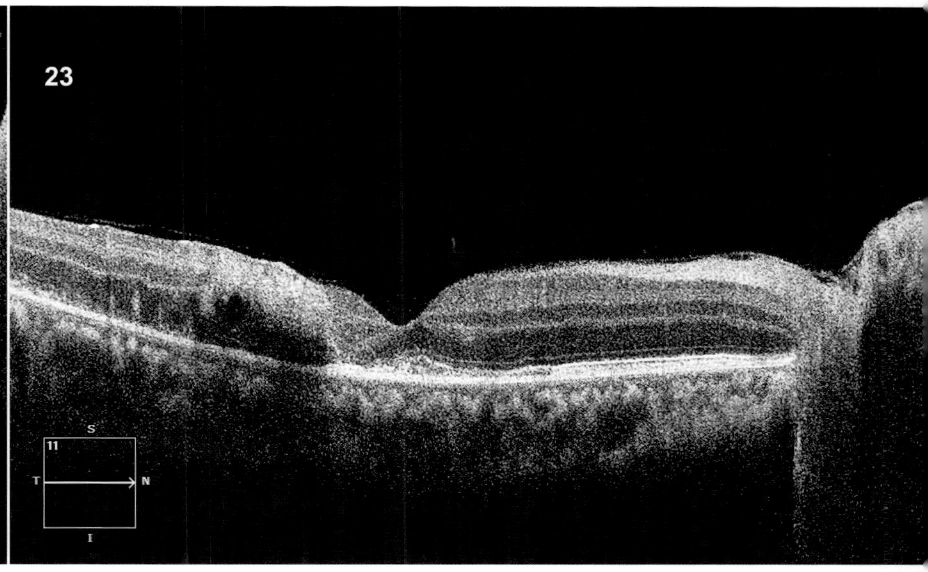


Figure 23 *Spectral domain OCT scan 3 days post-treatment demonstrating reduction in retinal thickness, with small patch of retinitis seen temporal to the foveal pit.*

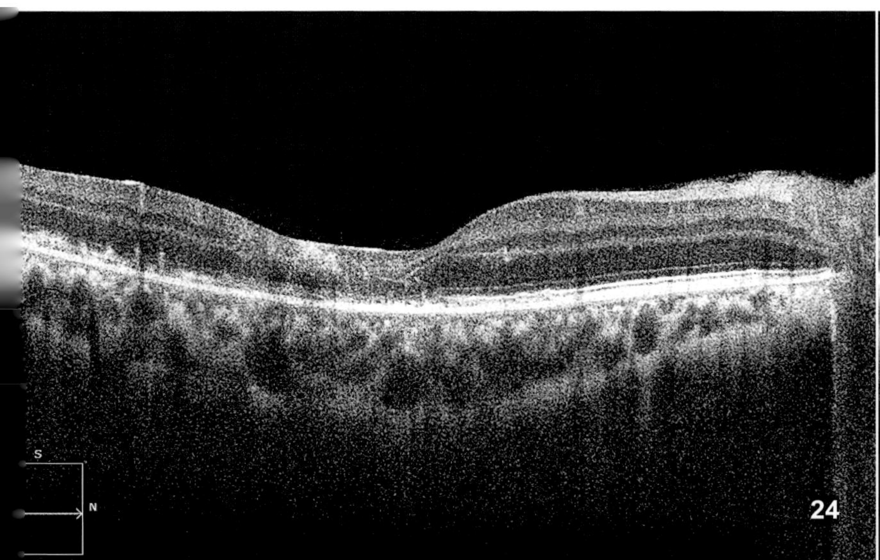


Figure 24 *Spectral domain OCT 1 month later demonstrating further reduction in the size of hyper-reflective retinitis patch with associated inner retinal damage.*

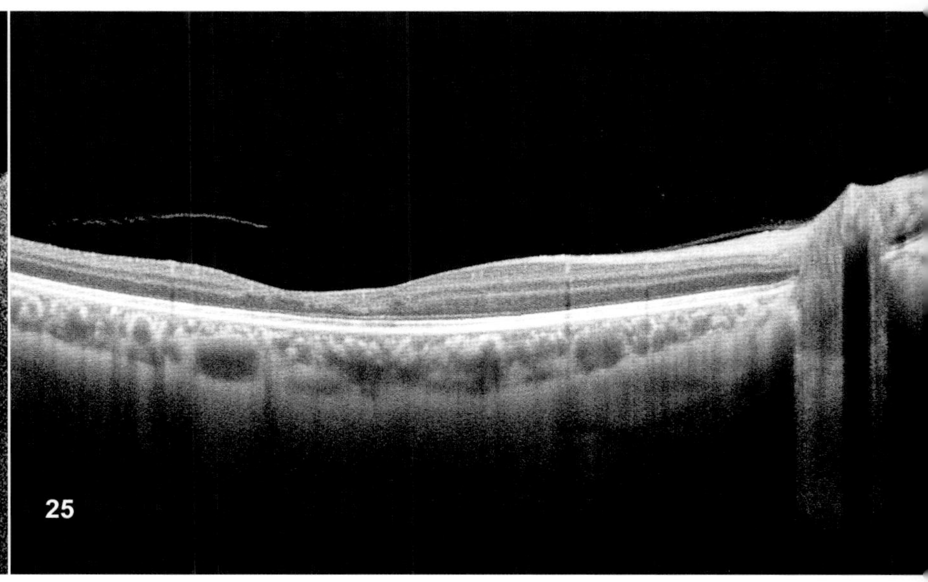


Figure 25 *Swept source OCT scan 1 year later demonstrating inner retinal layers atrophy at the site of original disease activity, fovea appears normal.*□

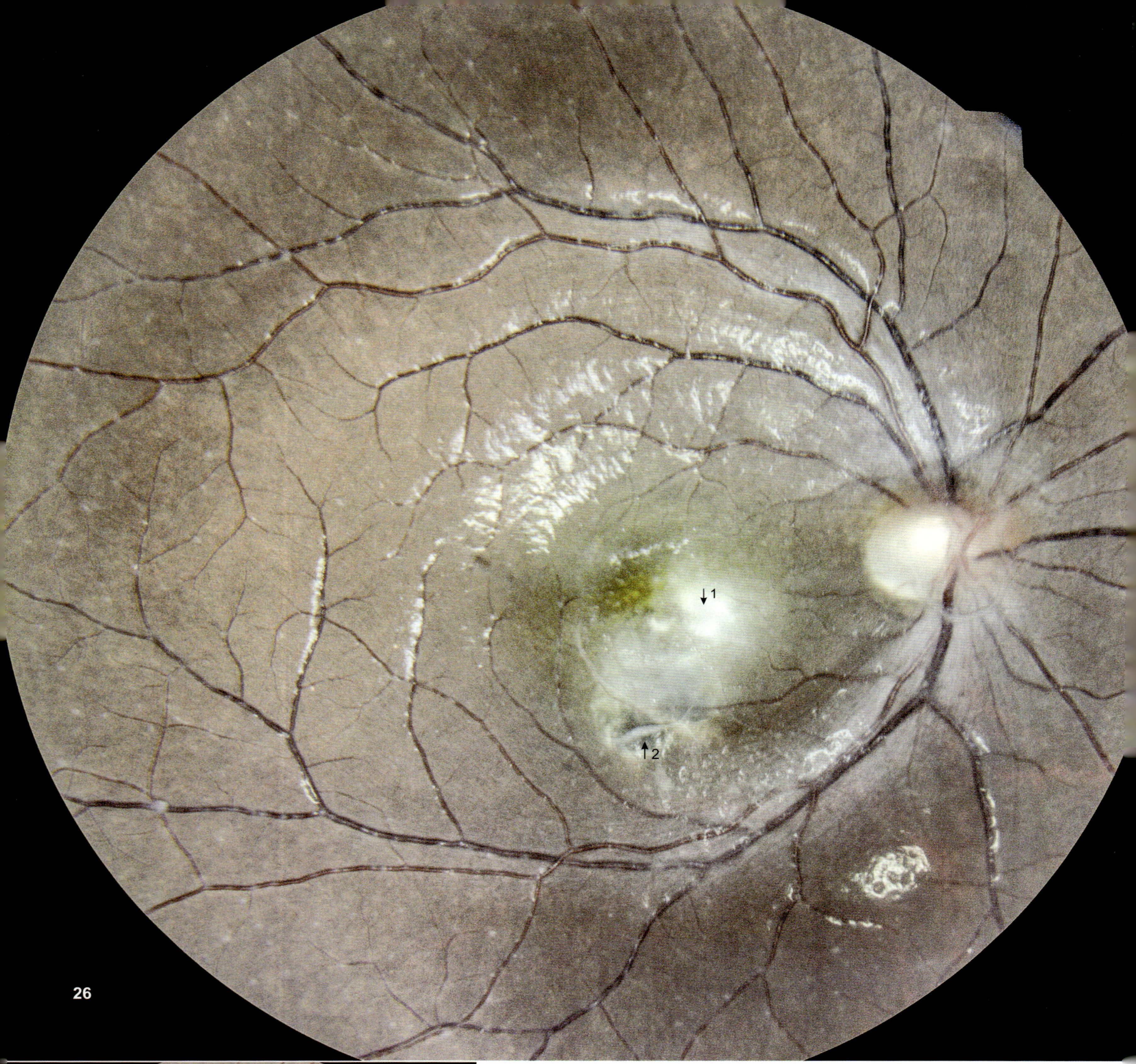


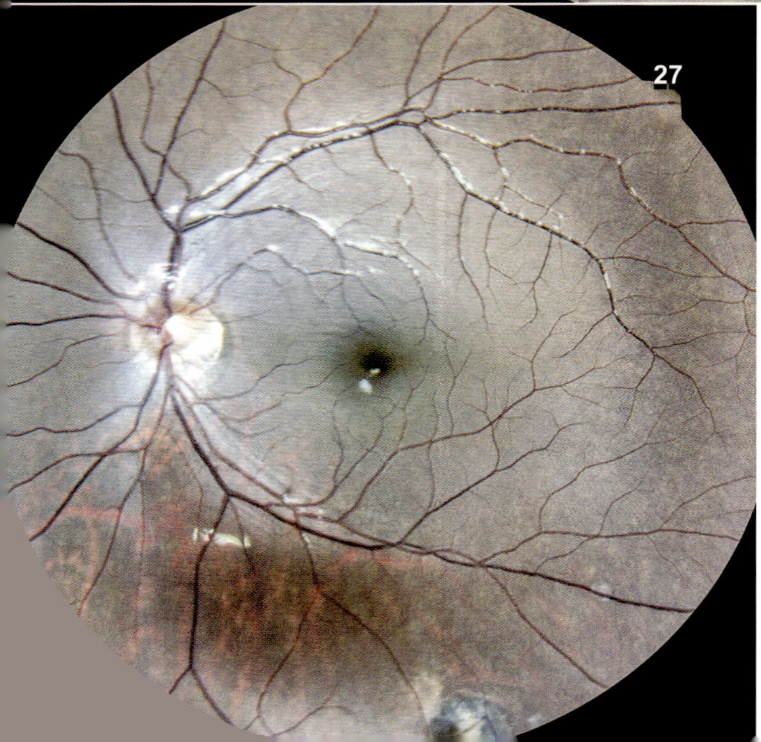


Figure 26 *Color fundus photograph demonstrating reactivation of toxoplasmosis retinochoroiditis in a 17-year-old boy. Note presence of whitish fluffy lesion with fuzzy borders (1) adjacent to an old toxoplasmosis scar (2).*

Patient had been investigated in the past and his aqueous tap had tested positive for toxoplasmosis. Since this was a recurrence that happened a year later, and clinical presentation was typical of reactivation, no further laboratory investigations were done. He was treated aggressively with single dose of intravitreal clindamycin and intravitreal dexamethasone injection as the lesions were threatening the fovea. Oral sepmax BD was given for 6 weeks. Three months later lesion shows complete healing seen with increasing pigmentation within the lesion and well-defined borders.

Figure 27 *Color fundus photograph of the left eye of the same patient demonstrates the presence of chorioretinal scar in the inferotemporal retina due to old toxoplasmosis.*

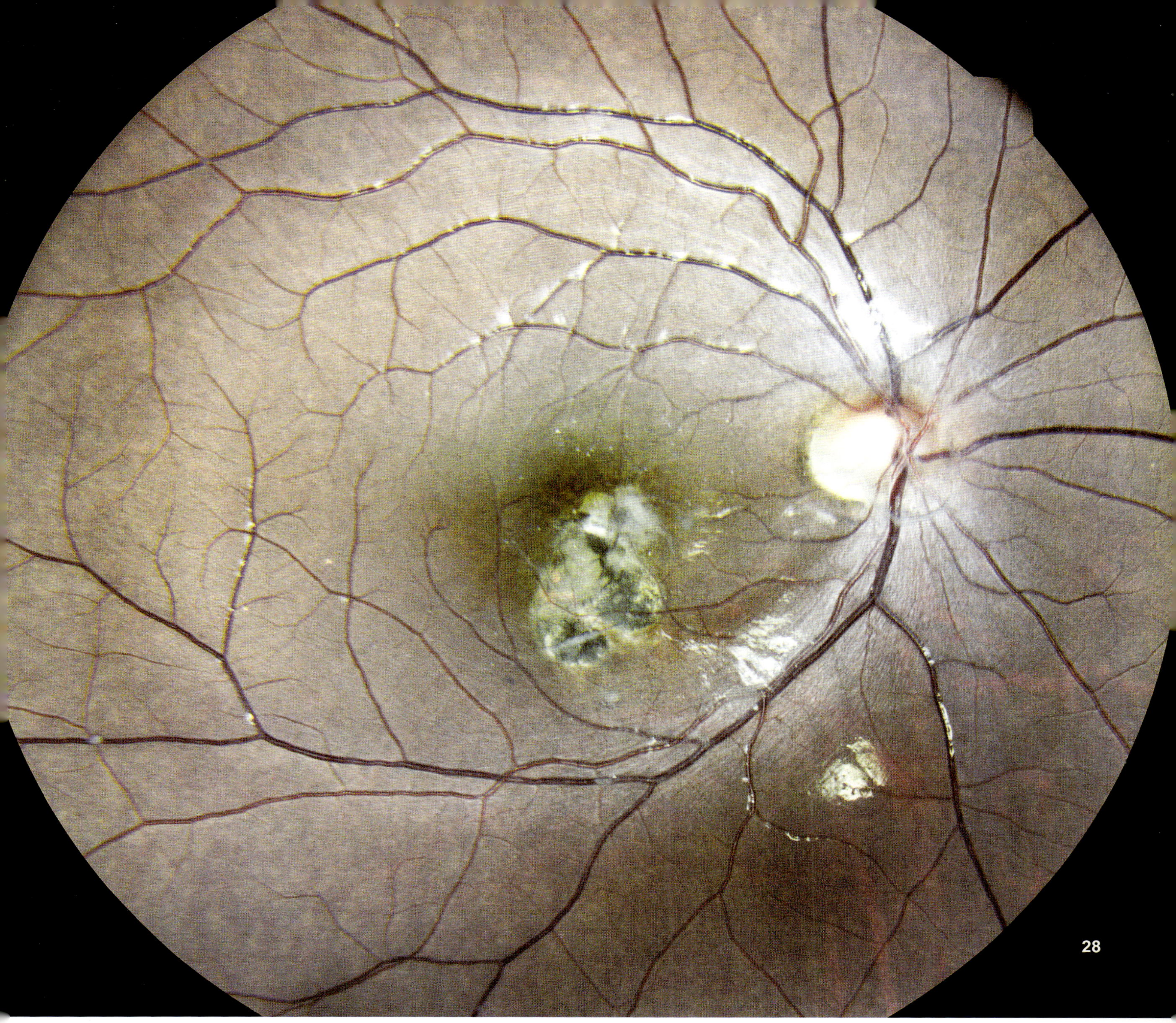


Figure 28 *Color fundus photograph 3 months after treatment shows healed toxoplasma retinochoroiditis.*

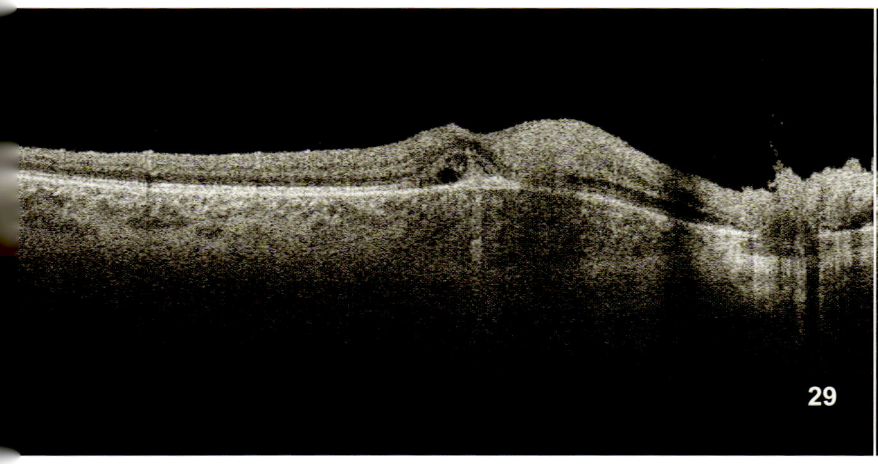


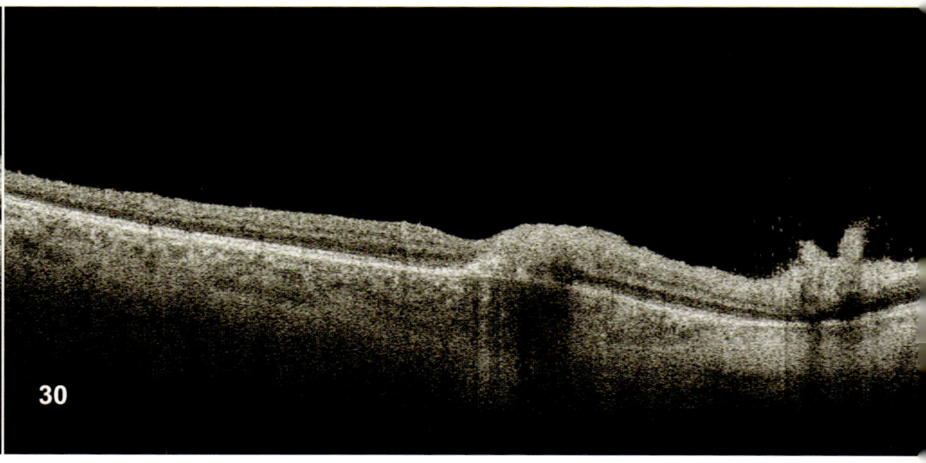


Figure 29 *Swept source OCT scan in active stage of toxoplasmosis showing inner retinal hyper-reflectivity corresponding to the patch of active retinitis, retinal thickening and choroidal shadowing with inflammatory fluid involving the fovea.*

Figure 30 *Swept source OCT scan 1 month later shows resolution of fluid, decreased retinal thickness' retinal architecture is still distorted in the area of disease activity.* □

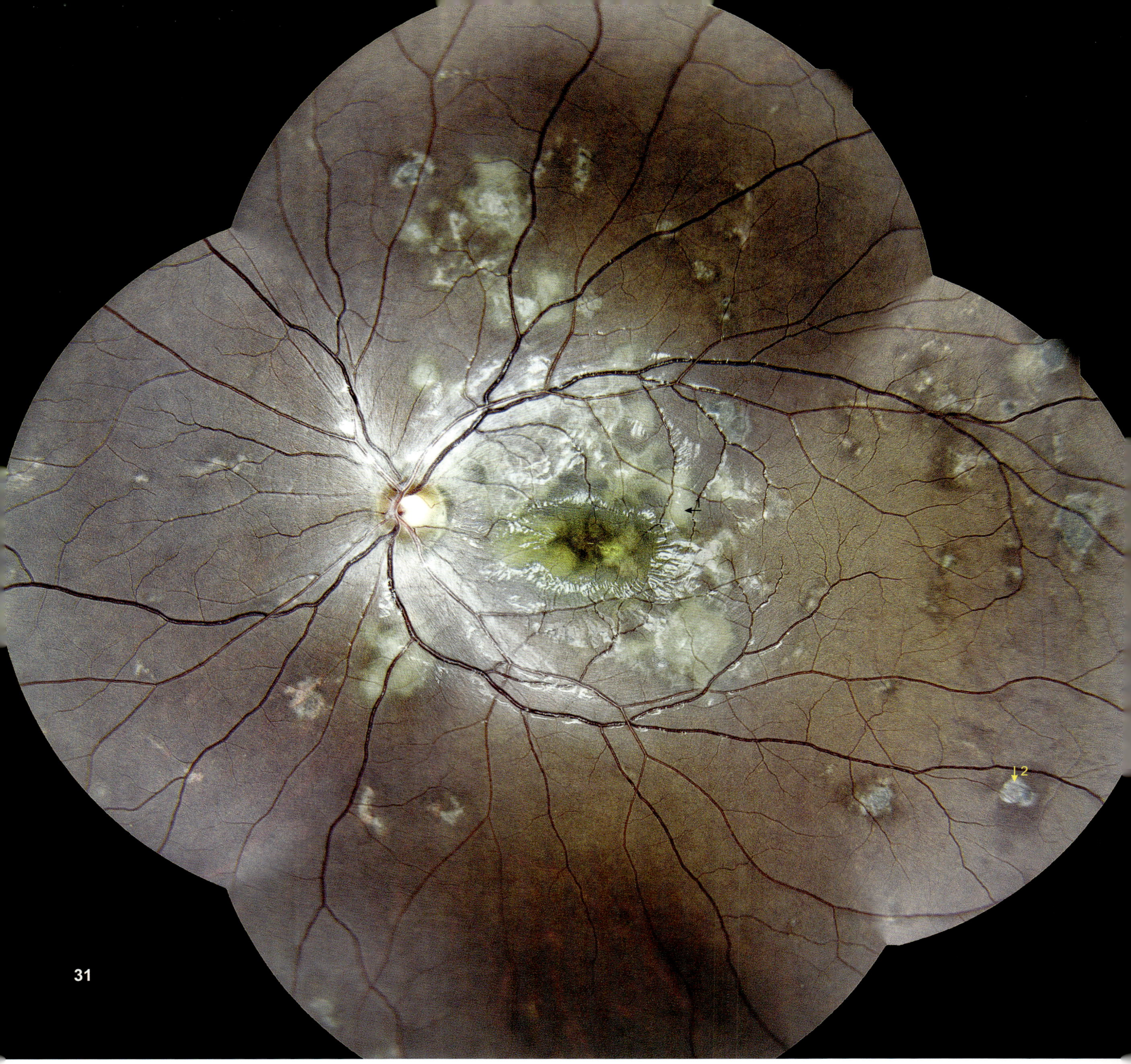


Figure 31 *Color fundus montage photograph of a young patient with multifocal choroiditis with lesions at various stages of healing. Note the presence of active patches of choroiditis that appears as yellowish fluffy lesions (1) at the macula with foveal involvement and also few scattered active lesions in the midperiphery and healed patches (2) that appears more pigmented with more discrete borders.*

A 25-year-old patient came with complaints of sudden onset floaters and blurred vision. Laboratory investigations tested positive for tuberculosis (Mantoux skin test positive, Quantiferon gold test). He was clinically diagnosed as multifocal serpiginoid type choroiditis of tubercular etiology. It is important to differentiate such cases from acute multifocal posterior pigment epitheliopathy (2), where lesions are also seen in various stages of evolution. However, AMPPE is limited to the posterior pole usually and there is no association with tuberculosis.

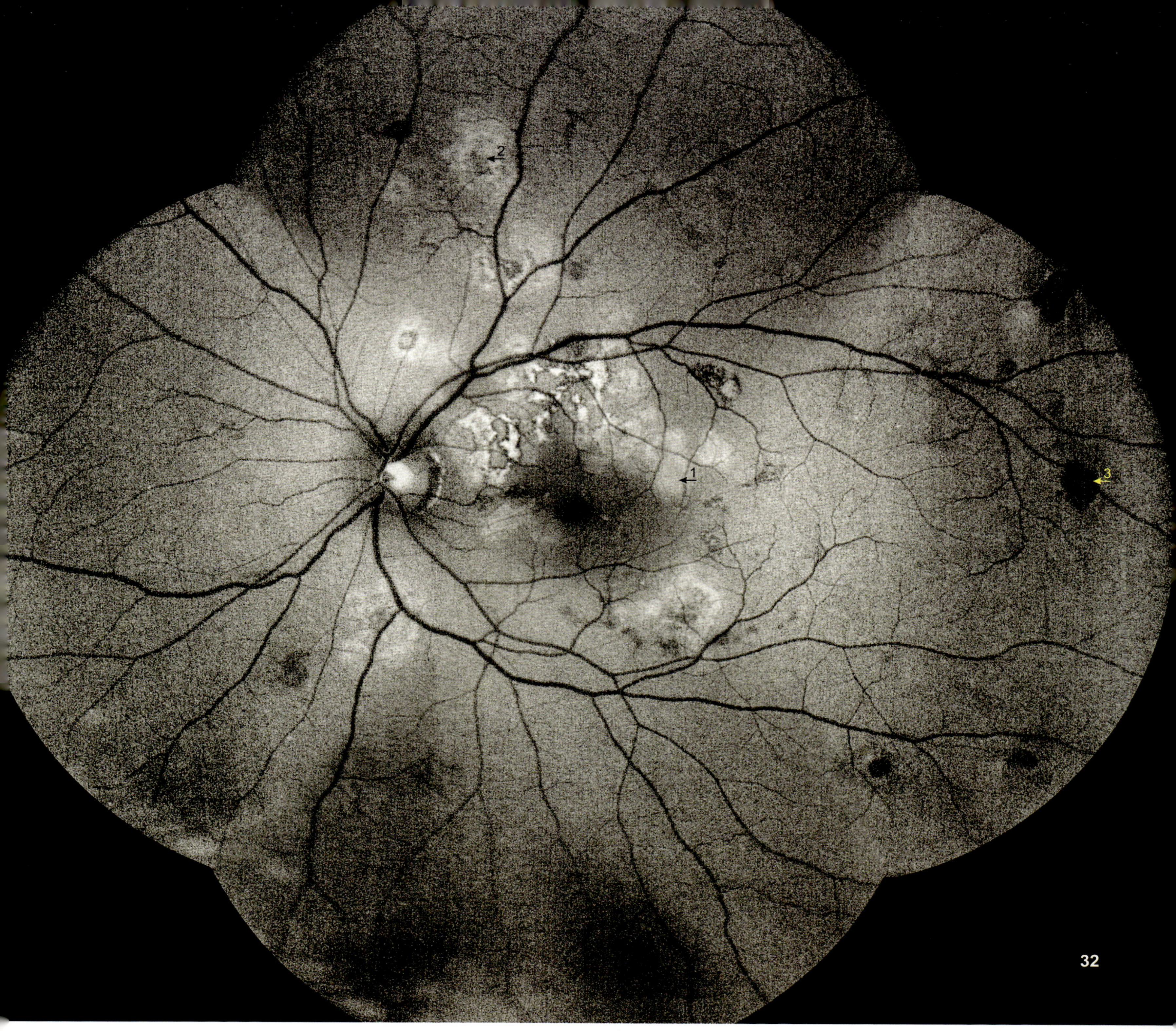


Figure 32 *Autofluorescence montage demonstrating lesions with various disease activity. Note the presence of active lesions that appear as hyperautofluorescent (1), healing lesions with hypo-autofluorescent center and ring of hyperautofluorescent at the edges (2) and healed lesions that appear completely hypo-autofluorescent (3).*

Figure 34 *OCTA wide field montage 12 mm × 12 mm slab at the level of superficial capillary plexus did not show any abnormality.* □

Figure 33 *OCTA montage at the level of choriocapillaris slab: Note that the active lesions appear hypo (1), due to capillary ischemic event or infiltration, as the lesions heal, they appear stippled with mixture of hypo and hyper, and healed lesions (2) show underlying large to medium choroidal vessels due to overlying RPE loss.*

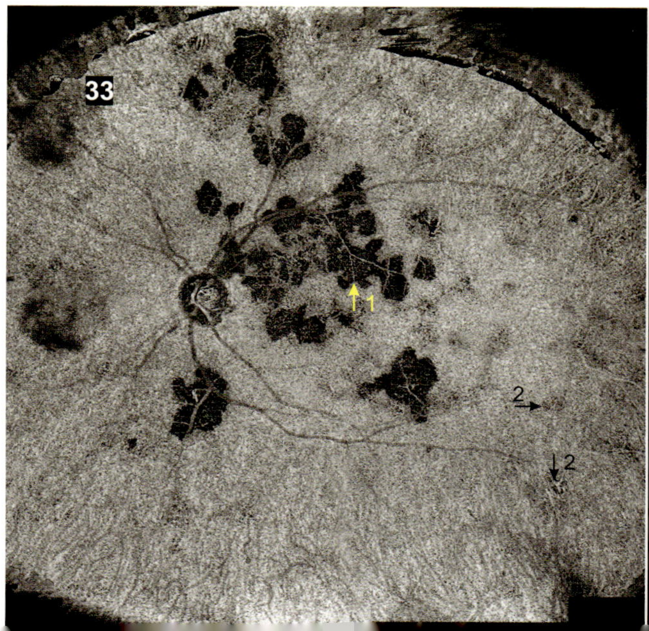


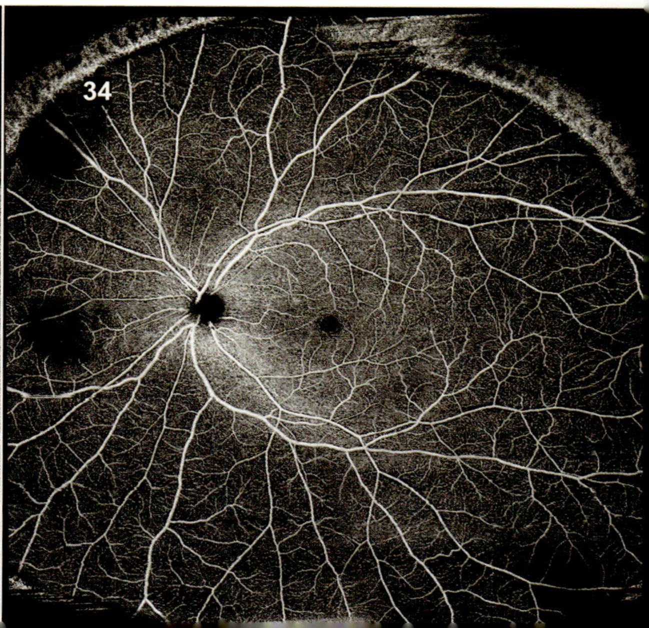

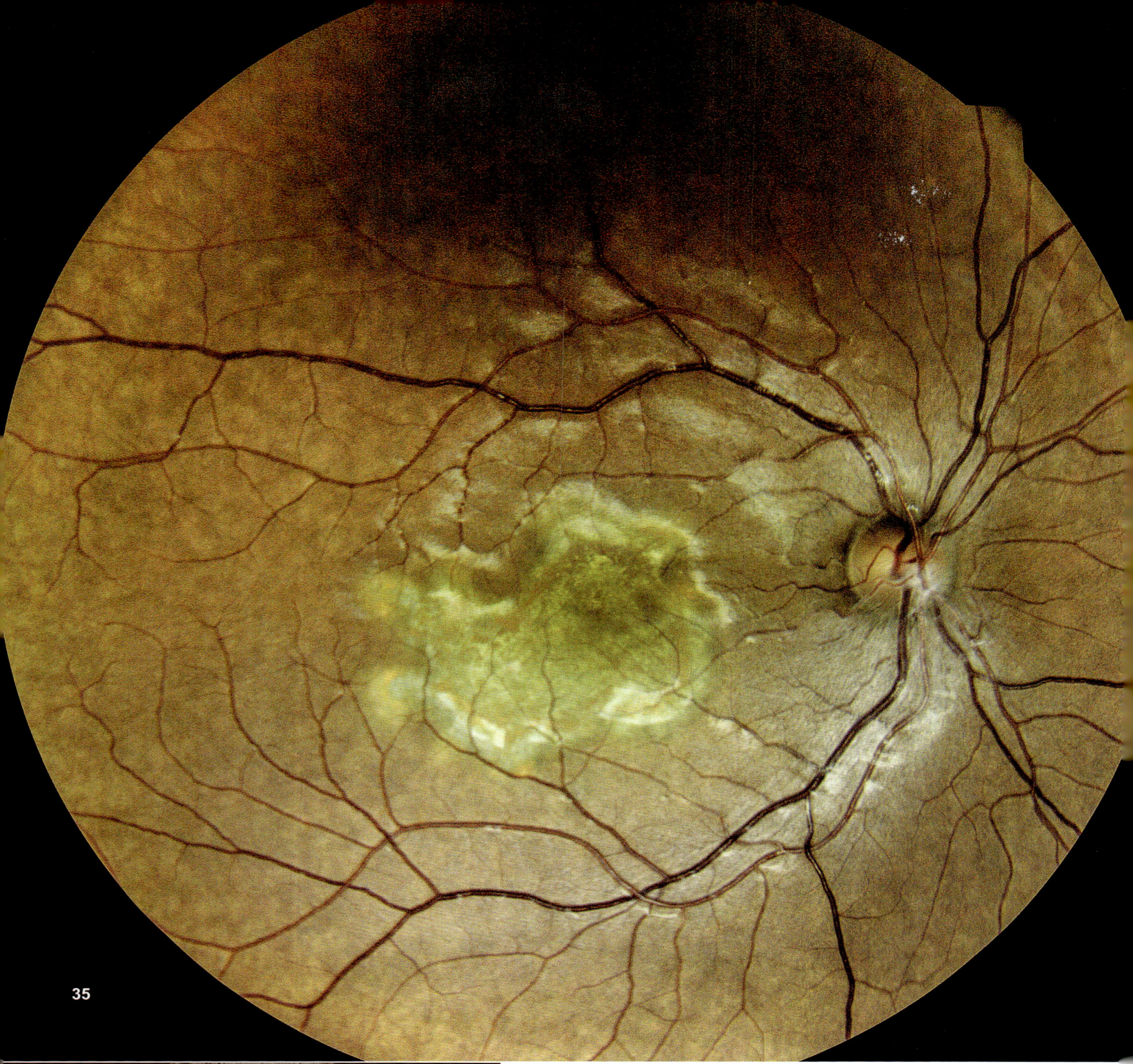

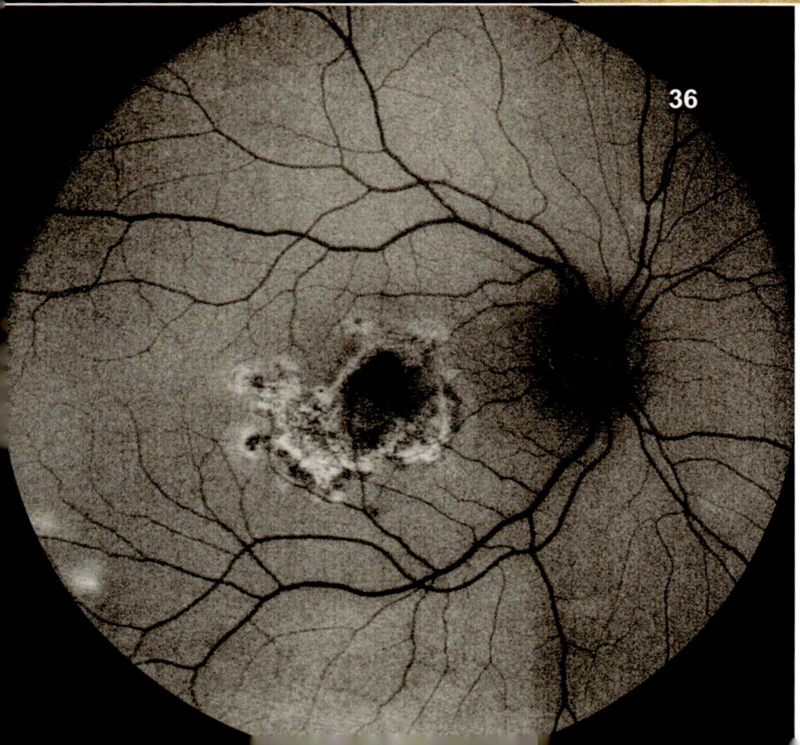

Figure 35 *Color fundus photograph of macular variant of serpiginous choroiditis.*

A 35-year-old young woman presented with sudden onset blurred vision in her right eye. Her best corrected visual acuity was 6/36. Color photograph demonstrates a large yellowish amoeboid-shaped patch of choroiditis at the macula. Margins of the lesion appear more fluffy than the center.

Serpiginous choroiditis also called geographic choroiditis is a chronic relentless inflammatory disorder of unknown cause that primarily involves the choroid and retinal pigment epithelium. Macular serpiginous choroiditis represents a variant of the disease, in which typical lesions are located initially or exclusively in the macular region. Individuals with macular variant may have poorer visual prognosis and accurate diagnosis and prompt treatment are of paramount importance.

Figure 36 *Autofluorescence of active choroiditis.*

In active choroiditis prominent hyperautofluorescence is seen at the active edges of the lesion due to increased metabolic activity at the level of retinal pigment epithelium.

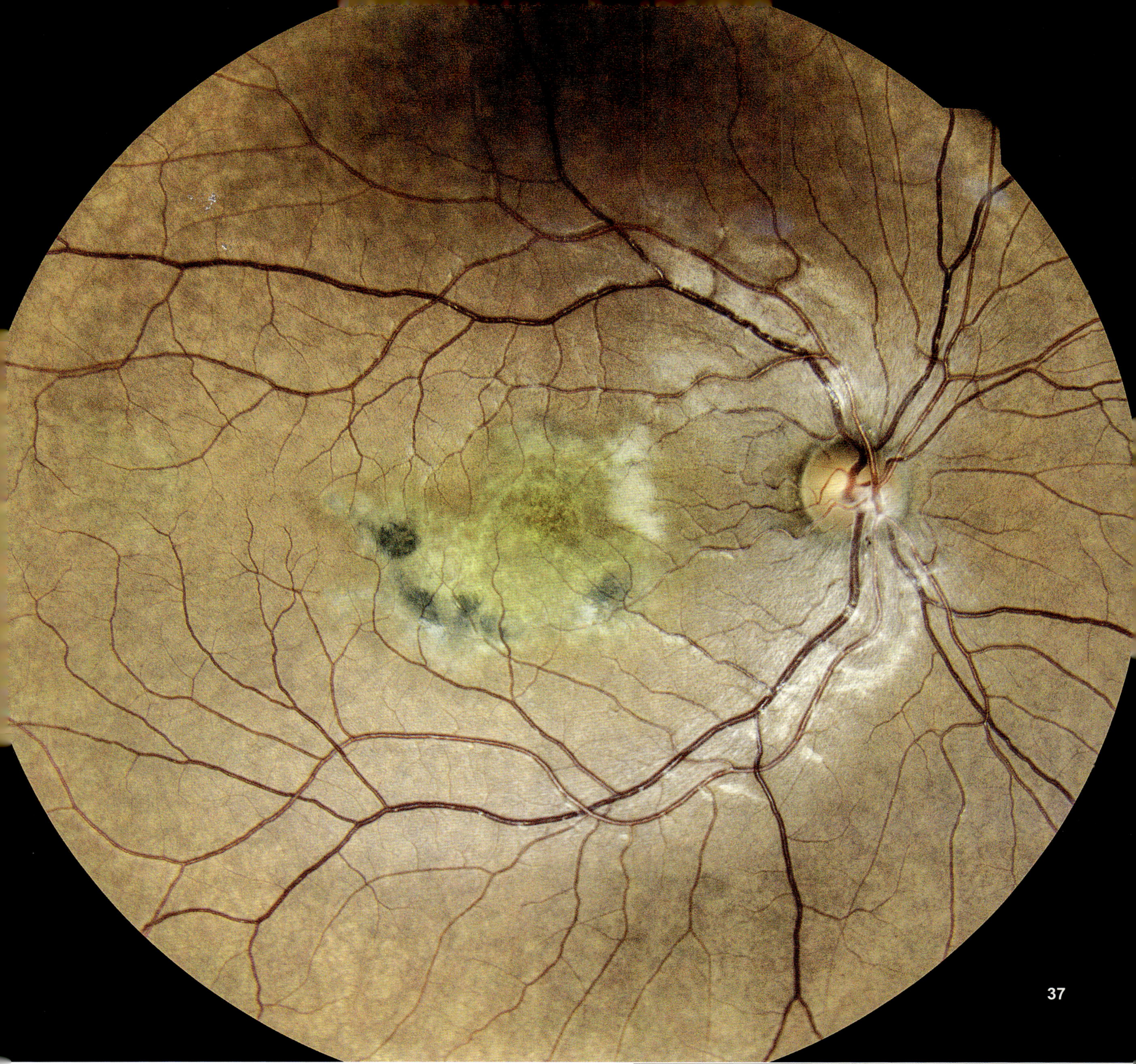

37

Figure 37 *Color fundus photo 6 months after treatment.*

She was thoroughly investigated to rule out infectious causes of uveitis. Complete laboratory investigations were done to rule out tuberculosis, syphilis and sarcoidosis. Autoimmune blood profile was also negative. She was started on oral steroids at the dose of 1 mg/kg body weight and nonsteroidal systemic immunosuppressives (tablet mycophenolate, mofetil) was added after 4 weeks. 6 months later, color photo shows patch of choroiditis has reduced in size with RPE hyperpigmentation visible at the temporal edge of the lesion. Her visual acuity has improved to 6/9.

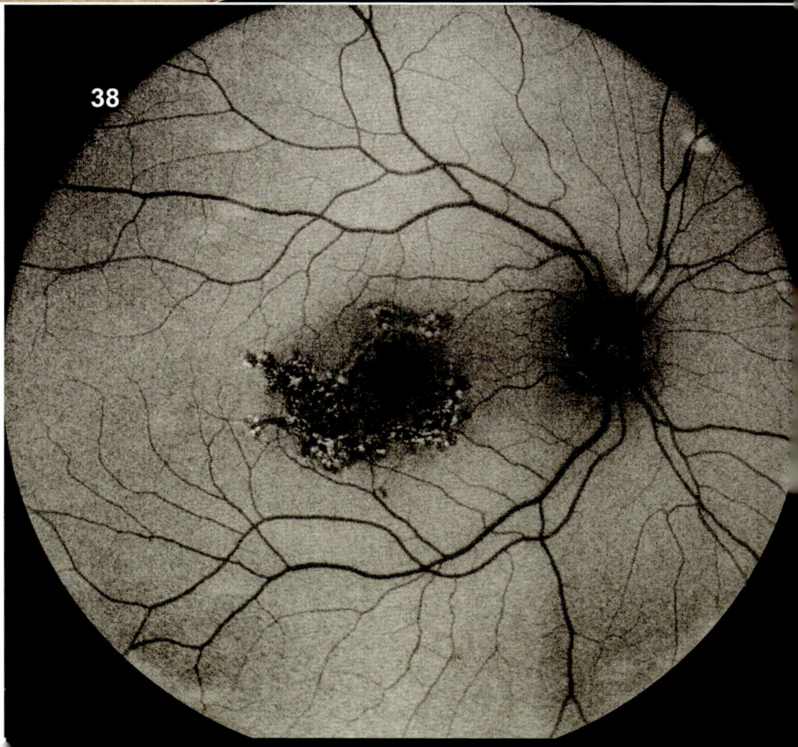

38

Figure 38 *Six months after treatment, there is predominantly hypoautofluorescence suggesting RPE damage due to healing. Also note absence of hyper-autofluorescent patch at the edges of lesion suggesting that the lesion is quiescent now (healed choroiditis).*□

Figure 39

*Case of serpiginous like choroiditis (SLC) of tubercular etiology.*

Color fundus photograph appears slightly blurred due to vitritis and posterior subcapsular cataract. Large yellowish patch of choroiditis is seen with active fluffy yellow edges (1).

Serpiginous-like choroiditis is a distinct form of serpiginous choroiditis characterized by multifocal choroidal lesions of varying size and shape which often coalesce to form diffuse choroiditis hence resembling serpiginous choroiditis in patients with presumed ocular tuberculosis.

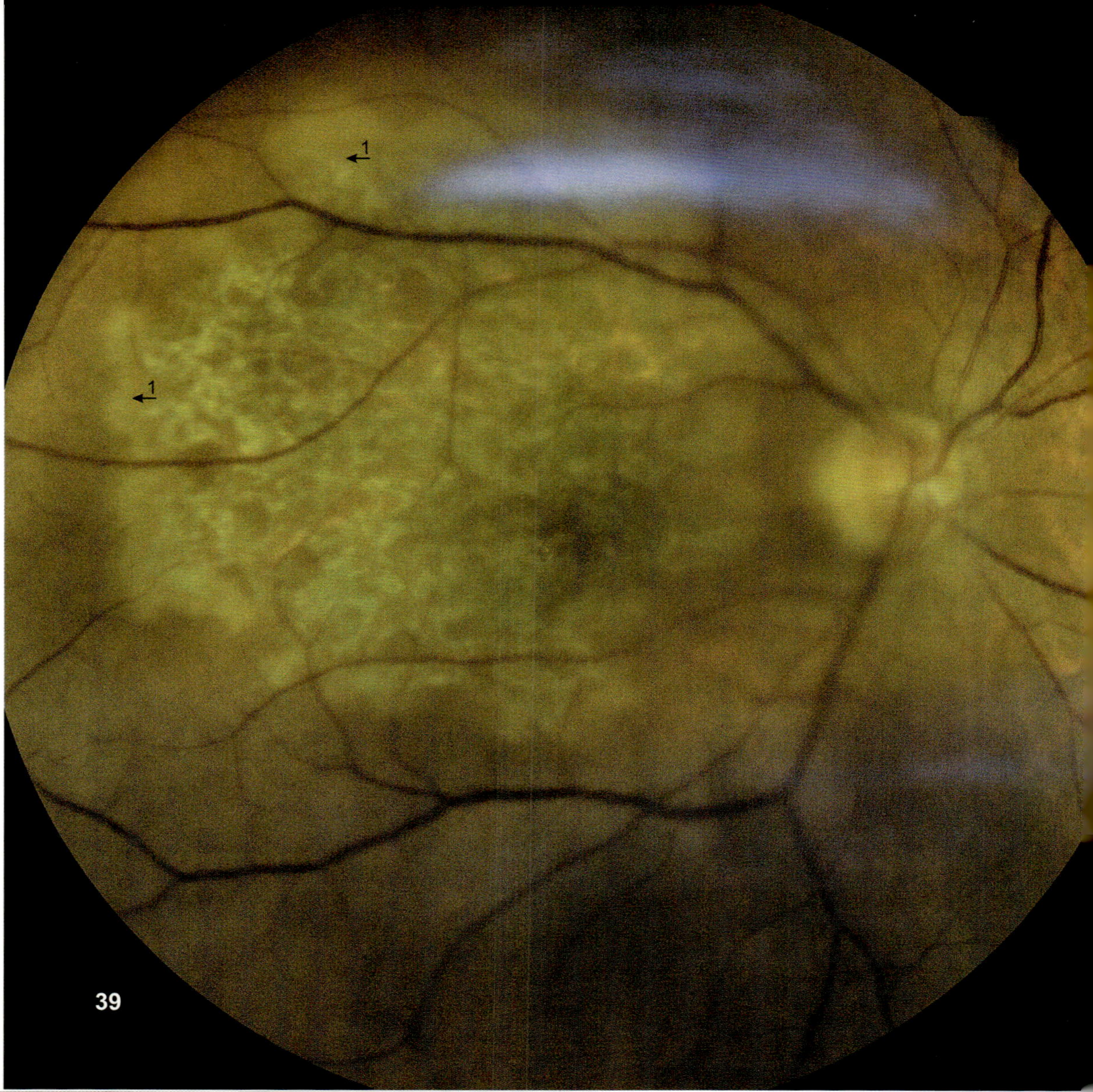


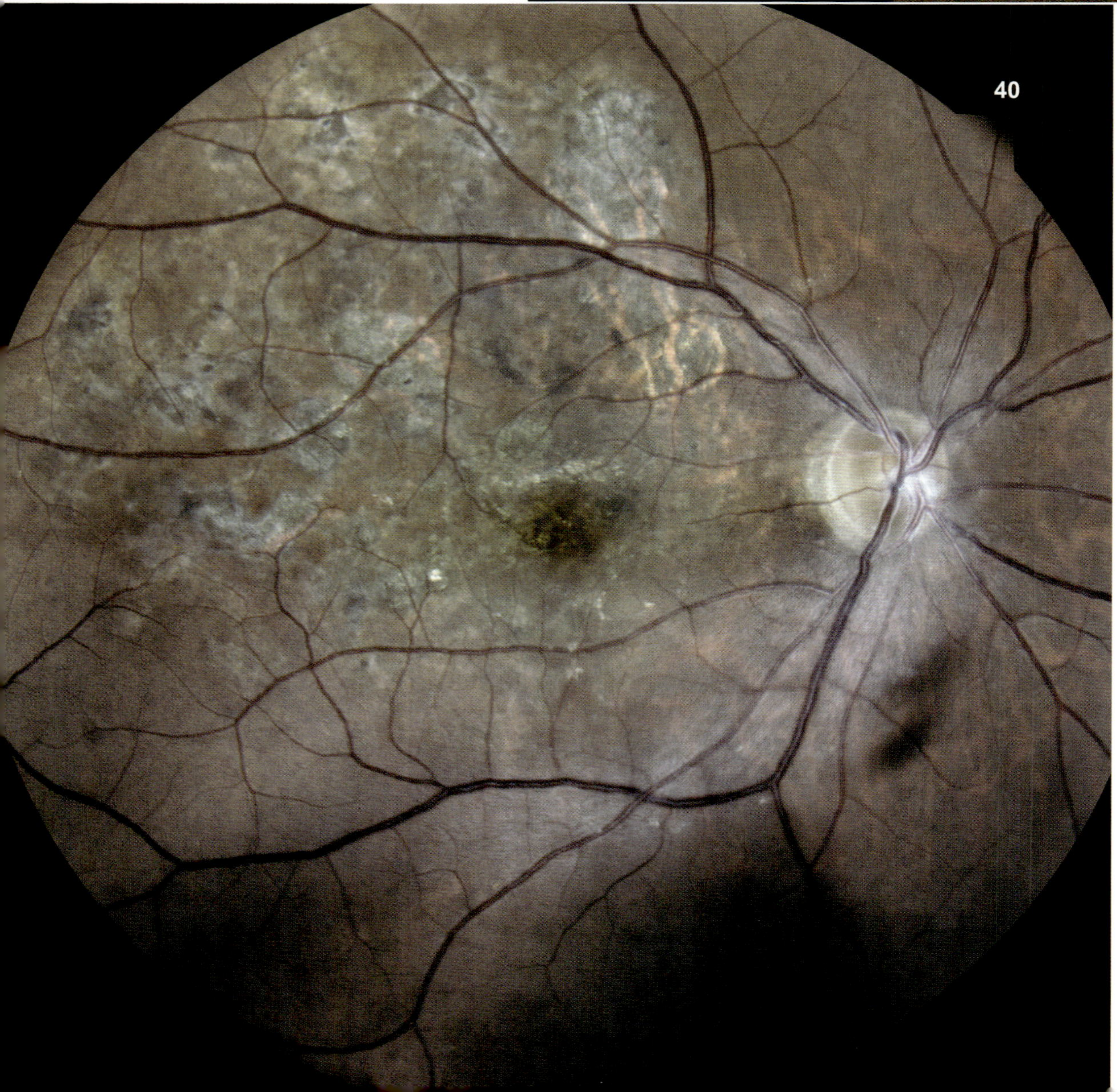


Figure 40

*Serpiginous-like choroiditis 1 year after treatment.*

Note areas of RPE atrophy and pigmentation. No new lesions have developed in the past 1 year and older lesions have healed.

She was 56-year-old female who presented with painless visual loss and floaters. Her Mantoux skin test was positive with induration of 25 mm, positive Quantiferon TB gold test and hilar lymphadenopathy on chest X-ray. Based on positive laboratory evidence and clinical picture she was advised 9 months course of antitubercular treatment along with oral steroids. She also underwent a cataract surgery during the course of treatment. □

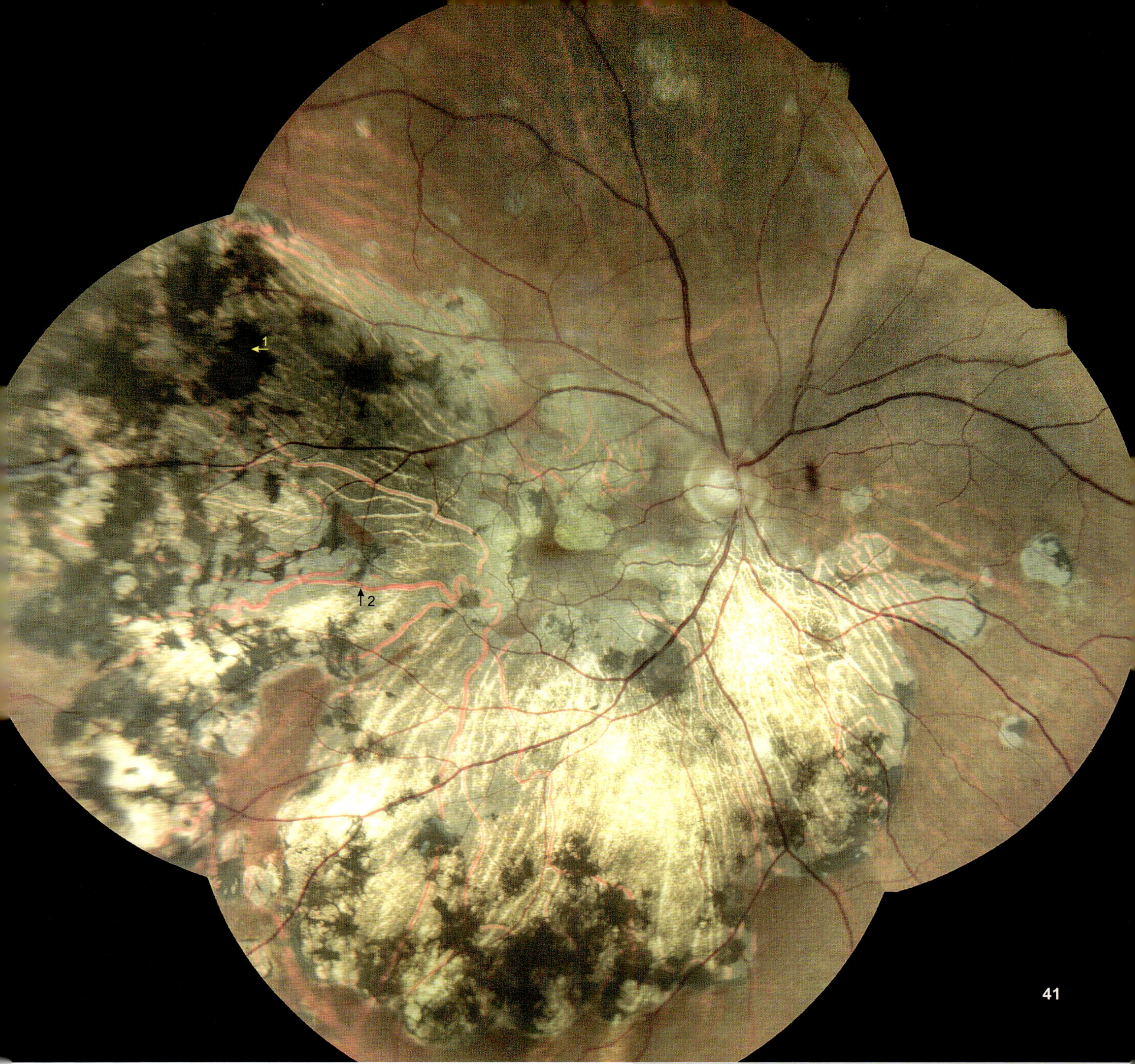


41

Figure 41 *Case of healed multifocal serpiginous choroiditis (tubercular etiology).*

Color montage photograph shows multiple discrete areas of retinal pigment epithelium atrophy and hyperpigmentation. Active lesions usually resolve within 6 to 8 weeks and are characterized by sharpening of the borders with irregular RPE hyperpigmentation (1), diffuse RPE and choriocapillary atrophy. Sometimes atrophy and destruction are so extensive that the large underlying choroidal vessels (2) are exposed. Sometimes whole of choroid up to sclera is disorganized.

42

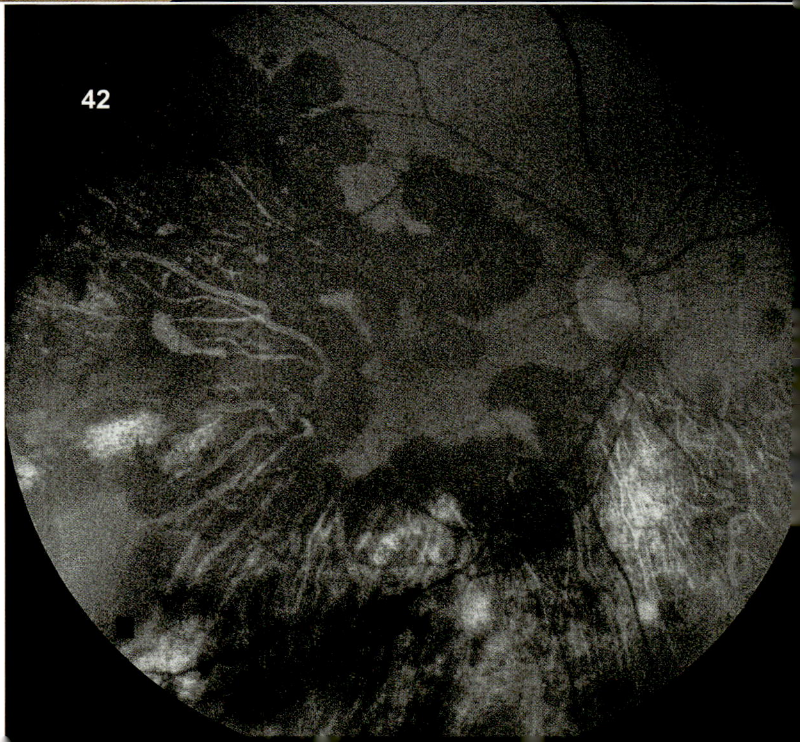

Figure 42 *Fundus autofluorescence reveals total hypoautofluorescent areas with sharp borders. At places there is complete loss of RPE layer exposing the underlying choroidal vessels.* □

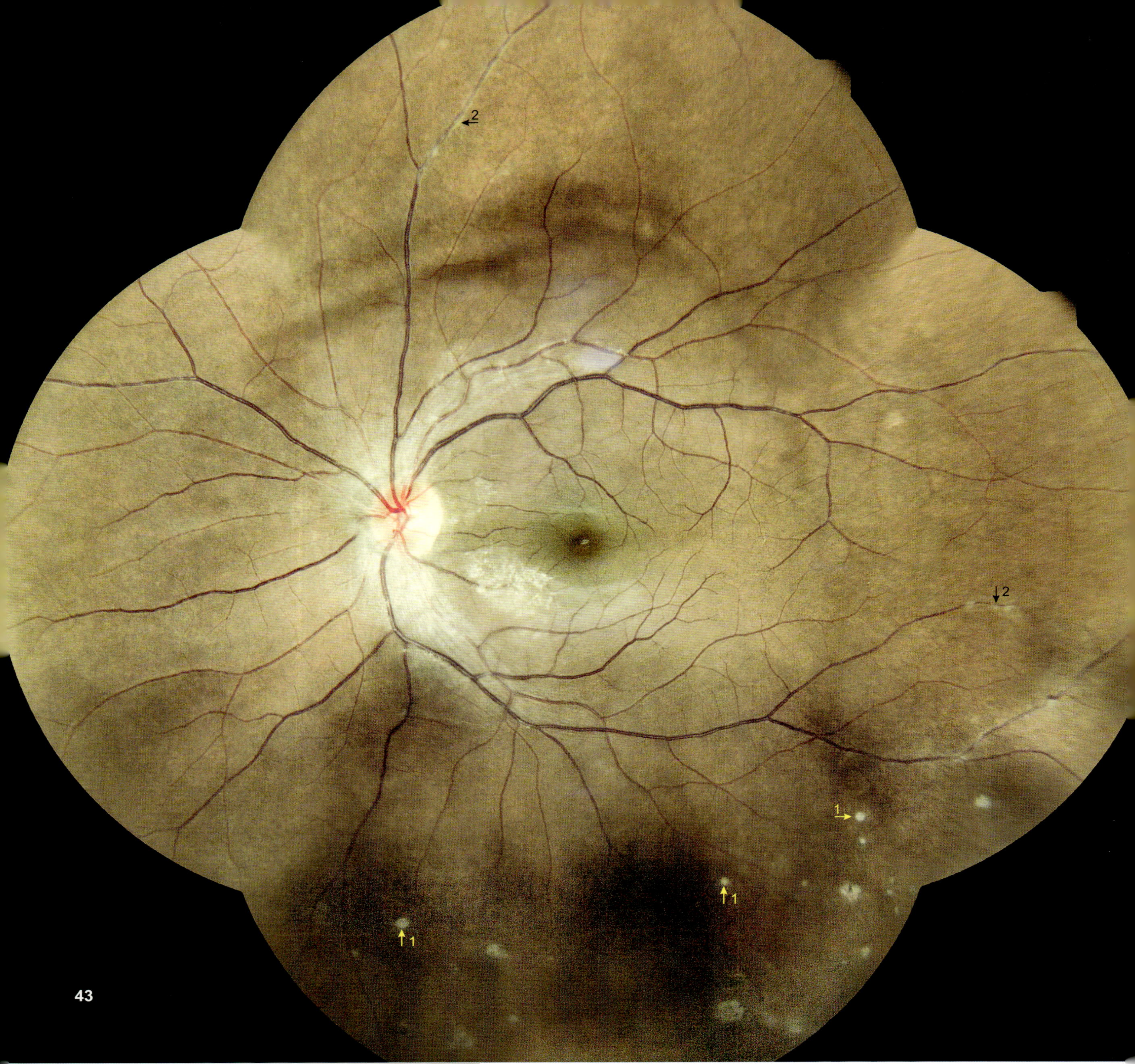

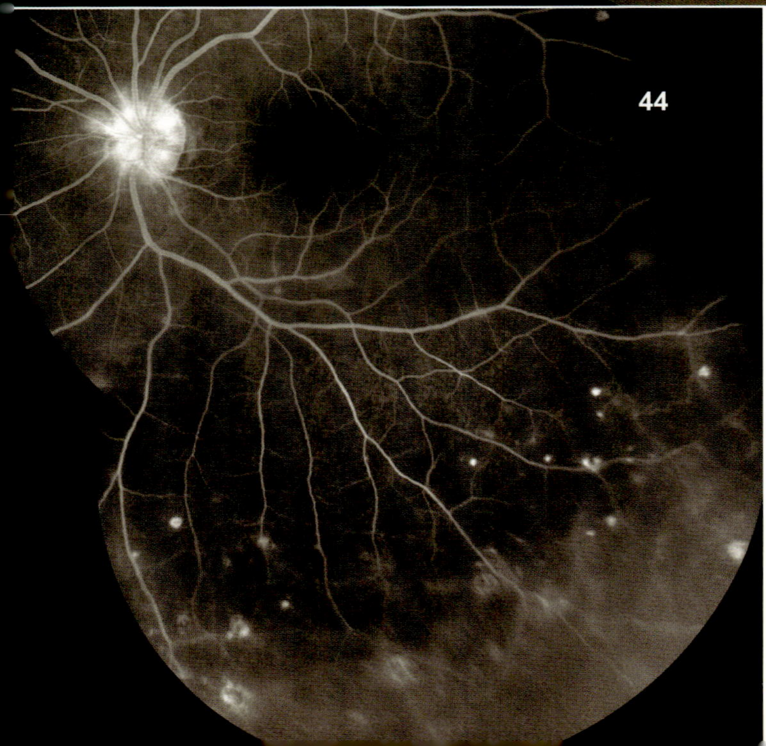

Figure 43 *A case of ocular sarcoidosis. White, small, round, multiple scattered chorioretinal lesions were seen in the peripheral retina (1). Note the presence of peripheral venous sheathing (2) along the retinal veins superiorly and temporally.*

Ocular involvement in sarcoidosis is seen in 15 to 25% of patients. Posterior segment manifestations occur in up to 28% of cases. Deeper chorioretinal lesions simulating Dalen Fuchs nodules have been reported. Perivascular sheathing occurs in 10–17% and is generally mid-peripheral without significant vascular occlusion.

Figure 44 *Fluorescein angiogram montage in case of ocular sarcoidosis.*

There is diffuse perivascular leakage predominantly along the inferior retinal veins. Few well-defined round hyperfluorescent dot like chorioretinal lesions are visible. Healed lesions appear more discrete whereas active lesions have fuzzy borders due to active fluorescein leak. □

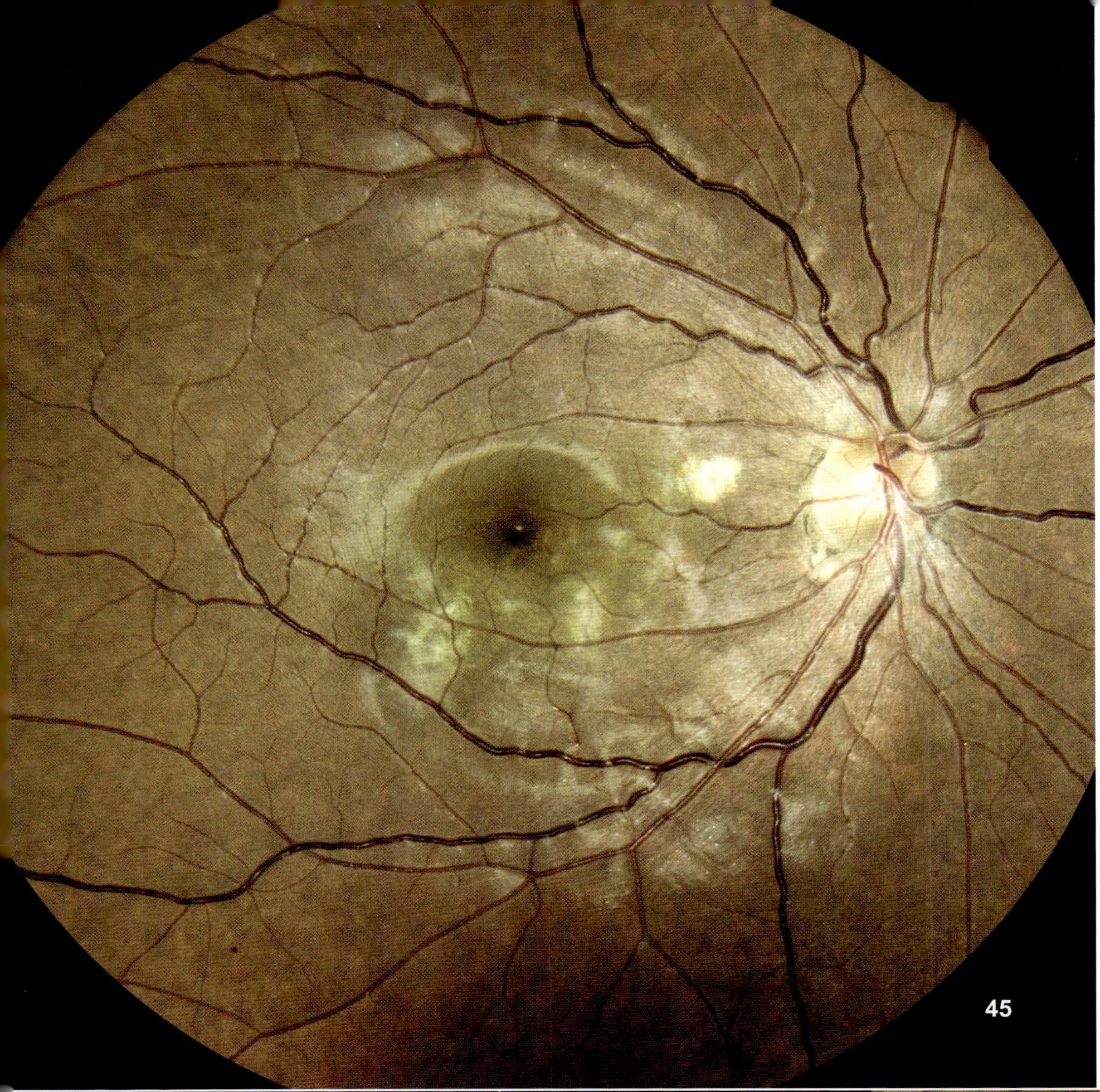

Figure 45

*A case of punctate inner choroiditis (PIC) right eye. Note presence of yellow spots with indistinct borders at the posterior pole in a 35-year-old young female.*

PIC has been described as a disease entity by Watzke et al in 1884. Its a form of choroiditis, that affects young healthy patients. These patients with PIC have no cells or other signs of inflammation and most of the PIC lesions are found in the posterior pole. Yellow spots usually measure between 100 and 300 micron and are located at the level of RPE and inner choroid.

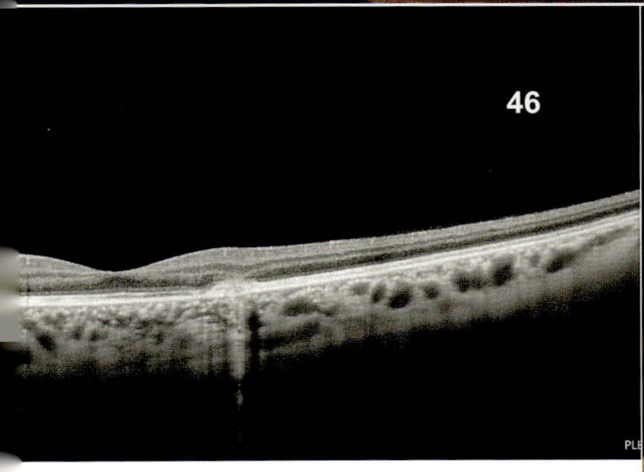

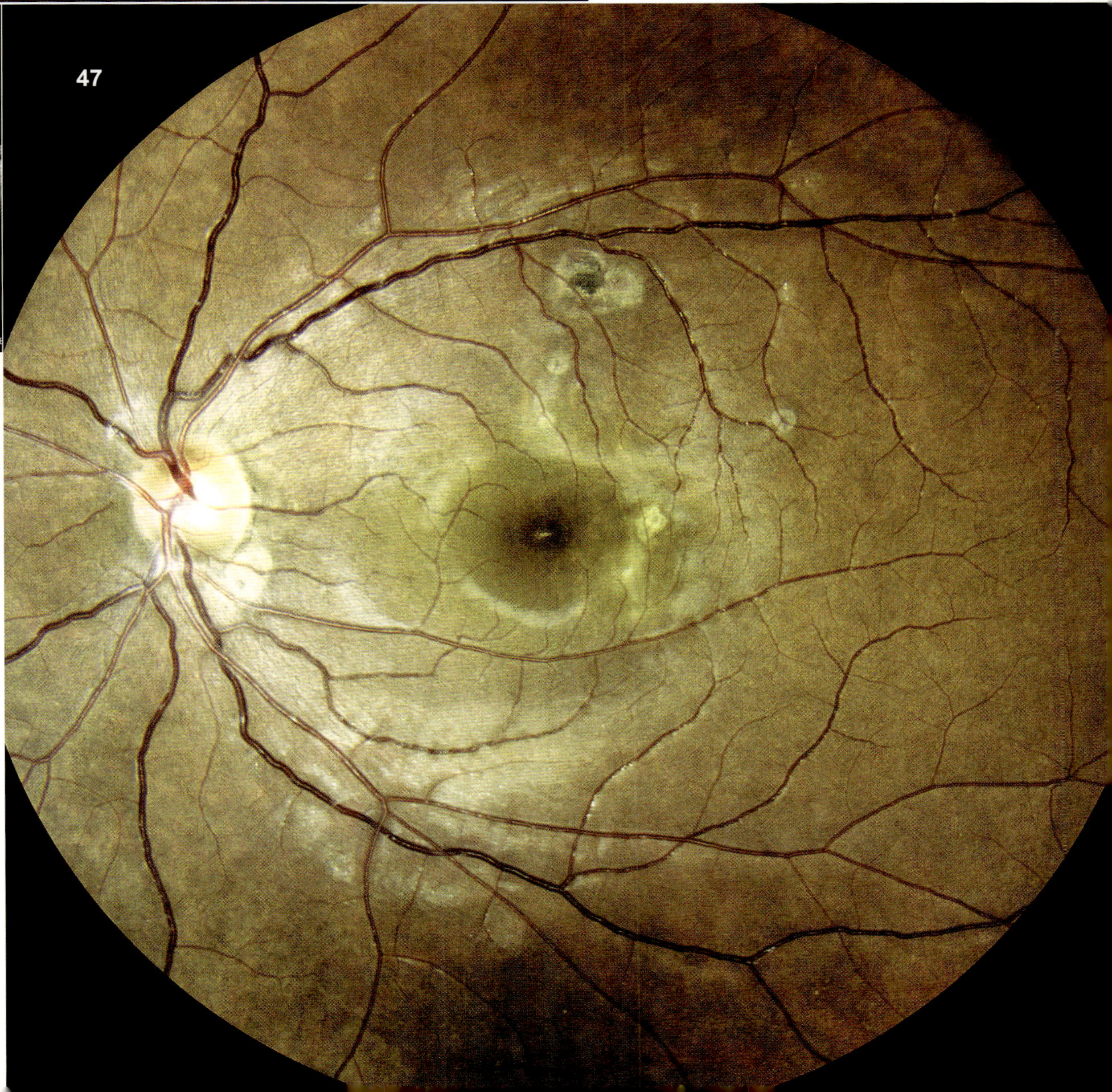

Figure 46

*Swept source OCT scan shows focal elevation of the retinal pigment epithelium, forming a chorioretinal nodule with corresponding disruption of inner segment/outer segment of photoreceptor interface.*

Figure 47

*Punctate inner choroiditis: Left eye of the same patient. Four tiny round irregular lesions of choroiditis is seen at the posterior pole. Large lesion near the superotemporal arcade is showing RPE hyperpigmentation.* □

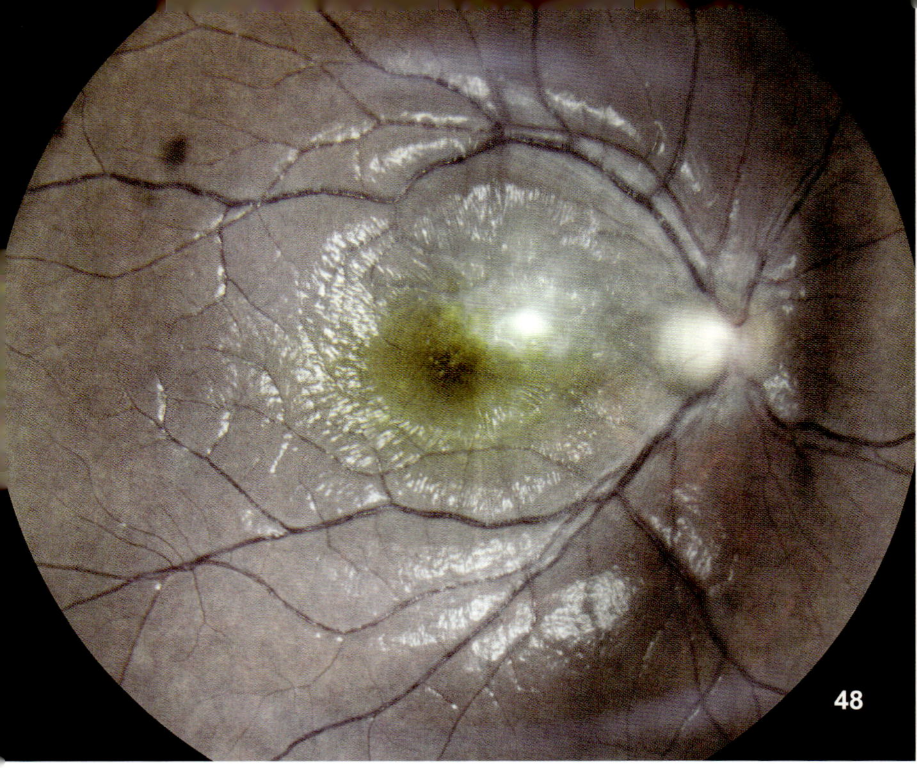


Figure 48 *Case of active ocular toxoplasmosis. Color fundus image shows a whitish patch of necrotizing retinitis just superior to the fovea.*

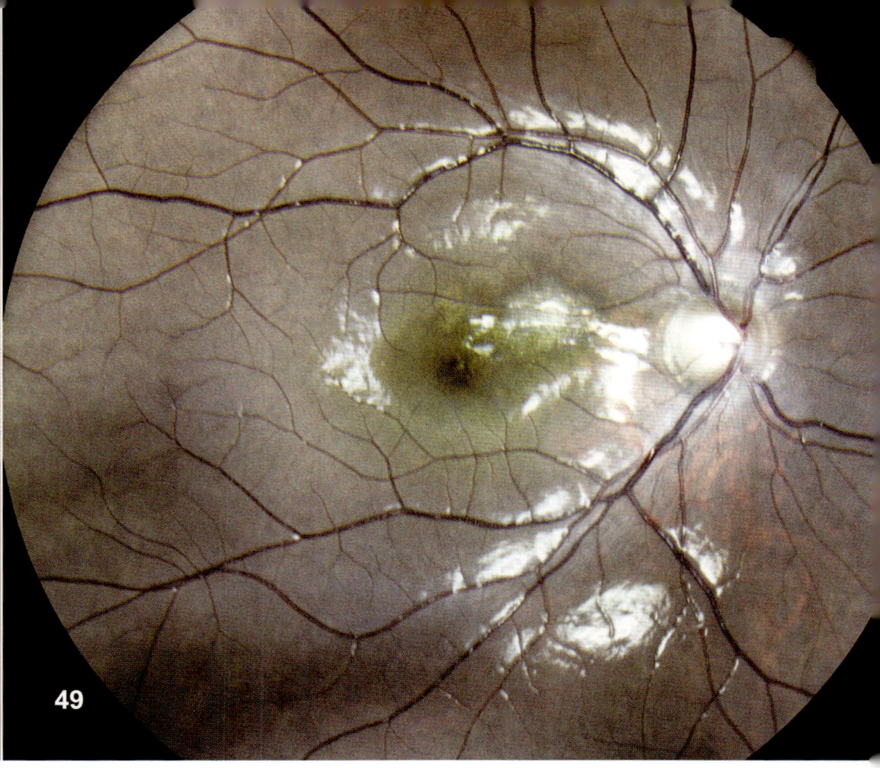


Figure 49 *Case of acute ocular toxoplasmosis-healed stage. Note the pigmentary changes that have developed at the site of active lesion due to RPE cell loss.*

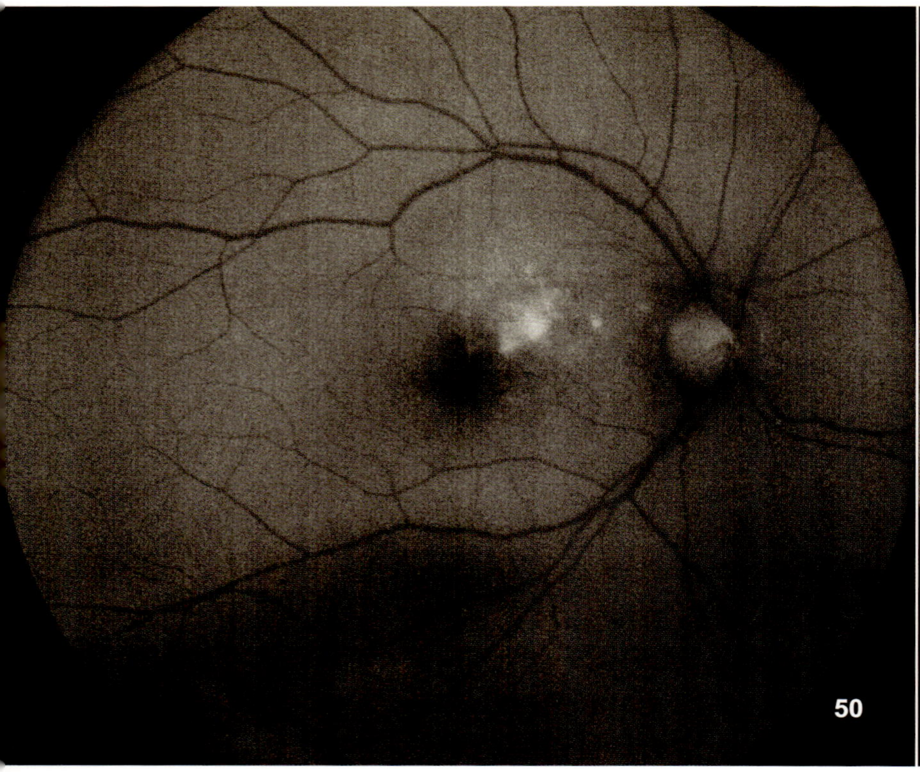


Figure 50 *Autofluorescence of central macula demonstrating hyper-autofluorescence from the active lesion of toxoplasmosis retinochoroiditis.*

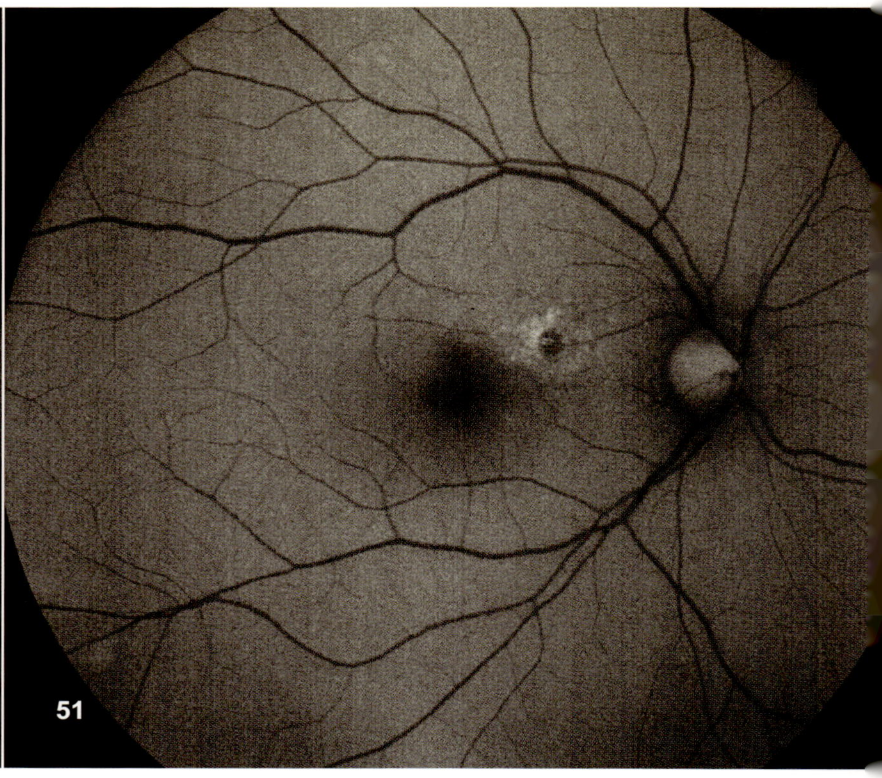


Figure 51 *Autofluorescence of central macula demonstrating hypoauto-fluorescence from the healed lesion of toxoplasmosis retino-choroiditis.*

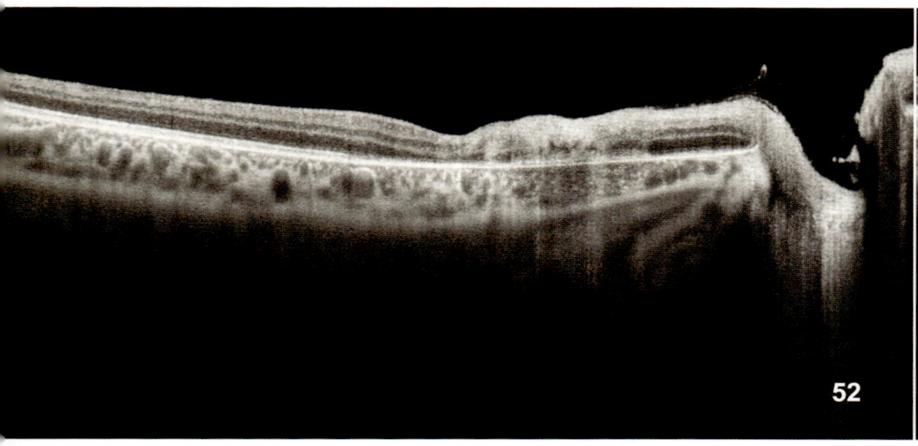


Figure 52 *Swept source OCT scan passing through the acute toxoplasmosis lesion shows disorganized inner retinal layers as a consequence to necrotizing retinitis.*

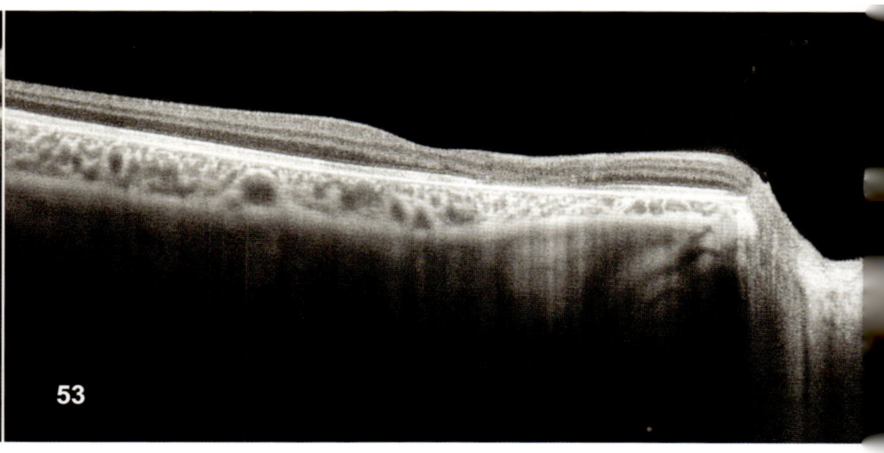


Figure 53 *Swept source OCT scan after lesion are healed. Note inner retinal layer architecture is better defined now, however outer retinal atrophy is seen due to RPE cell loss.* □

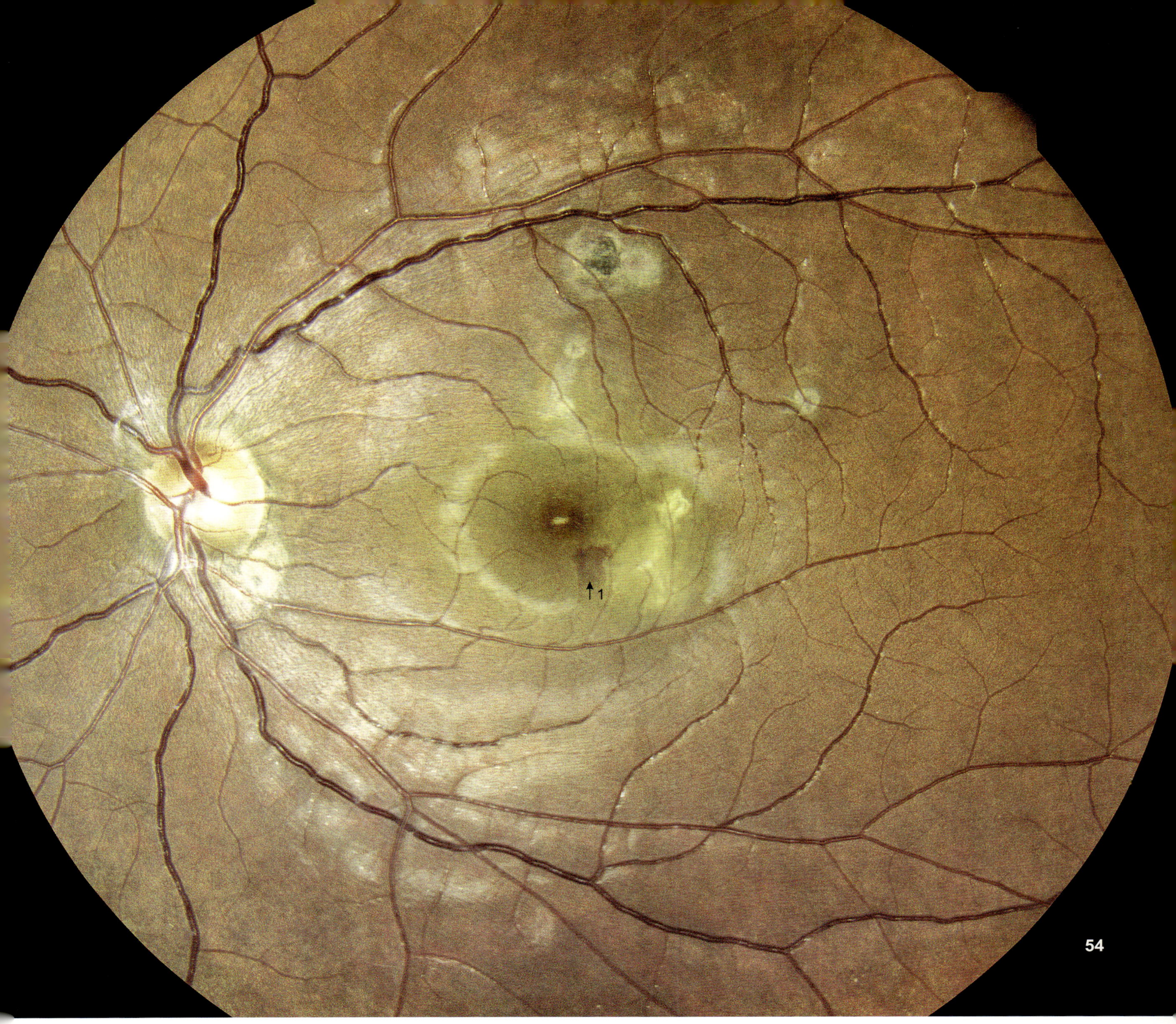


Figure 54 *Color fundus photograph of a patient with punctate inner choroiditis associated with inflammatory choroid neovascular membrane. Note the presence of multiple yellowish PIC lesions at the posterior pole. Small patch of subretinal hemorrhage is also seen at the inferior edge of the fovea (1).*

Figure 55 *Spectral domain optical coherence tomography scans passing through the fovea at baseline shows presence of subretinal fluid at the fovea and hyperreflective lesion (1) with fuzzy borders above the retinal pigment epithelium (type 2 CNVM) (2).*

Figure 56 *Spectral domain optical coherence tomography scans 1 month after treatment, shows resolution of subretinal fluid and CNVM complex. The borders have become more sharp and well-defined.*

Figure 57 *OCT angiography 6 mm × 6 mm scan shows frond of neovascularization (1) picked up in the outer retina choriocapillary slab (ORCC) at the site of retinal hemorrhage.* □

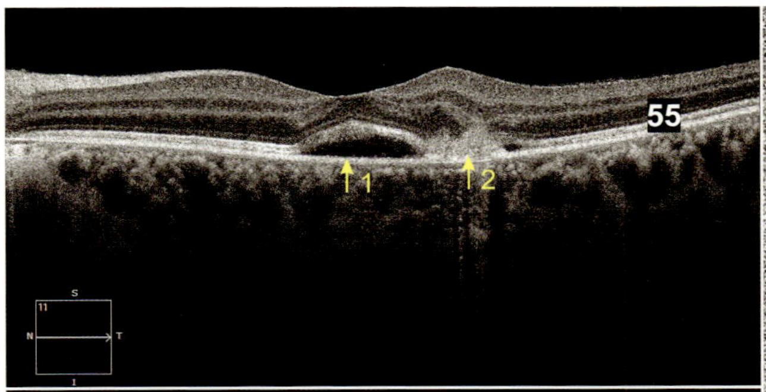


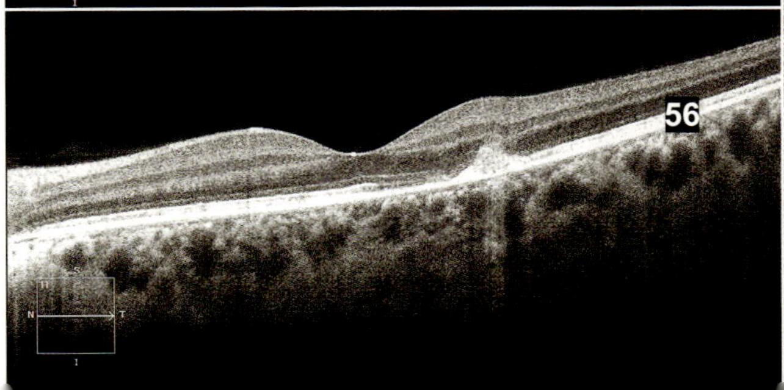


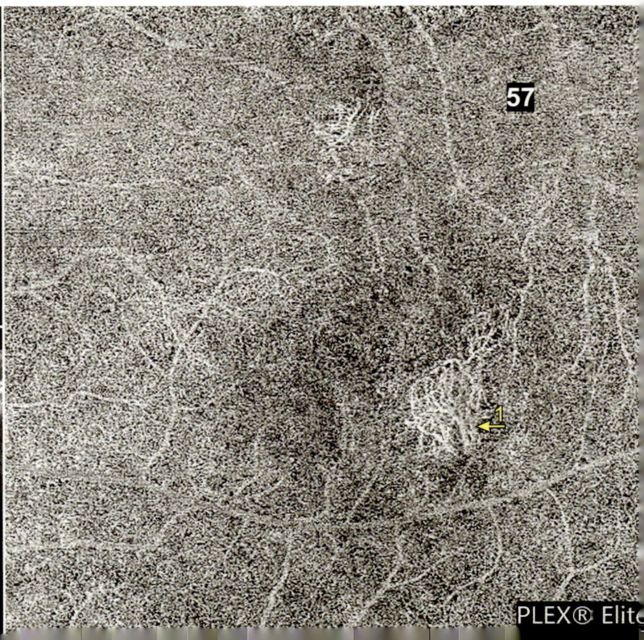

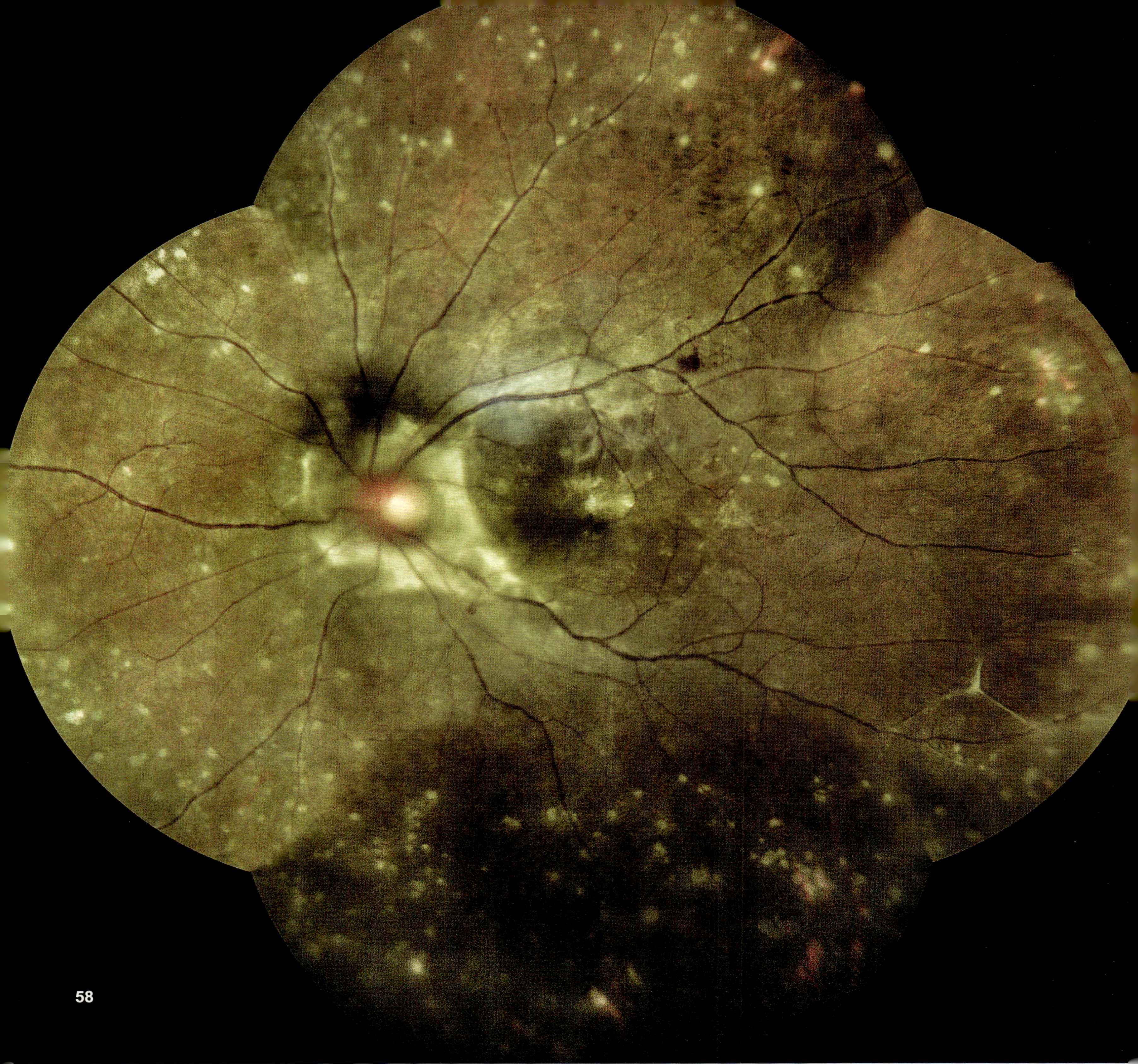

58

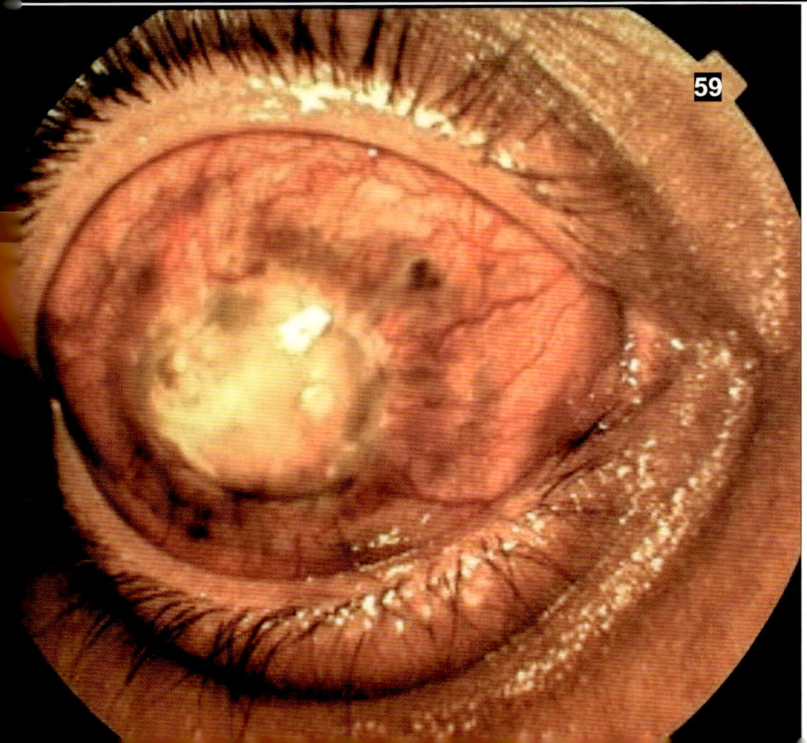

59

Figure 58 *Color fundus montage of a patient with sympathetic ophthalmia. Note the presence of multiple scattered yellowish appearing Dalen fuchs nodules involving all four quadrants of the retina with associated peripapillary fibrosis. There is a tiny retinal hemorrhage in superotemporal arcade.*

Sympathetic ophthalmia is a rare type of panuveitis that usually occurs in eye with history of trauma. Presentation could be within days or months of inciting injury but cases have been reported in the literature where disease develops year later after trauma. In our particular case sympathetic ophthalmia has developed 20 years after initial traumatic event. Few cases have also been reported to develop after complex ocular surgeries as well.

Figure 59 *External photograph shows the exciting blind right eye with no light perception following traumatic injury 20 years ago.*

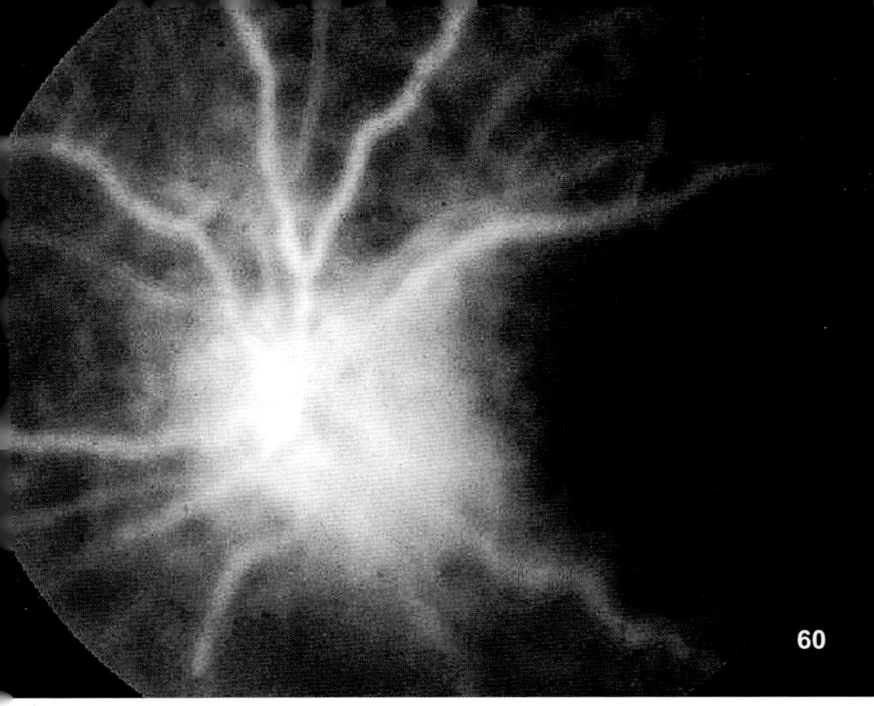


Figure 60 *Fluorescein angiography in the early frame shows early pinpoint hypofluorescent spots in the superior mid-peripheral area and early disk hyperfluorescence.*

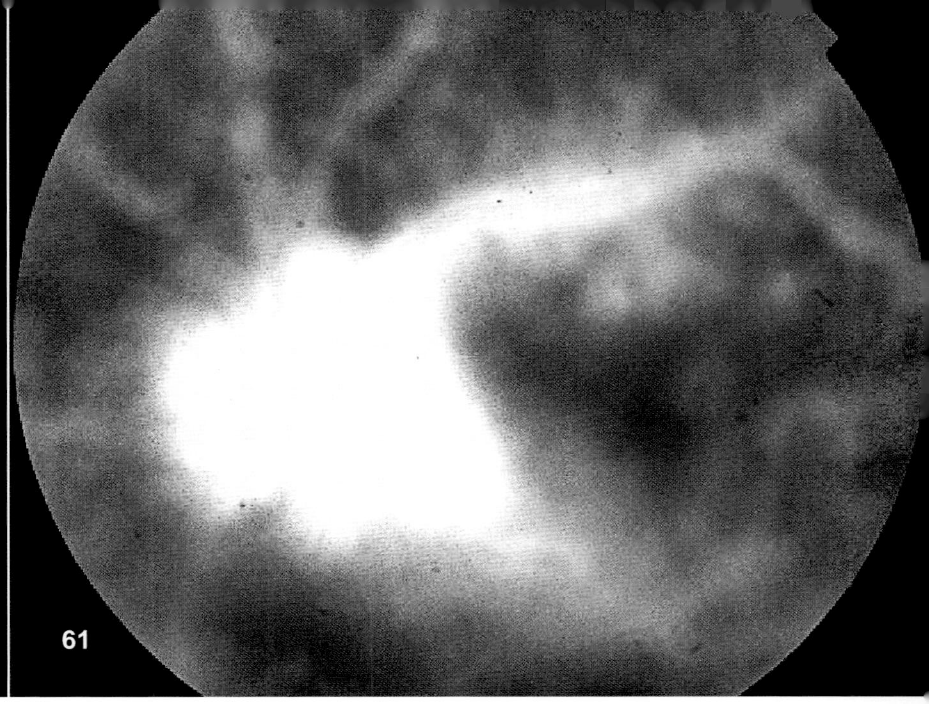


Figure 61 *In the late frame of the angiography, there is leakage at the disk and diffuse perivascular leakage.*

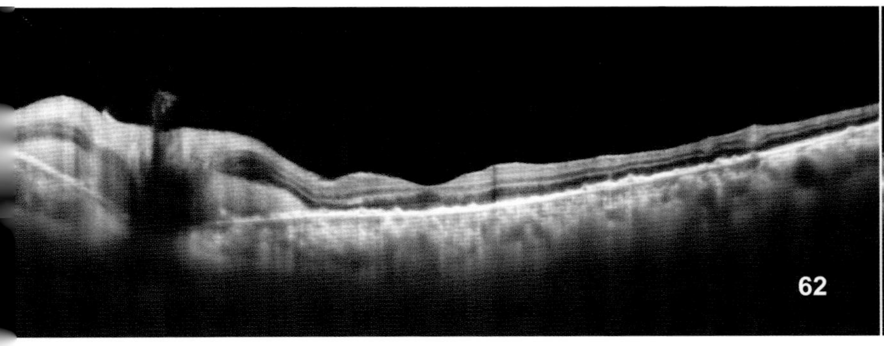


Figure 62 *Enhanced depth 16 mm horizontal OCT scans showing a very thickened choroid along with peripapillary subretinal hyperreflective material and multiple retinal pigment epithelium (RPE) drusen-like elevations in the macula at presentation.*

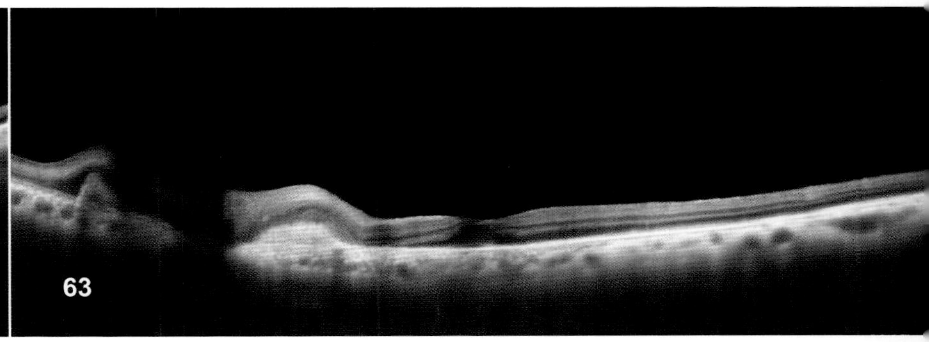


Figure 63 *OCT scan at 6 months demonstrates that there is near complete resolution of the RPE drusen-like elevations.*

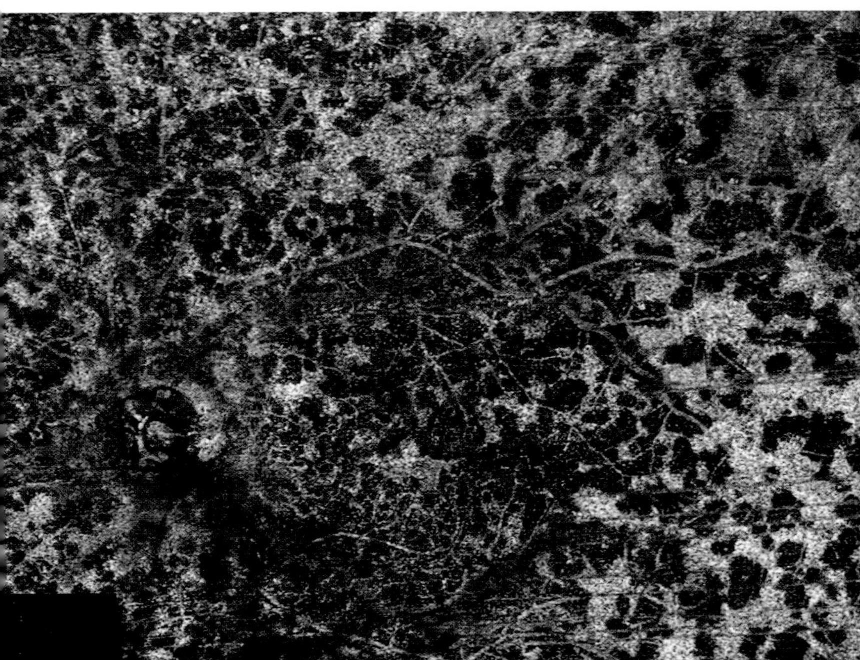


Figure 64 *Swept source optical coherence tomography angiography (OCTA) montage scans of 12 mm × 12 mm at level of choriocapillaris at presentation reveals multiple dark foci of flow voids of different shapes and sizes throughout the posterior pole consistent with likely choriocapillaris hypoperfusion at presentation.*

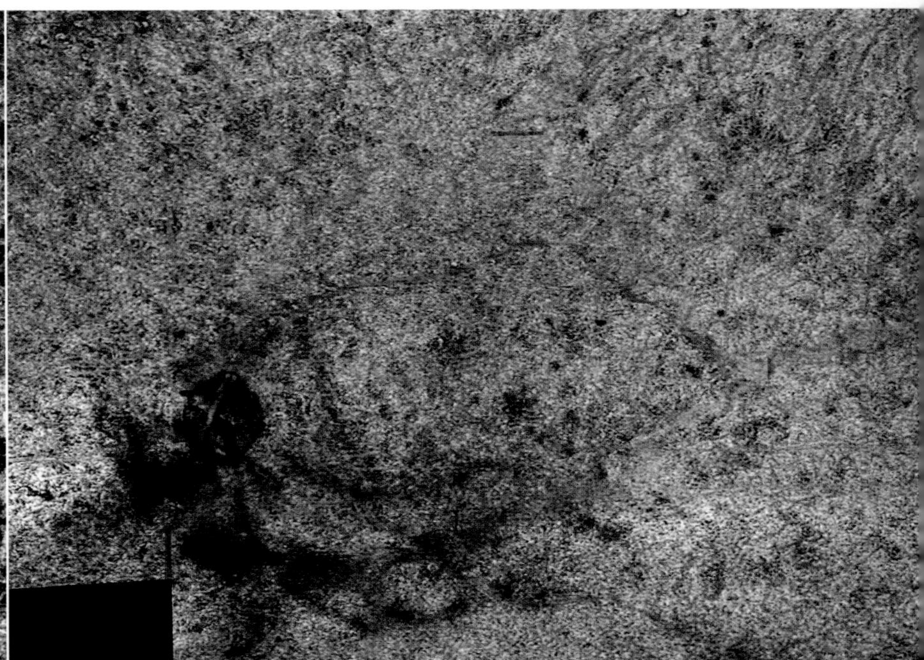


Figure 65 *OCTA scan at 6 months follow-up, there is near complete resolution, with only a few flow voids still visible. The optic nerve is darker due to a shadow artifact from overlying vitreous opacity.* □

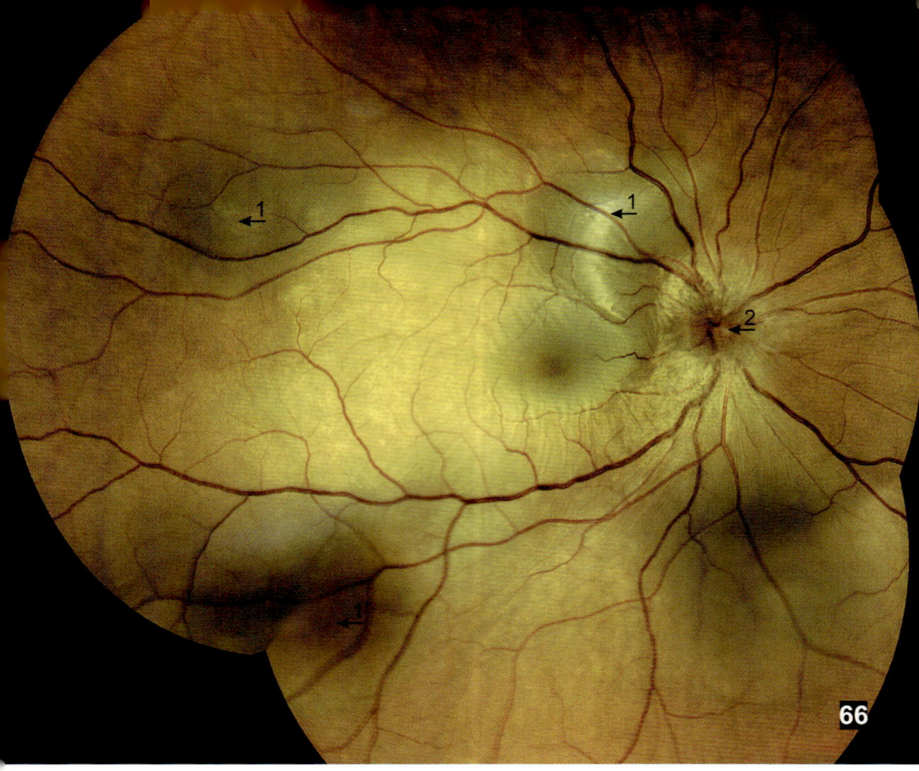


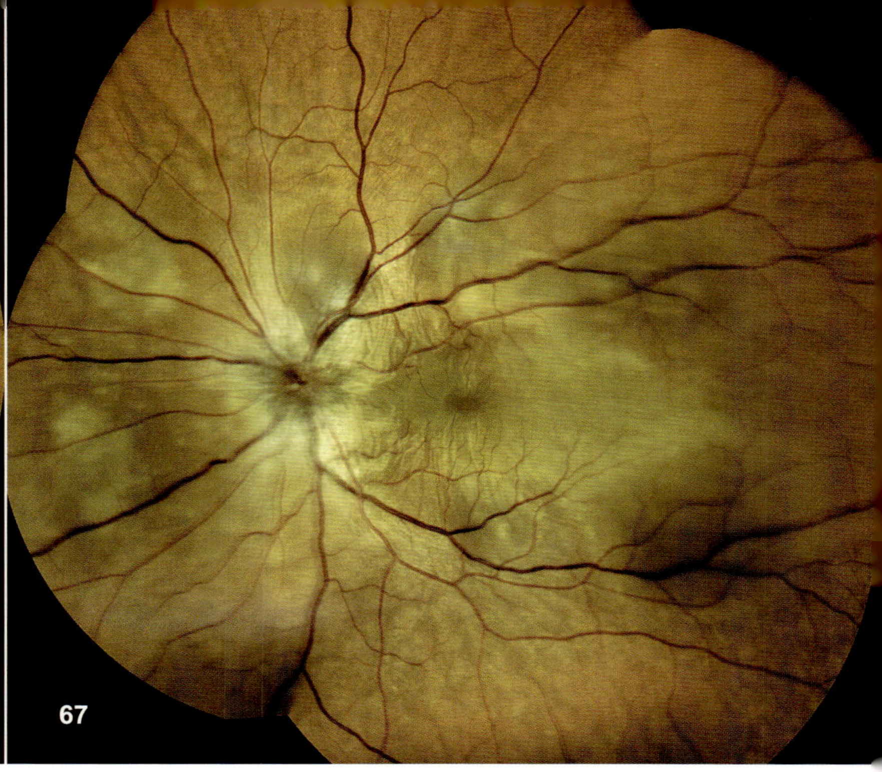


Figure 66 *A case of acute Vogt-Koyanagi-Harada disease in the right eye of a 38-year-old female. Multiple serous detachments (1) are associated with hyperemic optic disk (2).*

Figure 67 *Case of acute Vogt-Koyanagi-Harada disease in the left eye of the same patient demonstrating serous fluid pockets, elevated optic nerve with blurred margin.*

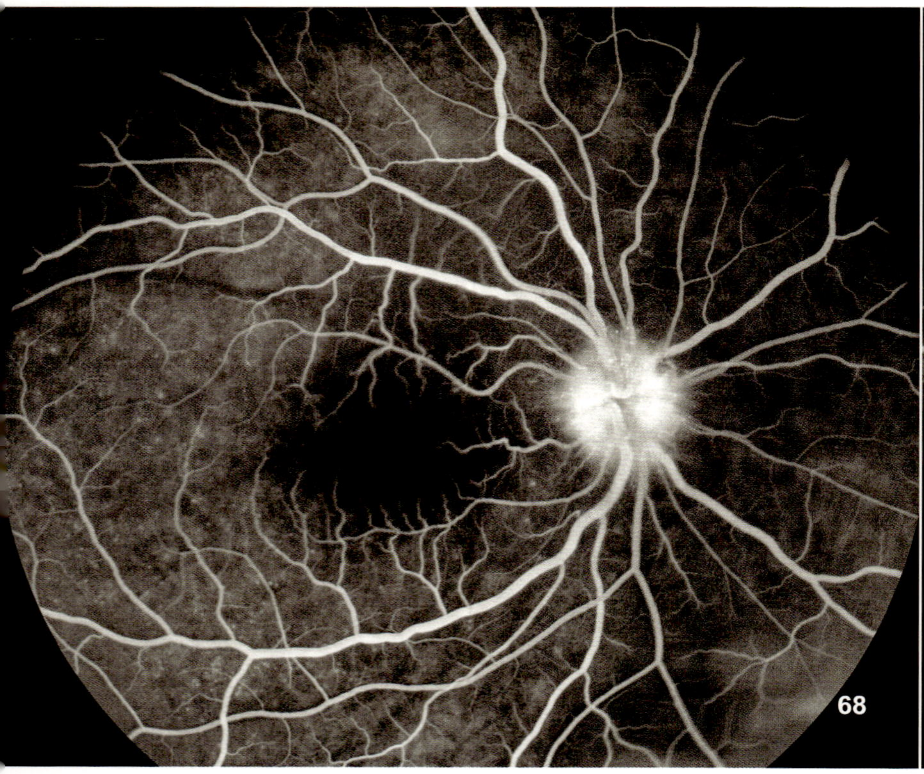


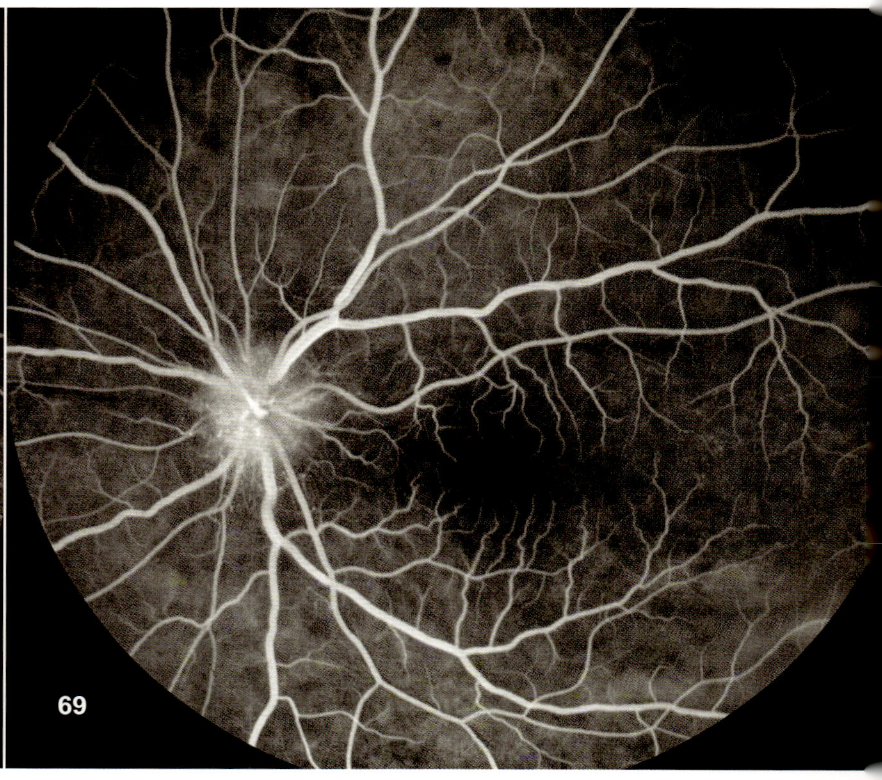


Figure 68 *Early phase angiogram of right eye demonstrates multiple hyperfluorescent dots at the level of retinal pigment epithelium and early disk hyperfluorescence.*

Figure 69 *Early phase of angiogram of the left eye demonstrating hyper-fluorescence at the optic disk.*

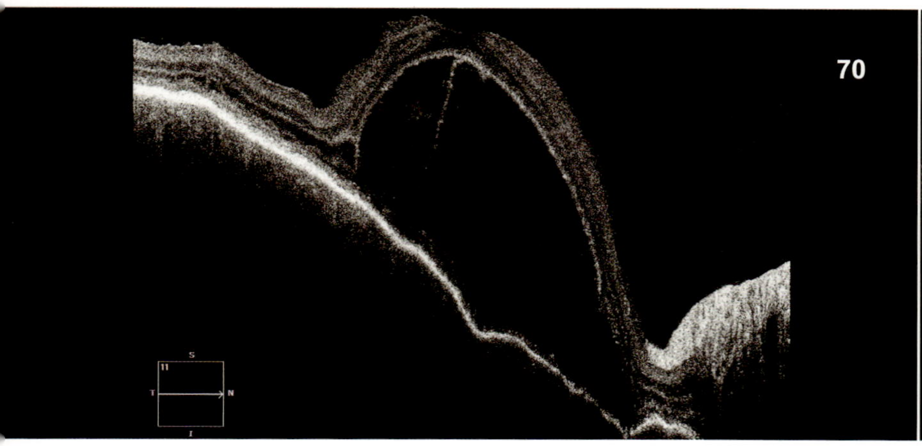


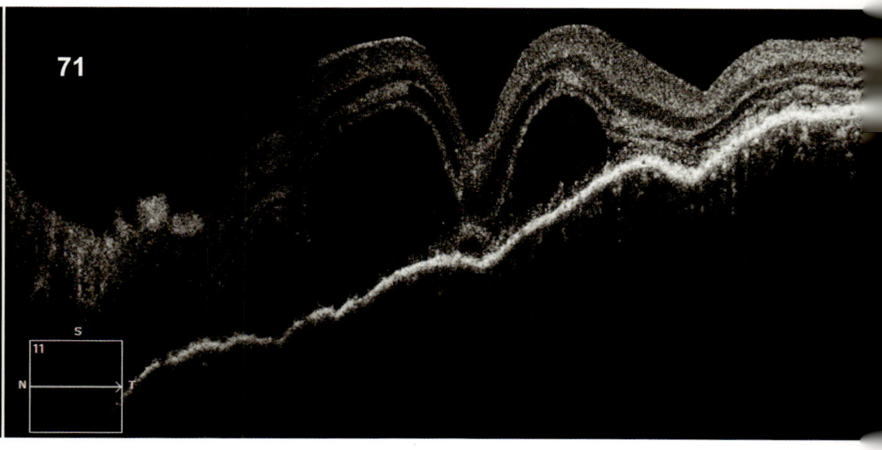


Figure 70 *OCT scan of the left eye demonstrating multiple pockets of subretinal fluid and undulating RPE.*

Figure 71 *OCT scan of the left eye demonstrating multiple pockets of subretinal fluid and undulating RPE.*

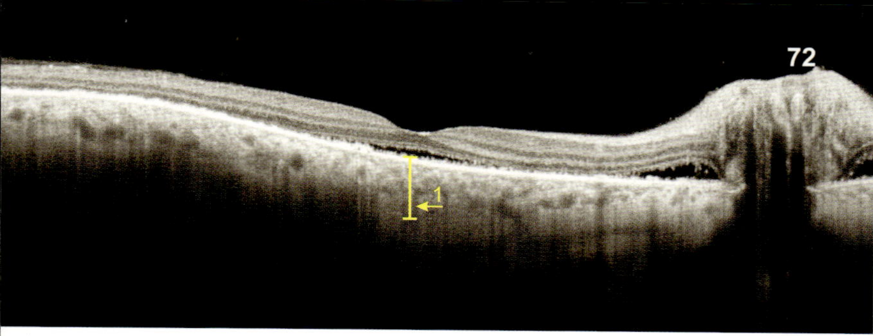


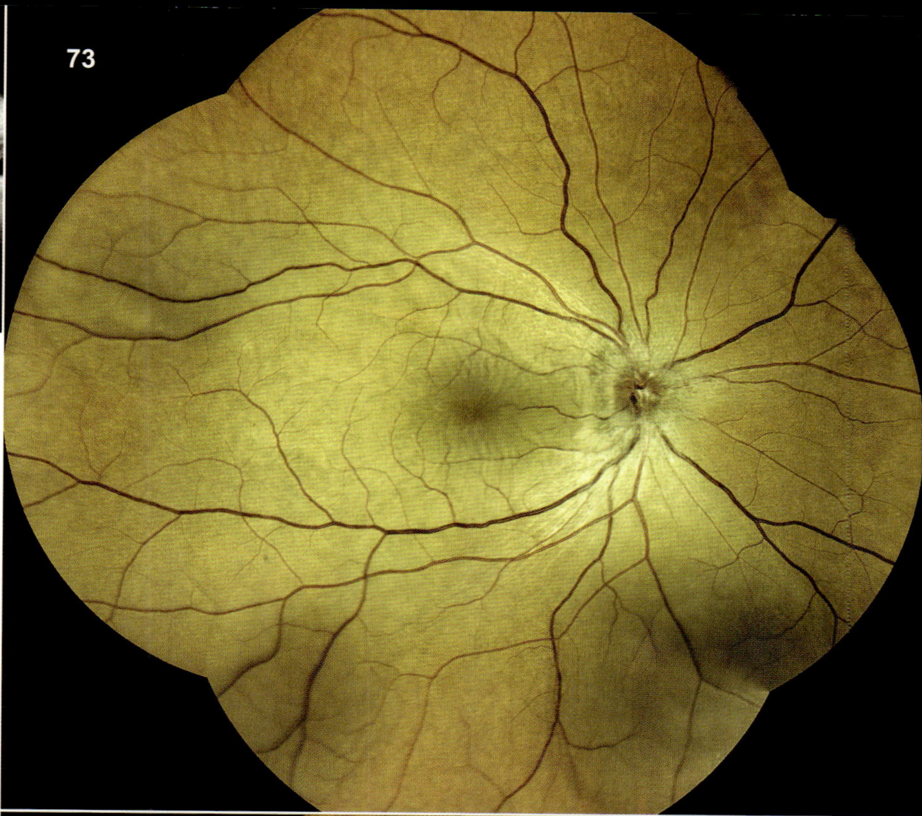


Figure 72

*OCT 3 days after initiation of treatment shows straightening of retinal pigment epithelial layer, disappearance of retinal fluid at the fovea. Shallow subretinal fluid persists in the peripapillary region. Choroid layer is still thickened (1).*

Figure 73

*Color fundus montage of the right eye 3 days after intensive intravenous pulse dose of methylprednisolone: Note the rapid resolution of serous detachments. It shows drastic reduction of serous macular detachment, retinal folds at the macula and optic disk is still hyperemic.*

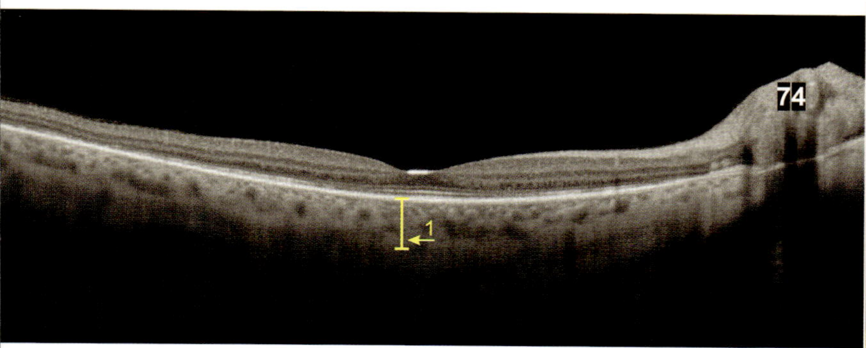


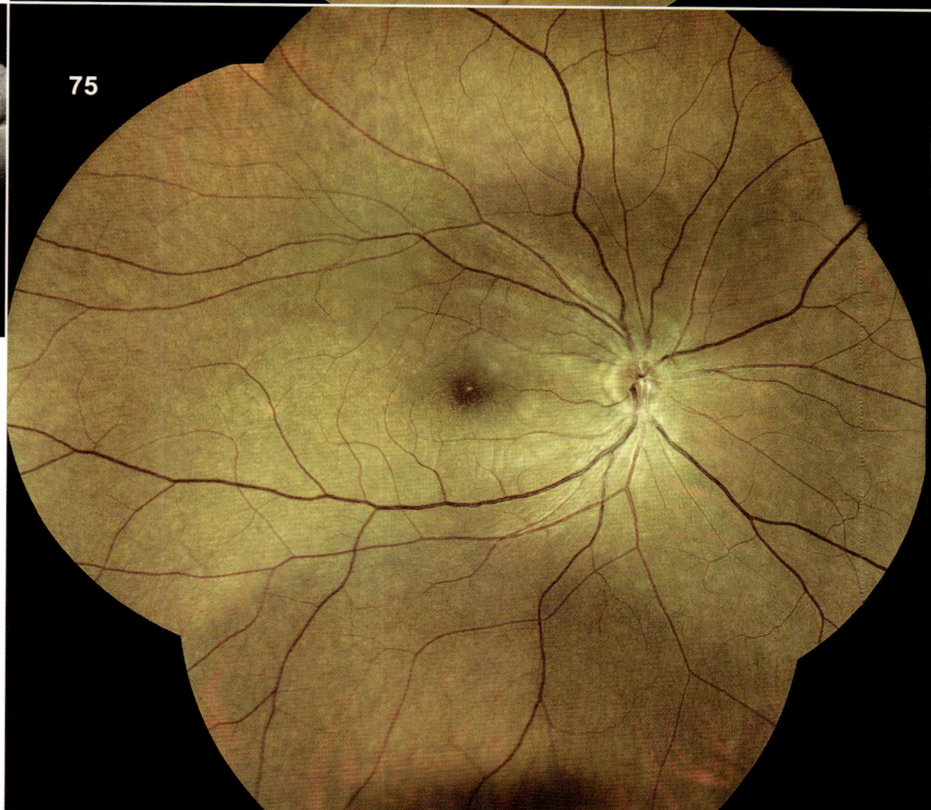


Figure 74

*OCT 1 month post-treatment demonstrating further reduction in the disk swelling and choroidal thickness (1).*

Figure 75

*Color fundus photo 1 month post-treatment: Patient was continued on high dose of oral steroids started at the dose of 1 mg/kg body weight with tapering dose every 2 weeks. Note complete disappearance of serous fluid from periphery and posterior pole and normal disk.*

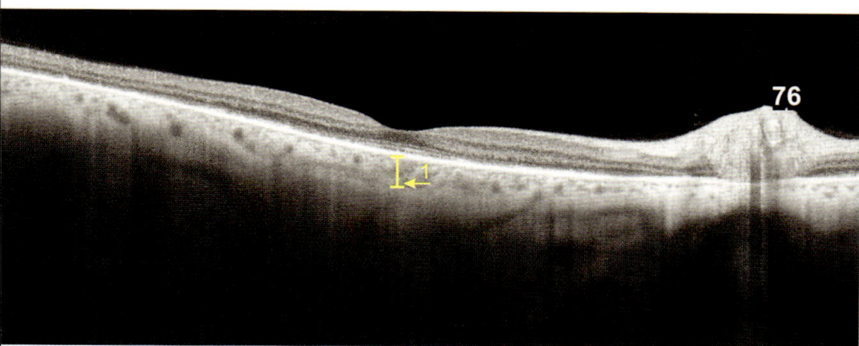


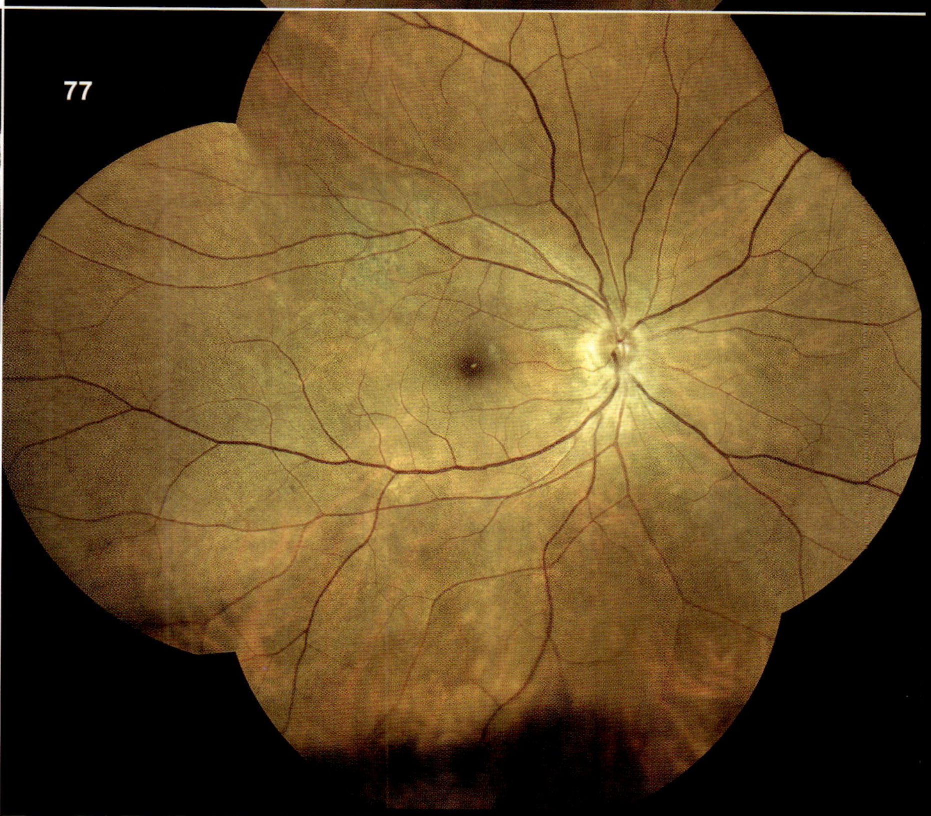


Figure 76

*OCT 9 month post-treatment demonstrating further reduction in the choroidal thickness (1).*

Figure 77

*Color fundus photo 9 months post-treatment: Note small area of RPE depigmentation in superotemporal region, rest of the fundus was unremarkable.* □

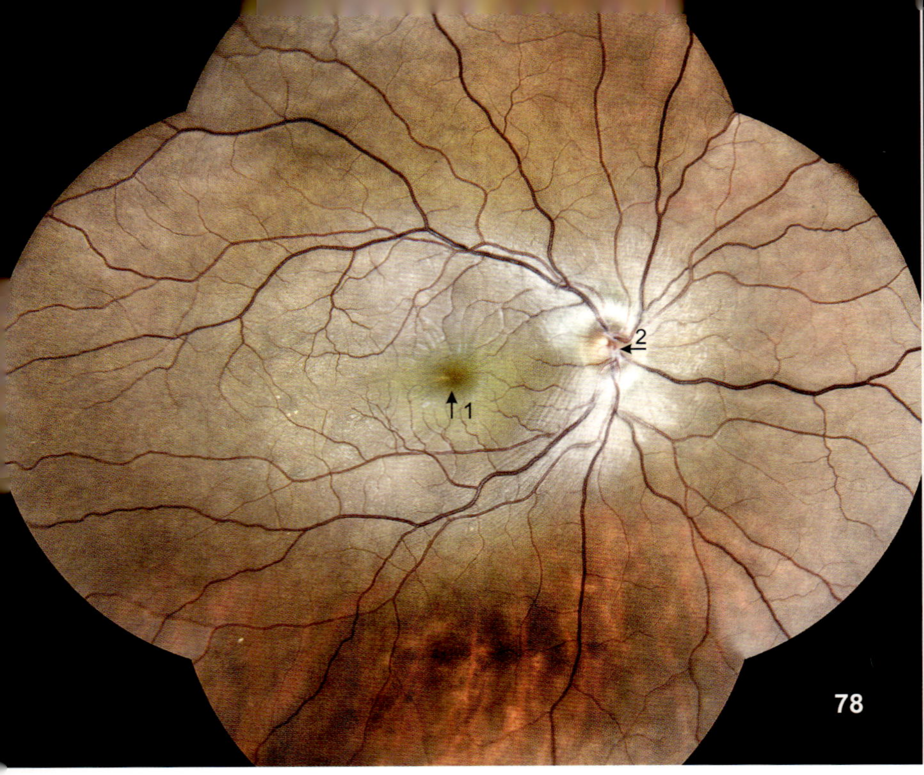


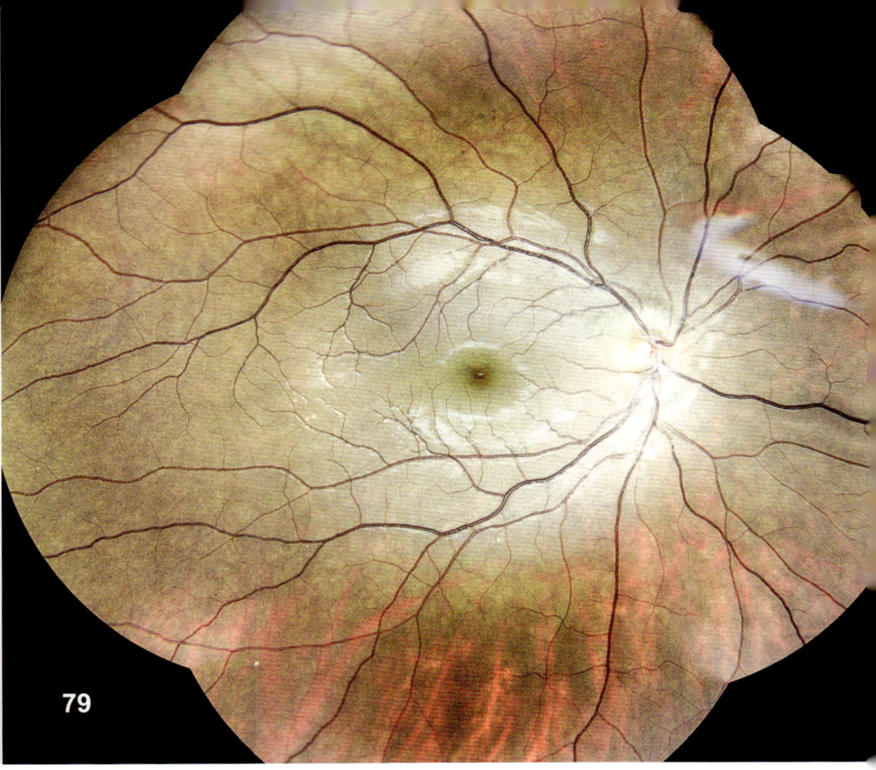


Figure 78 *Baseline color fundus montage of right eye in acute VKH. This 30-year-old female presented with typical history of headaches, tinnitus and blurred vision. Note the presence of serous elevation at the fovea (1), mild disk hyperemia (2), and few orange irregular patches of choroidal inflammation in the inferior retina.*

Figure 79 *Color fundus photograph 3 months after initiation of systemic immunosuppression demonstrating a good fovea reflex and normal appearance of the optic disk.*

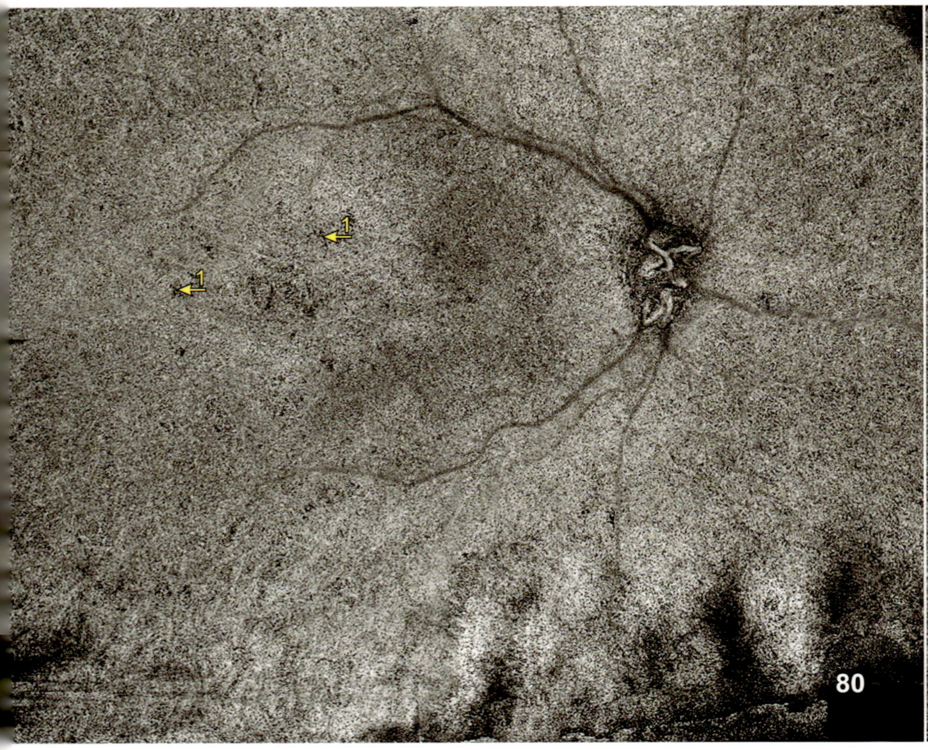


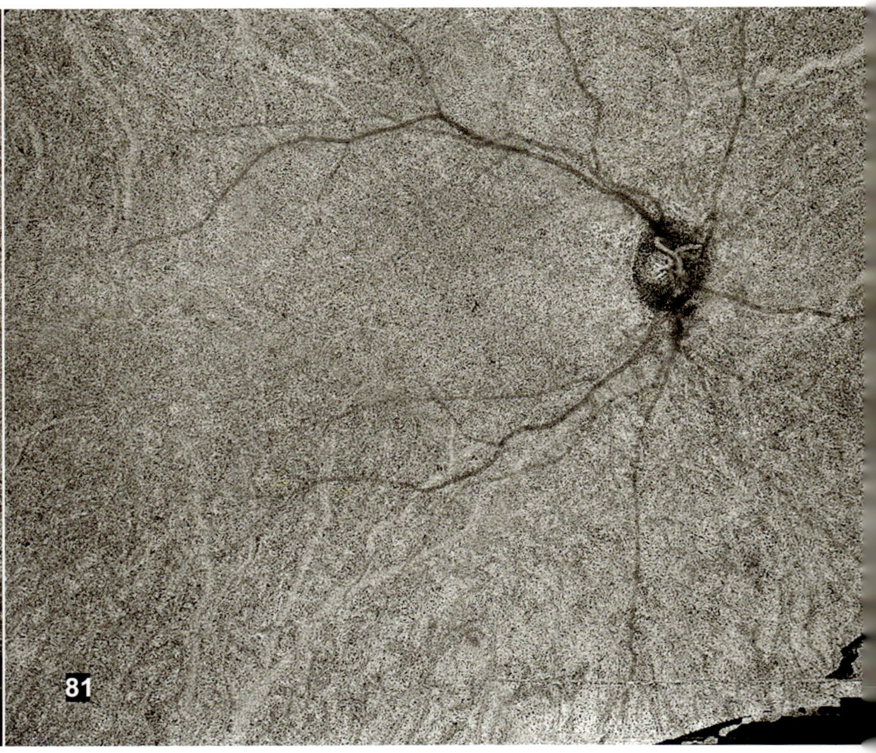


Figure 80 *Baseline OCT angiography choriocapillaris slab demonstrating multiple hypoflow void spots in the choroid (1).*

Figure 81 *OCT angiography at 3 months demonstrates significant reduction in hypofluorescent spots.*

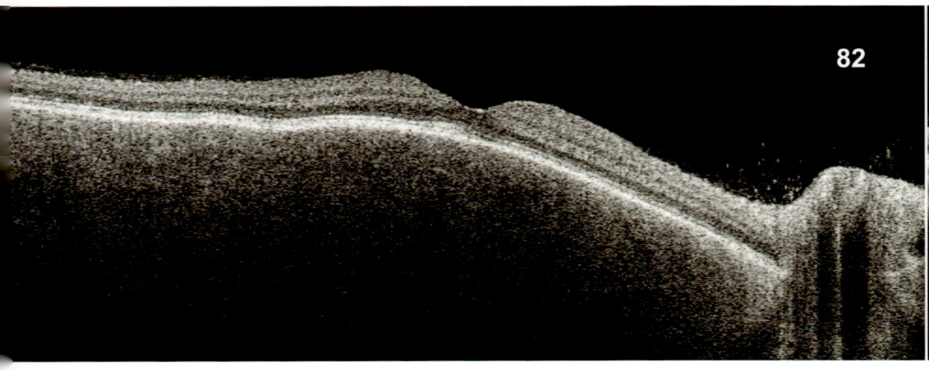


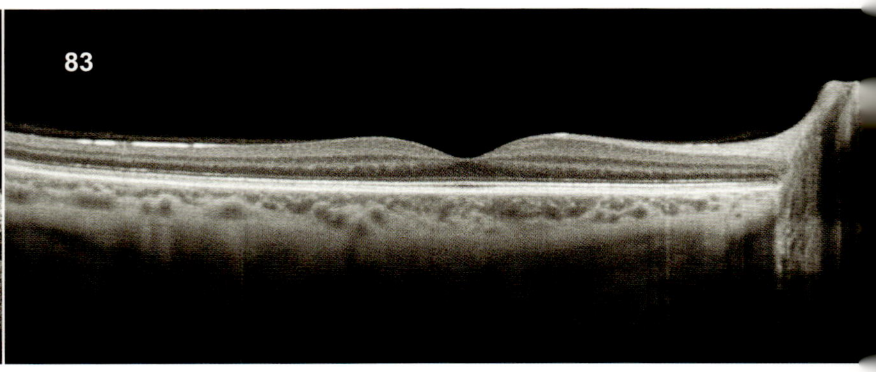


Figure 82 *Swept source OCT scan at baseline demonstrating elevation of macula with increased choroidal thickness.*

Figure 83 *Swept source OCT scan at 3 months demonstrated flattening of the macula with reduction in choroidal thickness.*

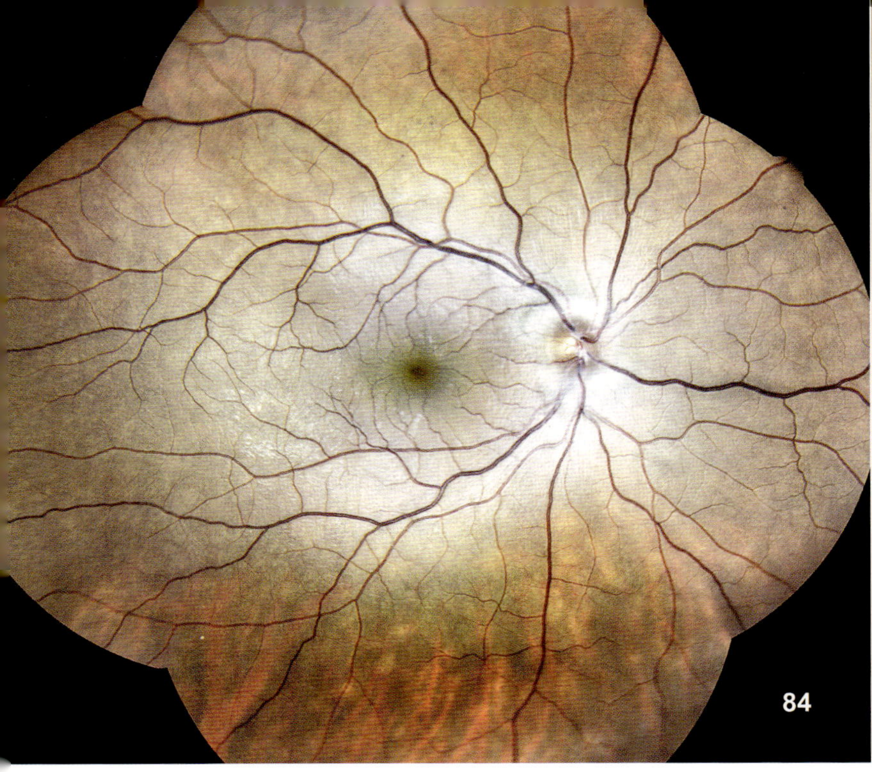


Figure 84 *Color fundus montage right eye 6 months after systemic immunosuppression (oral steroids stopped at 5 months, continued on azathioprine 100 mg/day)—relapse.*

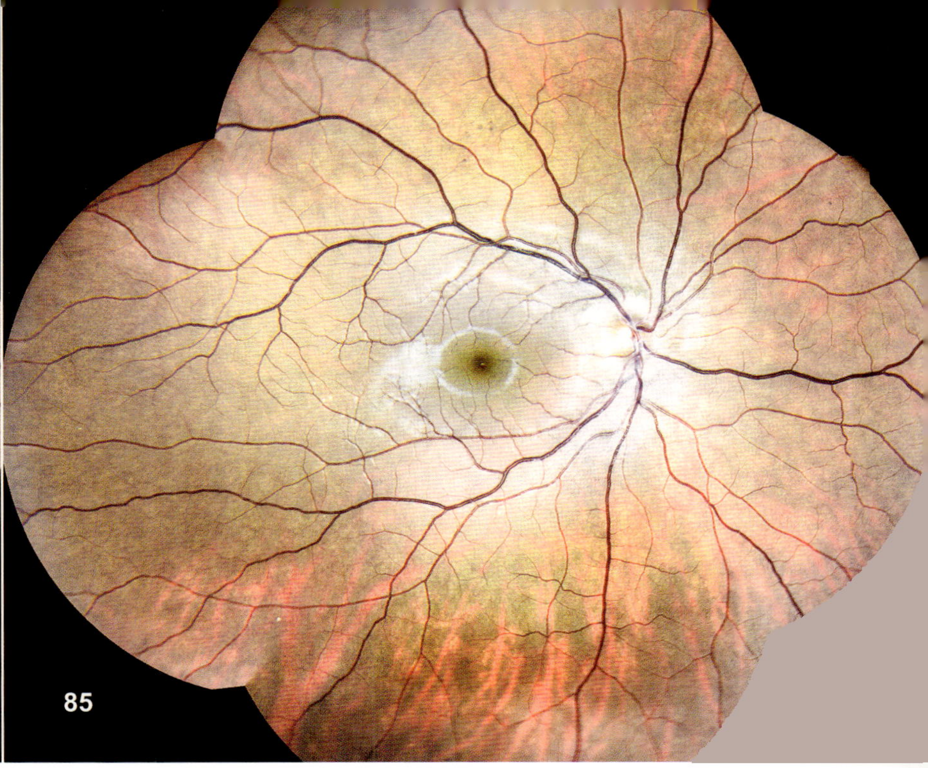


Figure 85 *Color fundus montage right eye 12 months after systemic immunosuppression.*

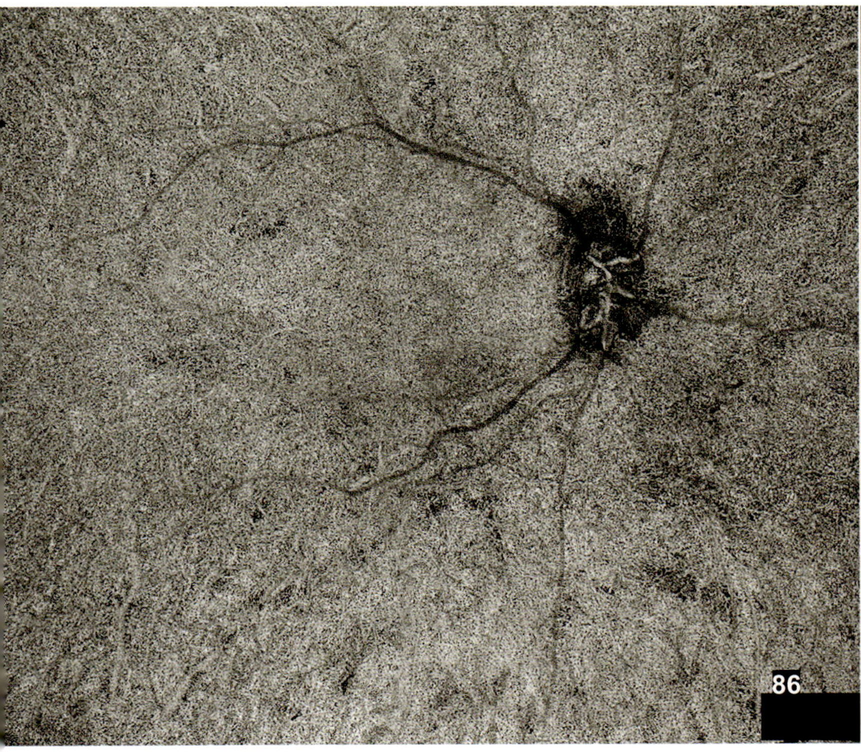


Figure 86 *OCT angiography montage 6 months post-treatment demonstrated reappearance of hypofluorescent spots.*

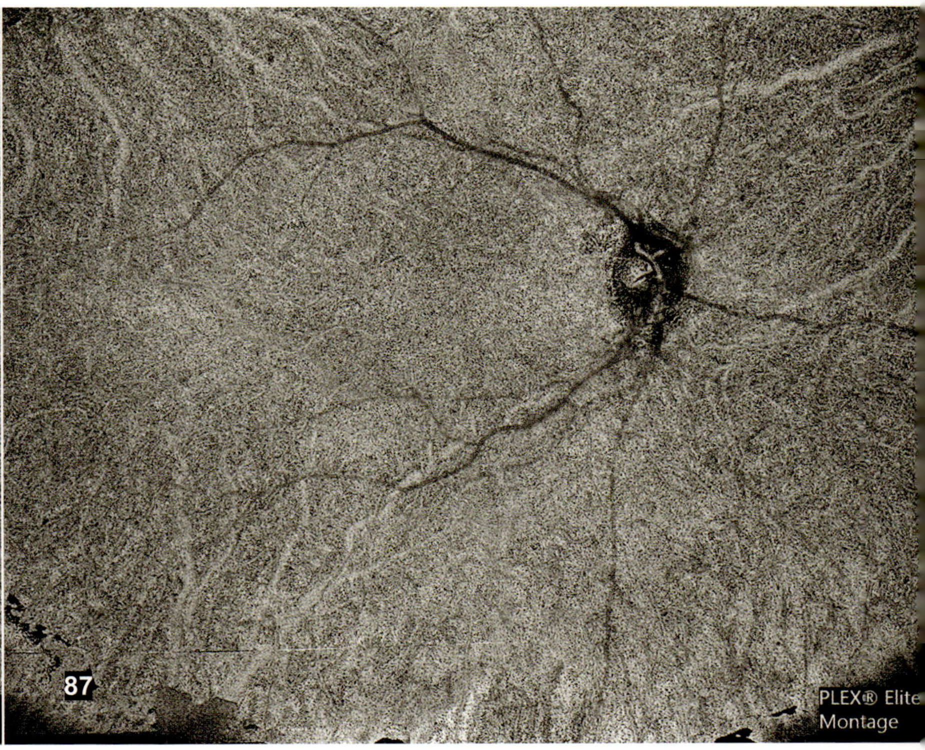


Figure 87 *OCT angiography montage 12 months post-treatment demonstrated disappearance of hypofluorescent spots suggesting disease in remission.*

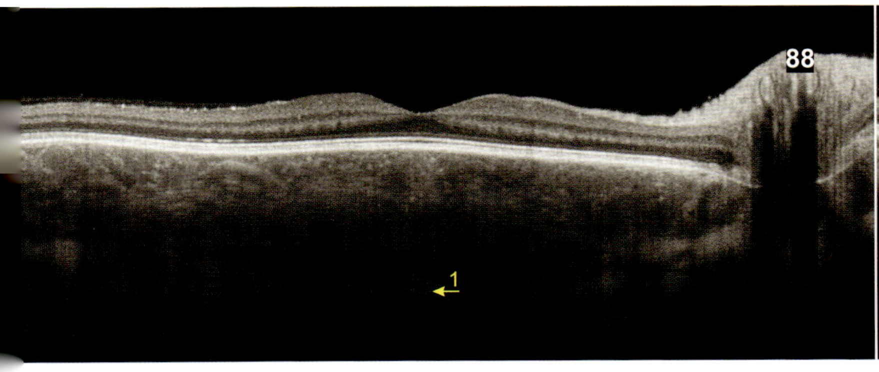


Figure 88 *Swept source OCT at 6 months reveals further increase in choroidal thickness (1) as compared to her OCT at 3 months indicating relapse of disease activity.*

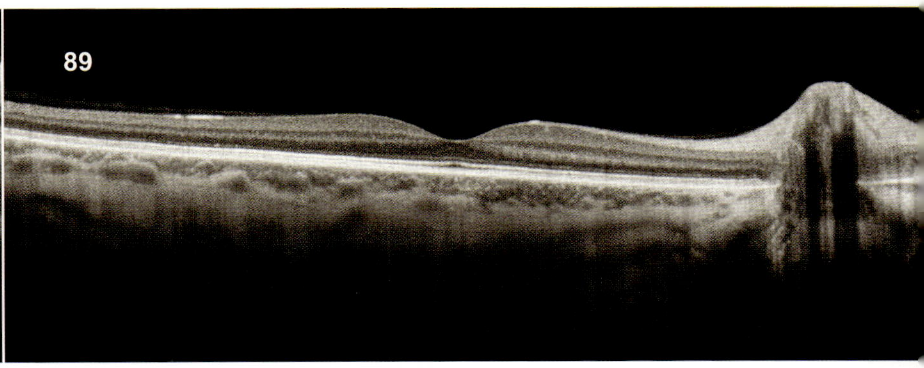


Figure 89 *Swept source OCT scan at 12 months demonstrating further reduction in choroidal thickness.* □

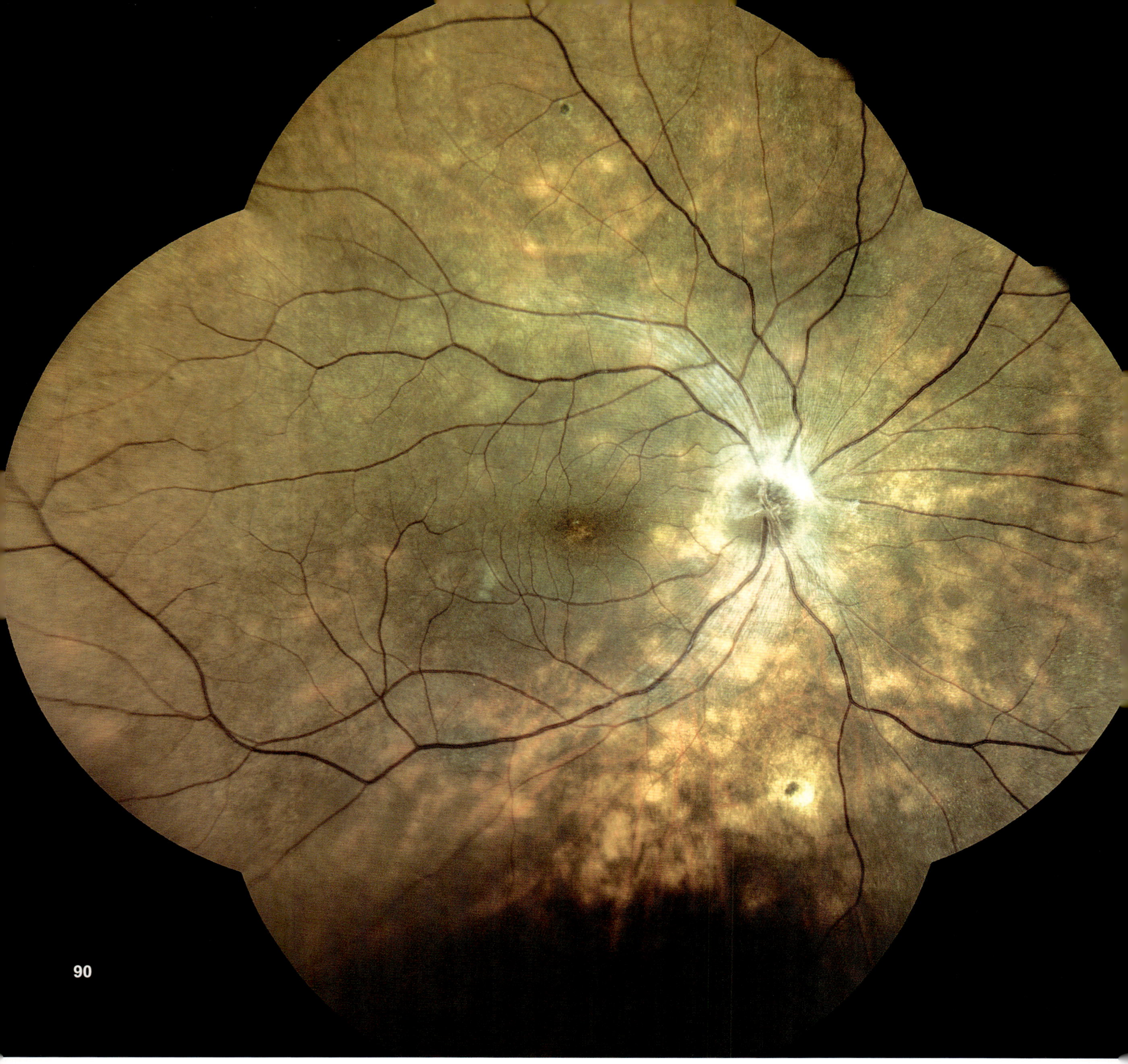

90

Figure 90 *Case of convalescent stage of Vogt-Koyanagi-Harada disease.*

Color fundus montage revealing sunset glow fundus. Note the presence of round to oval, irregular patches of RPE depigmentation more pronounced in the inferior mid-periphery, peripapillary atrophy is also seen.

During the convalescent stage, there is nongranulomatous inflammation, which consist histopathologically of a mild to moderate nongranulomatous inflammatory cell infiltrate with focal aggregates of lymphocytes and occasional macrophages. The loss of melanin granules of the choroidal melanocytes renders a pale, depigmented aspect to the choroid, known as 'sunset glow fundus'.

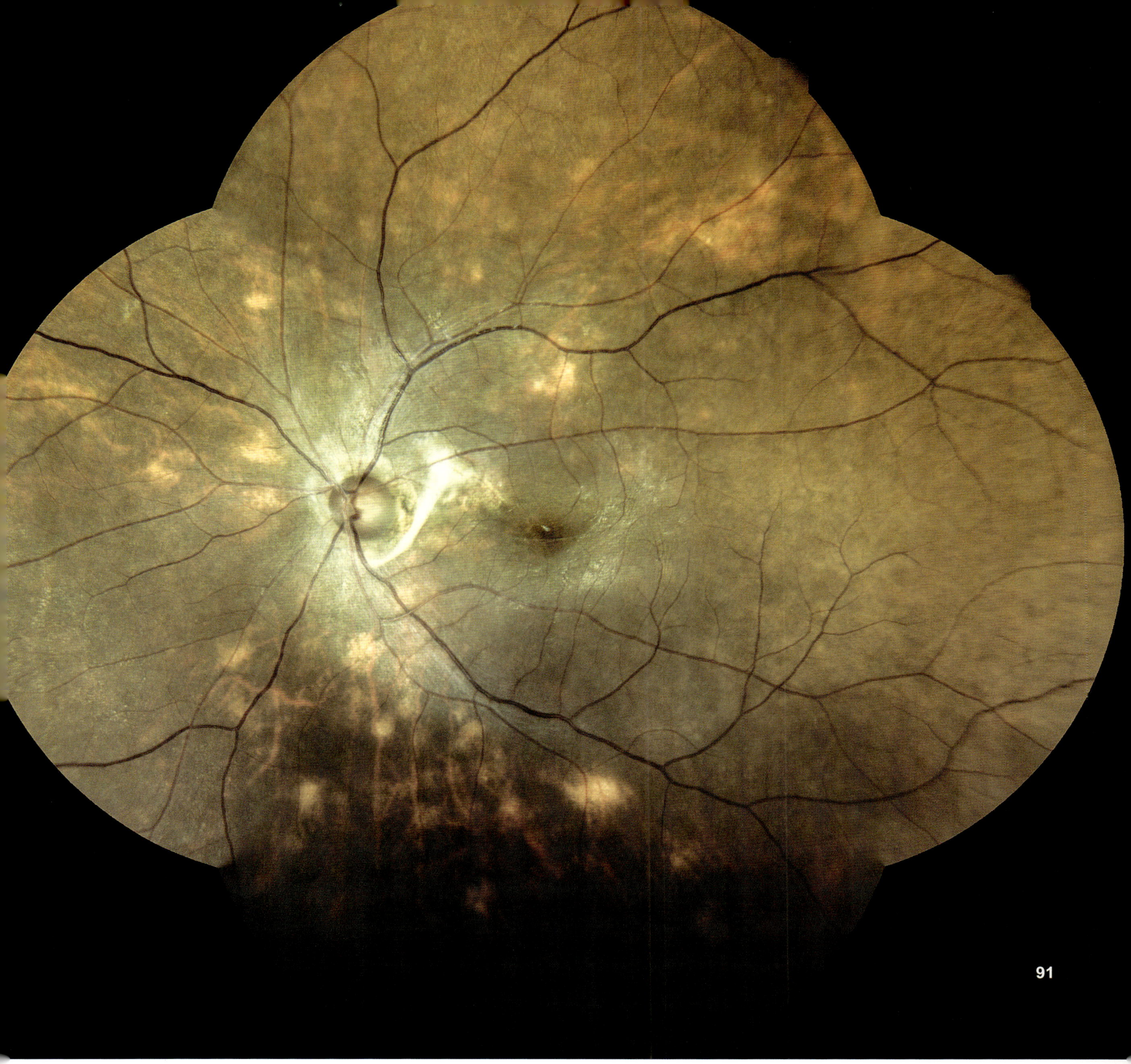

91

Figure 91 *Color fundus montage of left eye of the same patient demonstrating the convalescent stage of Vogt-Koyanagi-Harada disease. Depigmented RPE lesions, peripapillary subretinal fibrotic band, a cellophane reflex at the macula.*

Chronic or convalescent stage occurs several weeks after the acute uveitis stage and is characterized by the development of poliosis, vitiligo and depigmentation of the choroid. This leads to characteristic pale disk with bright orange red choroid known as sunset glow fundus. Juxtapapillary region also shows marked depigmentation. At this stage small yellow well-circumscribed foci of RPE depigmentation as a result of chorioretinal atrophy are also seen, mainly in the inferior mid-periphery. The convalescent phase may last for months and at times chronic recurrent smoldering panuveitis with acute exacerbation may also develop. □

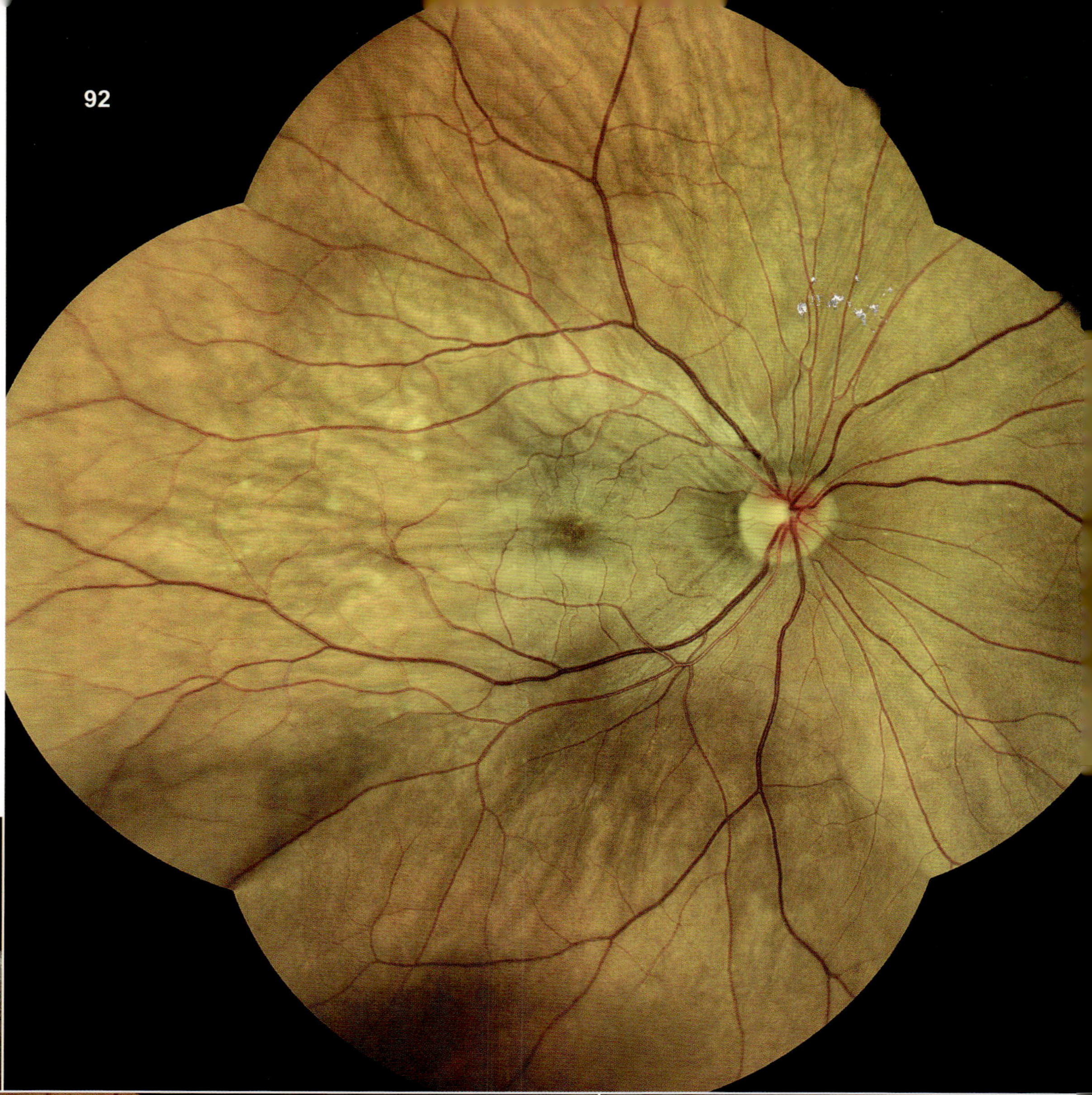

Figure 92

*Fundus montage photograph of right eye of a case of bilateral posterior scleritis.*

Color fundus montage of a 50-year-old female who presented with severe pain, headache and blurred vision of recent onset. Right fundus shows choroidal folds, few yellowish subretinal lesions and elevated macula due to serous detachment.

Figure 93

*OCT scan at presentation demonstrates retinal undulations due to choroidal folds and pockets of subretinal fluid in the peripapillary region.*

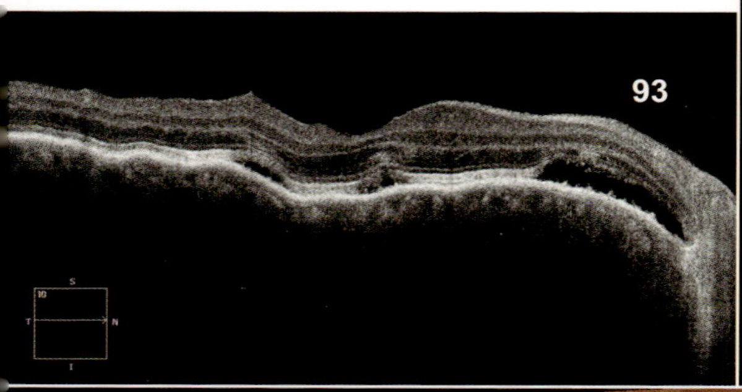

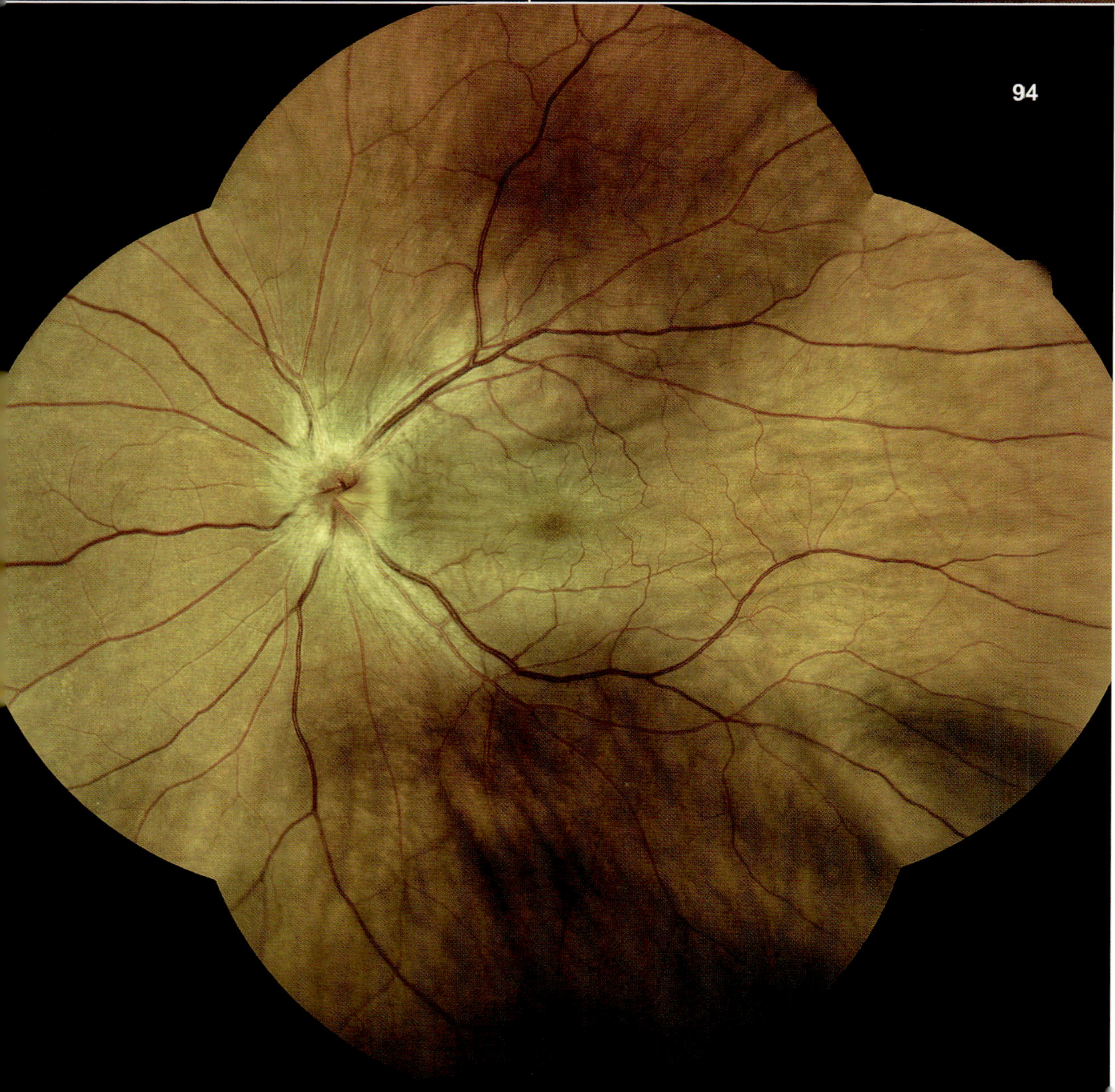

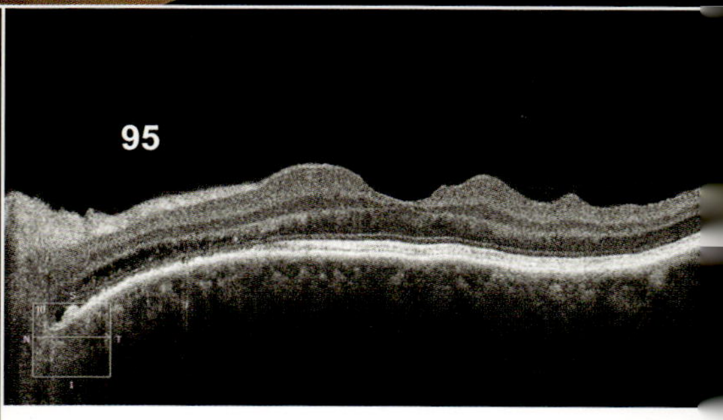

Figure 94

*Fundus montage photograph of left eye of a case of bilateral posterior scleritis.*

Left fundus photograph shows choroidal folds and elevated disk with blurred margins.

Figure 95

*Spectral domain optical coherence tomography scans of the left eye at presentation.*

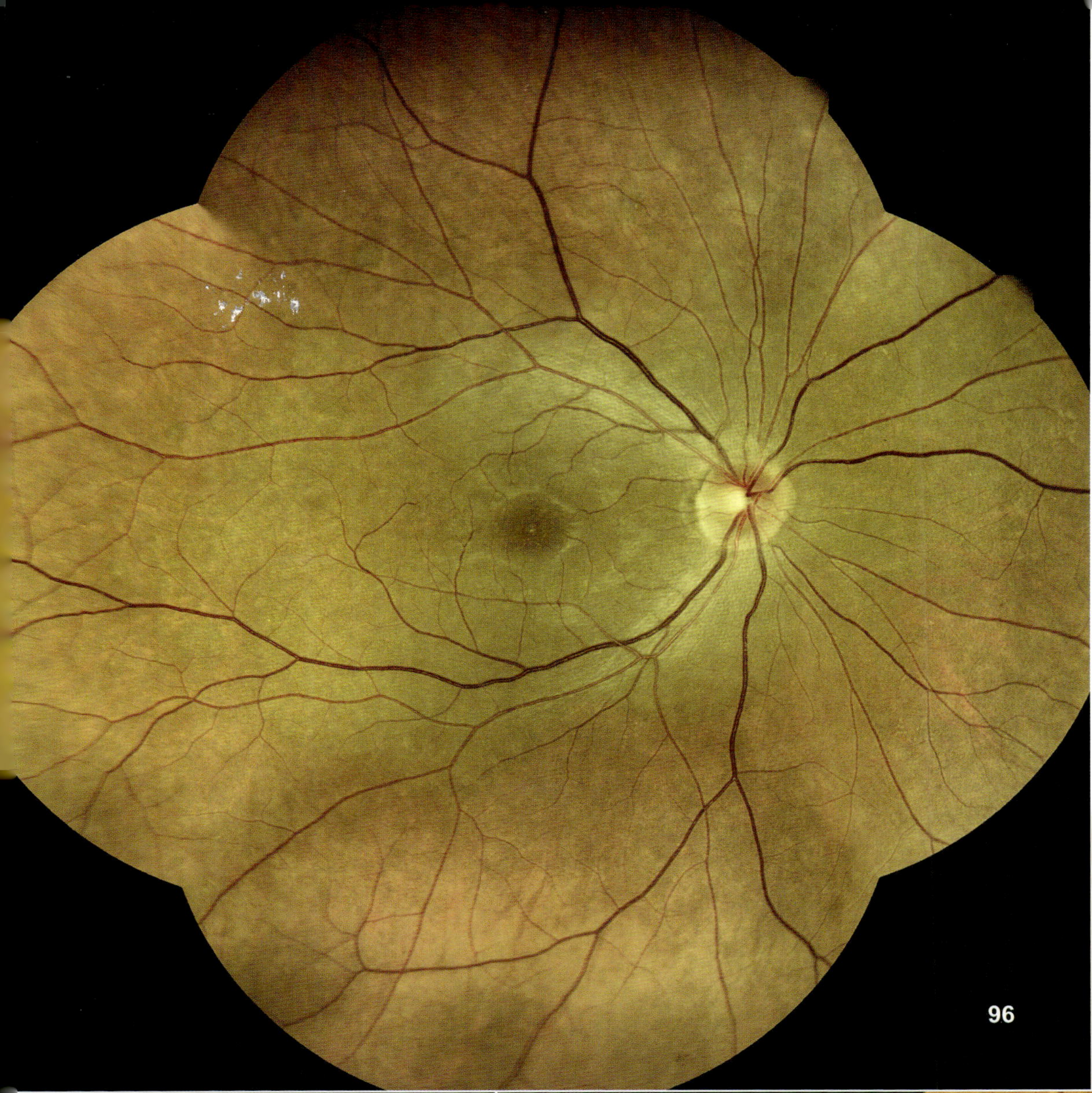

96

Figure 96

*Posterior scleritis: Right eye fundus montage 1 month post-treatment.*

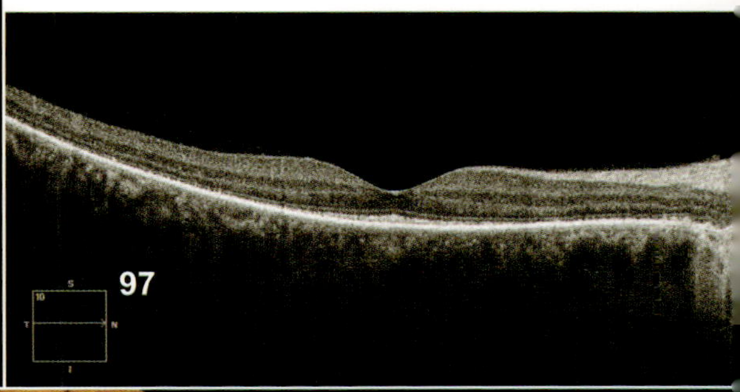

97

Figure 97

*Post-treatment optical coherence tomography scan shows disappearance of subretinal fluid and straightening of retinal pigment epithelial layer.*

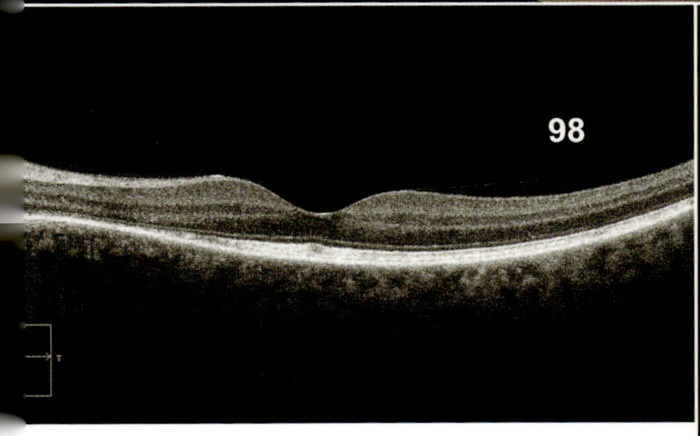

98

Figure 98

*Posterior scleritis: Left eye OCT scan 1 month post-treatment.*

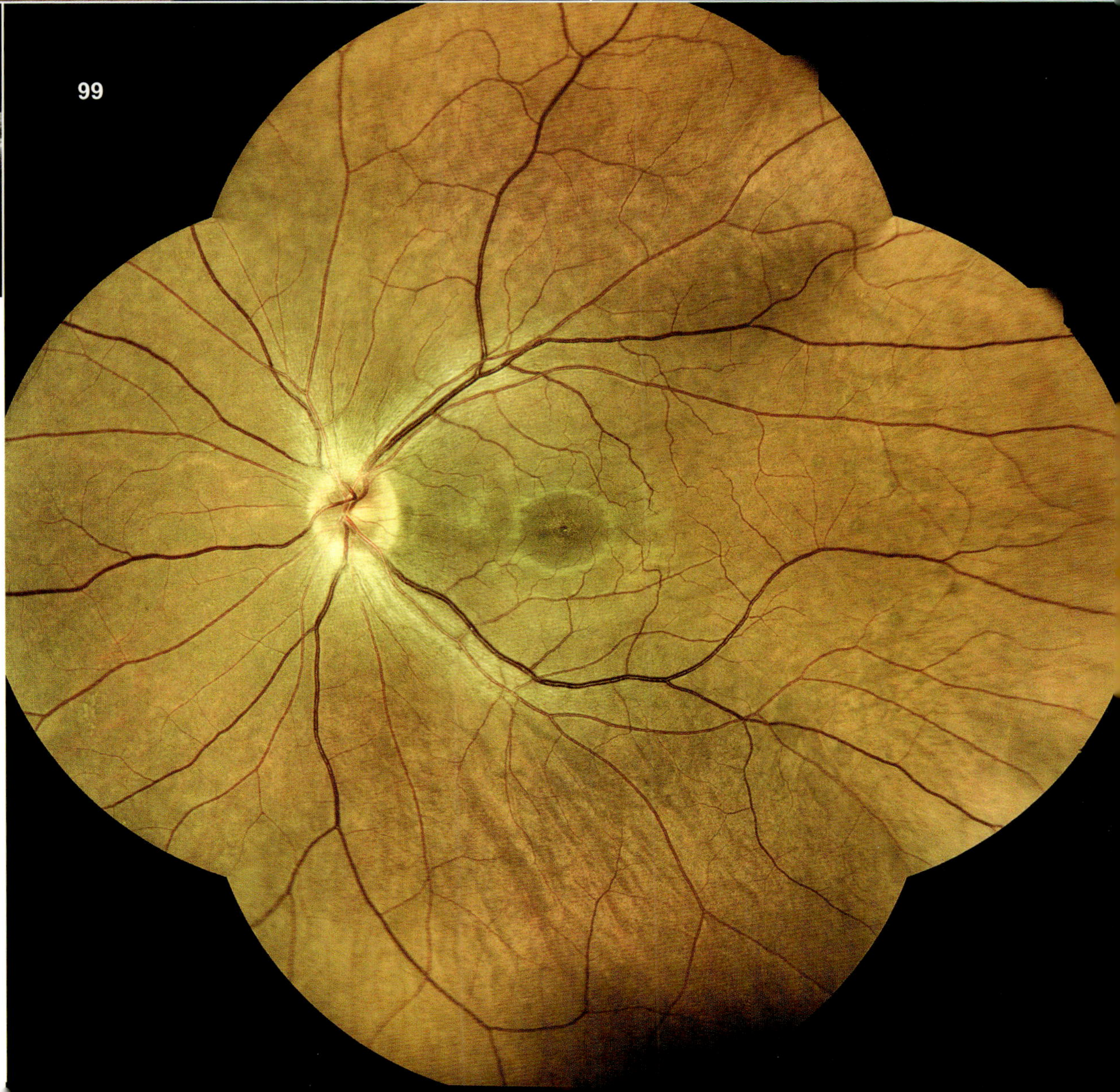

99

She underwent laboratory investigations to rule out systemic vasculitis, autoimmune or infective pathology. Her Mantoux skin test was highly positive, TB gold was also positive and chest X-ray abnormalities suggestive of tuberculosis. She under went 6 months course of ATT along with oral steroids. Fundus image at 1 month after initiation of treatment shows complete resolution of retinal changes and patient had no recurrence till 1 year follow-up.

Figure 99

*Posterior scleritis: Left eye fundus montage 1 month post-treatment.* □

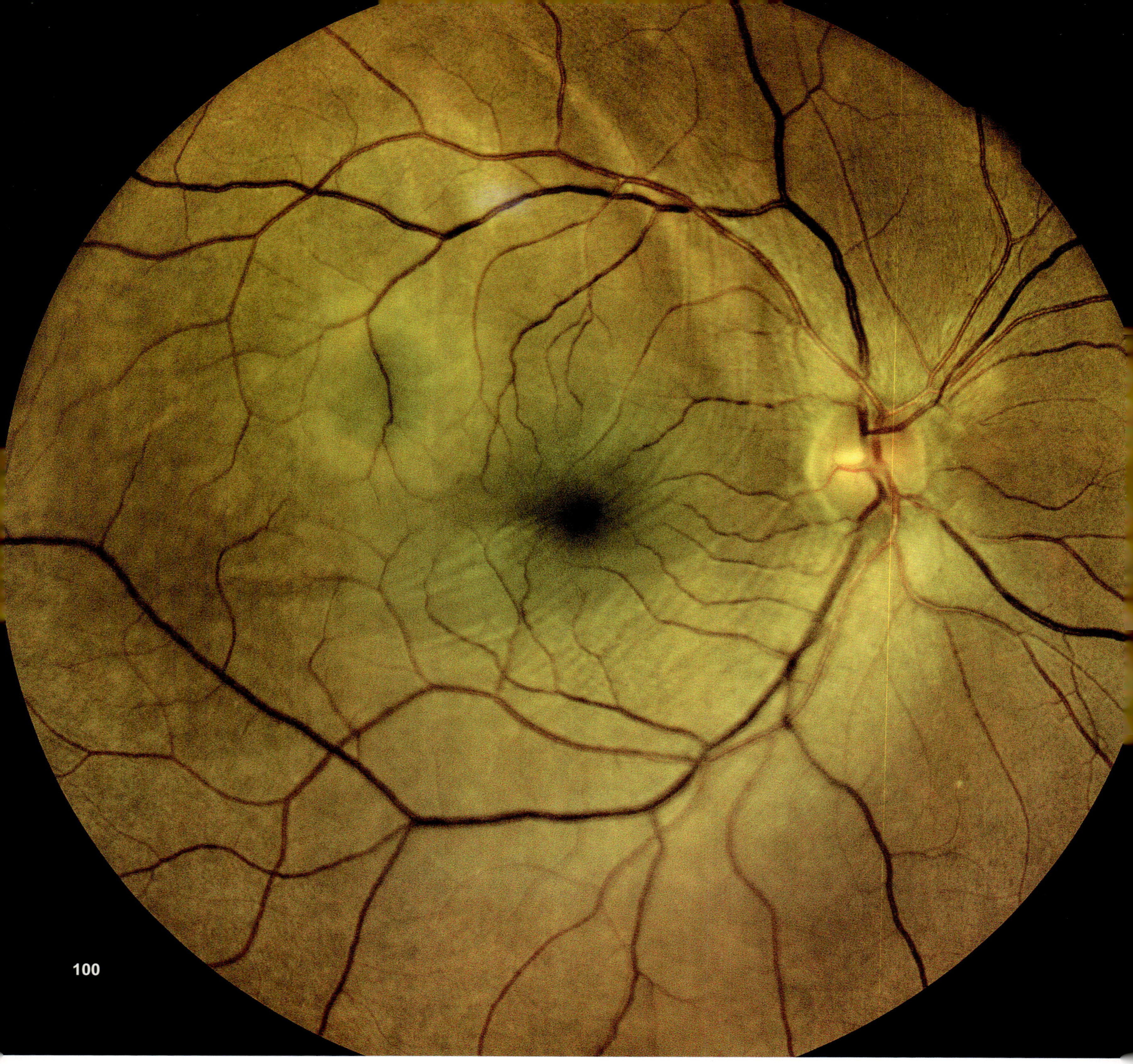

Figure 100 *Rare case of nodular posterior scleritis in HLA B51 positive patient.*

A 54-year-old lady with history of severe ocular pain and blurred vision in her right eye. Color fundus photograph shows single yellowish raised choroidal mass lesion temporal to the macula associated with serous detachment and retinal and choroidal folds.

Nodular posterior scleritis usually present as a circumscribed subretinal mass lesion which must be distinguished from primary and secondary choroidal neoplasm. Typical signs and symptoms of severe ocular pain and tenderness, presence of choroidal folds and absence of orange lipofuscin pigment favors diagnosis of posterior scleritis USG will help to confirm the diagnosis as it demonstrates the presence of tenons fluid (T-sign) that is characteristic of posterior scleritis. Other laboratory and systemic investigations should be done as required to confirm the diagnosis before initiating treatment.

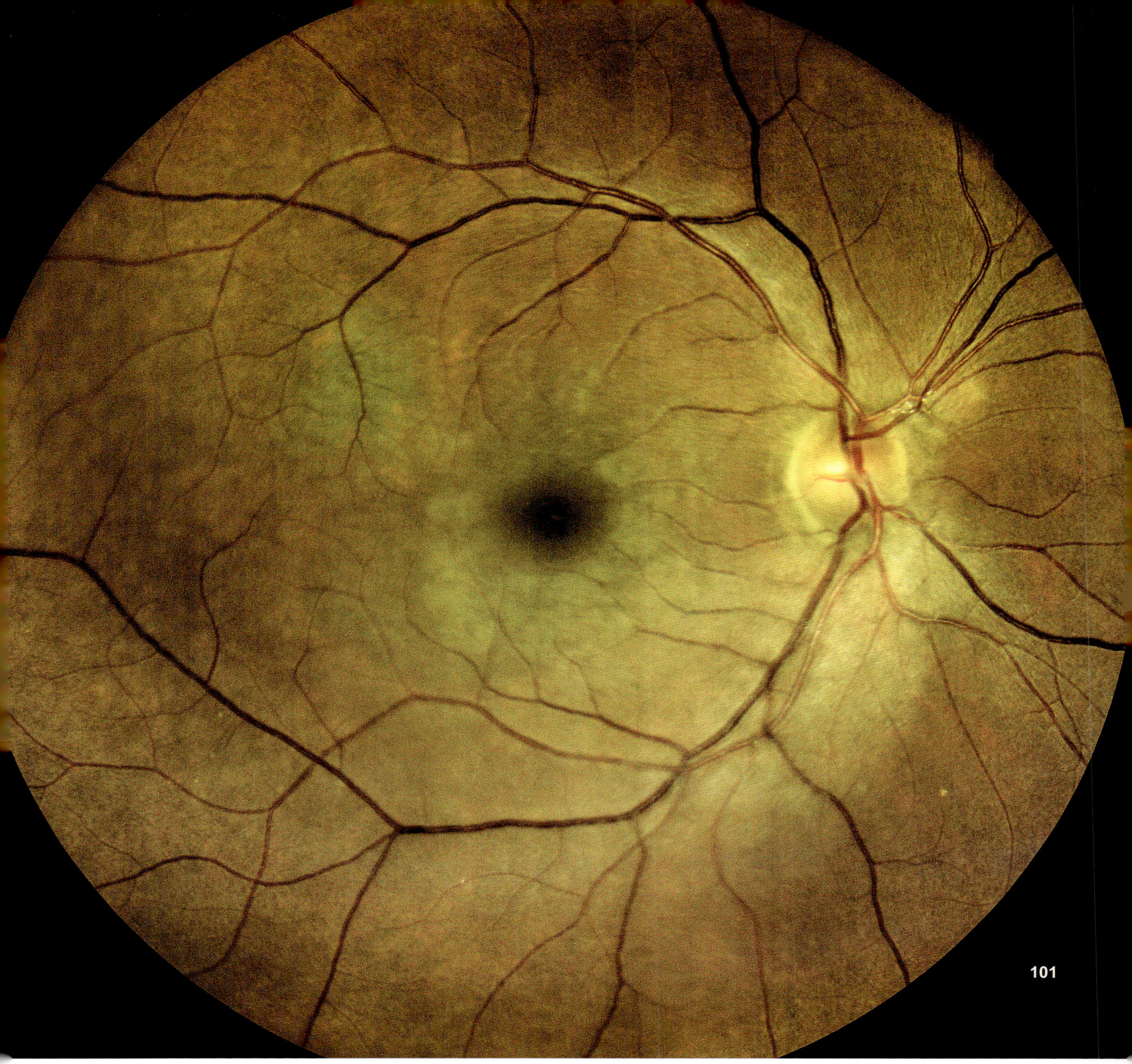


Figure 101 *Color fundus photograph 2 weeks after initiation of treatment: Patient underwent thorough systemic blood investigations. Blood test highlighted systemic vasculitis with raised ESR and HLA B 51 was positive. Mantoux skin test, TB gold, serum ACE and syphilis test were all negative. She was started on IV methylprednisolone three daily pulse dose followed by oral steroids. Color fundus photograph done 2 weeks later shows rapid resolution of the serous fluid with disappearance of yellowish mass lesion, altered pigmentary changes were seen at the site of lesion.*

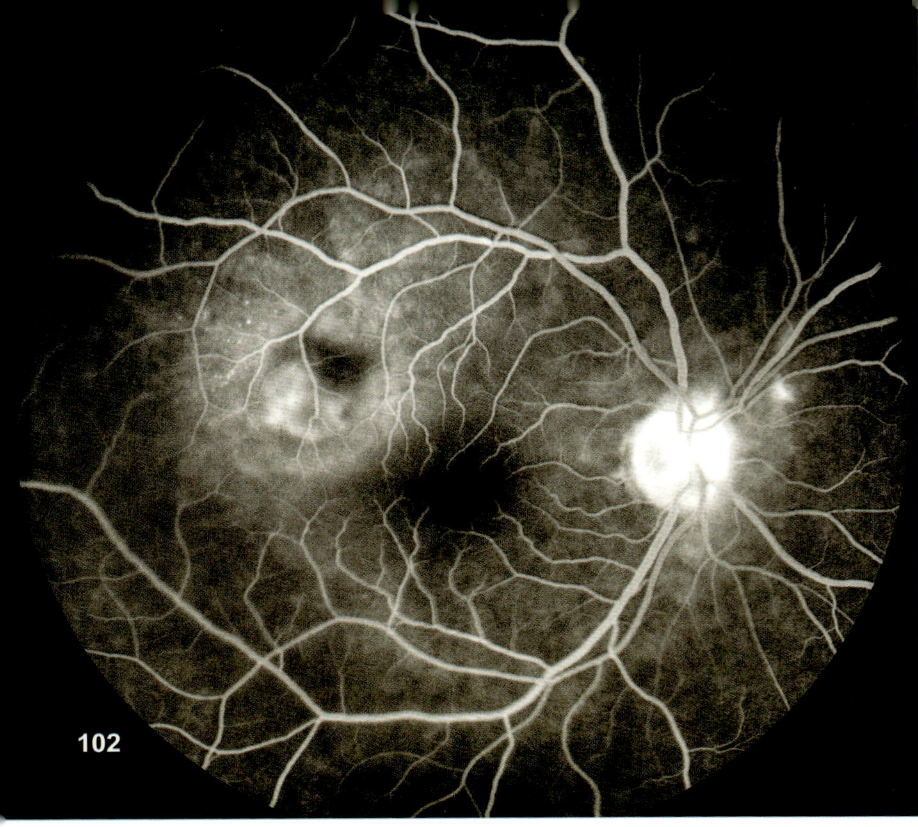


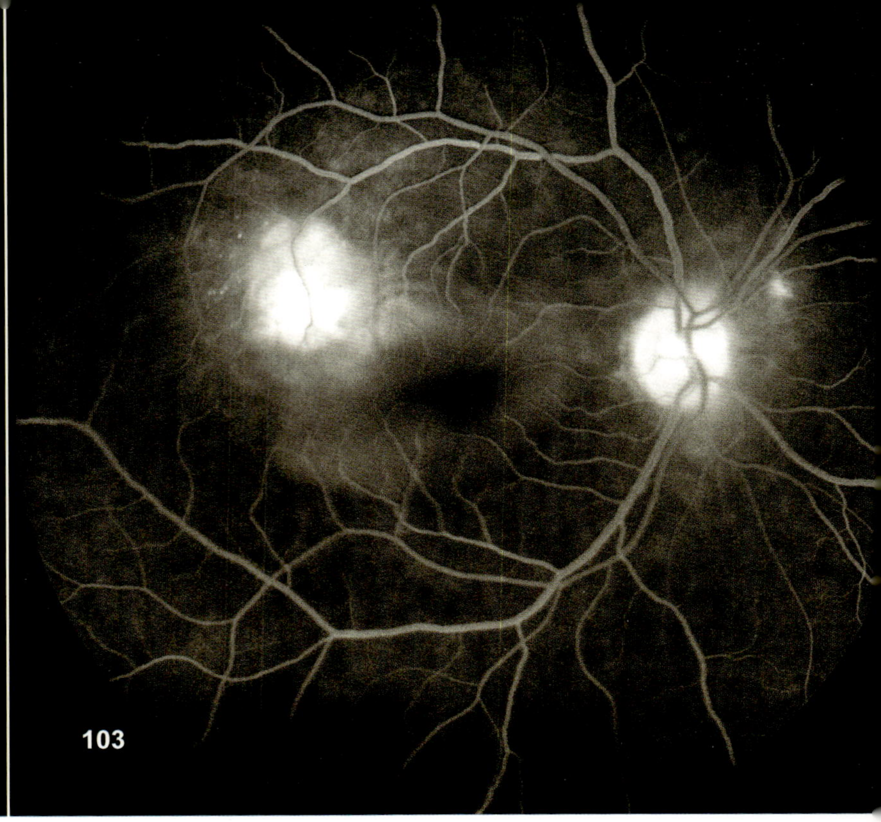


Figure 102 *Fluorescein angiogram of the early phase shows heterogeneous hyperfluorescence at the site of lesion with few pinpoint leaks surrounding it.*

Figure 103 *Late frame of the fluorescein angiogram depicts progressive increasing hyperfluorescence at the site of lesion with pooling of the dye in area of serous detachment.*

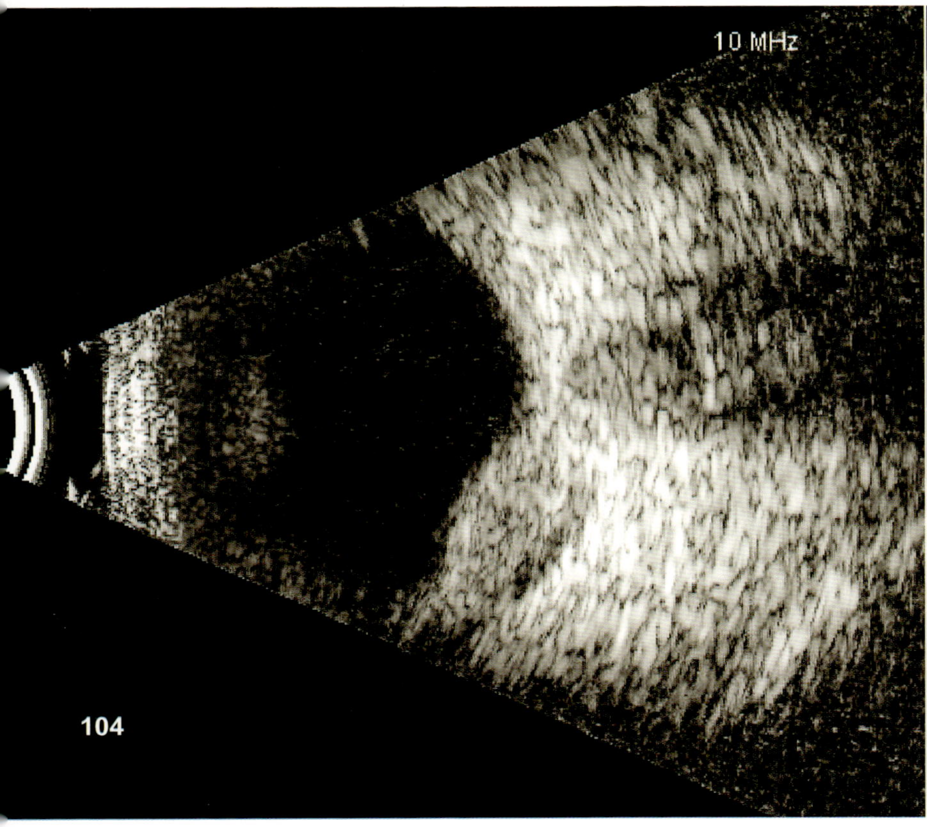


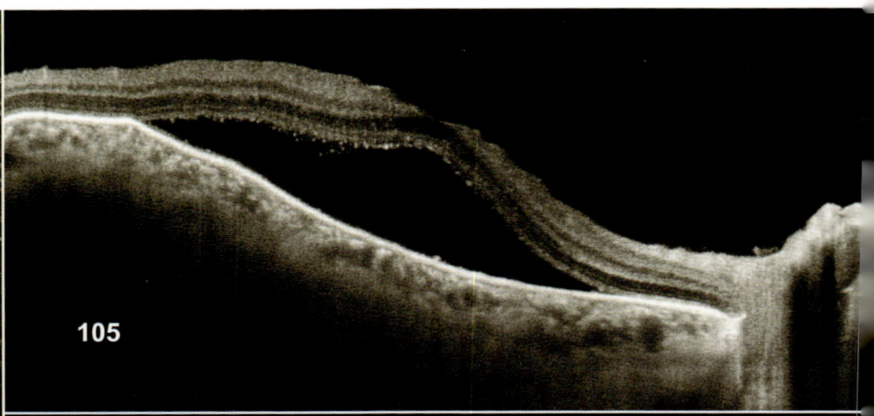


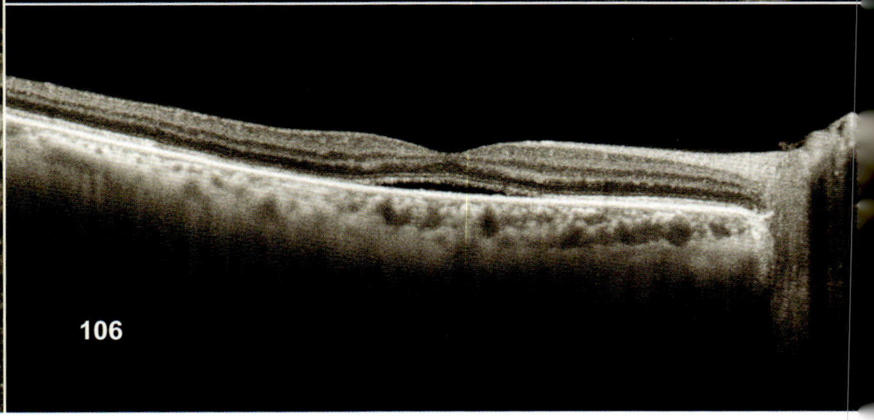


Figure 104 *Ultrasonography B-scan shows thickening of the ocular Coats associated with subtenon fluid (T-sign) adjacent to the mass. There is no orbital shadowing.*

Figure 105 *OCT scan shows subretinal fluid at the macula with elevation of the retina at the site of choroidal lesion.*

Figure 106 *Two weeks later the OCT scan shows flattening of RPE layer, reabsorption of subretinal fluid to a great extent. A small streak of subfoveal SRF is still persisting.* □

Figure 107 *Acute Posterior Multifocal Placoid Pigment Epitheliopathy (APMPPE)—color fundus montage image shown multiple yellowish white round chorioretinal lesions in nasal retina and at posterior pole (1). Few of these lesions have coalesced and ameboid-shaped yellowish lesion is formed temporal to the fovea (2).*

Figure 108 *Color fundus montage of case of APMPPE: 1 month after treatment. Note significant reduction in number of chorioretinal lesions in nasal retina and appearance of new lesions in temporal retina now (1). Chorioretinal lesions at posterior pole has also regressed after course of oral corticosteroids, initiated at 1g/kg body weight with weekly tapering. (This treatment is debatable, as the disease is known to be self-treatable).*

Figure 109 *Color fundus montage image of case of APMPPE 3 months after treatment showed complete disappearance of all chorioretinal lesions without scarring.* □

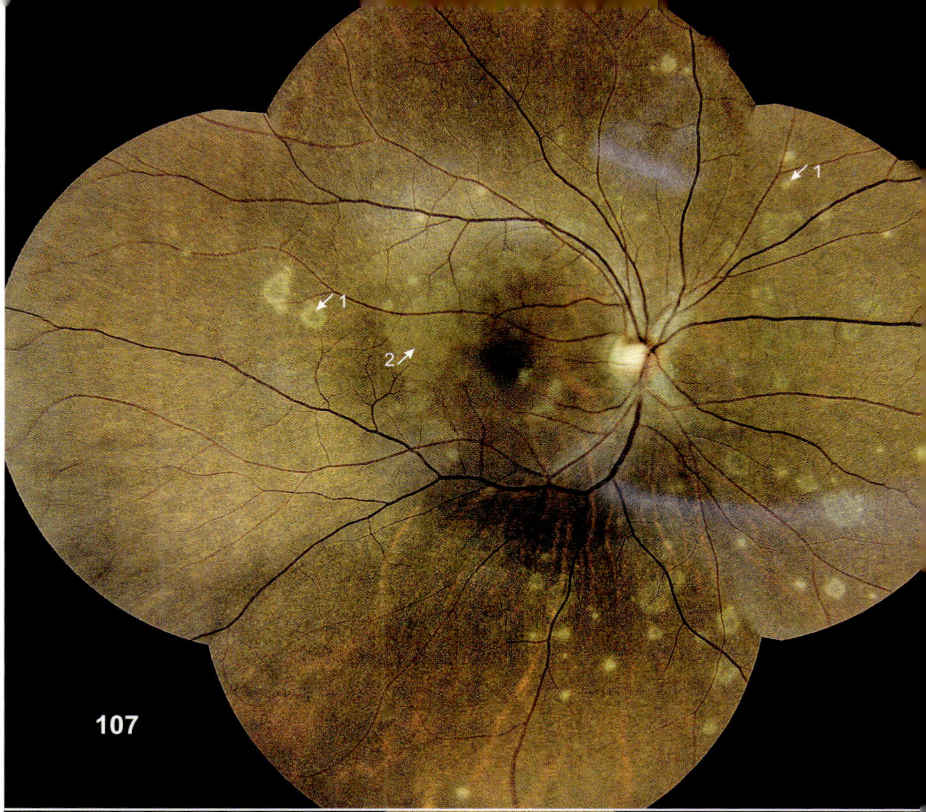


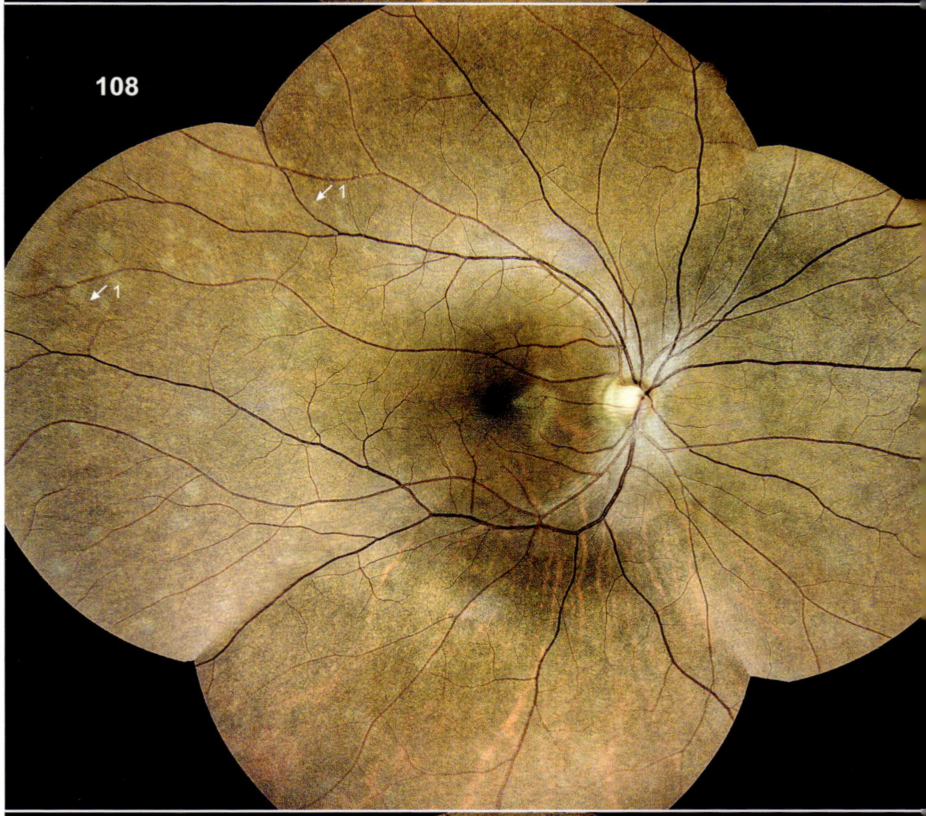


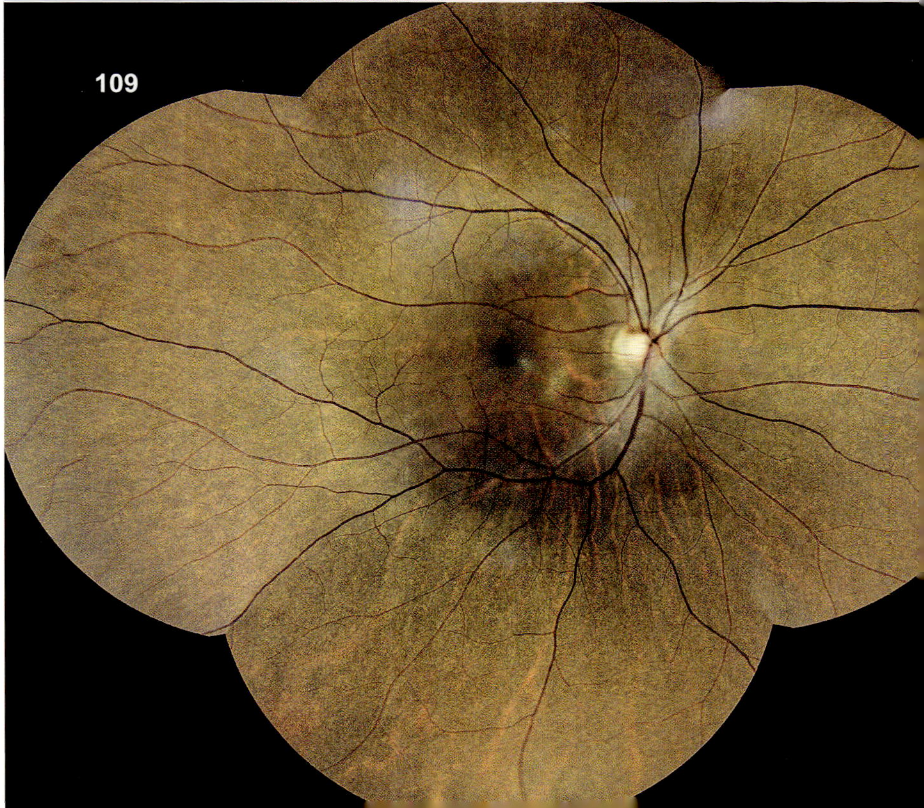

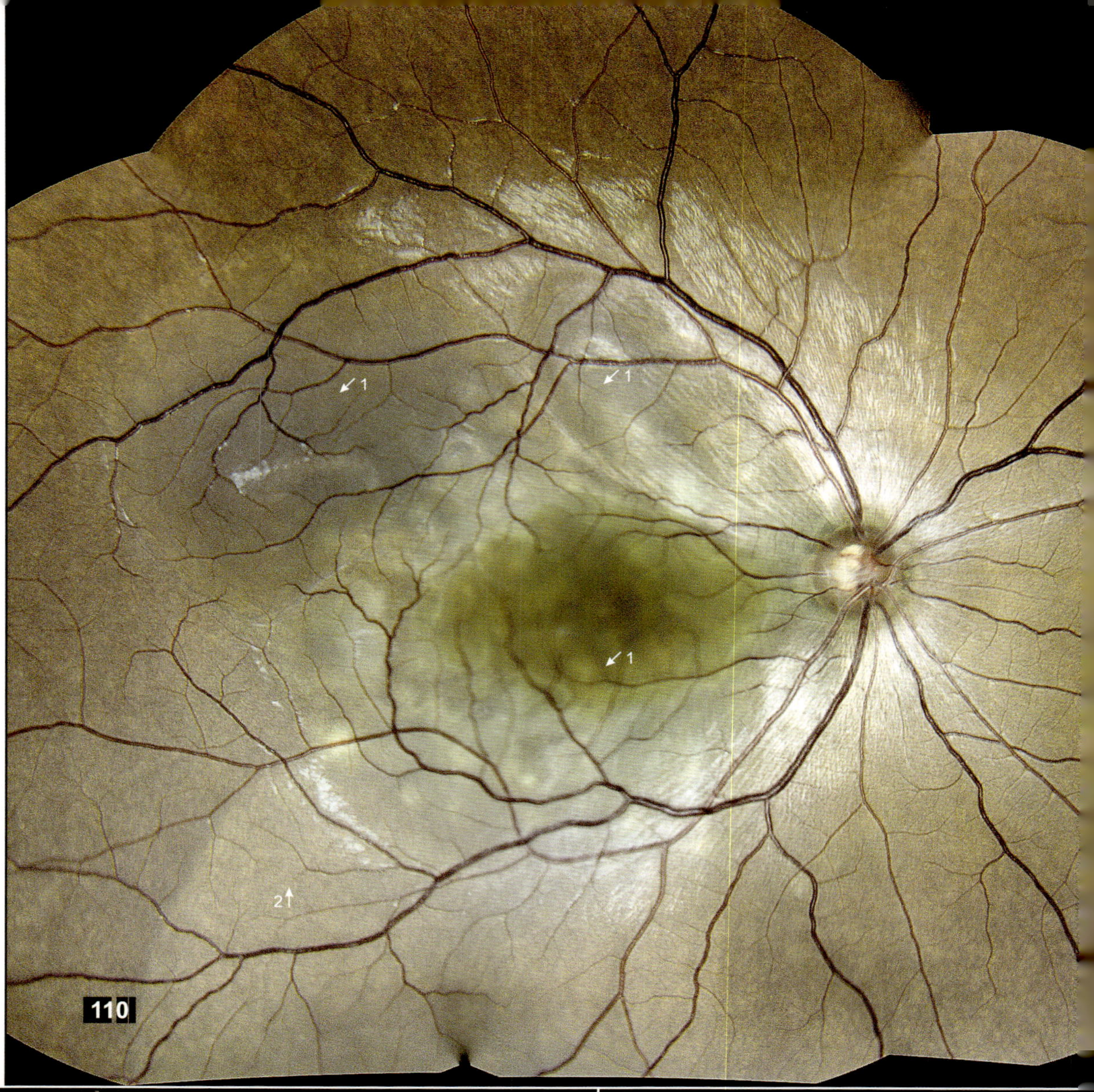

Figure 110

*Right fundus montage image in a case of acute Vogt-Koyanagi-Harada syndrome. Multiple areas of bullous exudative (1) fluid pockets at the posterior pole and extending up to mid-periphery retina inferiorly (2).*

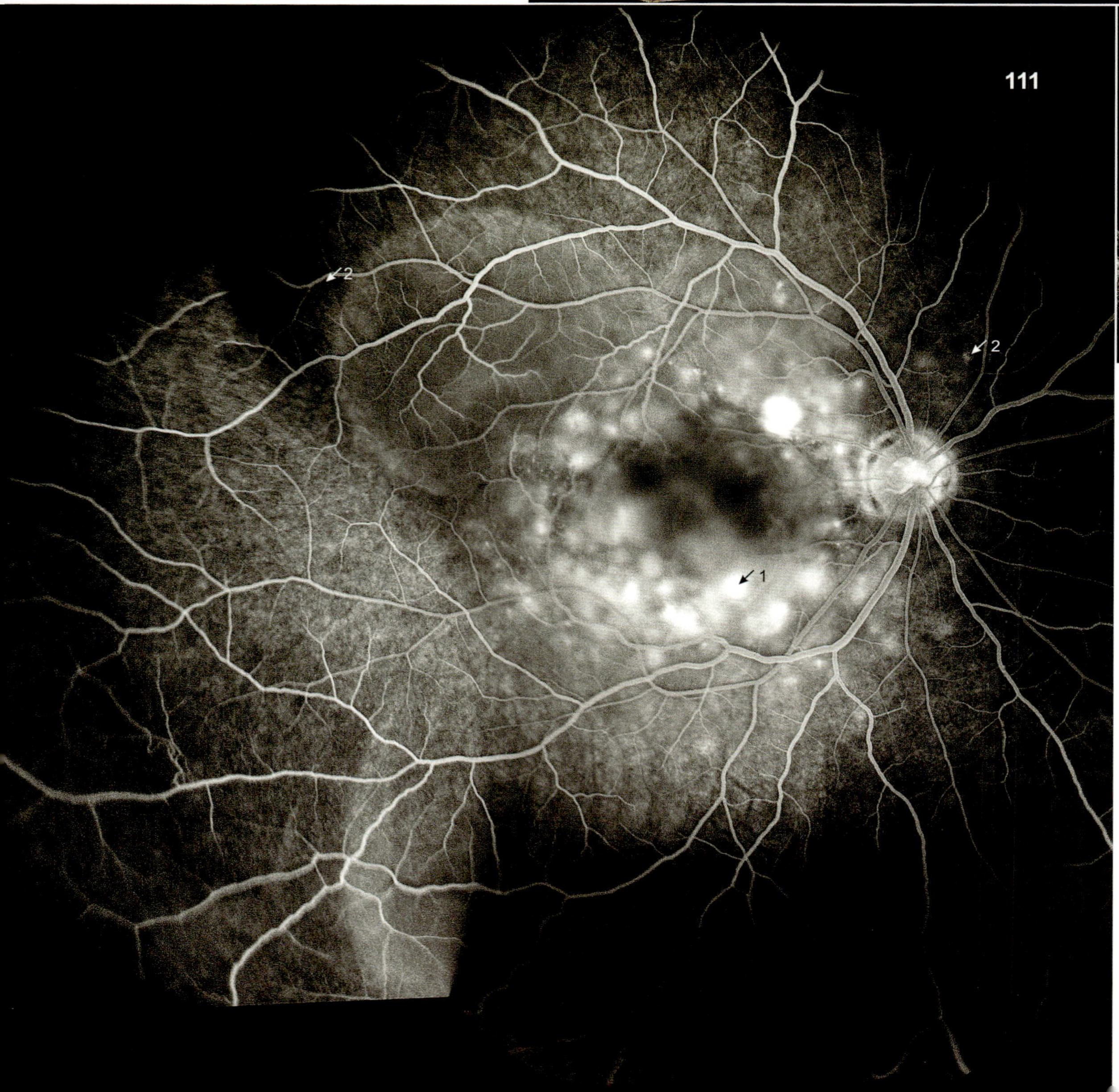

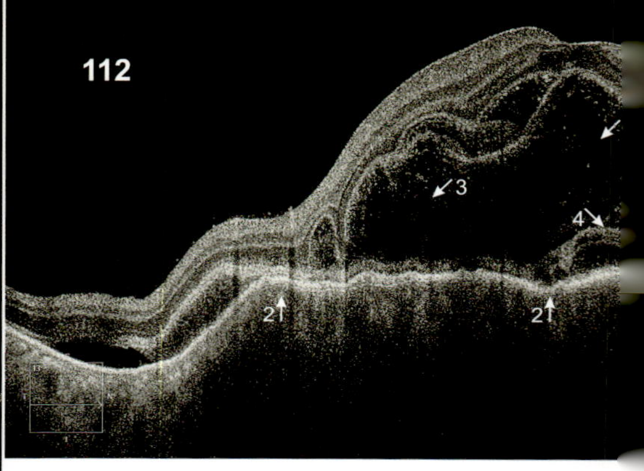

Figure 111

*FFA in mid-phase of dye injection showed multiple pinpoint RPE leaks (1) at the posterior pole extending beyond arcades also (2).*

Figure 112

*OCT image of right eye with acute Vogt-Koyanagi-Harada syndrome. Large serous detachment is seen at the fovea (1) with RPE undulations (2). Multiple hyper-reflective dots within subretinal space (3) and edematous photoreceptor layer (4).*

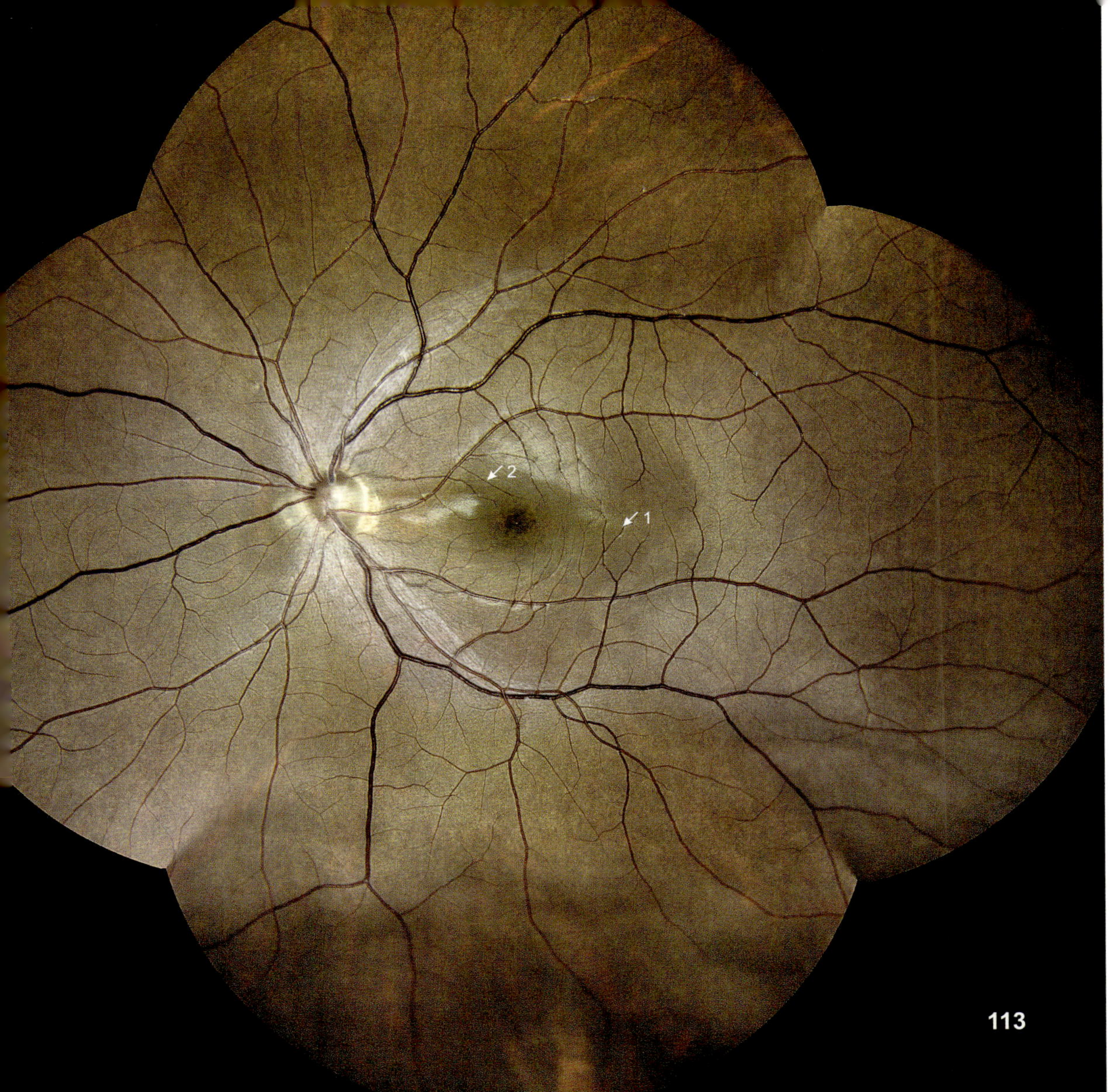


Figure 113

*Left fundus montage image of same patient with acute VKH shows two small pockets (1) (2) of serous fluid collection at the posterior pole.*

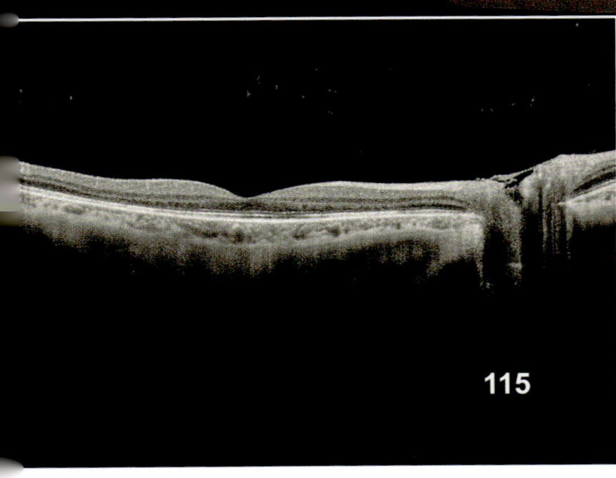


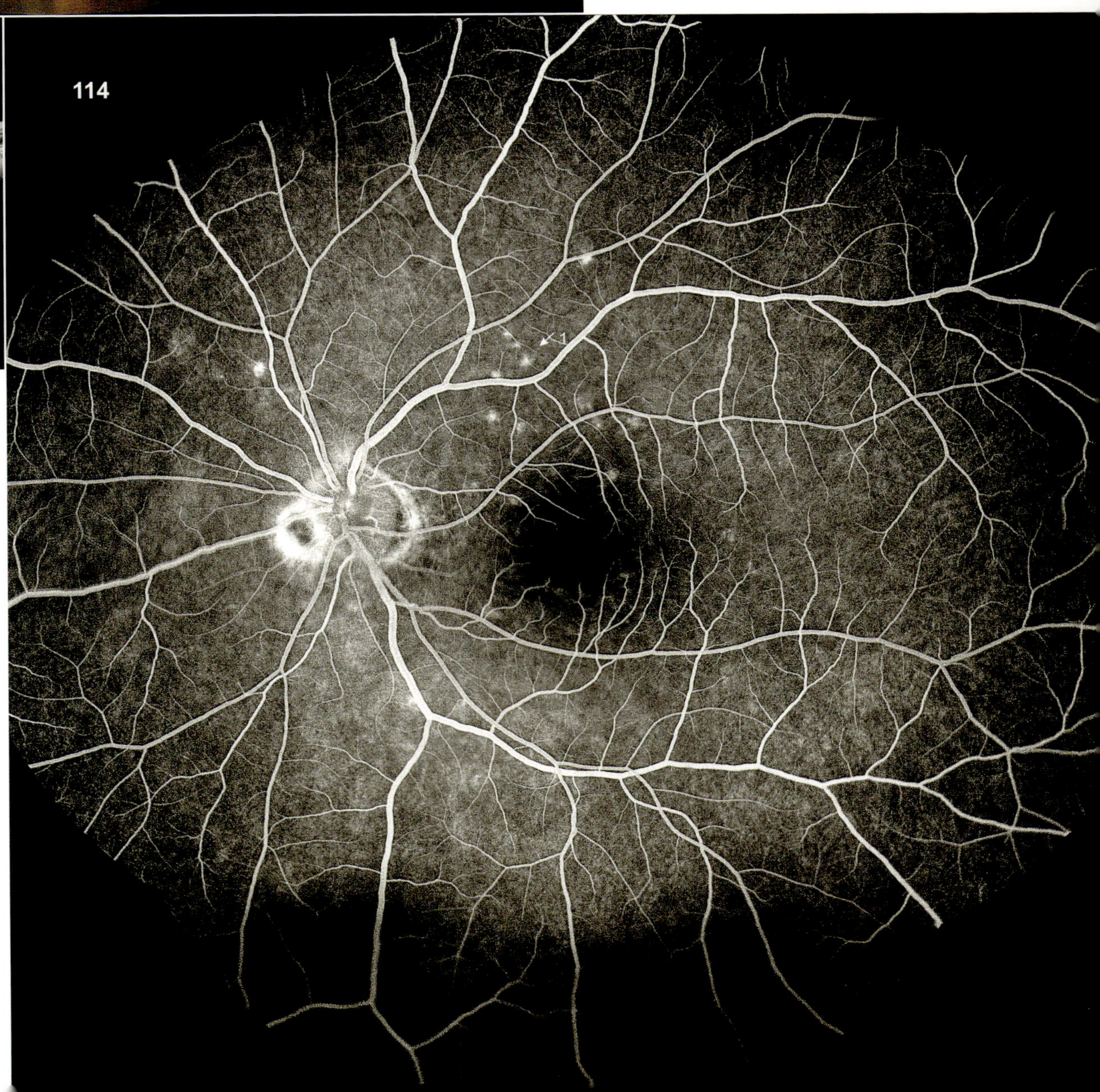


Figure 114

*FFA image of midphase of left eye with acute VKH demonstrating multiple round scattered pinpoint RPE peak points (1).*

Figure 115

*Left SD-OCT image is early stage of acute VKH, did not show any subretinal fluid collection.*□

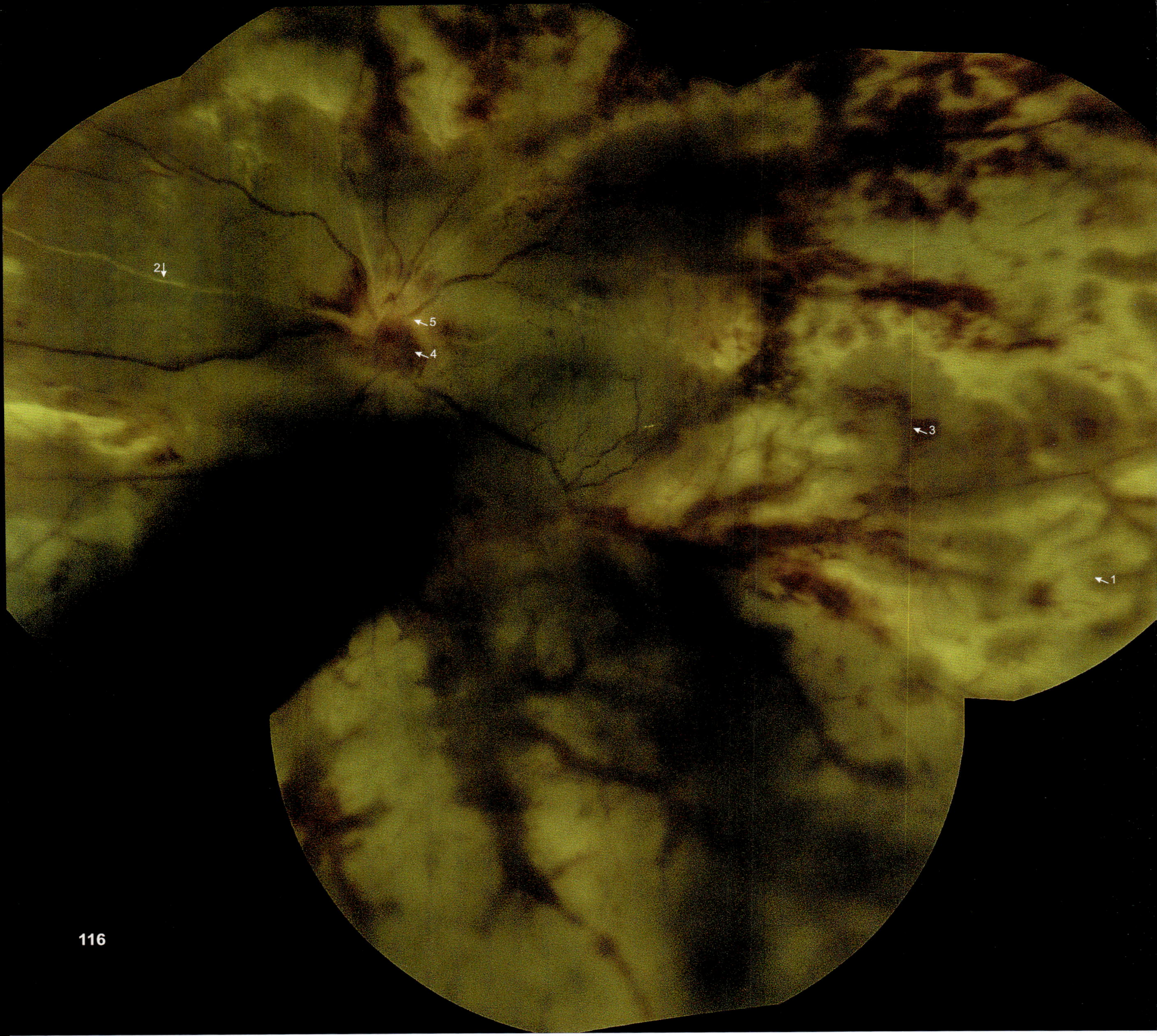


Figure 116 *A case of acute retinal necrosis: Color fundus montage image shows confluent areas of necrotizing peripheral retinitis that are seen as yellowish white patch of retinal opacification obscuring all other retinal details (1) also note the presence of occlusive vasculopathy of retinal vessels (2) scattered retinal hemorrhages (3) peripappilary hemorrhages (4) and disc edema is also seen (5).*

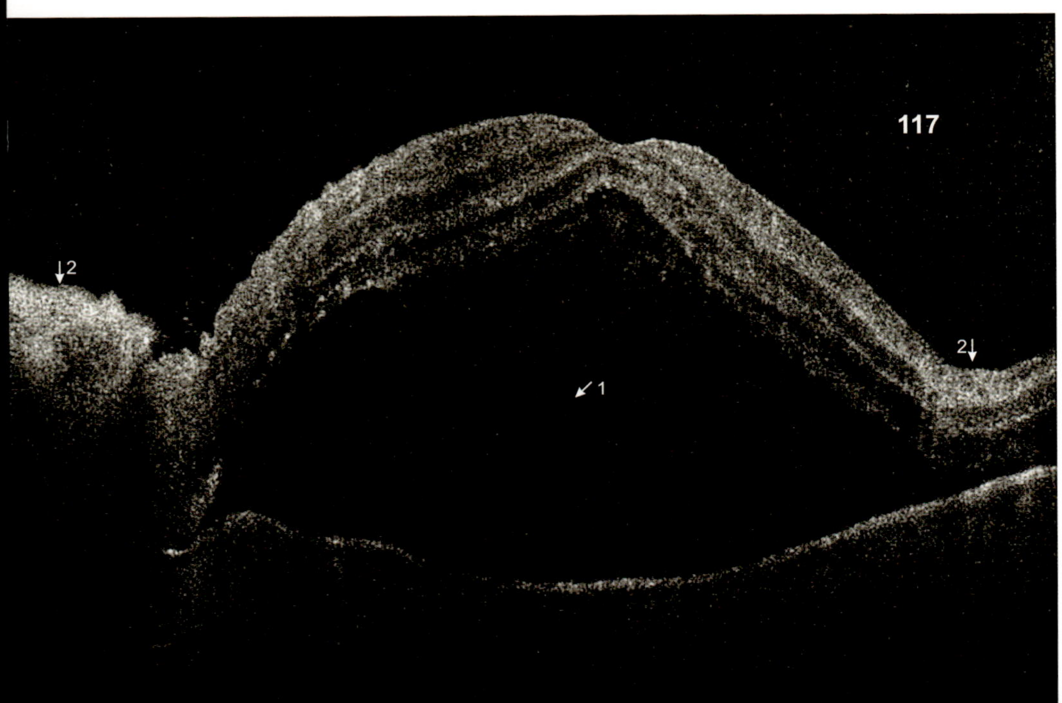


Figure 117 *SD-OCT scan in a case of acute retinal necrosis demonstrates macular serous detachment (1) and increased hyperreflectivity of inner retinal layers (2) suggestive of retinal ischemia/ necrosis.*□

# CHAPTER 7

## HEREDITARY

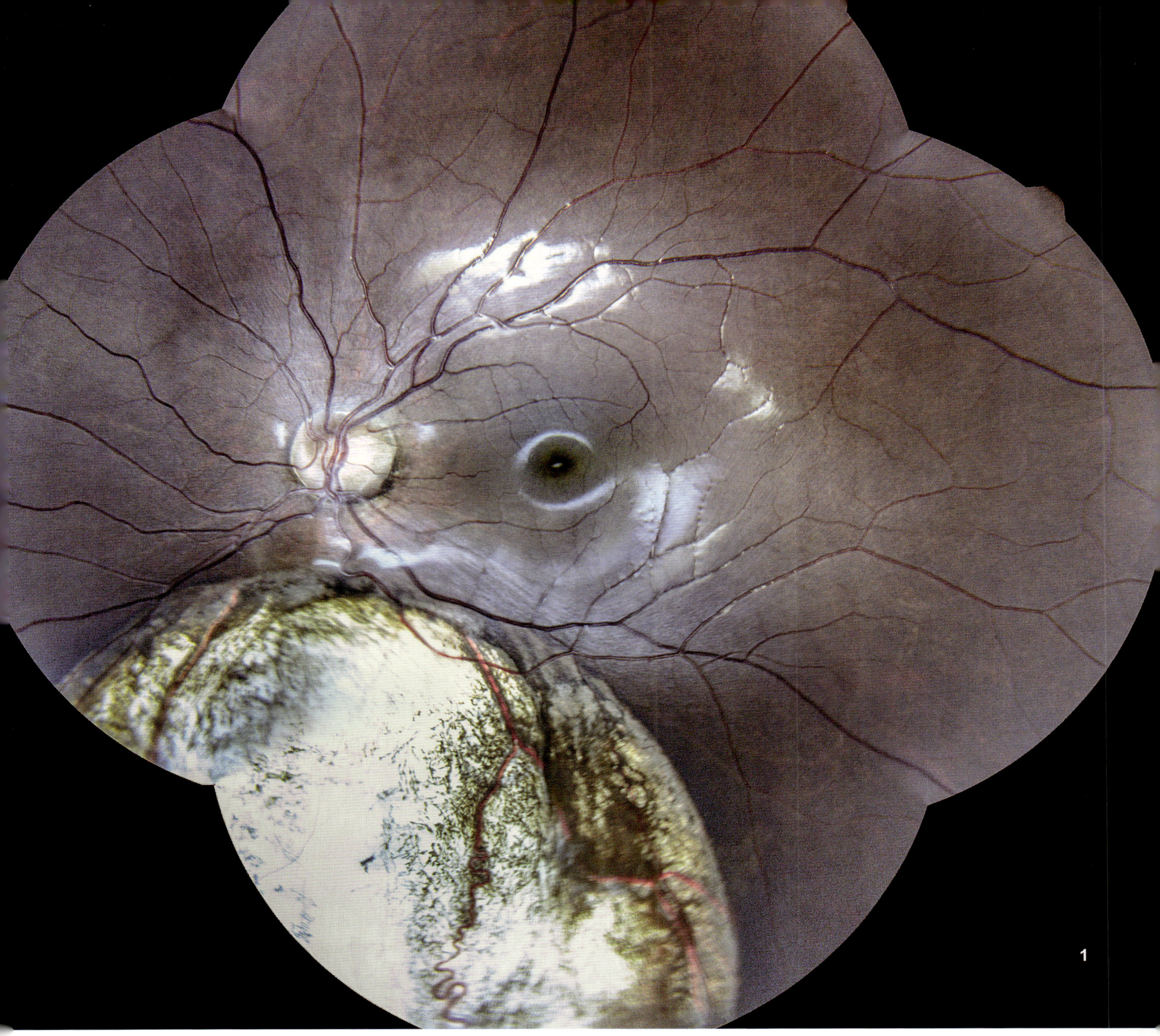



Figure 1 *Case of typical retinochoroidal Coloboma.*

Figure 2 *SS-OCT scan demonstrating a large excavation in the region of Coloboma. Retina is reduced to glial tissue with no differentiation of retinal layers, RPE or choroid.*

Color fundus montage photograph shows a dome-shaped area of retino-choroidal excavation that app-ears white with well demarcated sharp borders associated with pigment deposition at the junction of Coloboma and normal retina. Course of retinal blood vessels is also changed in the region of Coloboma.

It is a rare genetic developmental defect during embryogenesis characterized by partial absence of RPE and choroid. Inferonasal quadrant is the typical location 40% of the Coloboma develop retinal detachments. □

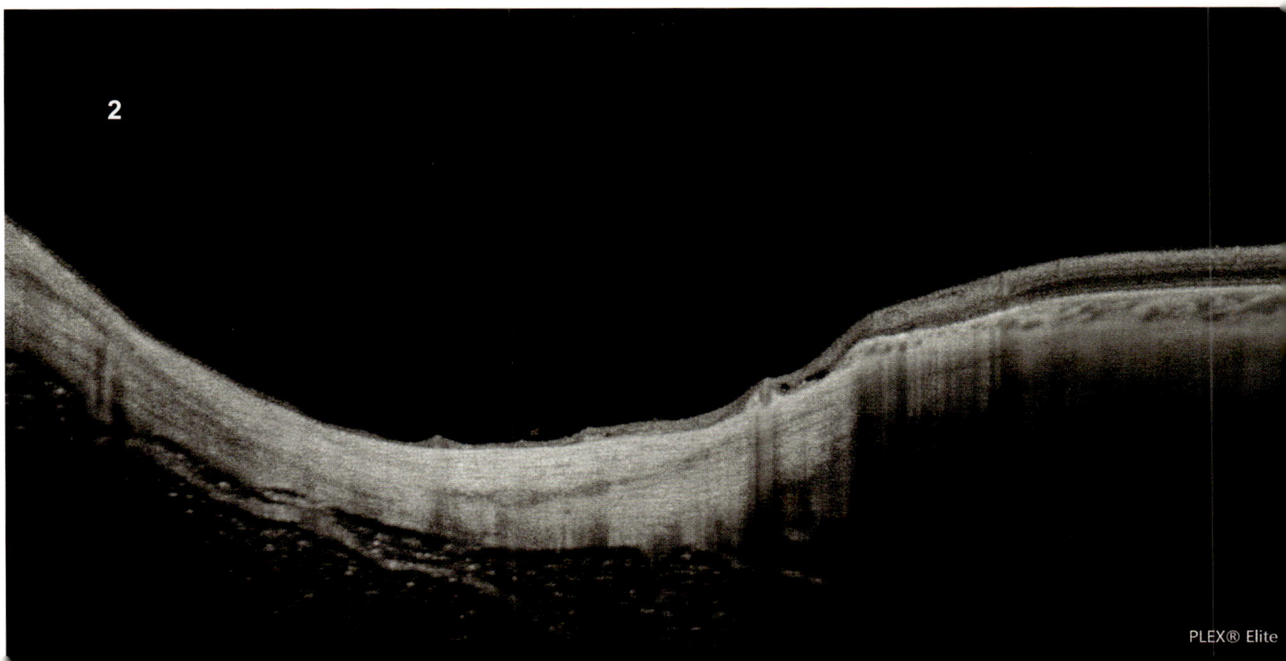

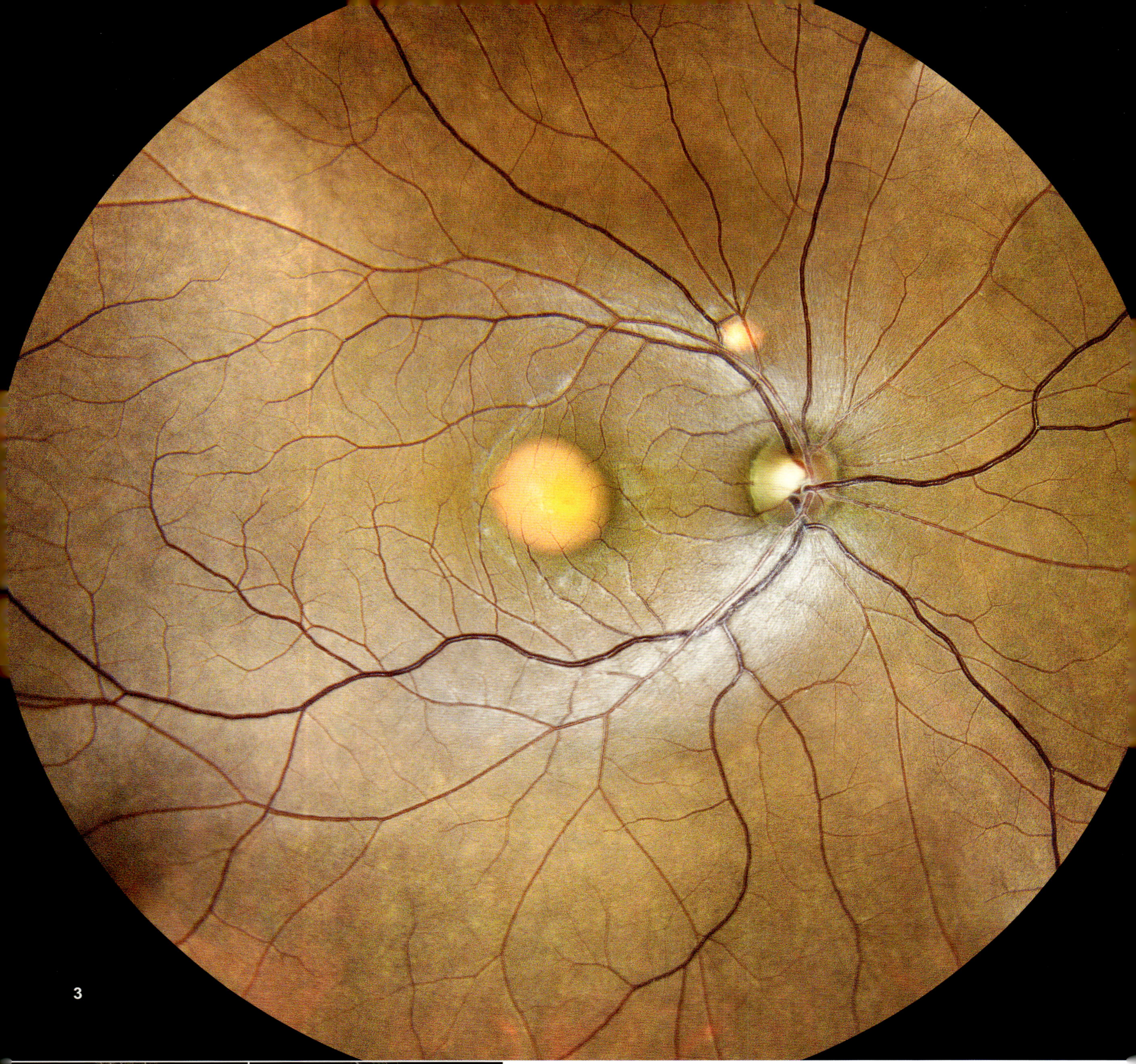

3

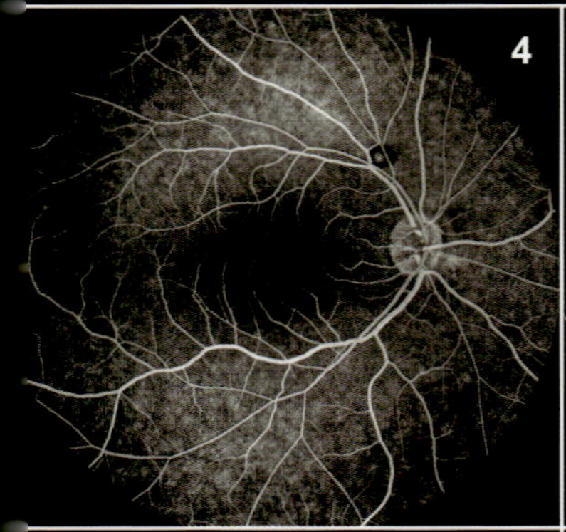

4

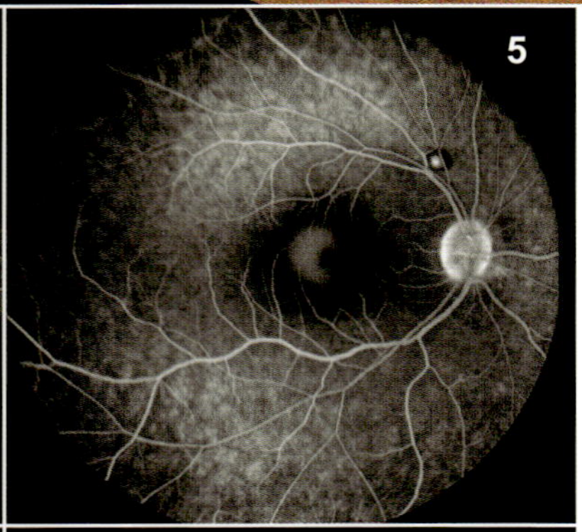

5

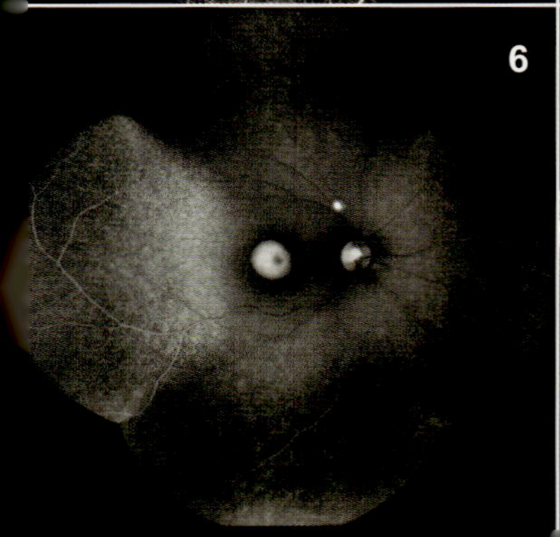

6

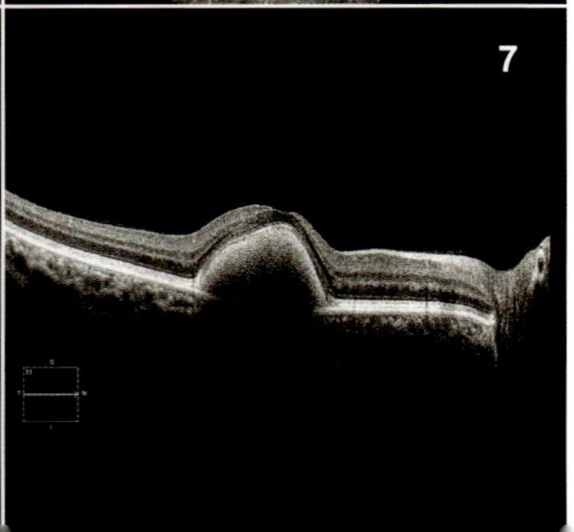

7

Figure 3 *Case of BEST disease with typical egg yolk lesions. BEST disease, also known as vitelliform dystrophy, is a bilateral AD disorder characterized by typical classic vitelliform lesions appearing as egg yolks-yellow, round, slightly elevated lesions at the macula.*

Figure 4 *Early frame of angiogram shows mixed pattern of hyperfluorescence and hypofluorescence at the site of the egg yolk lesion due to blocked fluorescence from the vitelliform material.*

Figure 5 *Late frame shows slight increase in the hyperfluorescence within the well-defined lesion boundaries.*

Figure 6 *Autofluorescence demonstrates excessive accumulation of lipofuscin in macular area with marked hyperautofluorescence.*

Figure 7 *OCT scan demonstrating well-defined hyperreflective vitelliform lesion with homogeneous hyper-reflectivity within it.*

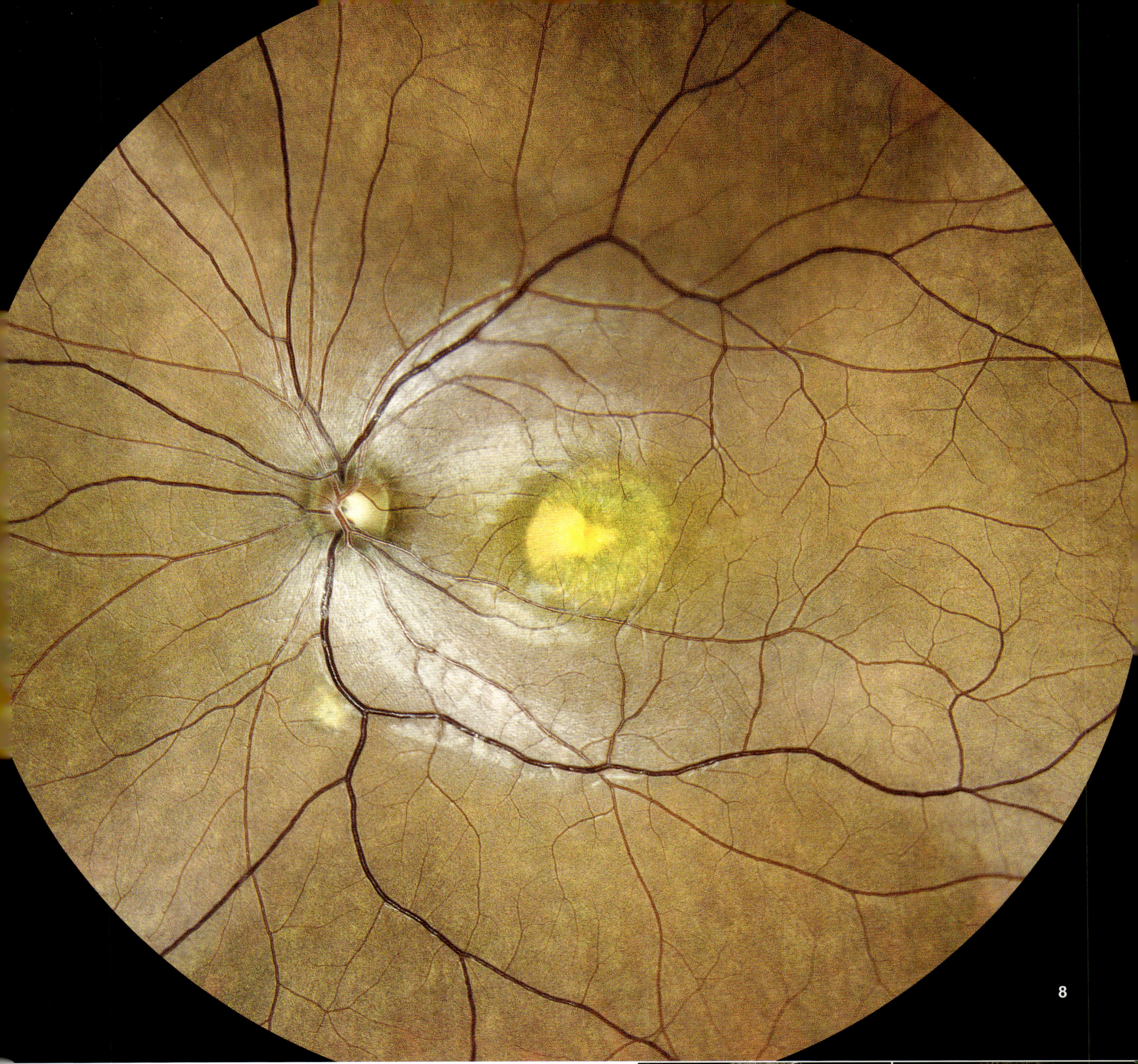


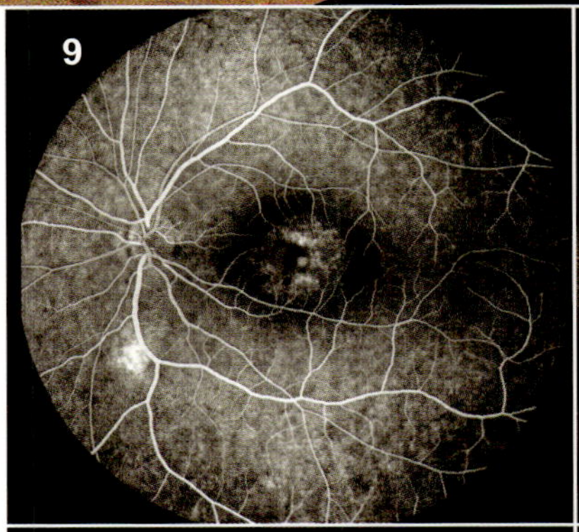


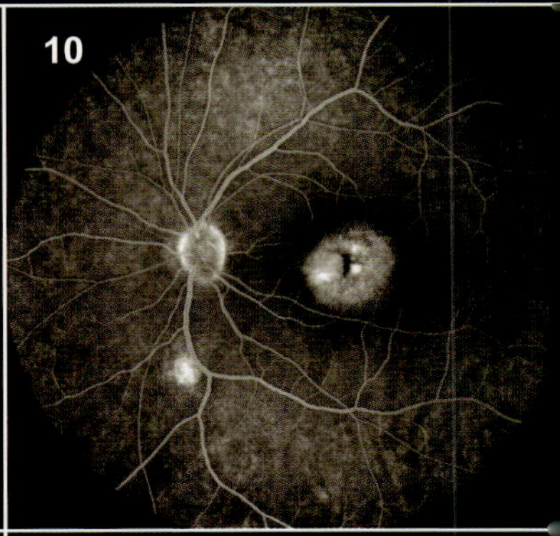


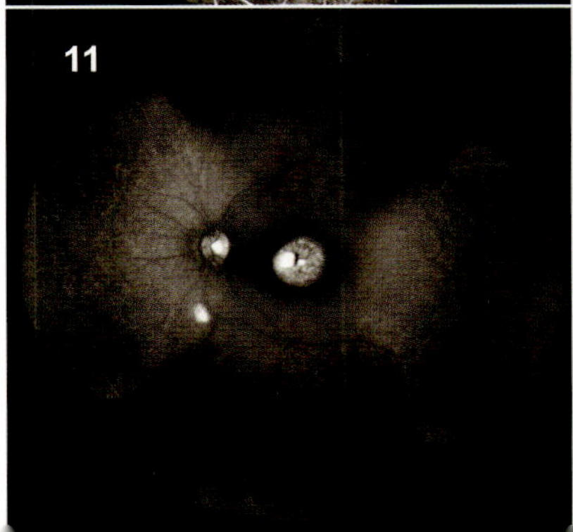


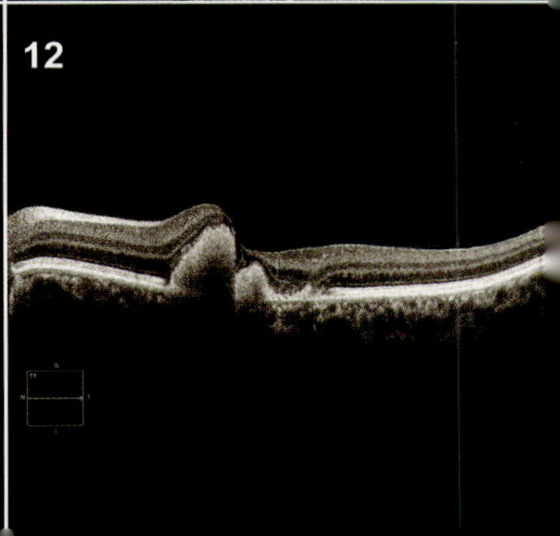


Figure 8 *Case of BEST disease with a scrambled egg appearance. As the disease progresses, yellowish material disintegrates and that results in a scrambled egg appearance which is often accompanied with a decrease in visual acuity.*

Figure 9 *Early frame of angiogram demonstrating areas of hyperfluorescence indicating RPE atrophy in the scrambled egg stage.*

Figure 10 *Late frame of angiogram demonstrating RPE staining.*

Figure 11 *Autofluorescence in scrambled egg appearance demonstrates areas of hyperautofluorescence interspersed with speckled areas of hypoautofluorescence corresponding to retinal pigment epithelium atrophy.*

Figure 12 *OCT scan demonstrating disrupted vitelliform lesion with associated outer retinal atrophic changes.* □

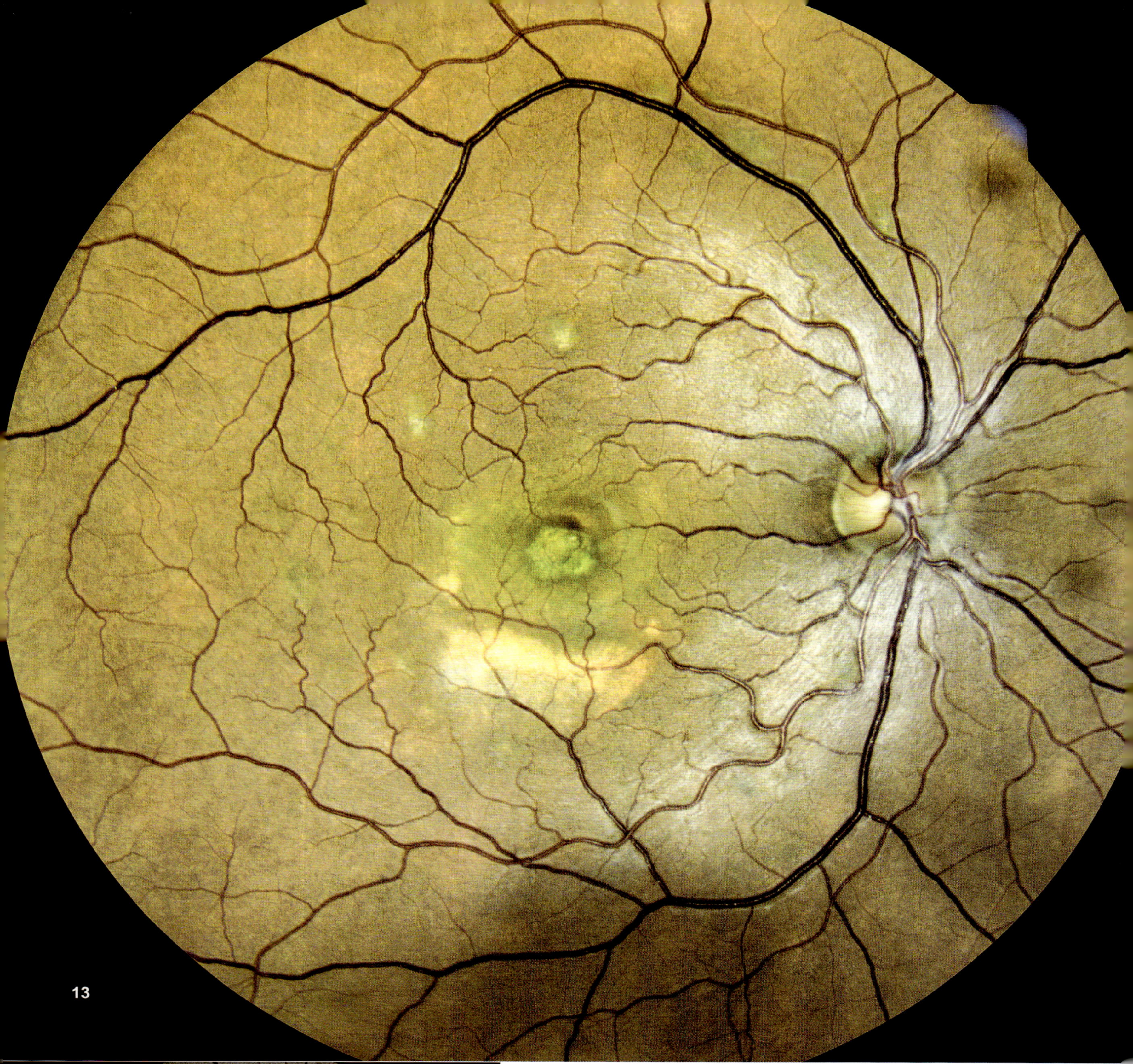

13

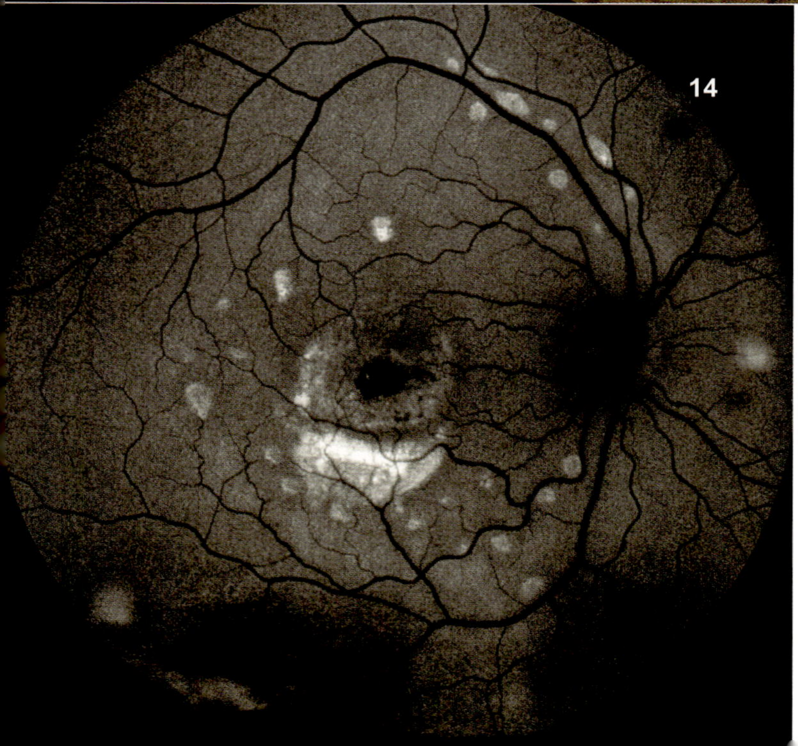

14

Figure 13 *Color fundus photograph of the left eye of the same patient with vitelliform macular dystrophy (BEST disease). Note the presence of a round well demarcated atrophic appearance of vitelliform lesion at the fovea center and a few atrophic RPE round lesions scattered at the posterior pole.*

It is an inherited autosomal dominant disorder caused by the mutations in the *BEST 1* gene that affects the macular region. Fundus findings are more dramatic than actual vision loss in the early stages of the disease. It is usually a bilateral abnormality characterized by the classic vitelliform structure, similar to an egg yellow, sometimes orange, round, slightly elevated structure surrounded by a somewhat darker border. One occasionally may see multiple vitelliform structures in the posterior pole. The ophthalmoscopy findings range from an exceedingly small, round, yellow dot at the fovea to a condition resembling the scar of a toxoplasmosis retinochoroiditis. Yellowish material in the disk may disintegrate, leaving a scrambled egg appearance as the disease progresses.

Figure 14 *Autofluorescence image demonstrating hypoautofluorescent changes at the fovea due to abnormal lipofuscin deposition at the level of RPE and disintegration of vitelliform lesions resulting in RPE atrophy appearing hyperautofluorescent in the inferior macula.*

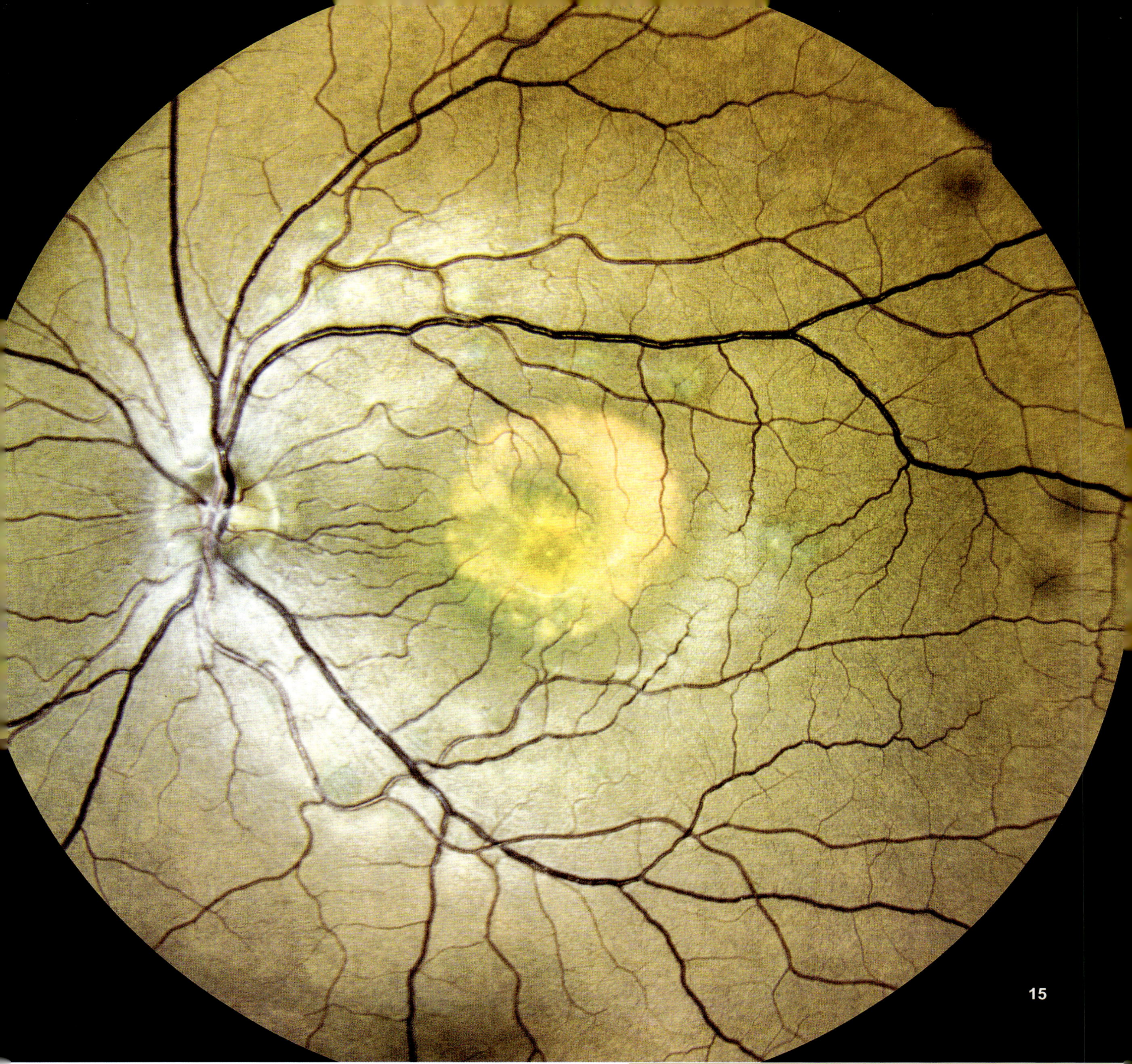

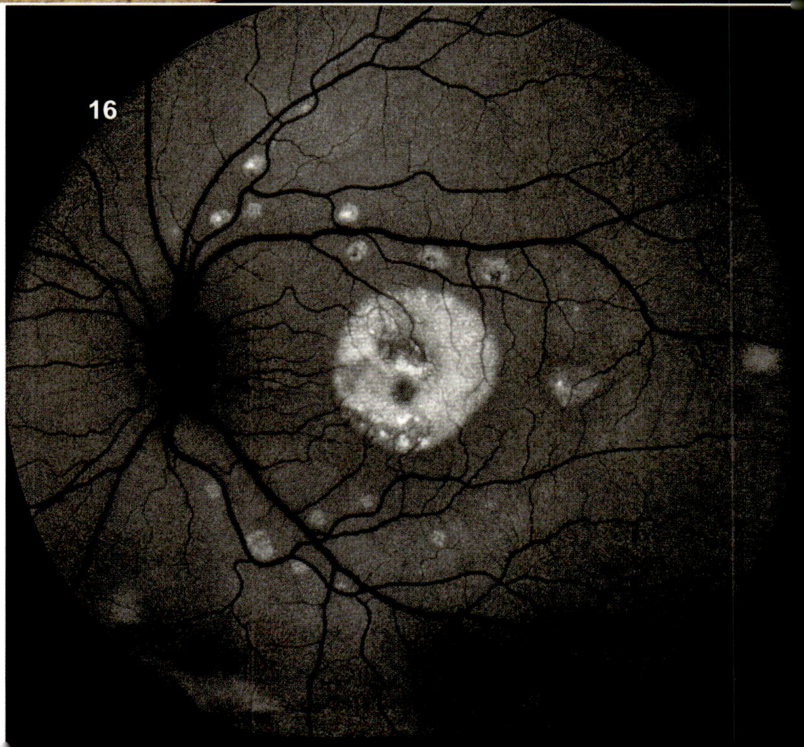

Figure 15 *Color fundus photograph showing pathognomonic "scrambled egg yolk" (Vitelliruptive lesion) appearance at the macula in a case of vitelliform macular dystrophy. Also note multiple small yellow vitelliform lesions scattered all around at the posterior pole.*

Figure 16 *Autofluorescence imaging demonstrating hyperautofluorescence from multiple vitelliform lesions due to RPE atrophy.* □

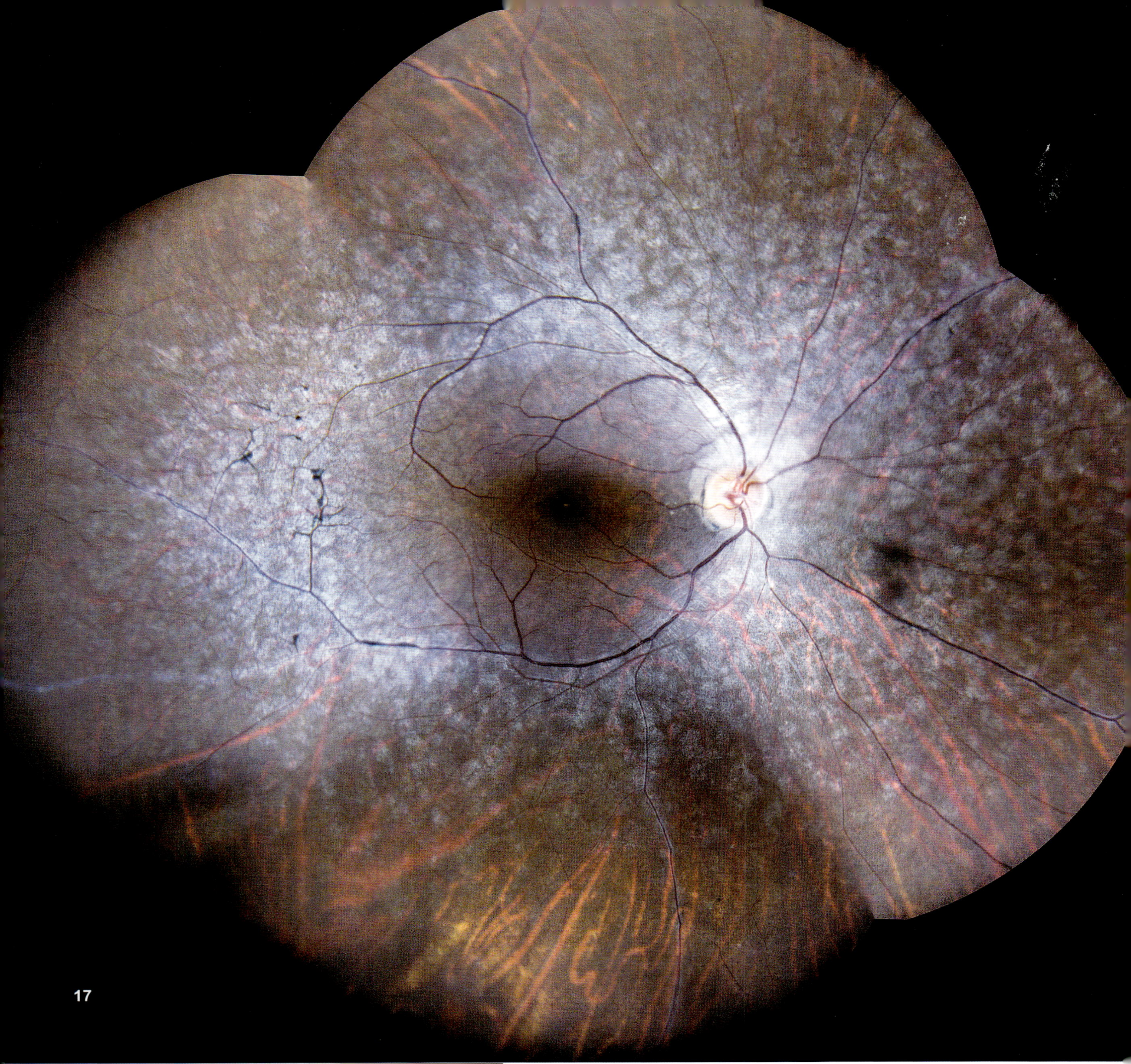

17

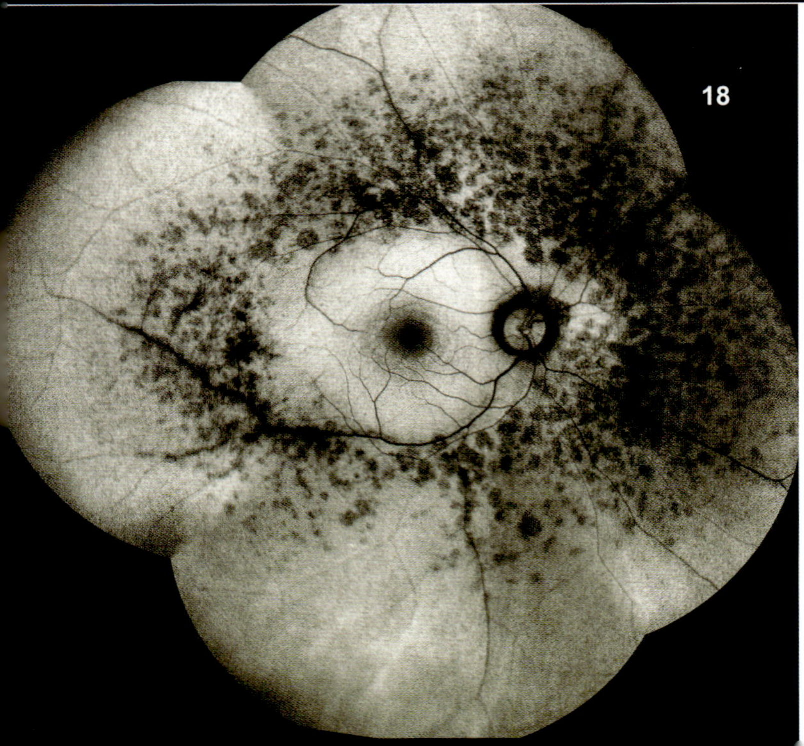

18

Figure 17 *Case of retinitis pigmentosa—right eye. Color fundus montage shows a bilateral symmetric disease characterized by the presence of characteristic mid peripheral distribution of RPE atrophy associated bony spicules and attenuation of retinal vessels in a case of retinitis pigmentosa. Macula and far periphery of retina appears relatively*

Figure 18 *Fundus autofluorescence again shows bilaterally symmetrical disease of RPE loss due to photoreceptor degeneration, distributed in the mid-peripheral retina, characteristically sparing the macula and periphery in a case of mild form of retinitis pigmentosa.*

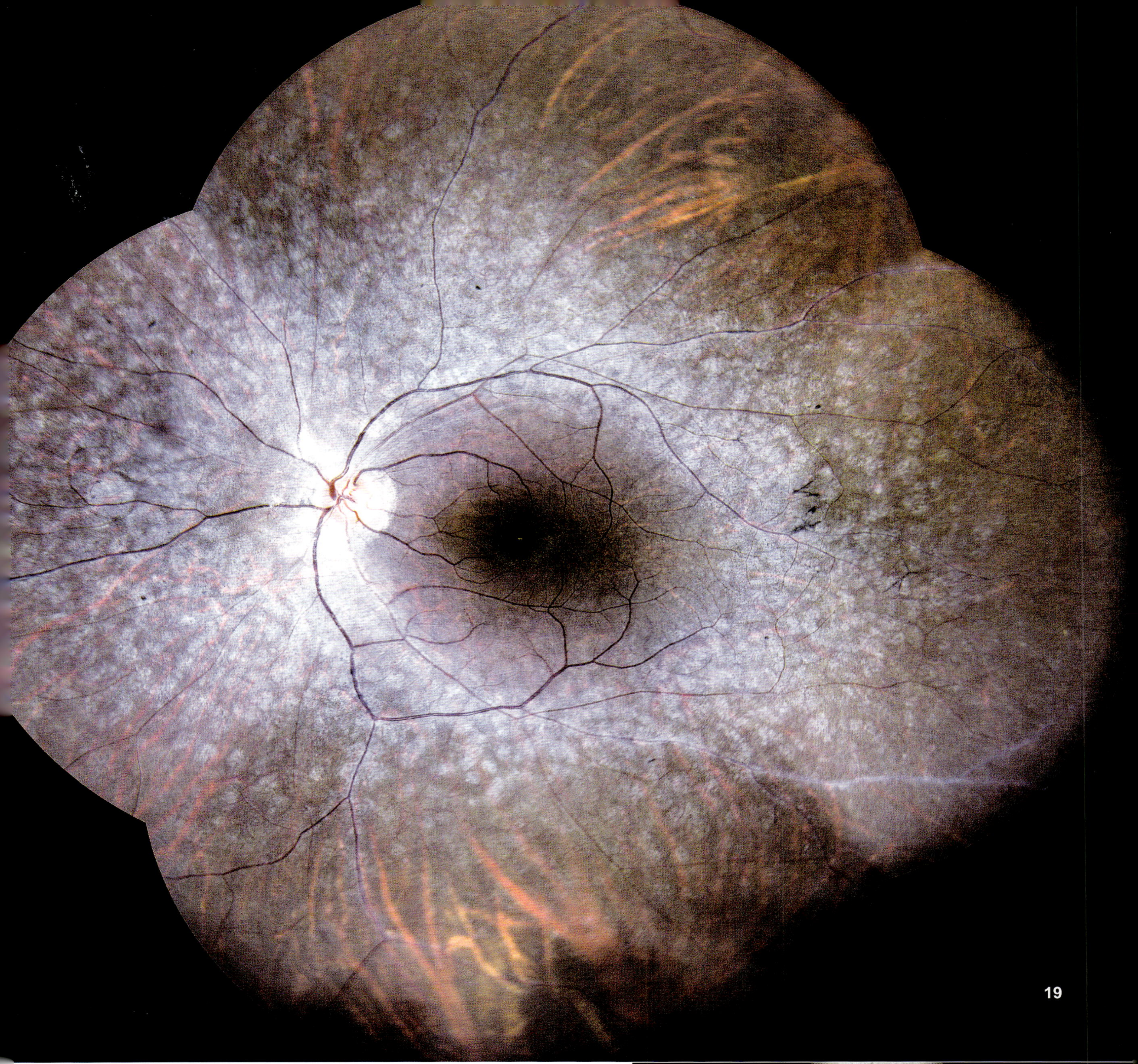

Figure 19 *Case of retinitis pigmentosa left eye of the same patient.*

Genetic mutations responsible for retinitis pigmentosa produce biochemical dysfunction specifically affecting the rod photoreceptors. Rod photoreceptors are distributed in high density as compared to the cones throughout the peripheral retina with a sharp decline in the fovea. Death of these rod photoreceptors have a deleterious affect on the retinal pigment epithelium resulting in RPE atrophy that is visible as fine mottling or granularity of RPE in the mid and far periphery. Intraretinal bony spicules represent migration of pigment into the retina.

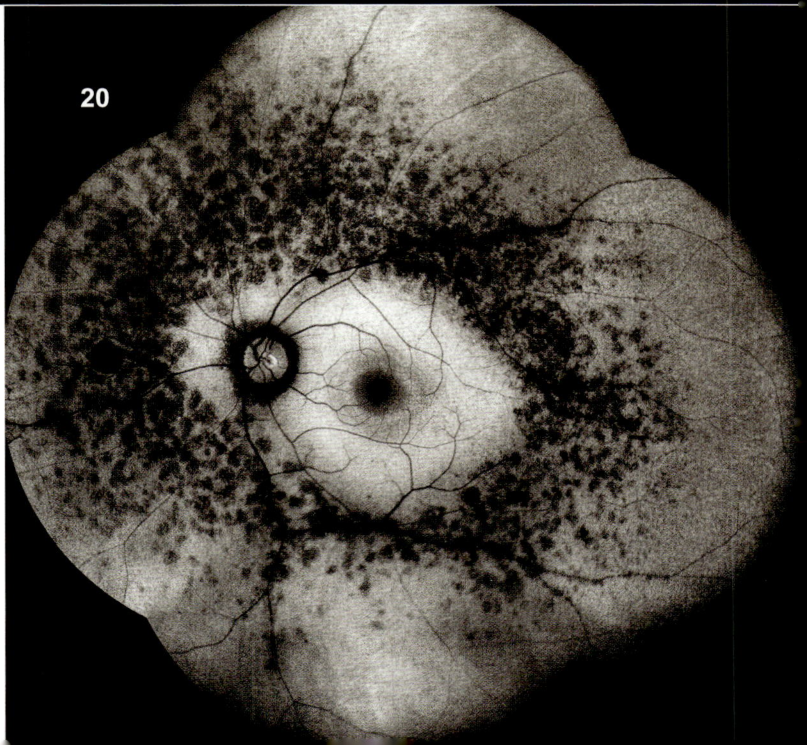

Figure 20 *Fundus autofluorescence montage image of left eye.* □

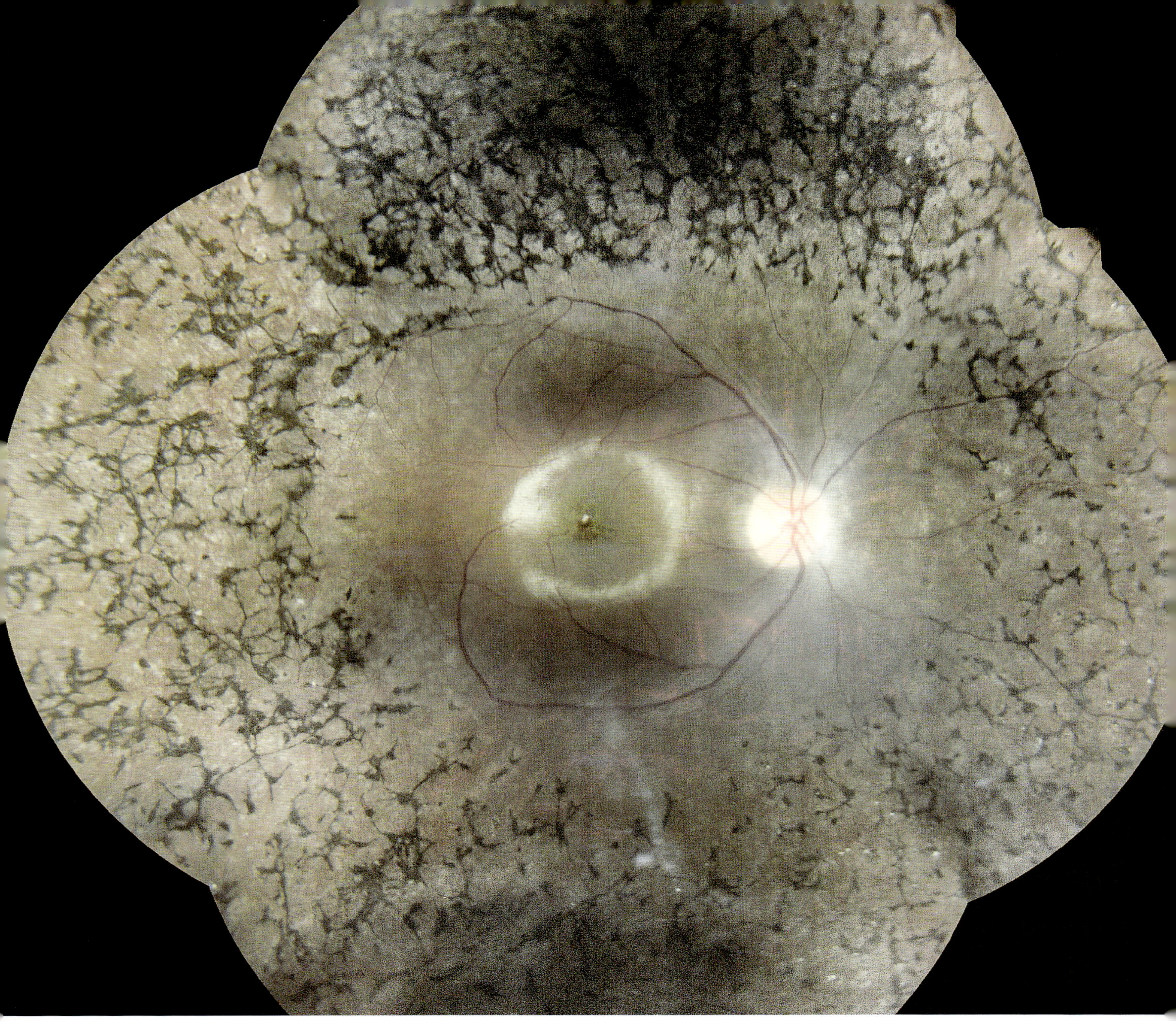

Figure 21 *Color fundus montage photograph of right eye of 28-year-old male with long standing history of night blindness came with complaints of blurred vision. Note the characteristic bone spicules involving all the four quadrants of fundus, sparing the fovea.*

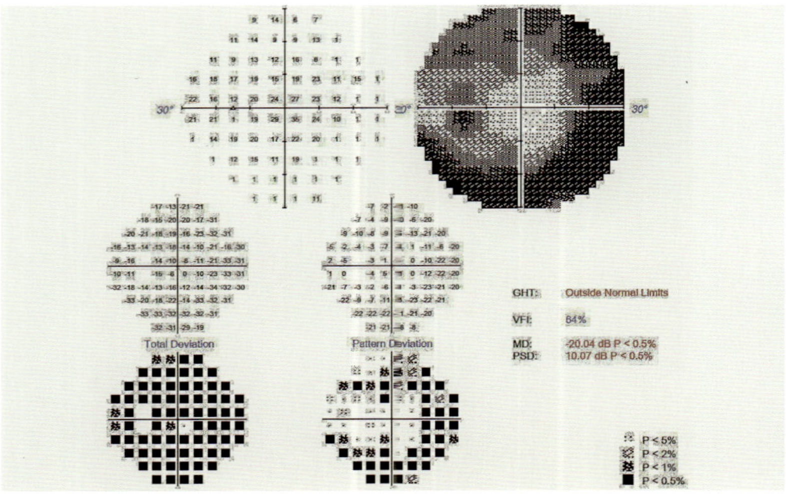


Figure 22 *Humphry visual fields 30° demonstrating gross construction of visual fields typically seen in cases of retinitis pigmentosa (RP) or pigmentary retinopathy.*

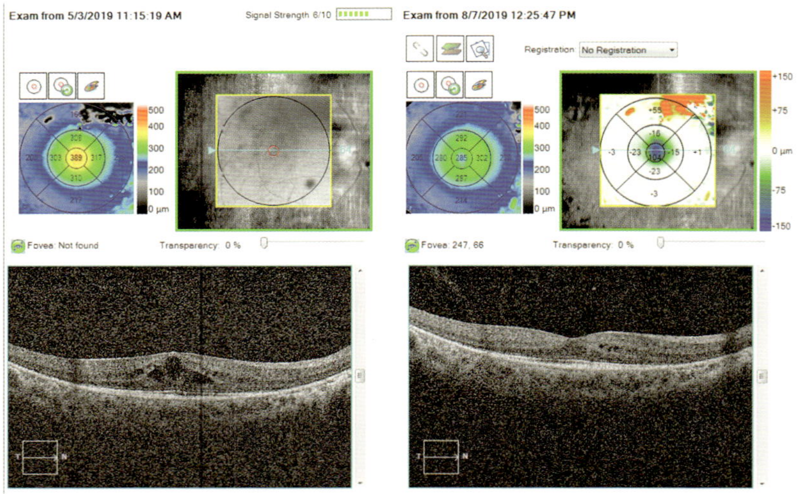


Figure 23 *OCT scan—macular thickness map of right eye shows macular edema with retinal thickening of 389 microns at presentation. He was prescribed topical dorzolamide eye drops to be used three times a day for 3 months. Macular thickness has reduced considerably at 3 months as seen on OCT macular thickness map (285 microns).*

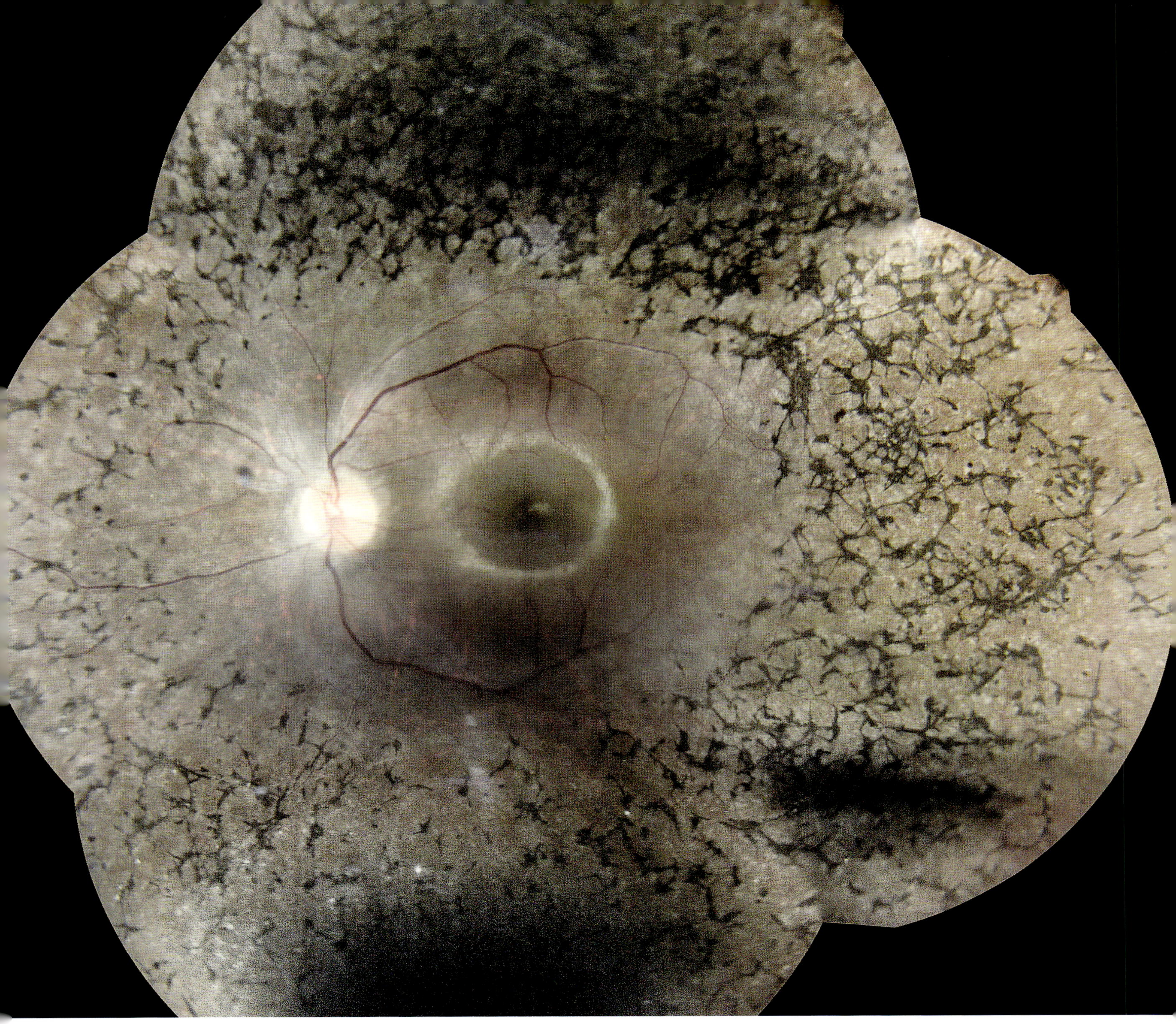

Figure 24 *Color fundus montage image of left eye of 28-year-old male with retinitis pigmentosa sparing the posterior pole.*

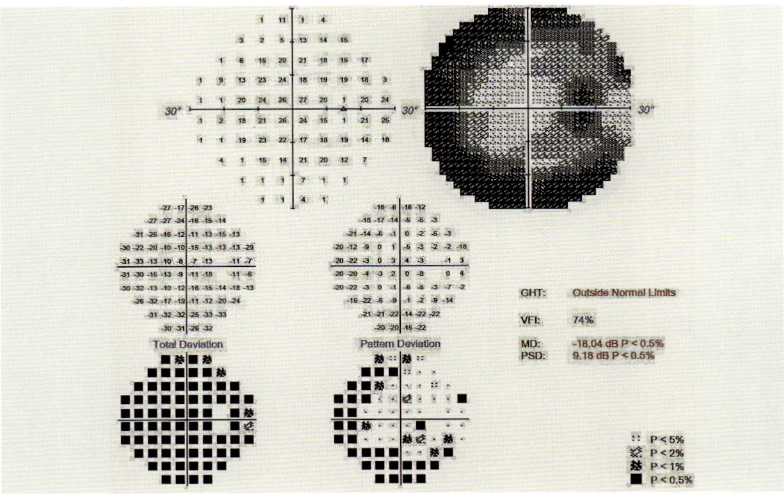

Figure 25 *Visual field of the right eye (30-2) shows mid-peripheral constriction.*

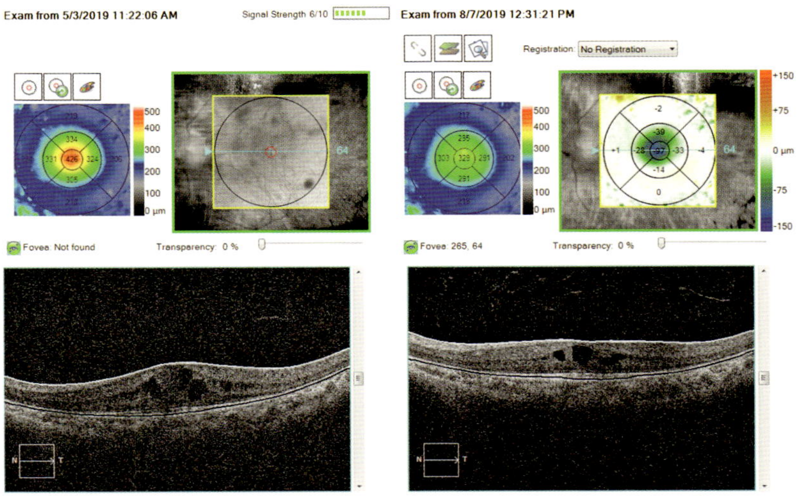

Figure 26 *Macular thickness map of the left eye at baseline and after 3 months of treatment. Macular thickness at baseline was 426 microns and has reduced to 329 microns at 3 months.* □

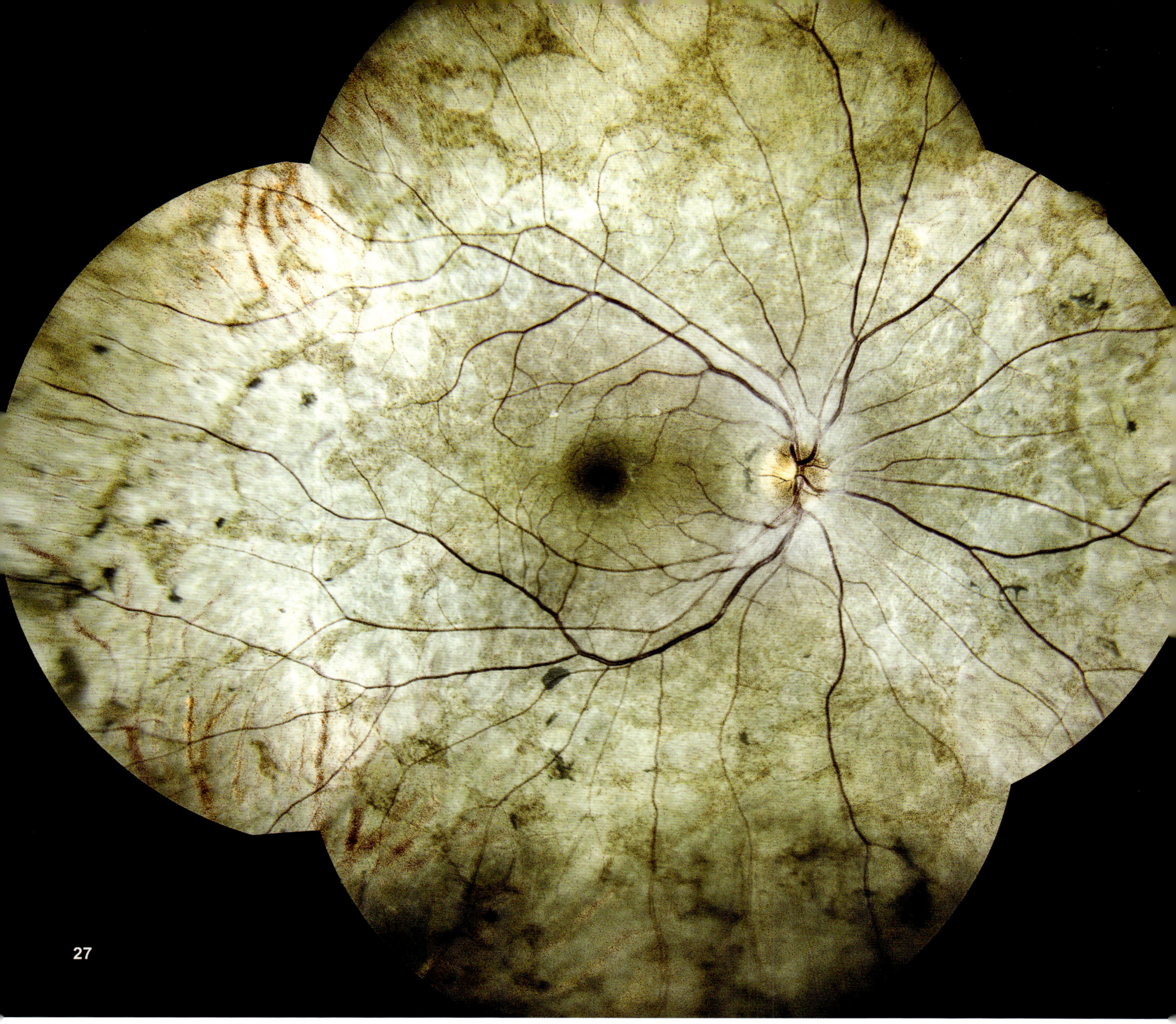

Figure 27 *Color fundus montage photograph of a patient with advanced gyrate atrophy. Gyrate atrophy is a rare autosomal recessive disease characterized by progressive chorioretinal degeneration which in the early stages is seen as well-defined circular patches of CRAO in the periphery, but as the disease advances atrophic lesions enlarge, coalesce and move centripetally correlating with progressive loss of peripheral vision.*

Gyrate atrophy is characterized by progressive vision loss. Over time field of vision continues to narrow resulting in tunnel vision. It is caused by deficiency of ornithine aminotransferase enzyme that leads to accumulation of excess ornithine levels in the plasma. The OAT enzyme converts ornithine into another molecule called P5C. Researchers have suggested that it is the deficiency of P5C that may interfere with the function of retina. So a subset of the patients who carry a genetic variant that is favorably responsive to supplementation with vitamin $B_6$ has been shown to partially restore the function of OAT enzyme.

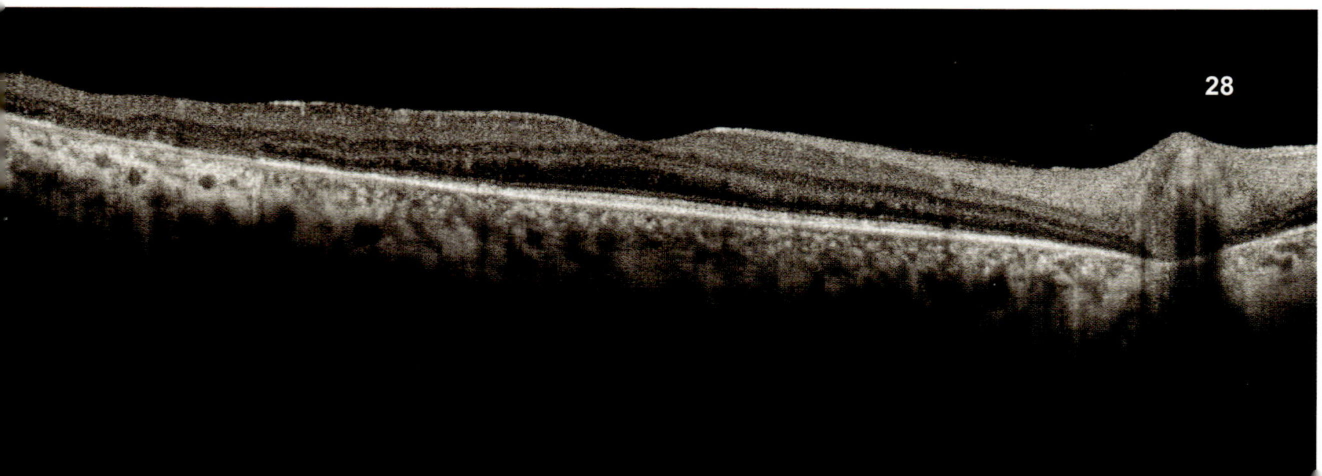

Figure 28

*Swept source OCT scan shows preserved IS/OS signal in and around the foveal region. At temporal edge of the scan note the presence of extensive loss of IS/OS layer, RPE and inner choroid reflectivity.*

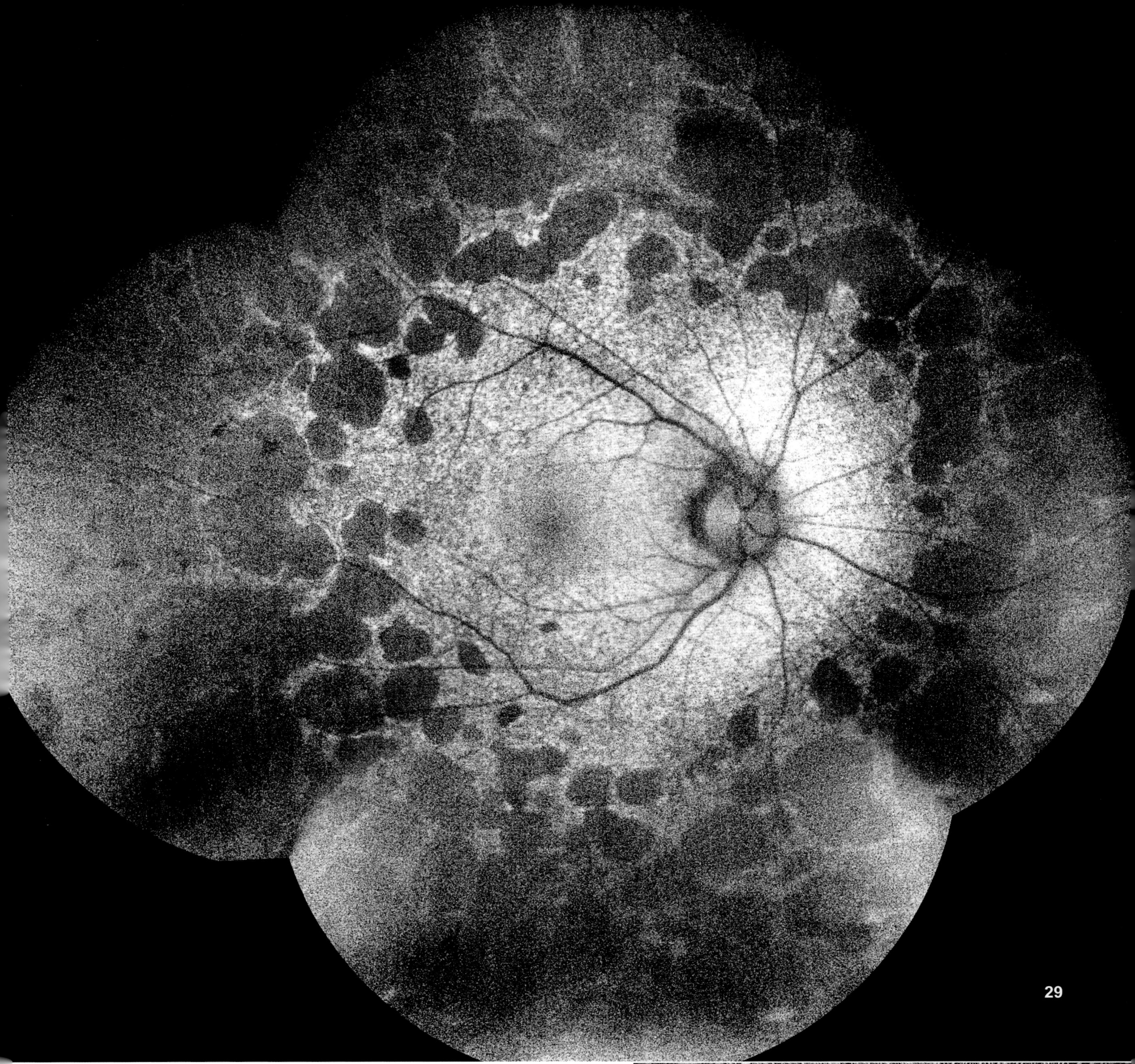



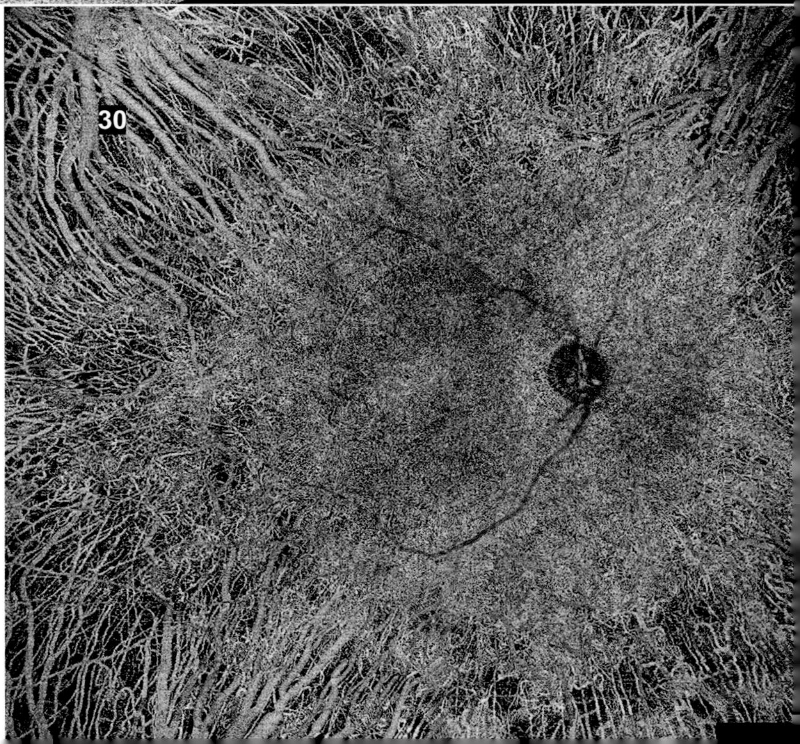



Figure 29 *Widefield autofluorescence montage in a patient with gyrate atrophy.*

Autofluorescence montage photograph shows focal and few confluent areas of absent autofluorescence which corresponds with the area of chorioretinal atrophy seen on fundus photograph.

Figure 30 *Widefield optical coherence tomography angiogram demonstrating visibility of large choroidal vessels in the mid-periphery secondary to atrophy of retinal pigment epithelium.*

Figure 31

*Color fundus montage image of a patient with advanced gyrate atrophy.*

Color image shows bilaterally symmetrical distribution of large patches of chorioretinal atrophy with small islands of preserved retina in between and at the macula.

Figure 32

*Swept source OCT scan in gyrate atrophy.*

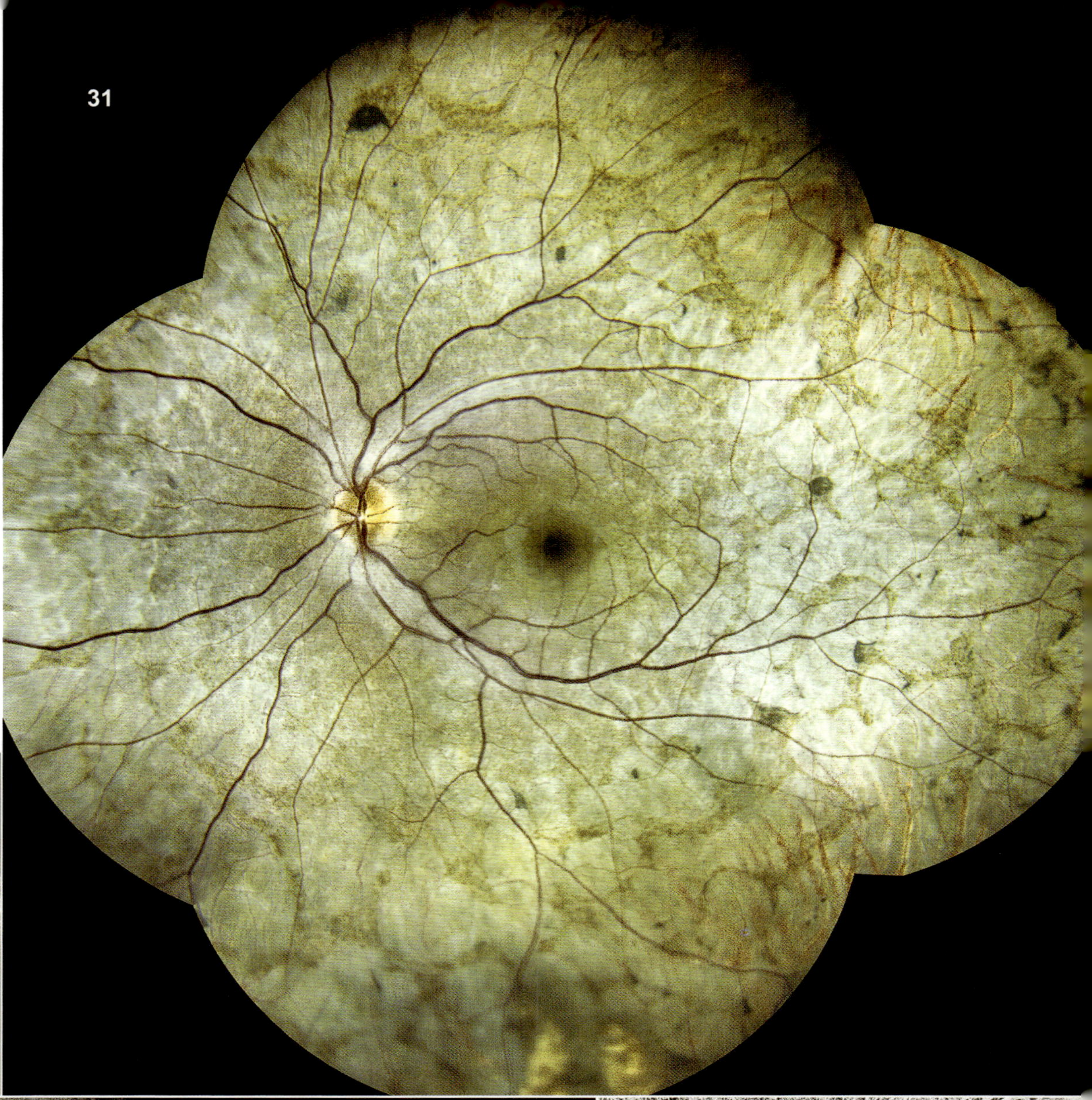


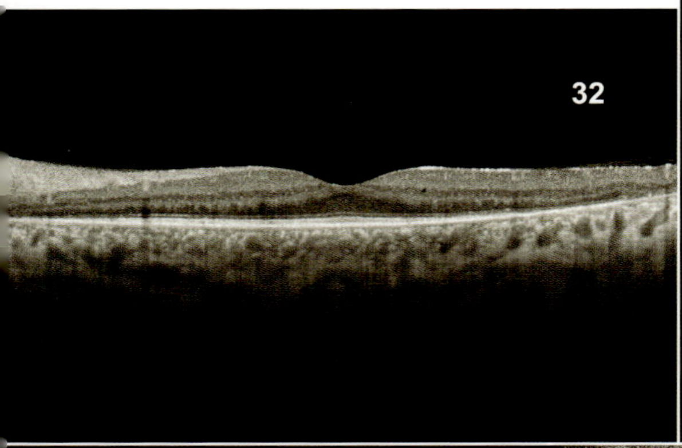


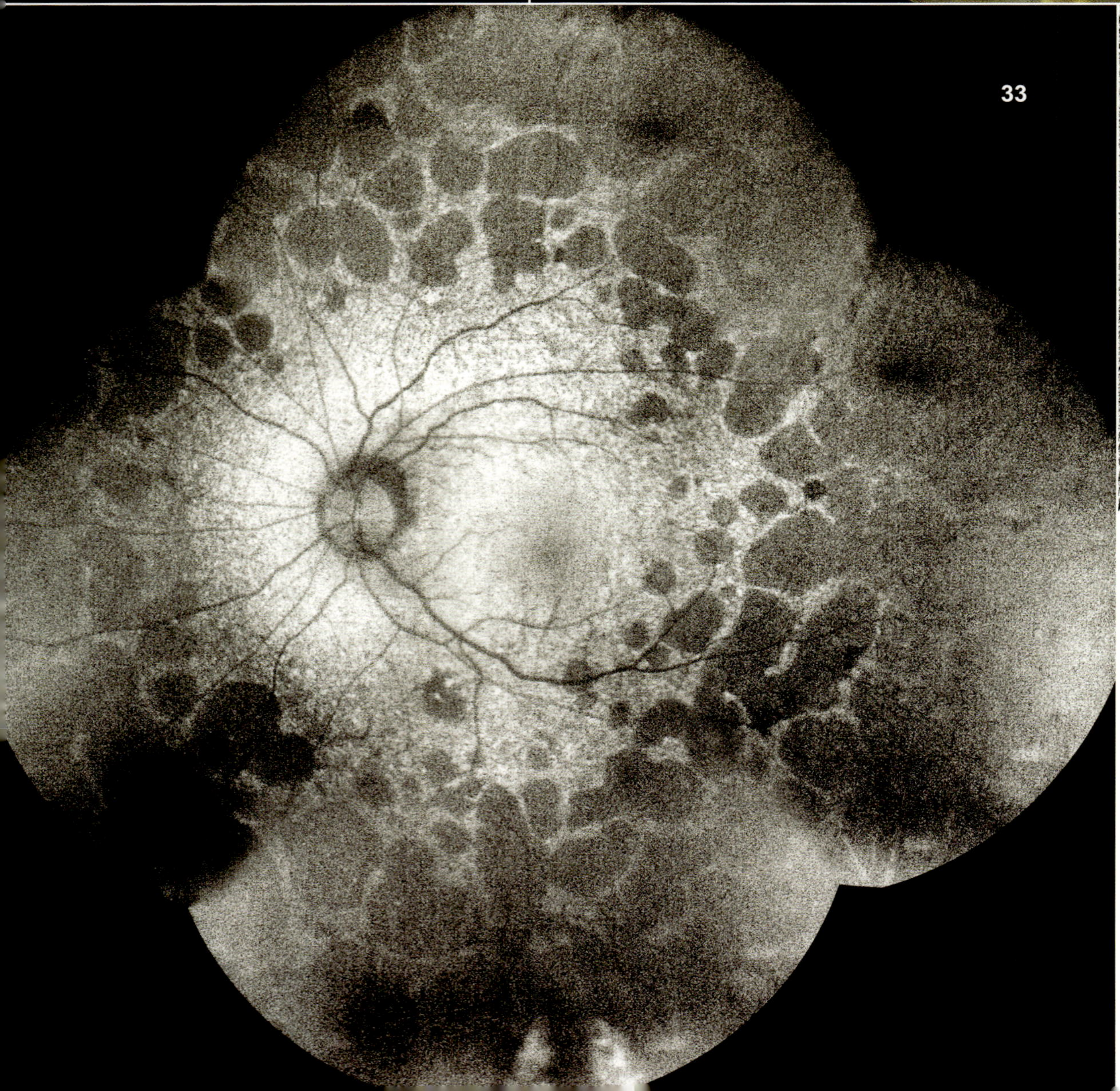


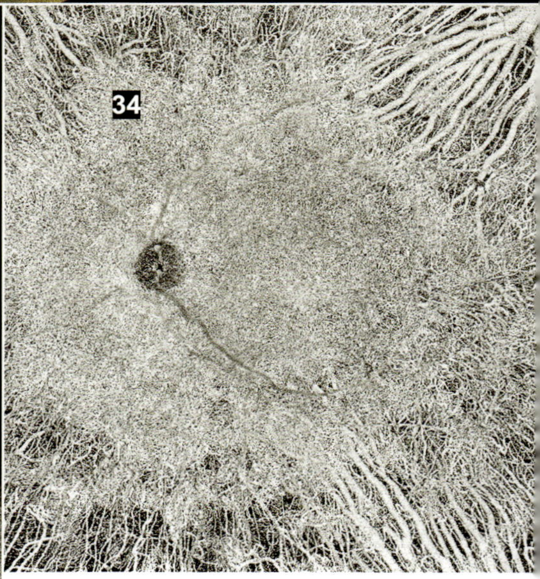


Figure 33

*Widefield autofluorescence montage in a patient with gyrate atrophy.*

Figure 34

*Widefield optical coherence tomography angiogram demonstrating visibility of large choroidal vessels in the mid-periphery secondary to atrophy of retinal pigment epithelium.*□

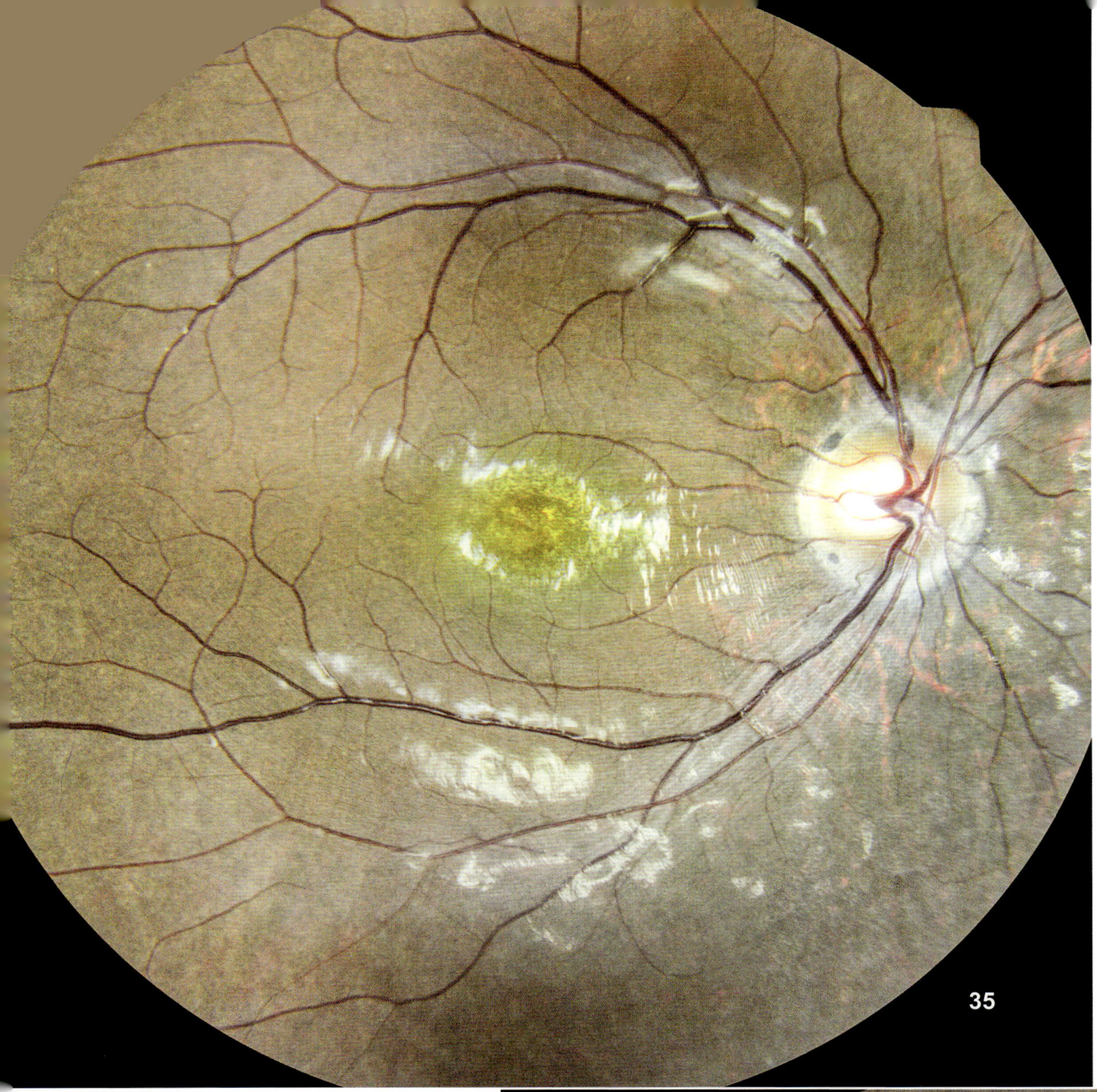

Figure 35

*Case of hereditary macular dystrophy.*

Abnormal yellowish sheen is seen at the fovea due to underlying RPE atrophy. Rest of the retina, vessels and optic nerve appears normal.

Macular dystrophy is characterized by abnormal changes restricted to the posterior pole. Patients usually present in their childhood with complaints of difficulty in reading/reading a book too close to the face. Disease usually progresses slowly over time but visual impairment is restricted to fine visual tasks only. Thus, it is important to have a confirmatory diagnosis and right counseling after excluding other progressive rod cone retinal dystrophy's which usually have a much worse prognosis and could cause complete blindness in few advanced stages of dystrophy's.

Figure 36

*Case of hereditary macular dystrophy—left eye of the same patient.*

Note the symmetrical presentation with macular involvement only. Fovea is showing granular appearance. □

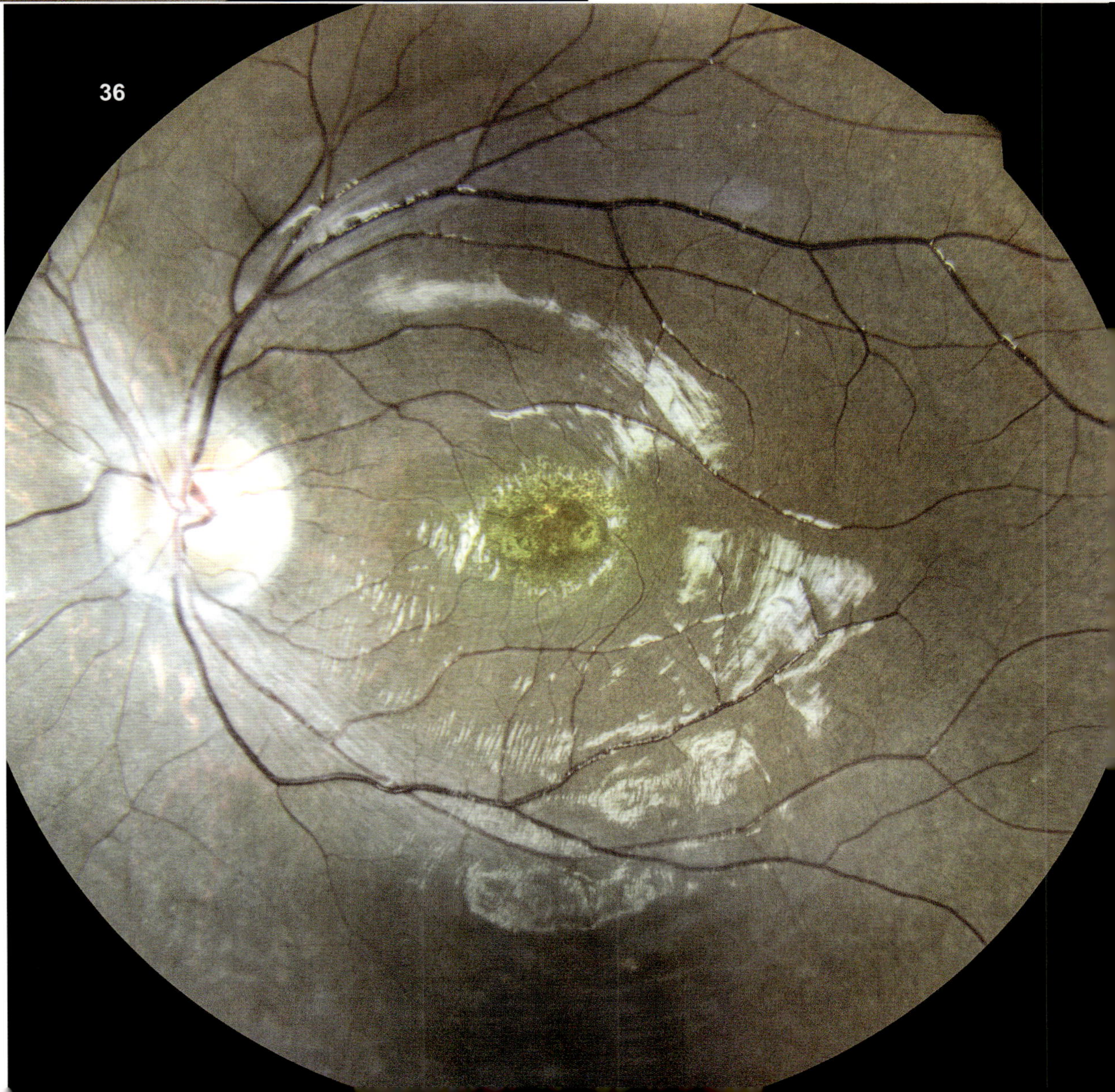

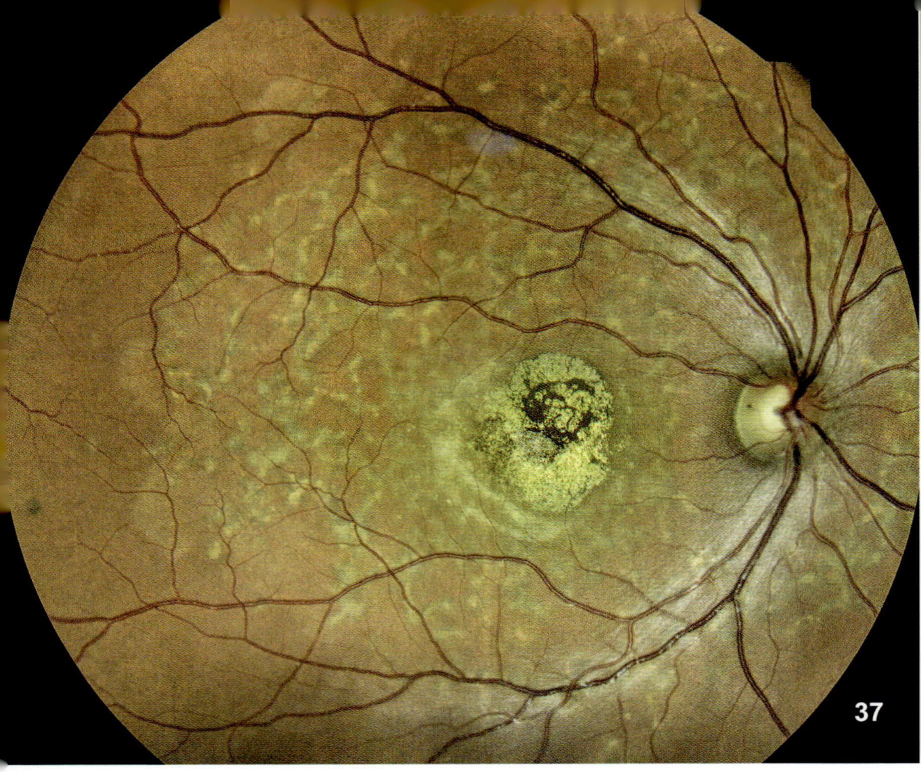

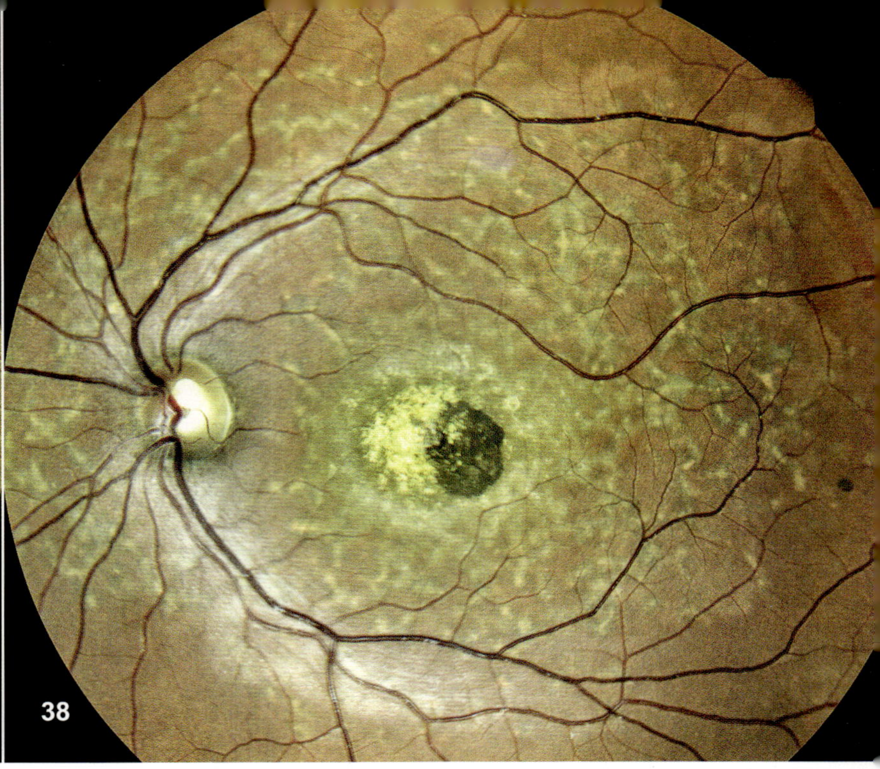

Figure 37 *Case of atrophic macular dystrophy with fundus flavimaculatus. Stargardt's disease. Posterior pole of both eyes show a virtually symmetric fundus picture consisting of yellowish spots below the level of retinal vessels. These yellow spots are ill-defined and shaped like a crescent, shark fin or fish tail. They are forming garlands around the fovea. Fovea appears yellowish atrophic with RPE hyperpigmentation.*

Figure 38 *Case of atrophic macular dystrophy with fundus flavimaculatus (left eye).*

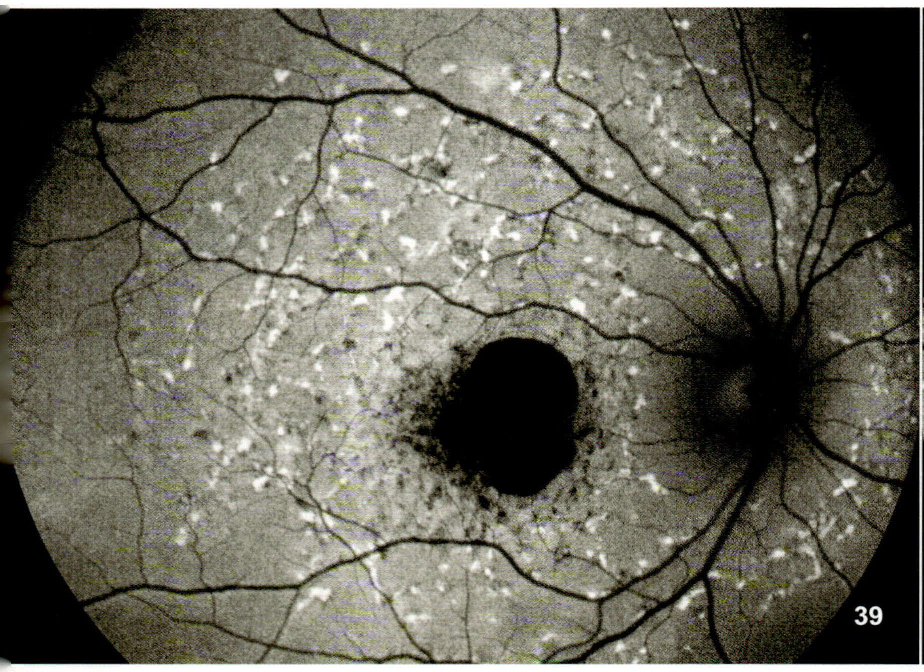

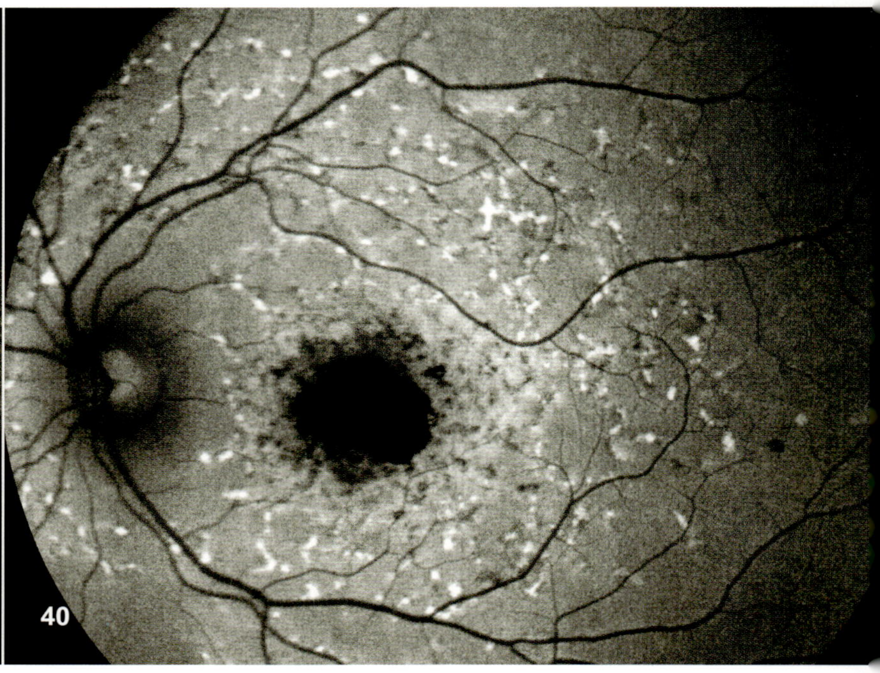

Figure 39 *Fundus autofluorescence photograph of the right eye demonstrating complete loss of autofluorescence at the fovea and hyperautofluorescence from the flecks.*

Figure 40 *Fundus autofluorescence of the left eye shows similar abnormalities of RPE loss at the fovea resulting in well-defined patch of hypoautofluorescent at the fovea.*

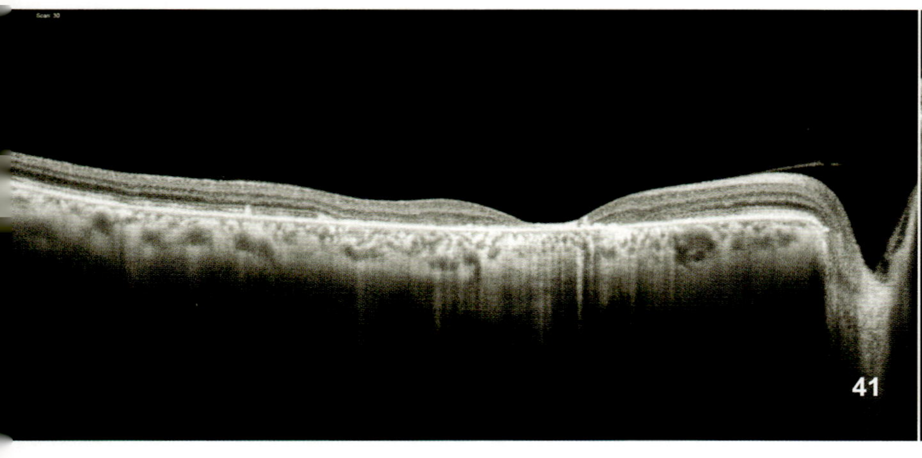

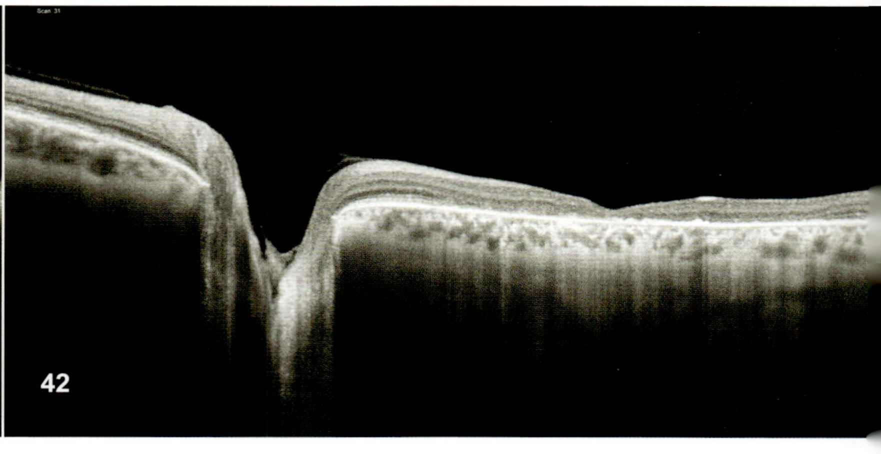

Figure 41 *Swept source OCT scan of the right eye demonstrating outer retinal atrophy at the fovea.*

Figure 42 *Swept source OCT scan of the left eye in a patient with advanced Stargardt's disease.* □

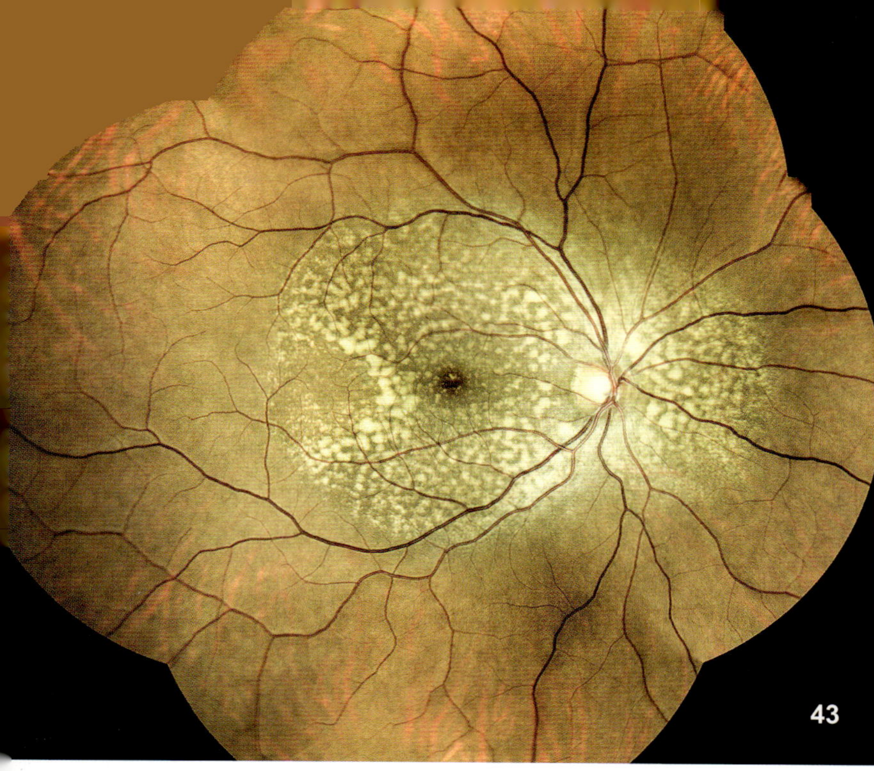


Figure 43 *Color fundus montage photograph of a case of familial (hereditary) drusen in a 44-year-old female.*

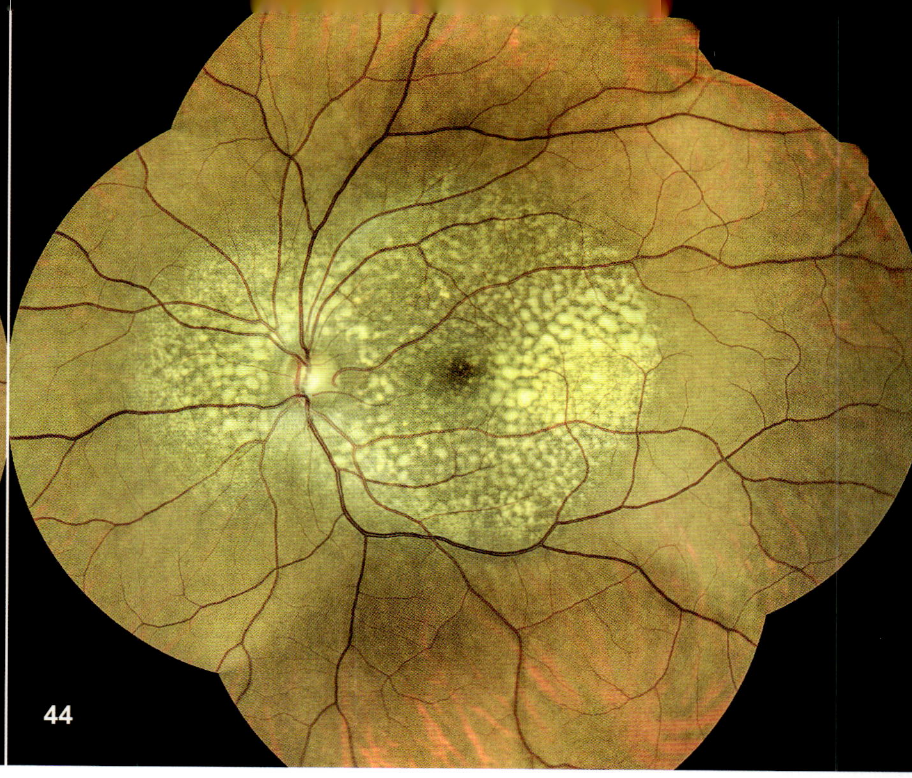


Figure 44 *Left eye color fundus montage photograph of a case of familial drusen.*

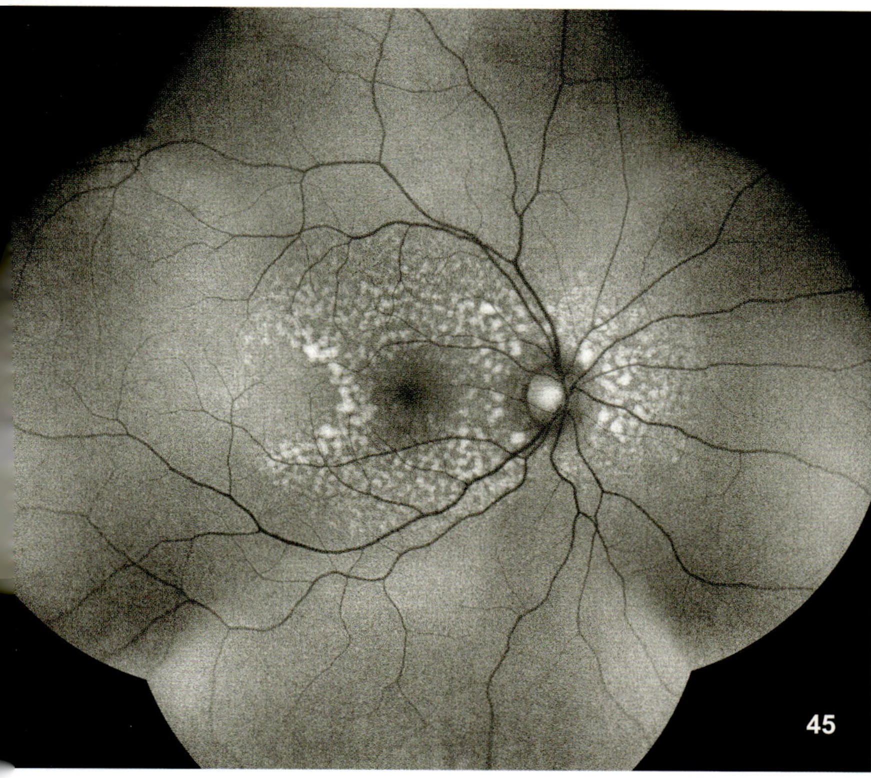


Figure 45 *Hyperautofluorescent dots corresponding to the drusens are seen on the autofluorescence montage image.*

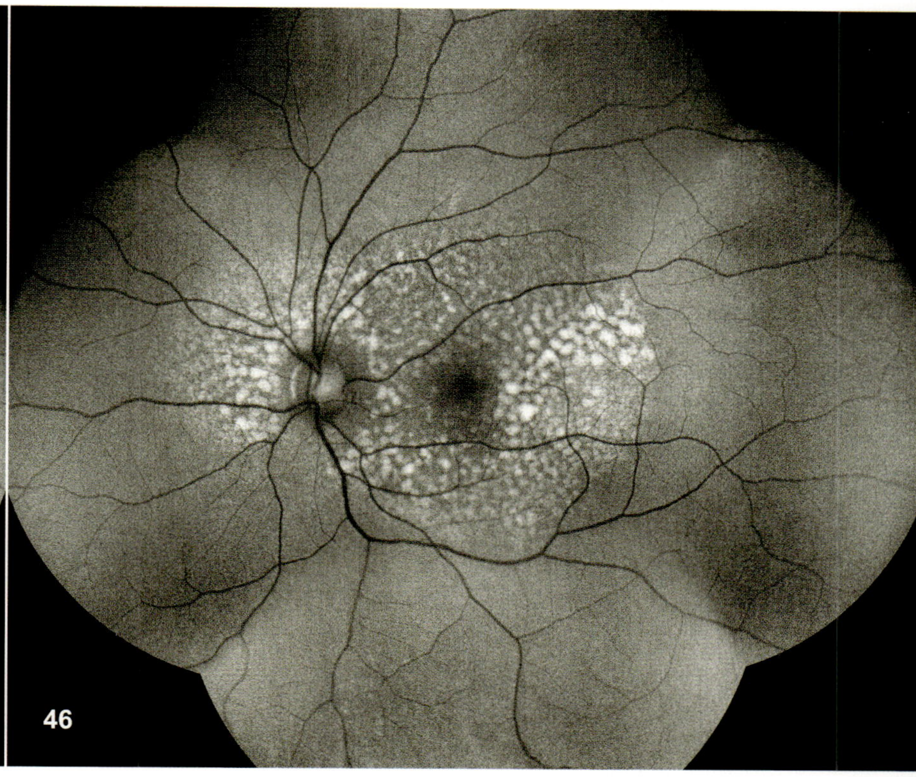


Figure 46 *Hyperautofluorescent dots corresponding to the drusens are seen on the autofluorescence montage image.*

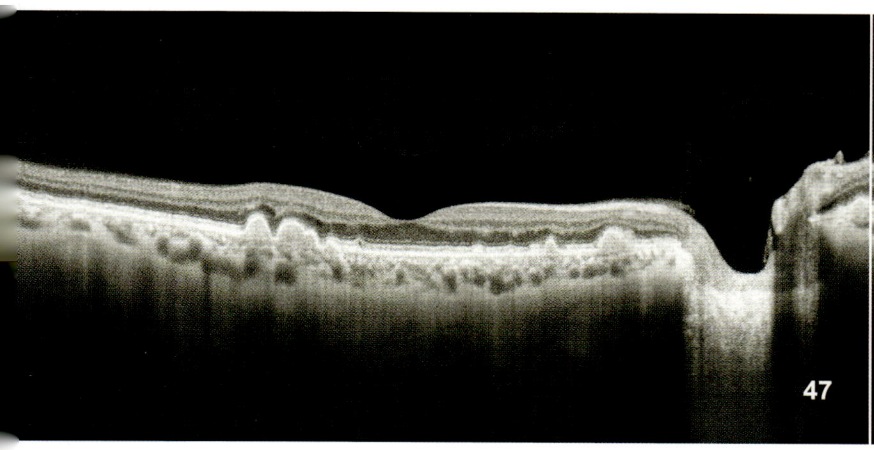


Figure 47 *OCT scans demonstrating drusens seen as RPE layer irregularities.*

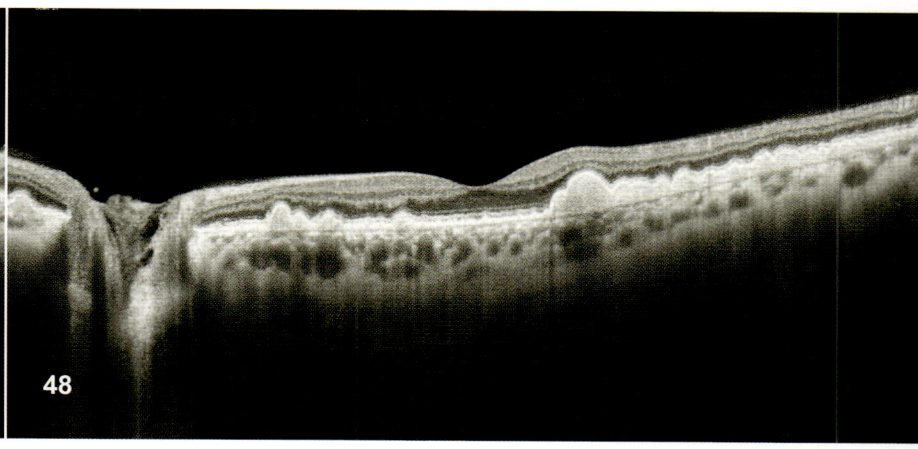


Figure 48 *Small dome-shaped drusenoid deposits at the level of retinal pigment epithelium in a case of familial drusen.* □

Figure 49

*Oculocutaneous albinism—left eye fundus photograph.*

Albinism refers to a group of genetic disorder that involves an abnormality of melanin synthesis in conjunction with characteristic visual and ocular pathway abnormalities. Oculocutaneous albinism involves hypopigmentation of skin, hair and eyes. Ocular clinical features include refractive errors. Pendular nystagmus, foveal hypoplasia, iris transillumination defect, strabismus, poor vision and abnormal decussation of visual pathways. Management involves optimizing the visual function by correction of refractive errors, nystagmus, squint and through medical examination to evaluate for the presence of systemic syndrome and such patients are strongly encouraged to limit the sun exposure through avoiding outdoor occupations and use of sun protective agents.

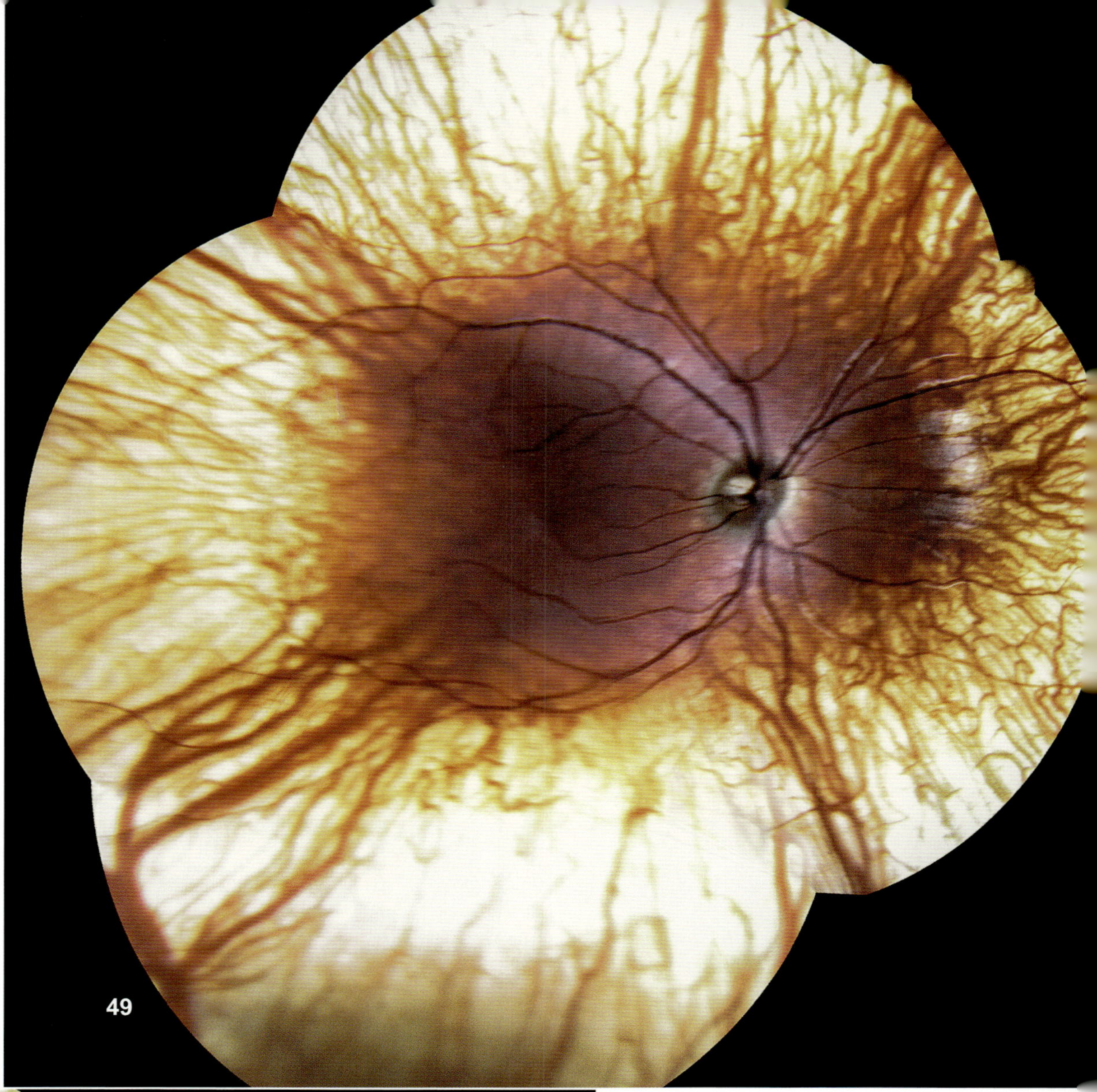


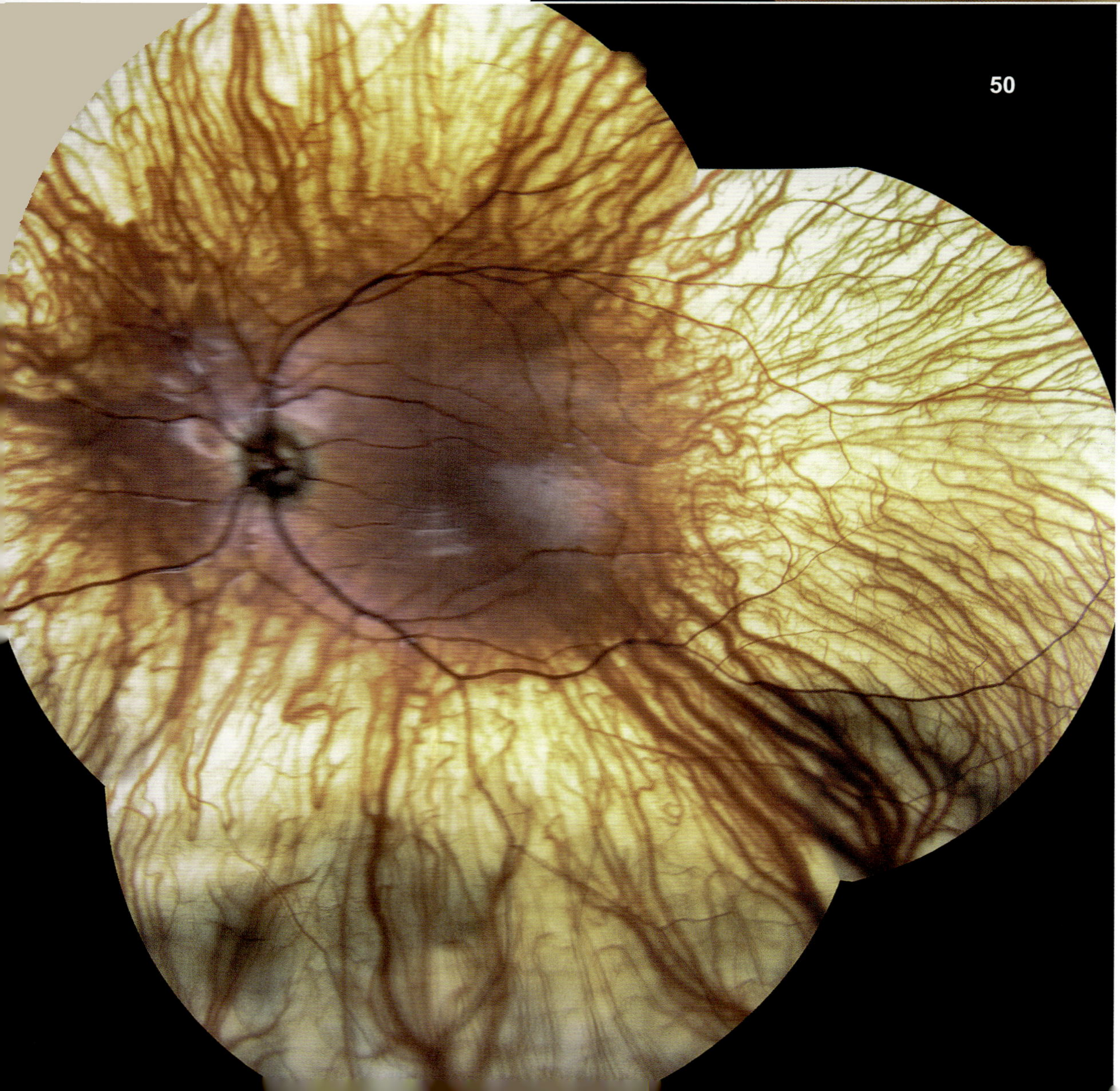


Figure 50

*Oculocutaneous albinism—right eye fundus.*

Fundus photographs of a 14-year-old boy with oculocutaneous albinism showing pigmentation sufficient to mask the choroidal vessels at the posterior pole, but with peripheral hypopigmentation described as "mud splattered appearance" due to areas of hypopigmentation interdigitating with normal pigmentation. Note foveal reflex is absent in both eyes.□

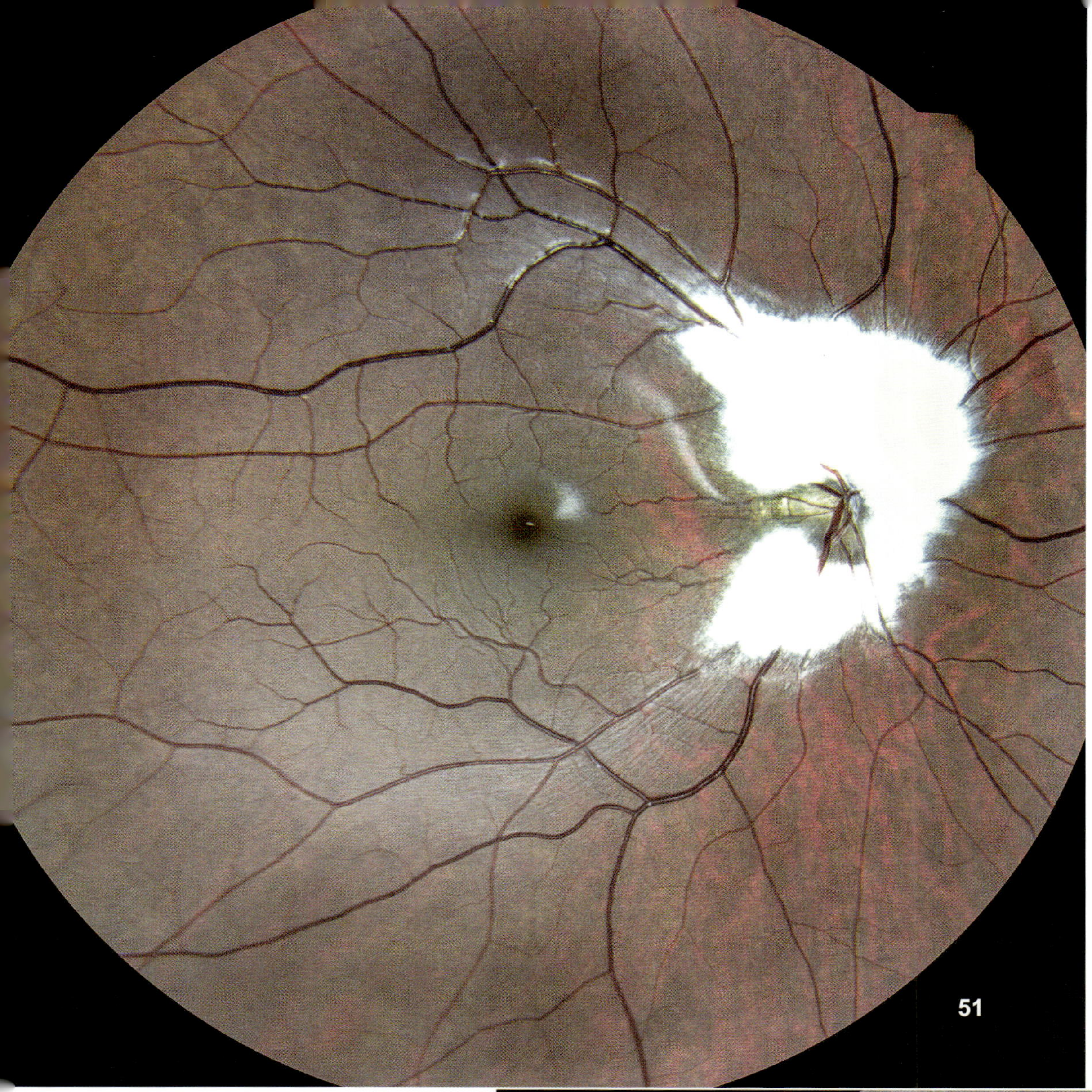


Figure 51

*Myelinated nerve fibers:gray white well demarcated feathery patches along the retinal nerve fiber layer obscuring the retinal vessels is seen in right eye and left eye.*

It is a rare congenital anomaly in which retinal nerve fibers are mistakenly myelinated. The exact pathogenesis is not known.

Oligodendrocytes are responsible for the myelination of ganglion cell axons which normally began at the lateral geniculate body and proceeds anteriorly to end at the lamina cribrosa, which is thought to act as a barriers to the anterior migration of myelination of retinal nerve fibers.

It has been postulated that myelinated retinal nerve fibers results from an imbalance between the formation of lamina cribrosa and the process of myelination. This imbalance is more likely to occur in myopia due to the enlarged eyeball. Myelinated nerve fibers in majority of the cases does not affect the patients vision, however it may be associated with myopia, strabismus which causes poor vision.

Figure 52

*Color fundus photograph demonstrating myelinated nerve fiber at the optic disk margin in the left eye.* □

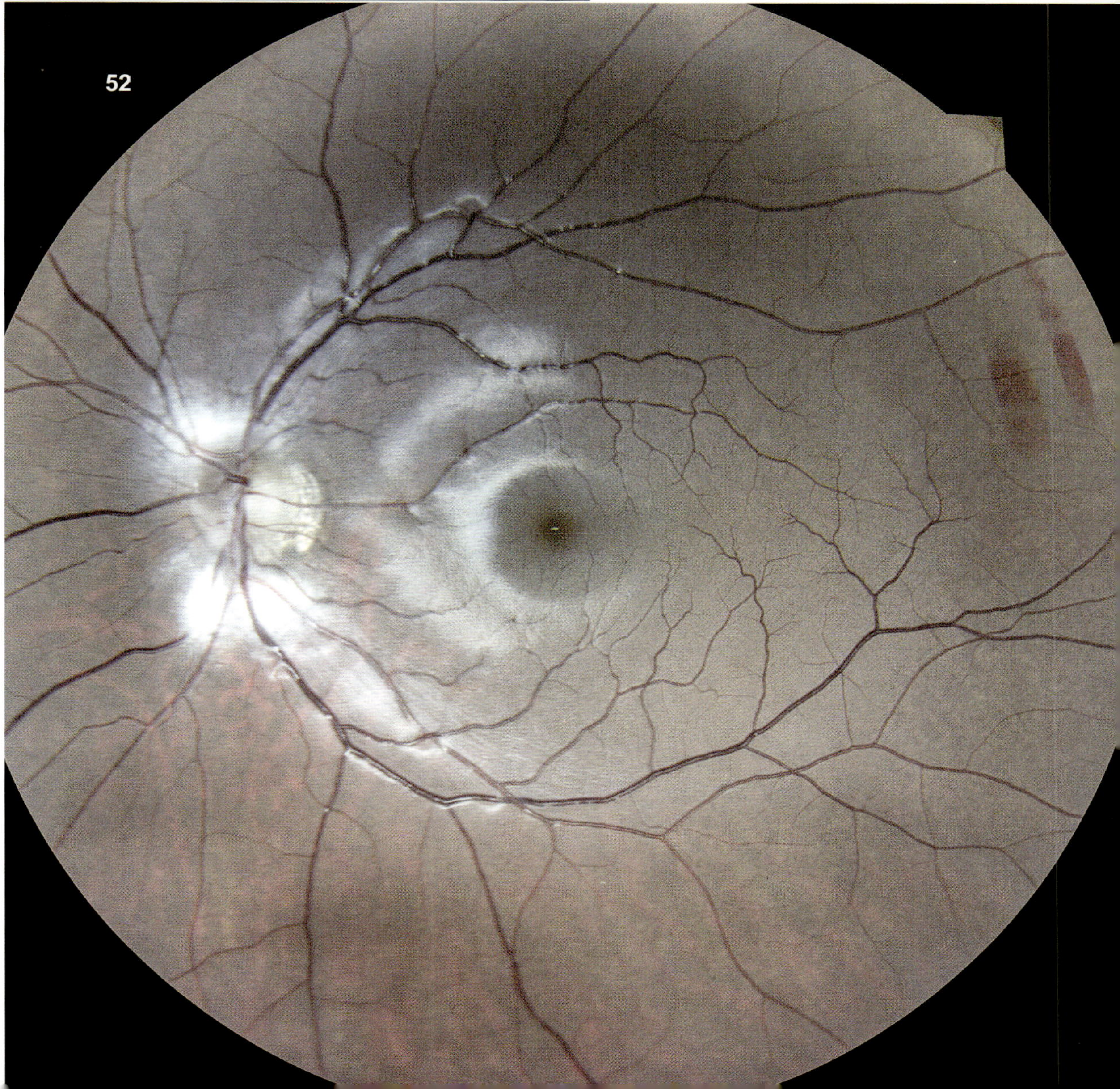

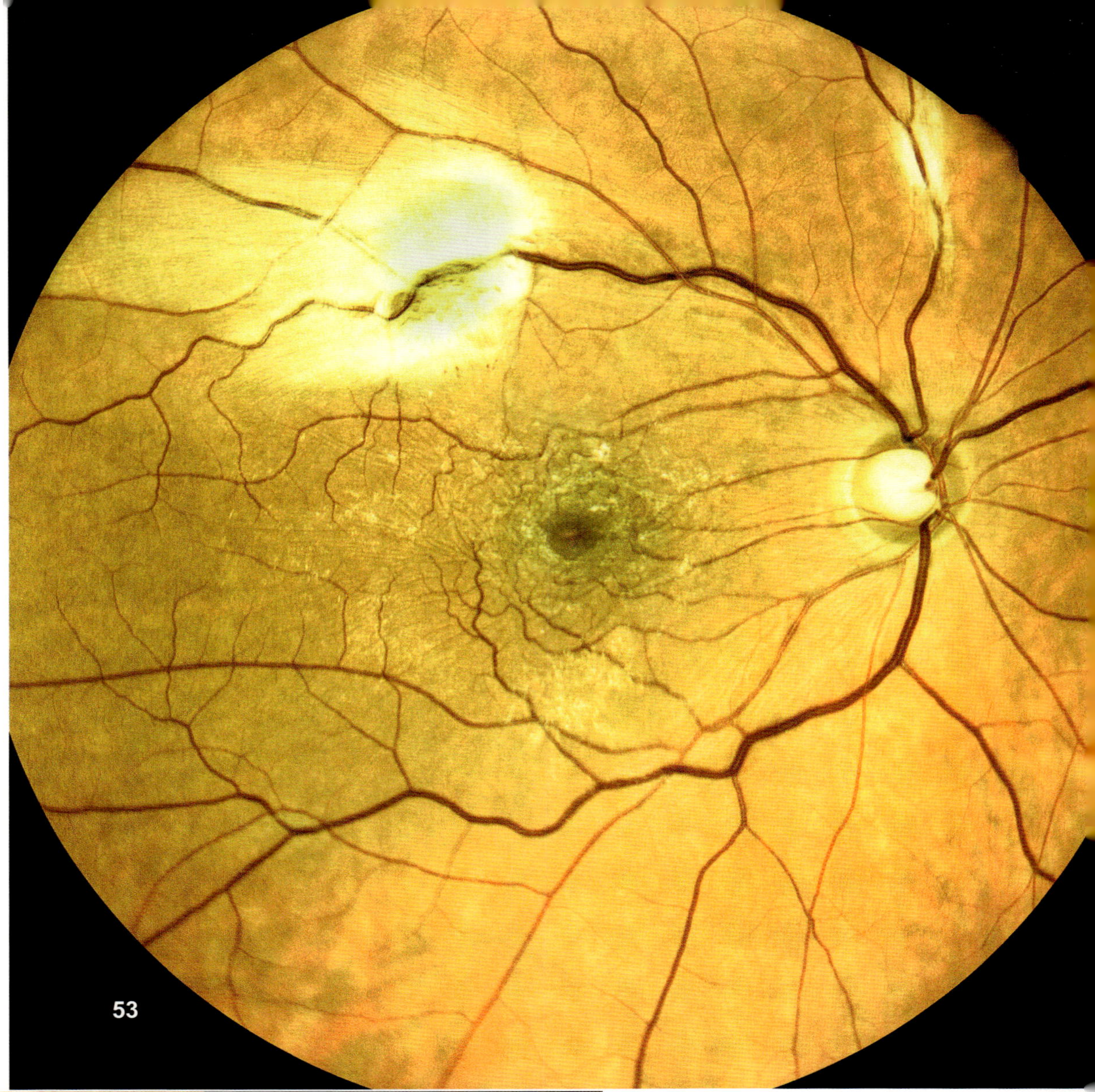

53

Figure 53

*A case of myelinated nerve fiber with epiretinal membrane in both eyes.*

A 52-year-old male came for routine eye examination, BCVA was 6/9 both eyes. Color fundus photo shows gray white well demarcated patches with frayed borders along retinal nerve fiber layer obscuring underlying retinal vessel suggestive of myelinated retinal nerve fiber (MRNF) which is discontinuous form the optic nerve head. Grayish white cellophane reflex at macula suggestive of epiretinal membrane can be seen.

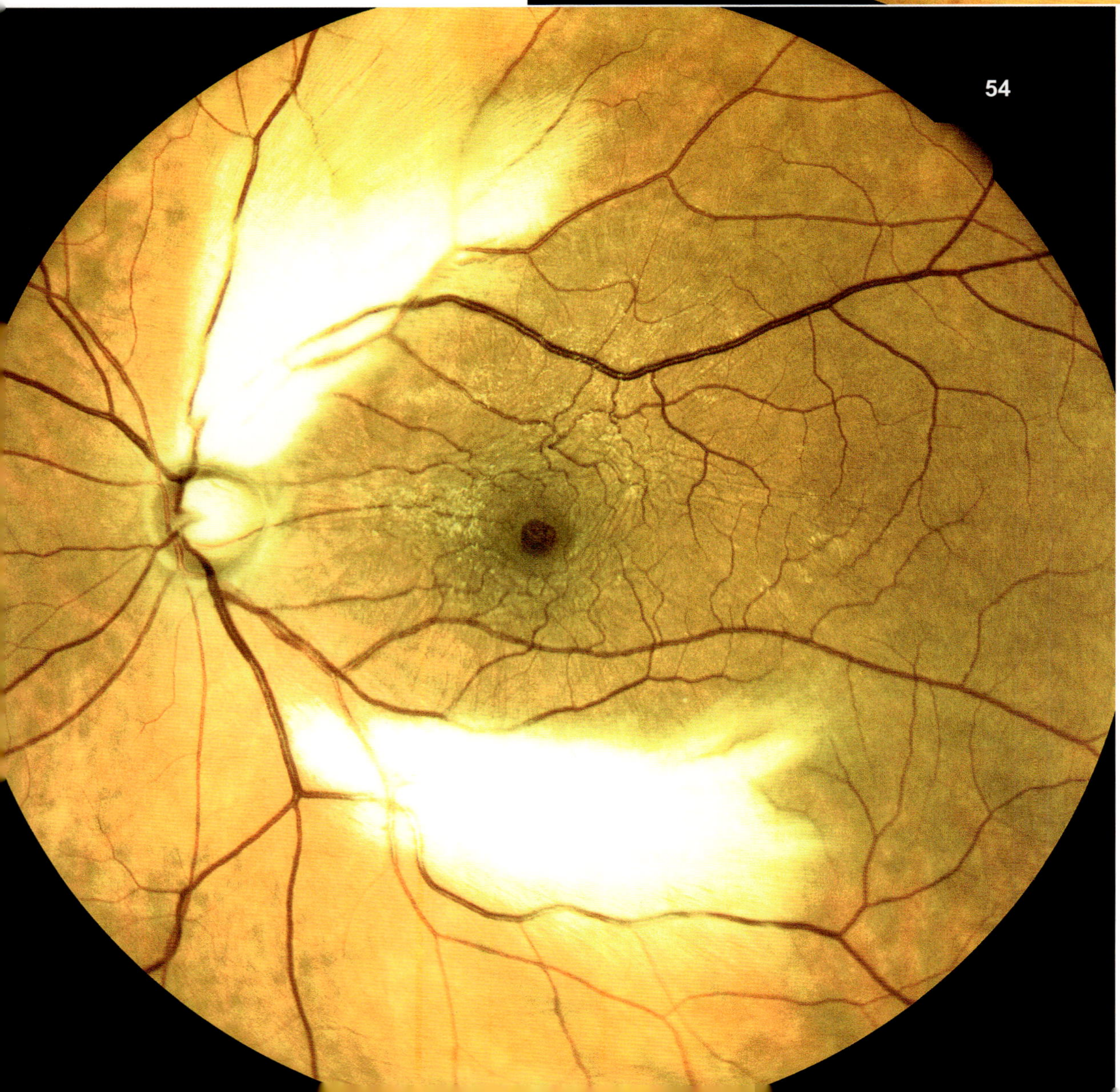

54

Figure 54

*Color fundus photo shows gray white well-demarcated patches with frayed borders along retinal nerve fiber layer obscuring underlying retinal vessel suggestive of myelinated retinal nerve fiber (MRNF) which is continuous form the optic nerve head unlike the other eye. Cellophane reflex at macula suggestive of epiretinal membrane can be seen. MRNF are typically present at birth and are static lesions, they can occur bilaterally in around 7% of cases. Most patients are asymptomatic.* □

# CHAPTER 8

## OCULAR TUMORS AND OPTIC NERVE DISORDERS

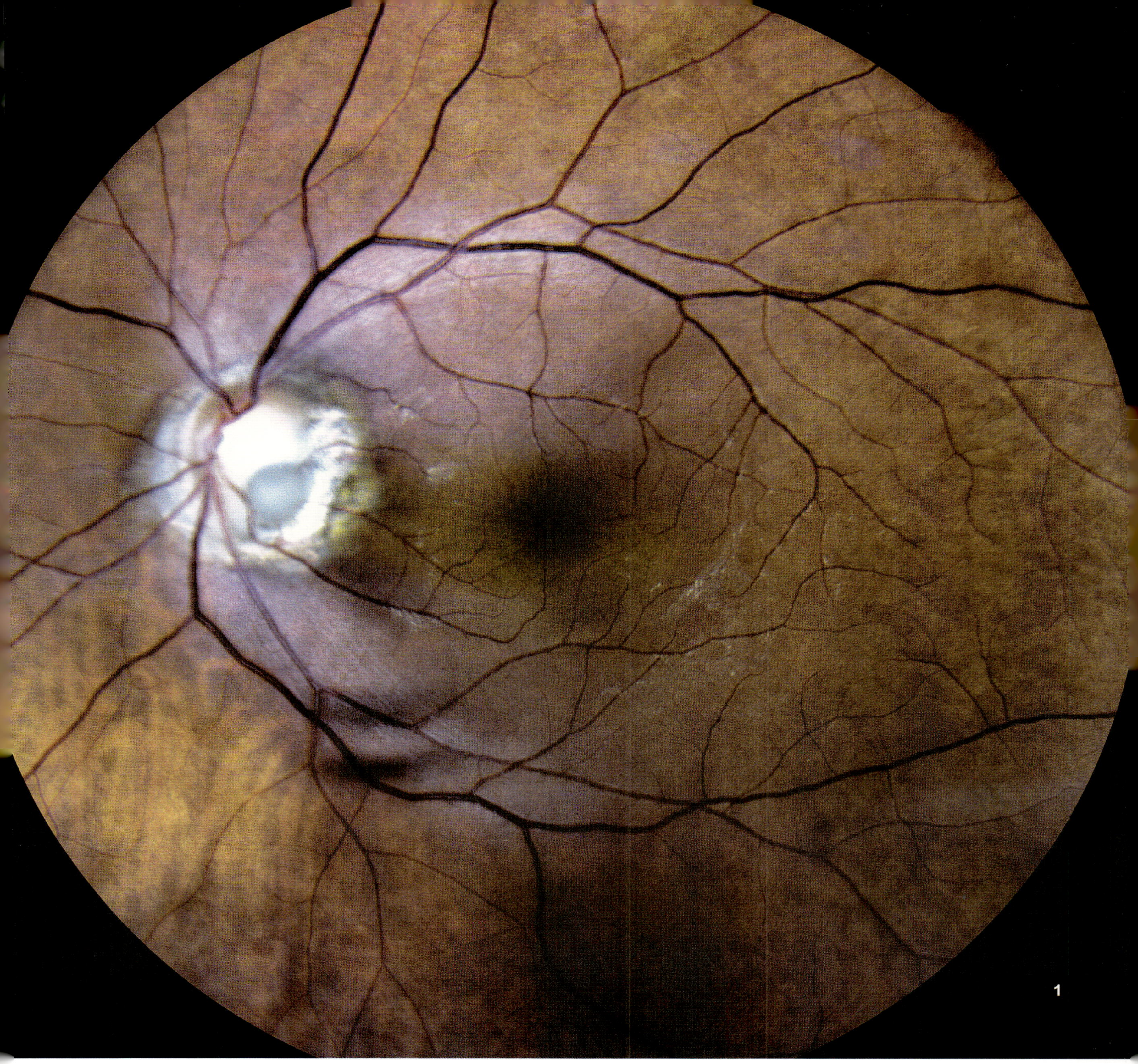

Figure 1 *Color fundus photograph demonstrating an optic disc pit. Note the presence of a grayish oval depression at the inferotemporal aspect of the optic disc.*

Optic disc pits are considered as a part of the spectrum of congenital cavity anomalies. Histologically, optic disc pit is herniation of the dysplastic retina into the collagen rich excavation that extends into the subarachnoid space through the defect in lamina cribrosa. Optic pits are usually unilateral in 85% of the cases. They may cause visual symptoms if they are complicated by a maculopathy.

Figure 2 *Horizontal optical coherence tomography scan through the optic pit shows communication between the pit and schisis cavity in the outer retina.* □

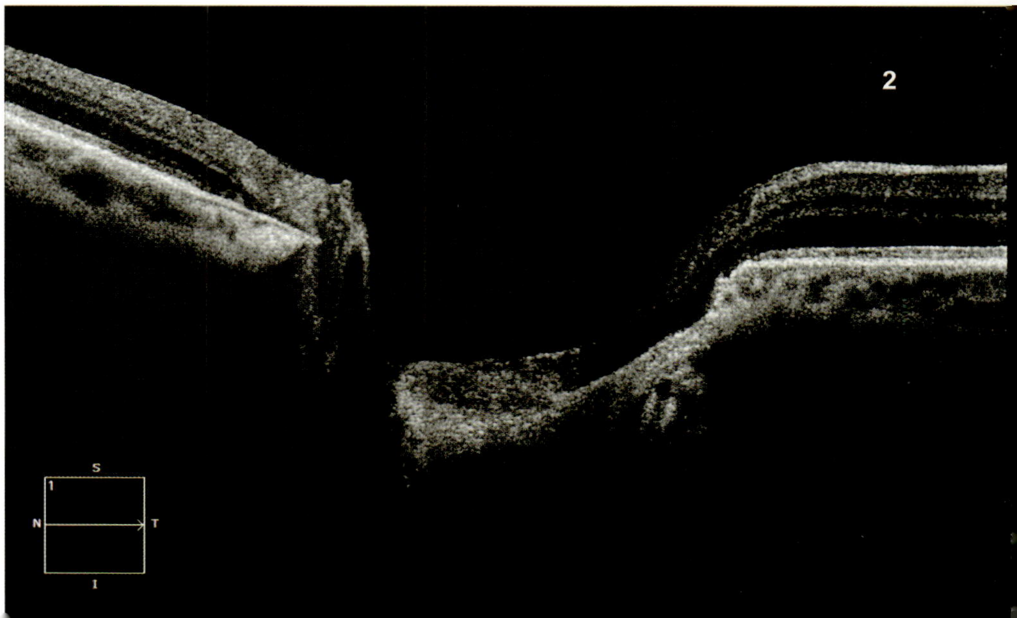

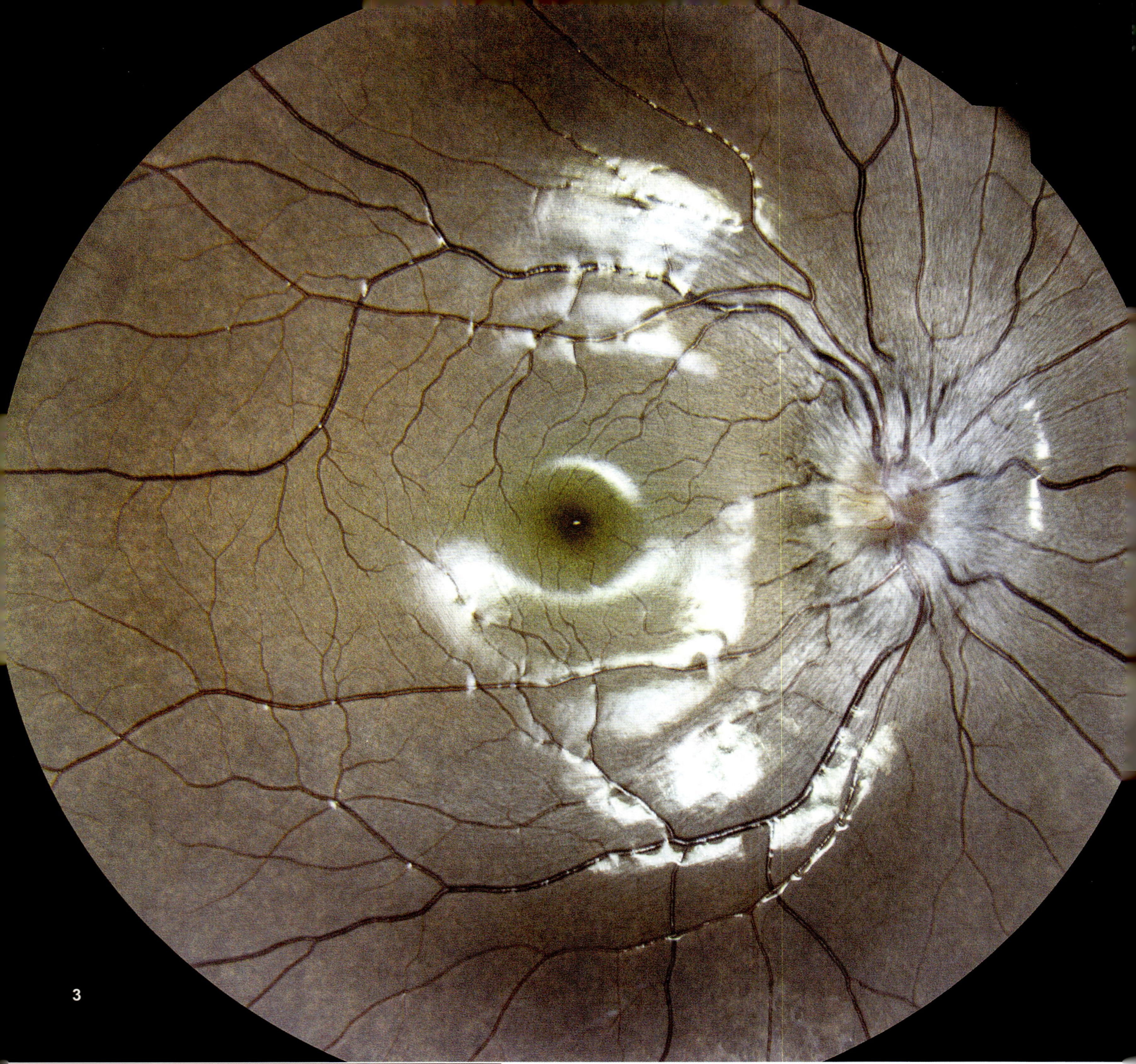

3

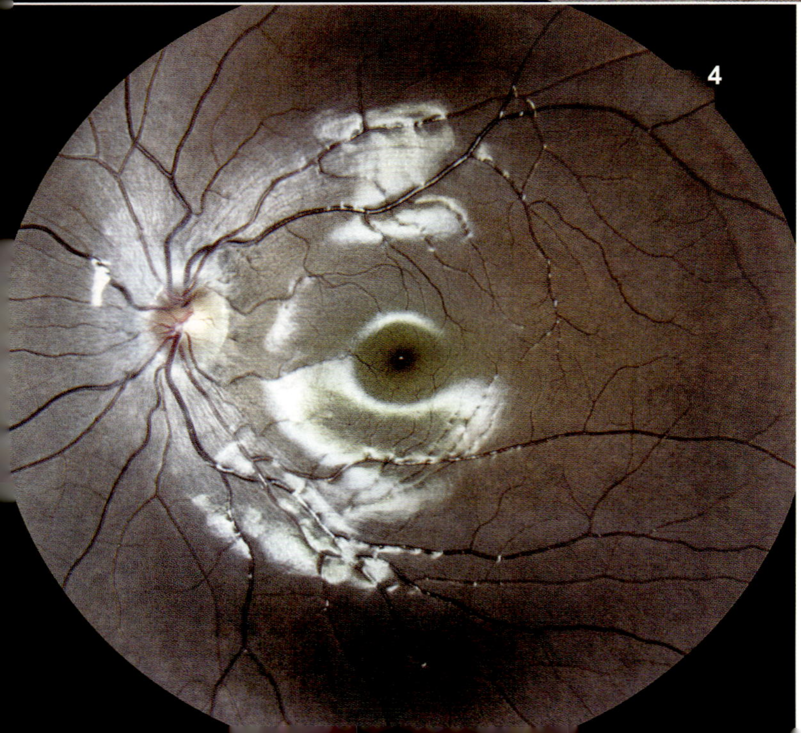

4

Figure 3 *Case of unilateral disk edema.*

Color fundus photograph of the right eye demonstrates edematous optic disk with blurred margins. Retinal vessels appear tortuous as they exit from the optic disk.

This is a case of 15-year-old young girl who was recently diagnosed with ovarian torsion cyst and started on oral contraceptive pills by her gynecologist. She presented to ophthalmological clinic with complaints of blurred painless vision loss in her right eye. Left eye was asymptomatic. She was diagnosed as a unilateral disk edema and underwent magnetic resonance imaging of her brain and was diagnosed with cerebral venous thrombosis (sagittal, straight and lateral sinus thrombosis). She was then started on oral warfarin and oral acetazolamide.

Figure 4 *Normal appearance of the optic disk in the left eye of the same patient.*□

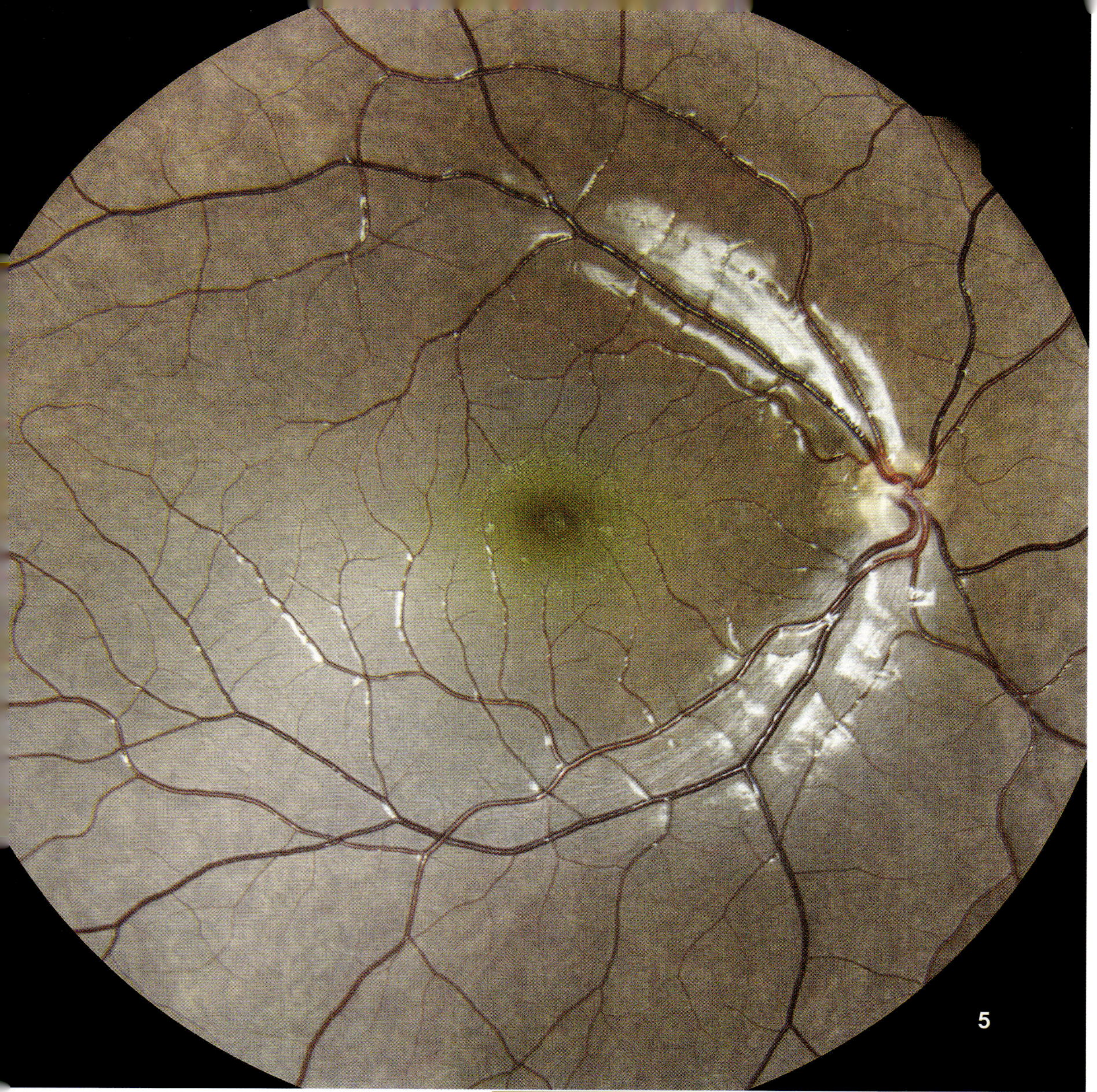

Figure 5

*A case of optic nerve hypoplasia (ONH) which is a congenital anomaly of the optic disk that might result in moderate to severe vision loss.*

A 14-year-old female presented with complaints of diminished vision in both eyes since childhood. Color fundus photo of both eyes demonstrates a small disk which is pale with peripapillary double-ring sign, vascular tortuosity, and thinning of the nerve fiber layer.

A patient with ONH should be assessed for presence of neurologic, radiologic, and endocrine associations. There may be maternal associations like premature births, fetal alcohol syndrome, and maternal diabetes. Systemic associations in the child include endocrine abnormalities, developmental delay, cerebral palsy, and seizures. Besides the hypoplastic optic nerve and chiasm, neuroimaging shows abnormalities in ventricles or white- or gray-matter development, septo-optic dysplasia, hydrocephalus, and corpus callosum abnormalities.

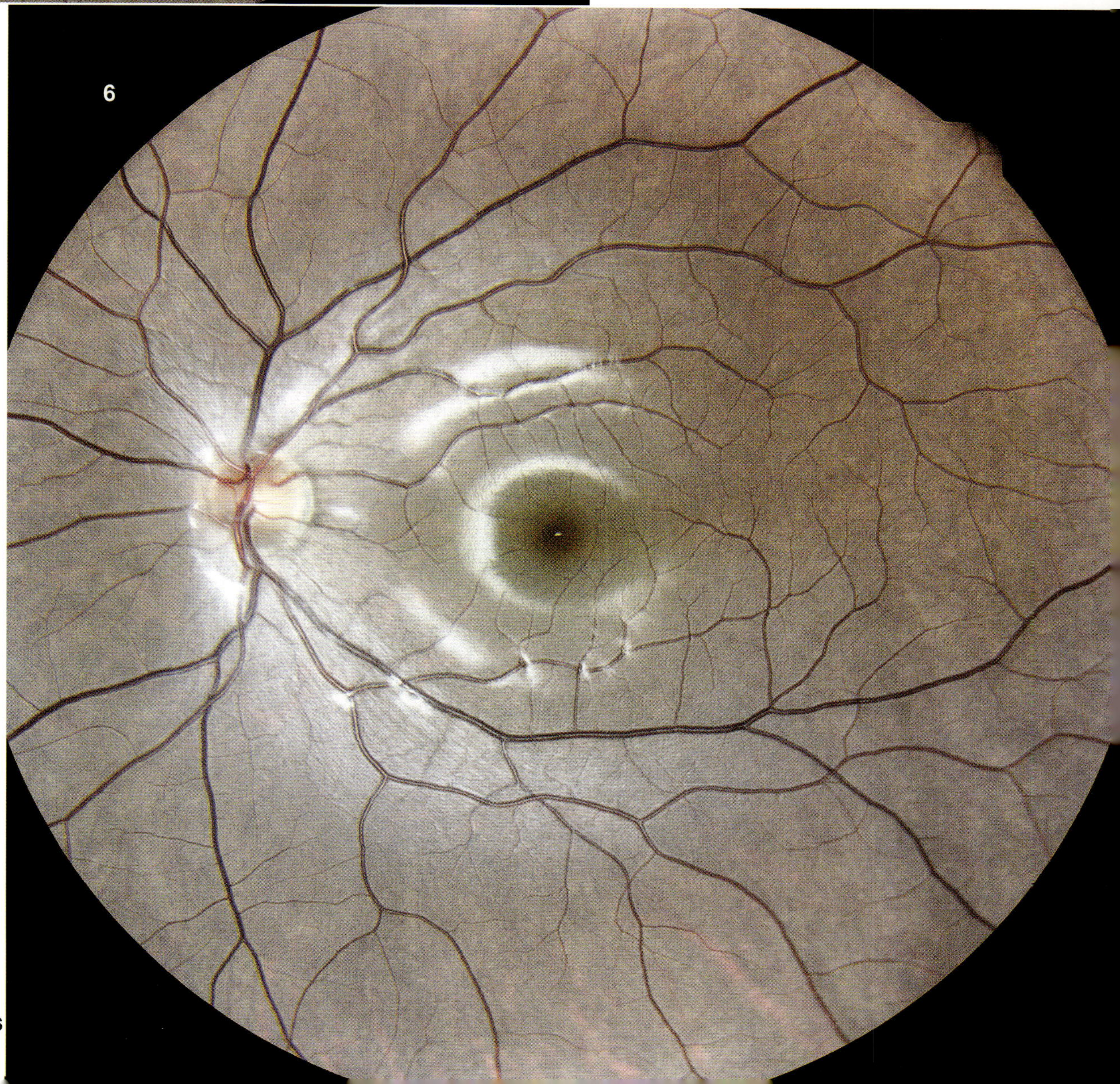

Figure 6

*A case of optic nerve hypoplasia (ONH) which is a congenital anomaly of the optic disk that might result in moderate to severe vision loss.* □

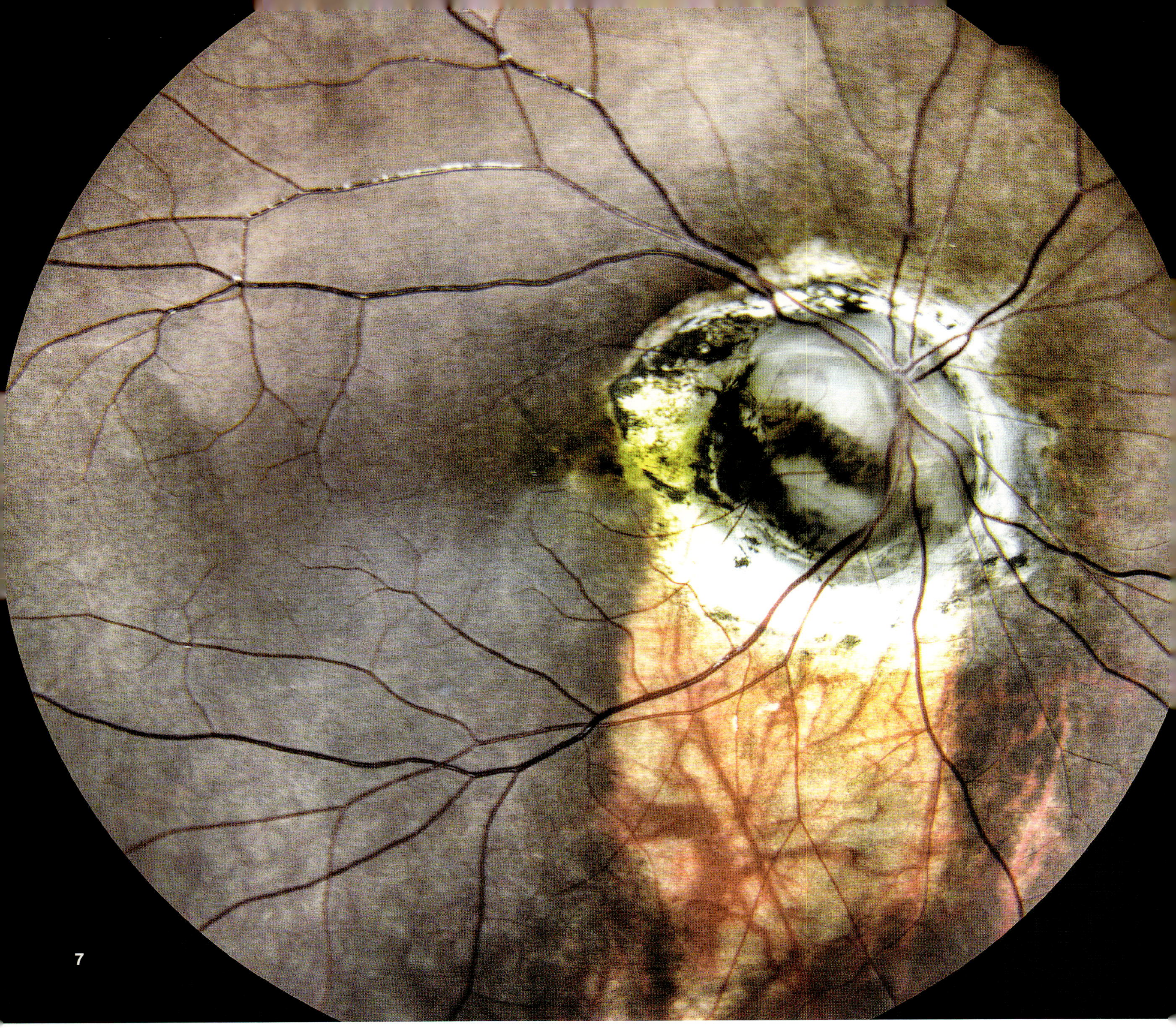


Figure 7 *Case of optic disk coloboma: Large optic nerve excavation is seen in the inferior half of the optic nerve with surrounding abnormal hyperpigmentation.*

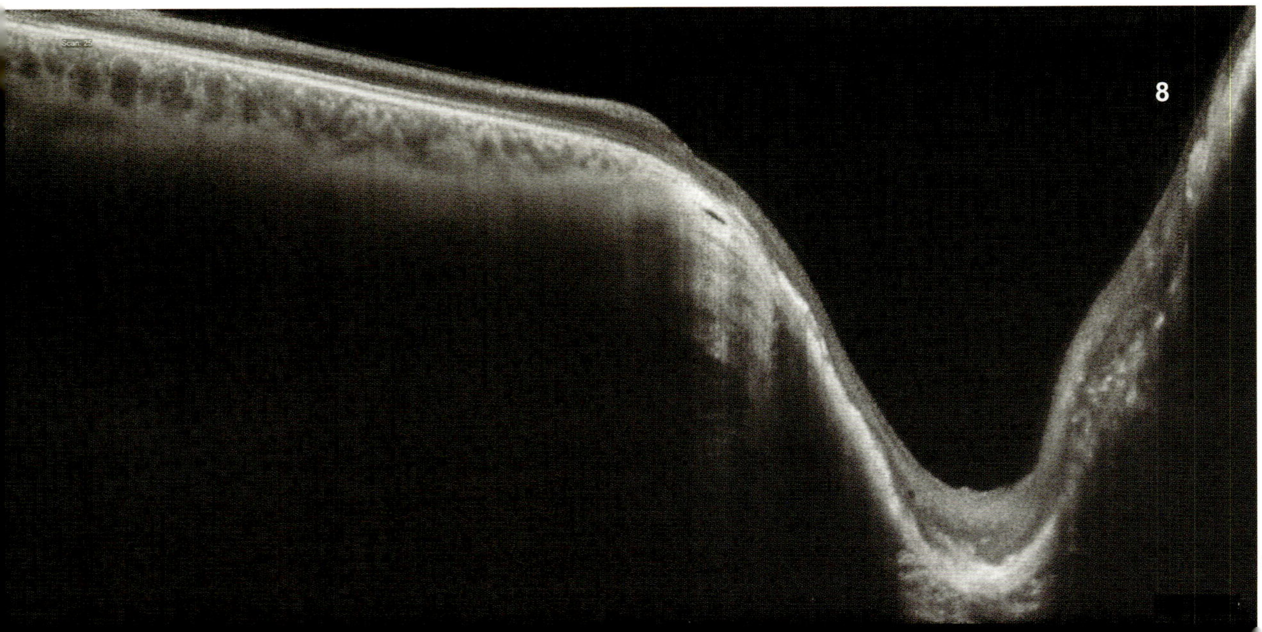


Figure 8 *Swept source OCT scan shows retinochoroidal-scleral excavation of the nerve.*

Optic disk coloboma is a congenital defect that has been thought to be due to incomplete fusion of proximal ends of the optic cup or another theory points out to the defective migration of neural crest cells and/or due to *PAX2* gene mutation. The associated complications are retinal detachments, peripapillary CNVM. Systemic associations are seen in 30% of the cases (CHARGE, Dandy Walker, Aicardi syndromes). □

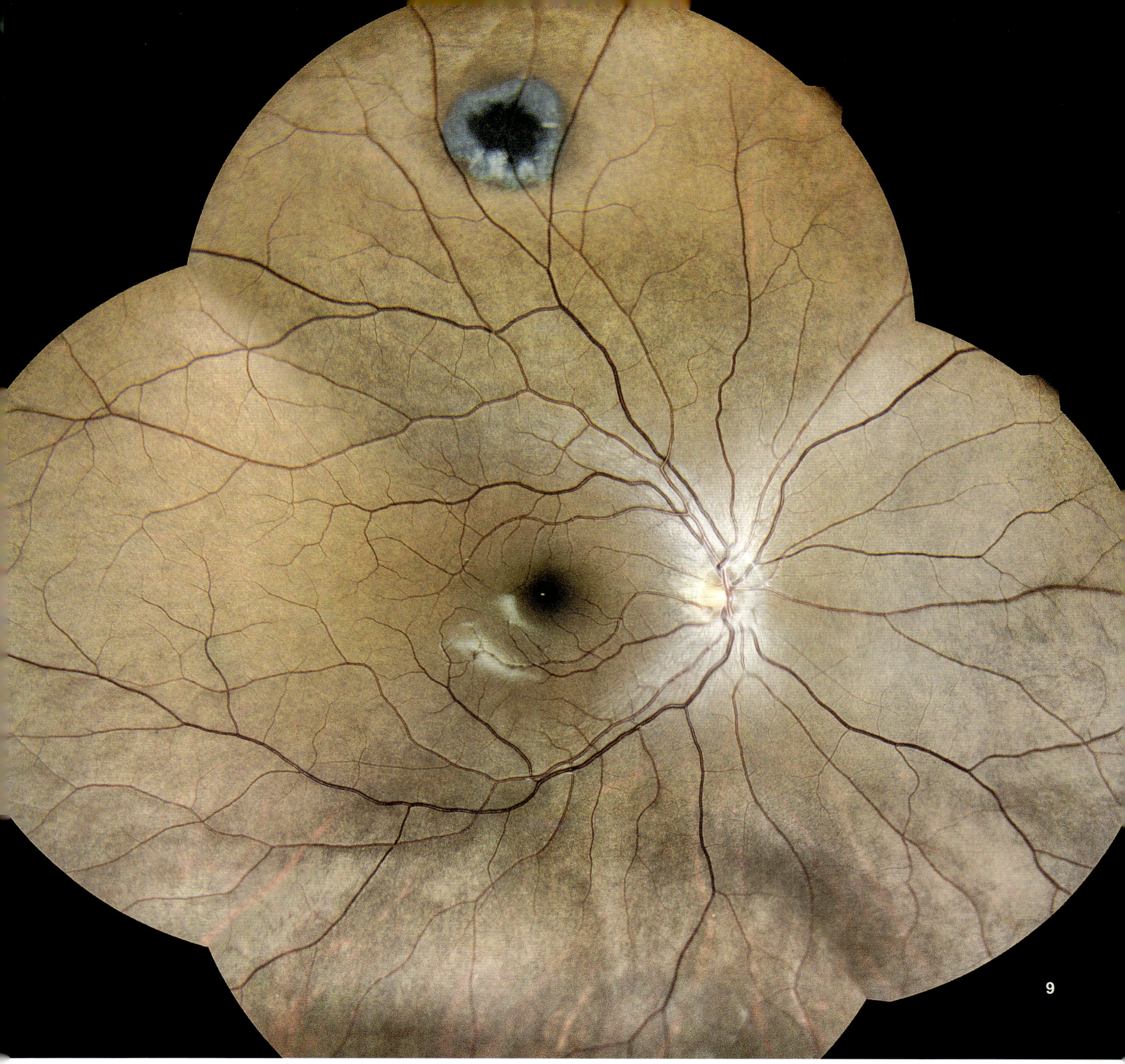

Figure 9 *A case of choroidal melanocytoma which was incidentally picked up on routine fundus examination.*

A 23-year-old female came for routine fundus evaluation prior to refractive surgery. BCVA was 6/6. Color fundus photo demonstrates a well-defined deeply pigmented circular well-defined lesion in the superior part of retina overlying a retinal blood vessel and masking it suggestive of ocular melanocytoma. Gross features of malignant tumors such as subretinal fluid and orange lipofuscin pigment were absent.

Intraocular melanocytomas are rare, benign tumors. These tumours usually do not affect vision, are slow growing and rarely undergo malignant transformation. Follow-up can be done at 3 monthly intervals initially and yearly thereafter if no change is documented. Color fundus photography is an excellent tool for monitoring these lesions. Melanocytomas can undergo spontaneous necrosis causing inflammation and pain. They can also cause vasoocclusion, especially at the optic disk with the development of neovascular glaucoma. Other potential complications of melanocytomas include ischemic retinopathy and melanocytic glaucoma from pigment dispersion.□

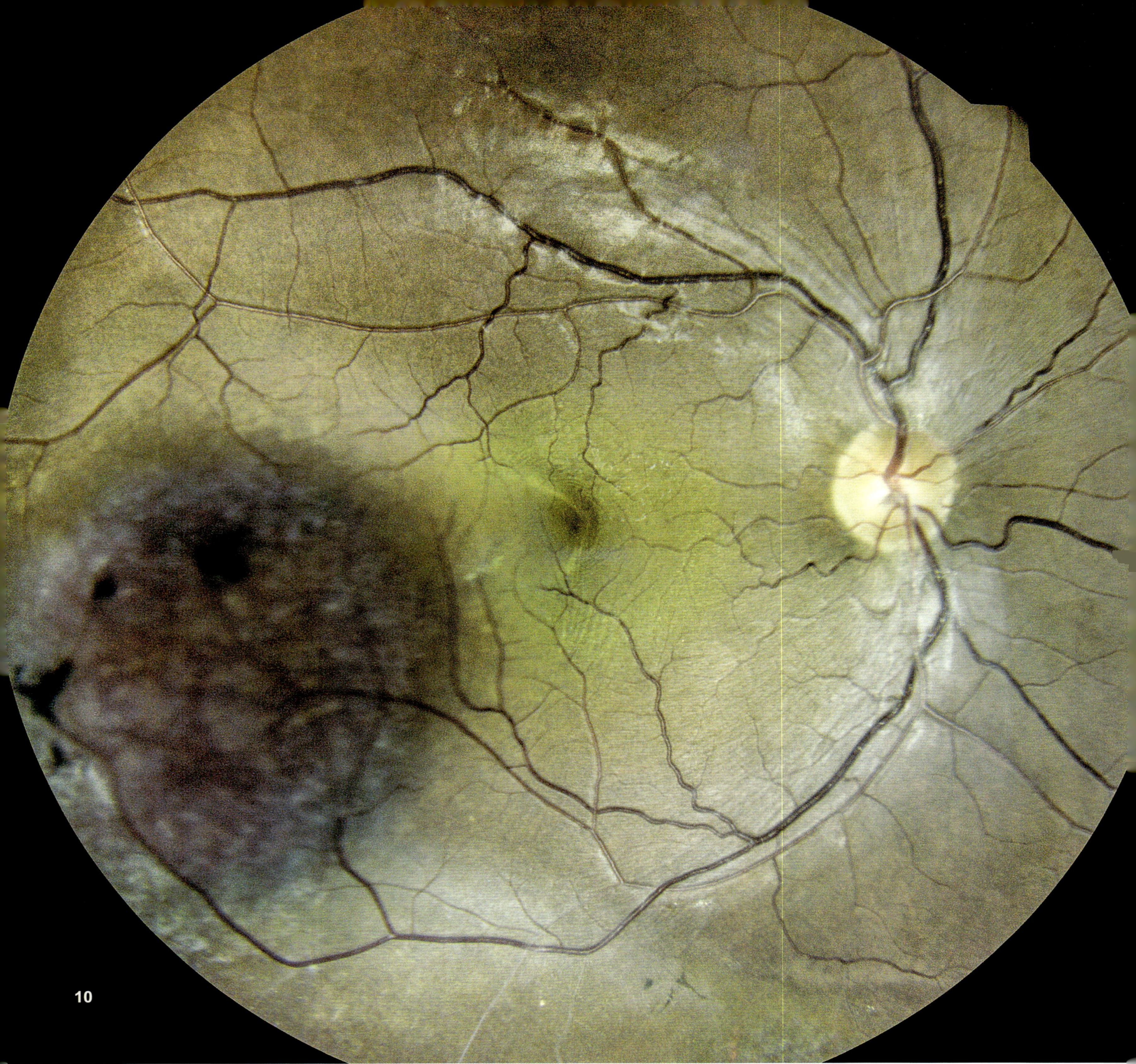

10

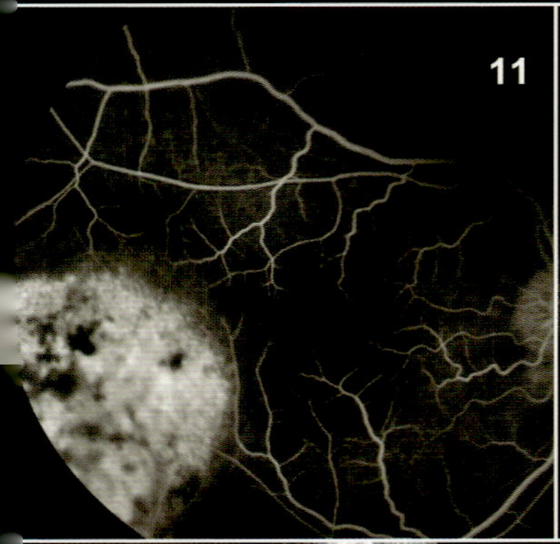

11

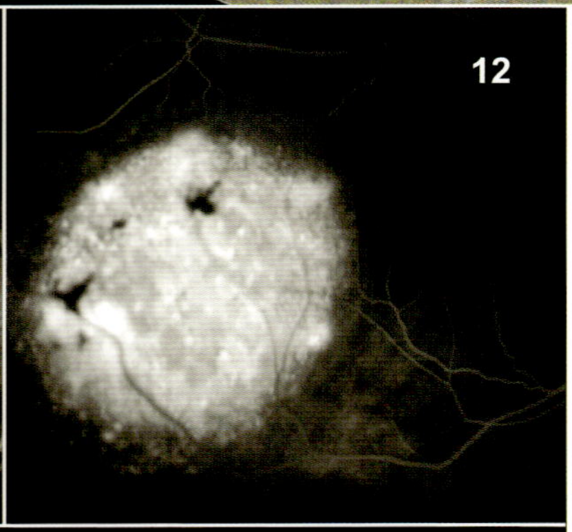

12

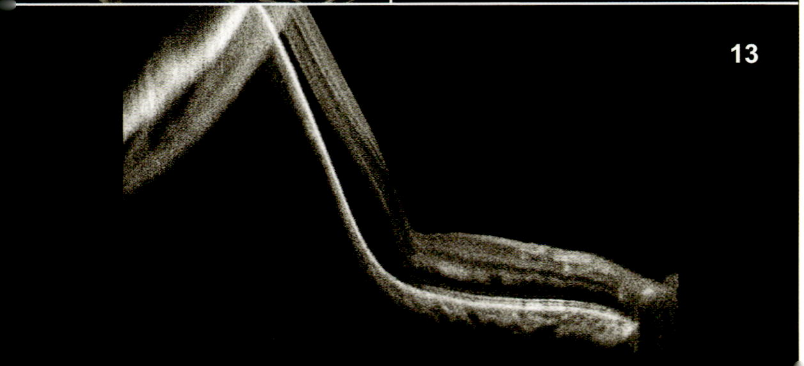

13

Figure 10 *Case of a circumscribed choroidal hemangioma.*

Color fundus photograph shows a well circumscribed, raised, reddish round mass lesion in the inferotemporal macula with associated neurosensory detachment extending to the inferior retina. Foveal reflex is absent. Circumscribed choroidal hemangioma is a benign vascular tumor of the choroid, is sporadic and unilateral in presentation. Visual acuity is likely to be affected due to the submacular fluid. If left untreated, eventually total retinal detachment may occur.

Figure 11 *Early frames of fluorescein angiogram demonstrate characteristic early hyperfluorescence due to filling up of the large choroidal blood vessels.*

Figure 12 *Late frames of fluorescein angiogram demonstrating increasing hyperfluorescence within the tumor and pooling of the dye in the region of neurosensory detachment.*

Figure 13 *OCT scan documented an elevated choroidal mass associated with subretinal fluid reaching up to the fovea.*□

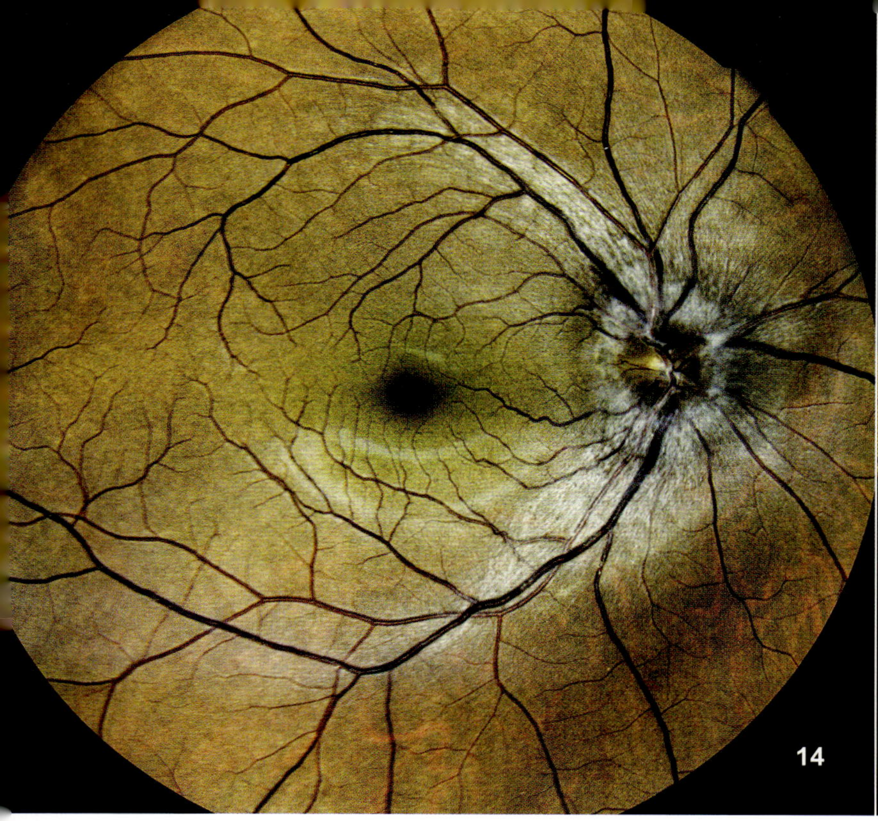

Figure 14 *Color fundus photograph demonstrating disc edema in a 45-year-old male with diagnosis of optic neuritis.*

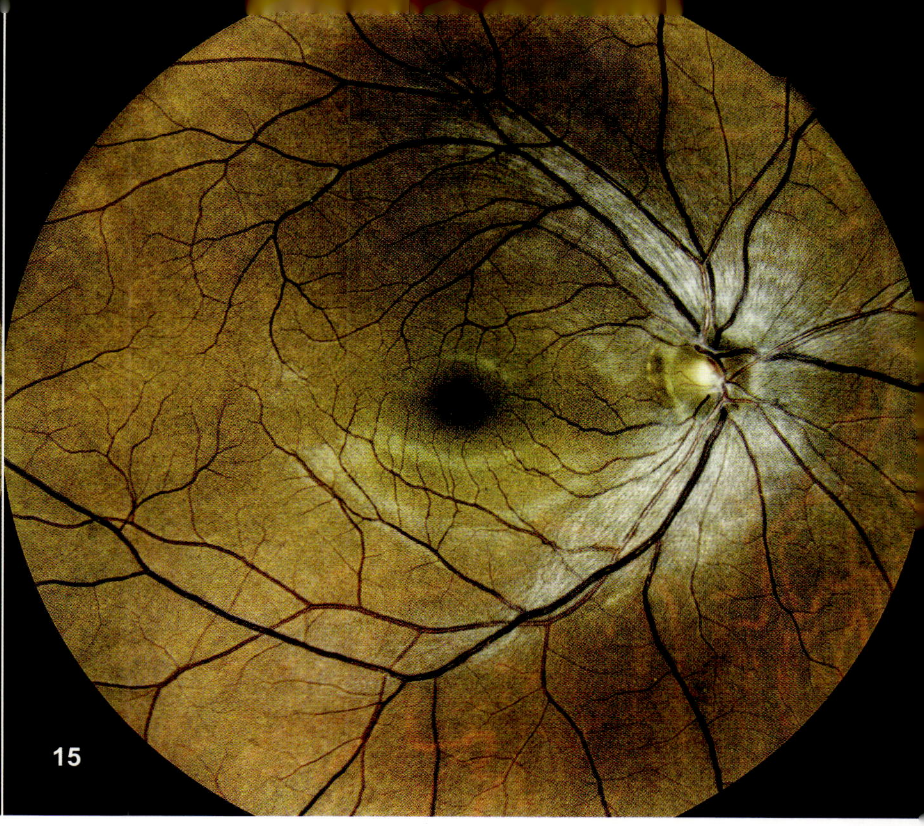

Figure 15 *Color fundus photograph 6 weeks post-treatment: Note the resolution of disc edema after oral steroids.*

Patient presented with sudden onset blurred vision. At presentation his VA was 6/12. Clinical fundus examination shows swelling of the optic disc. MRI brain and orbit were done to rule out space occupying lesion and to see for demyelination of the optic nerve. IV steroids were given for 3 days followed by oral steroids for 15 days as per ONTT trial.

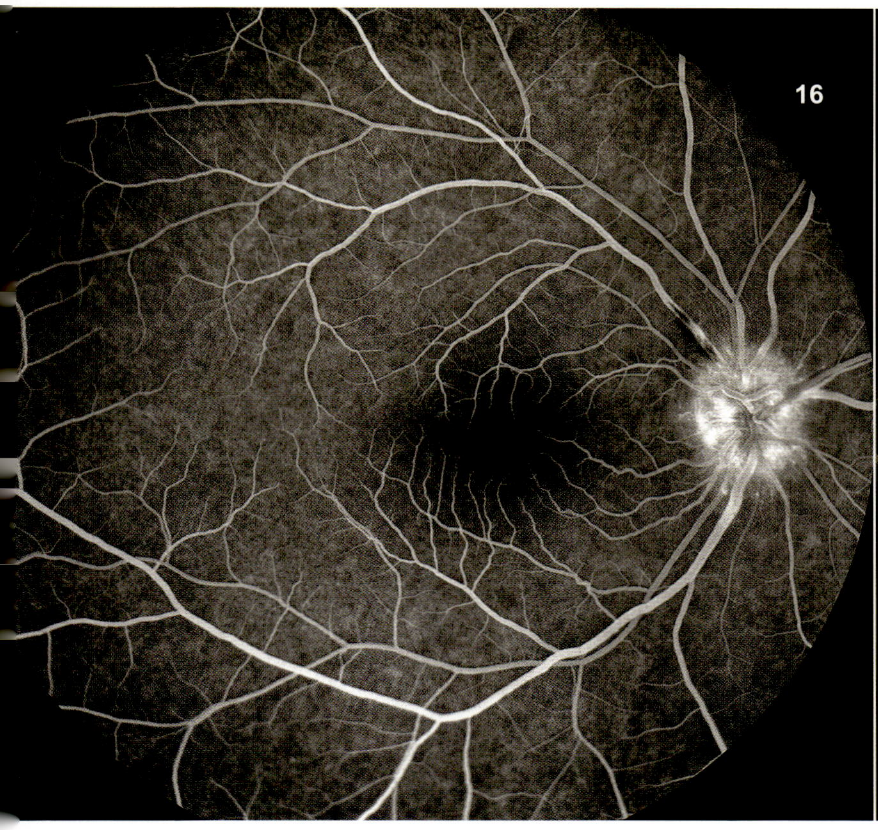

Figure 16 *Early phase of fluorescein angiogram shows disk hyperfluorescence.*

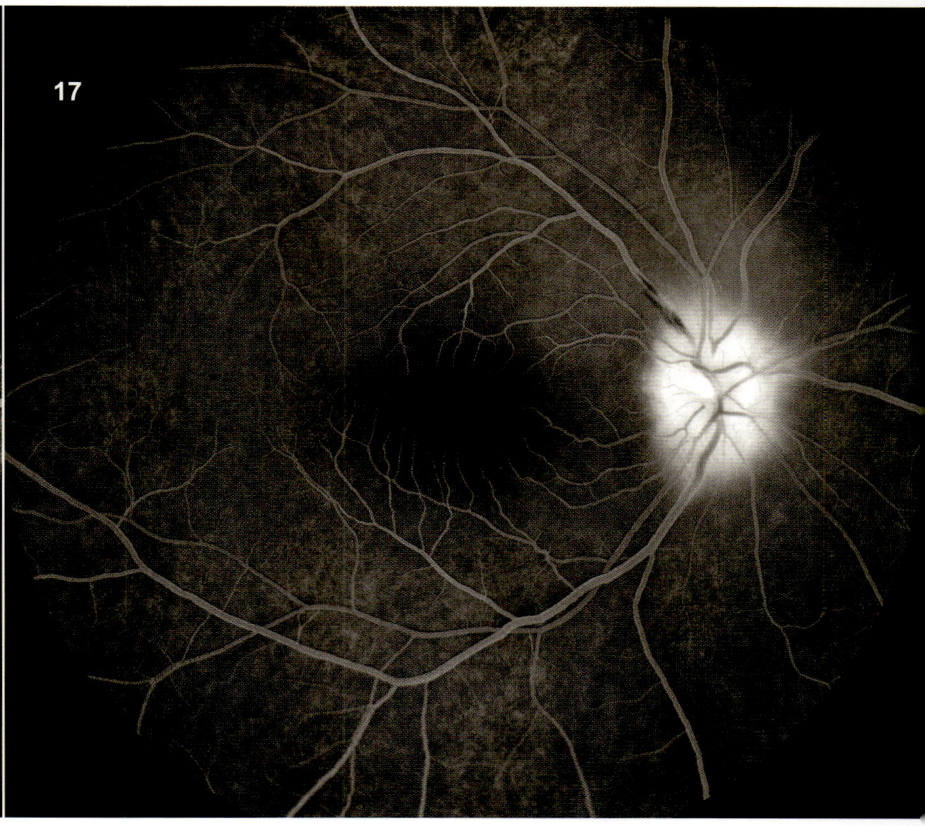

Figure 17 *Late phase of fluorescein angiogram demonstrating increased hyperfluorescence at the disk.* □

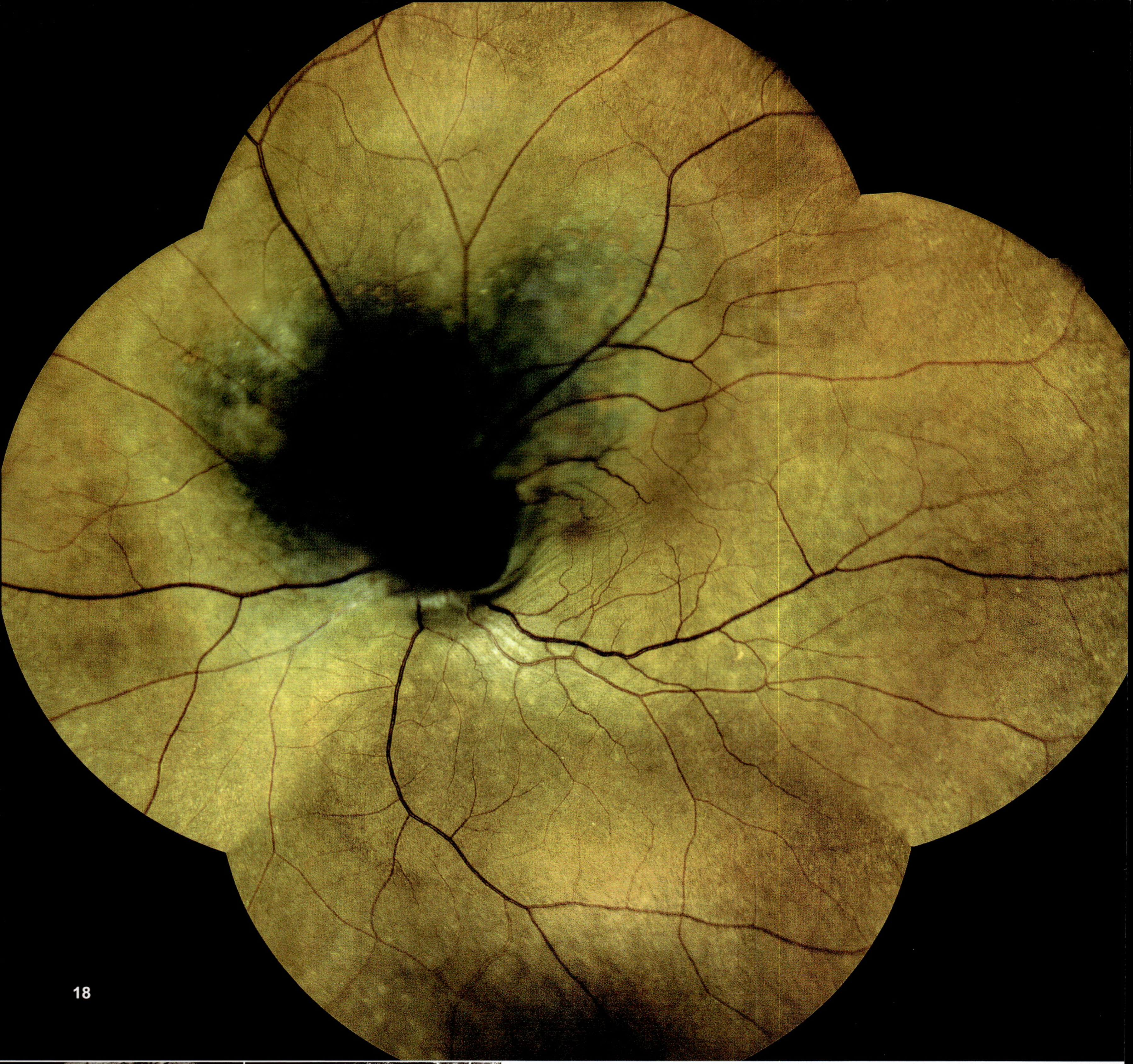

18

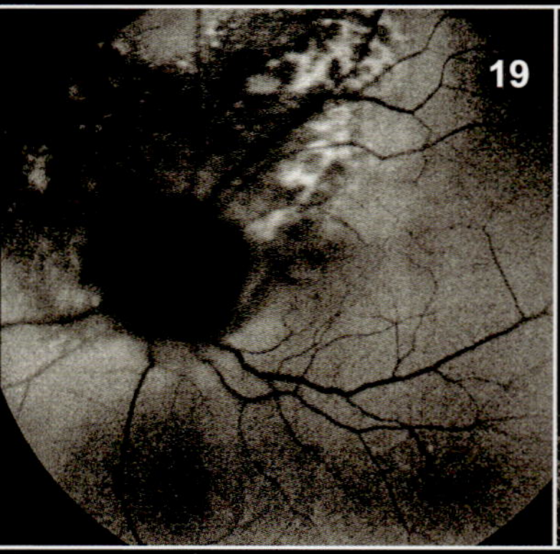

19

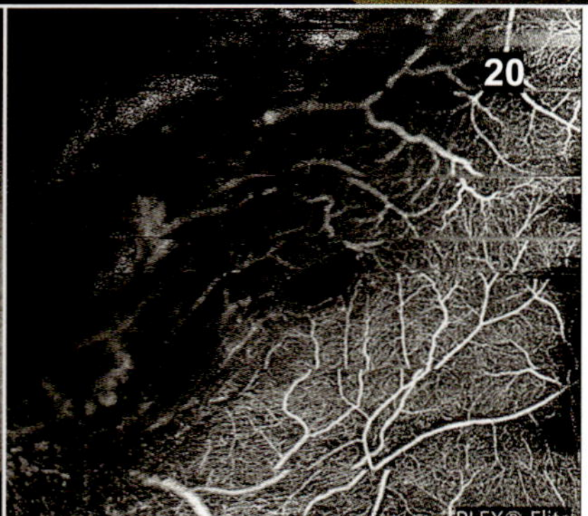

20



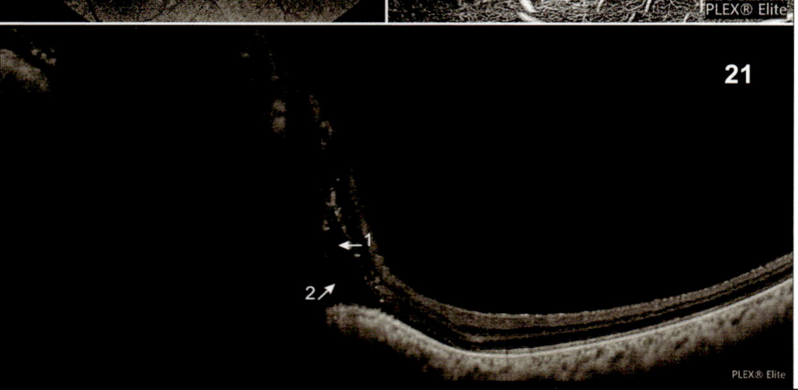

21



Figure 18 *A rare case of congenital oculodermal melanocytosis.*

A 23-year-old female complained of blurring of vision. There is deeply pigmented black to bluish discoloration of the optic nerve head. It is extending nasally, superiorly and temporally to involve the macula. Fovea is spared. Nevus of Ota (Oculodermal Melanocytosis) is a dermal melanocytic hamartoma that presents as bluish hyperpigmentation along the first or second divisions of trigeminal nerve. It is usually unilateral (90%). A small number of patients have only ocular involvement, sometimes termed as ocular melanocytosis.

Figure 19 *Fundus autofluorescence of the left eye shows dense hypoautofluorescence of at the disk and in areas corresponding to the lesion owing to masking effect of melanin in the lesion.*

Figure 20 *OCT angiogram of central macula demonstrated the hyporeflectance corresponding to the lesion and partially visualization of choroidal vessels.*

Figure 21 *Swept-source OCT scan shows a dome-shape mass with a dense posterior shadowing and multiple hyper-reflective dots overlying the lesion continuous with the retinal inner layers (1). Note the presence of serous fluid adjacent to lesion (2).* □

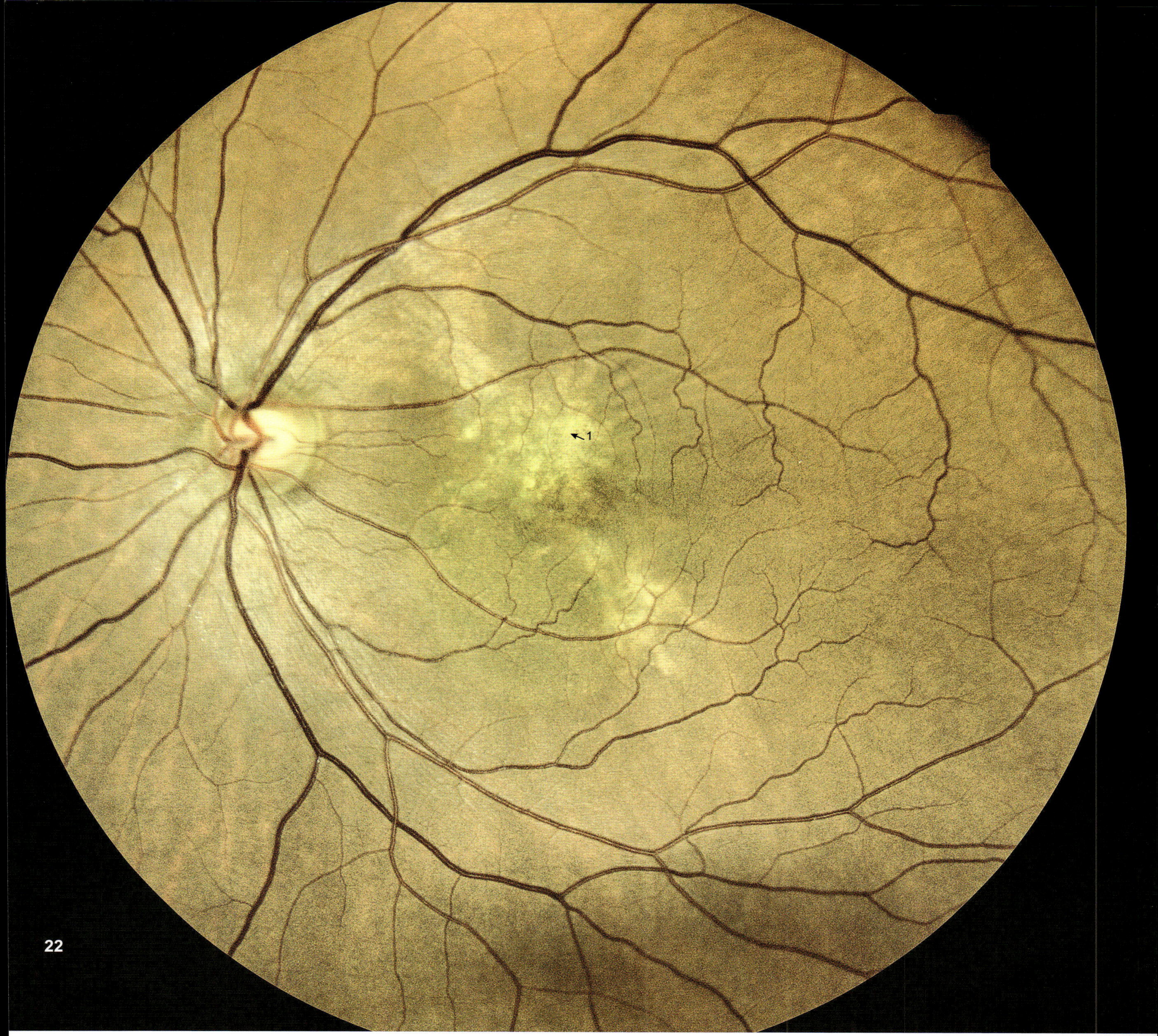

Figure 22 *Color fundus image of 45-year-old with subfoveal choroidal osteoma in her left eye. It appear as slightly elevated whitish in color irregular patches seen at superior macula (1).*

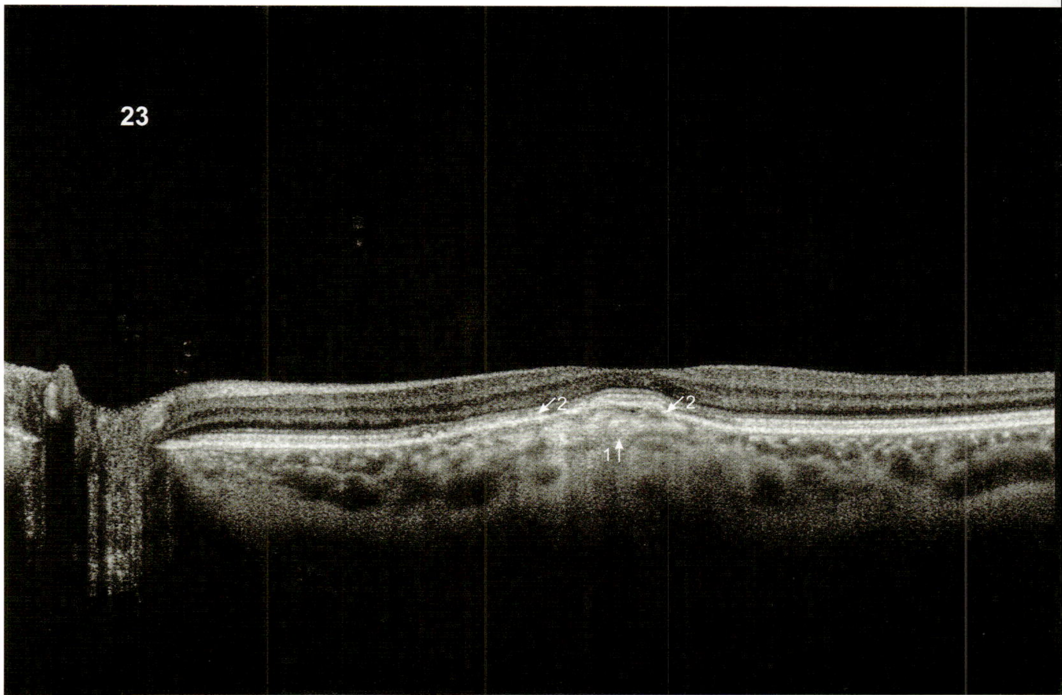

Figure 23 *Enhanced depth image (EDI)—OCT demonstrating subfoveal choroidal osteoma. Note the presence of elevated choroidal lesion at fovea with hetrogeneous hyperreflectivity (1) with overlying irregularities in photoreceptor layer (2).*

Choroidal osteoma is a rare benign tumor of choroid, typically unilateral and found in healthy young female in 2nd or 3rd decade of life. Diagnostic test like OCT provides important information about stage of choroidal osteoma and also help to detect presence of CNVM, if any. □

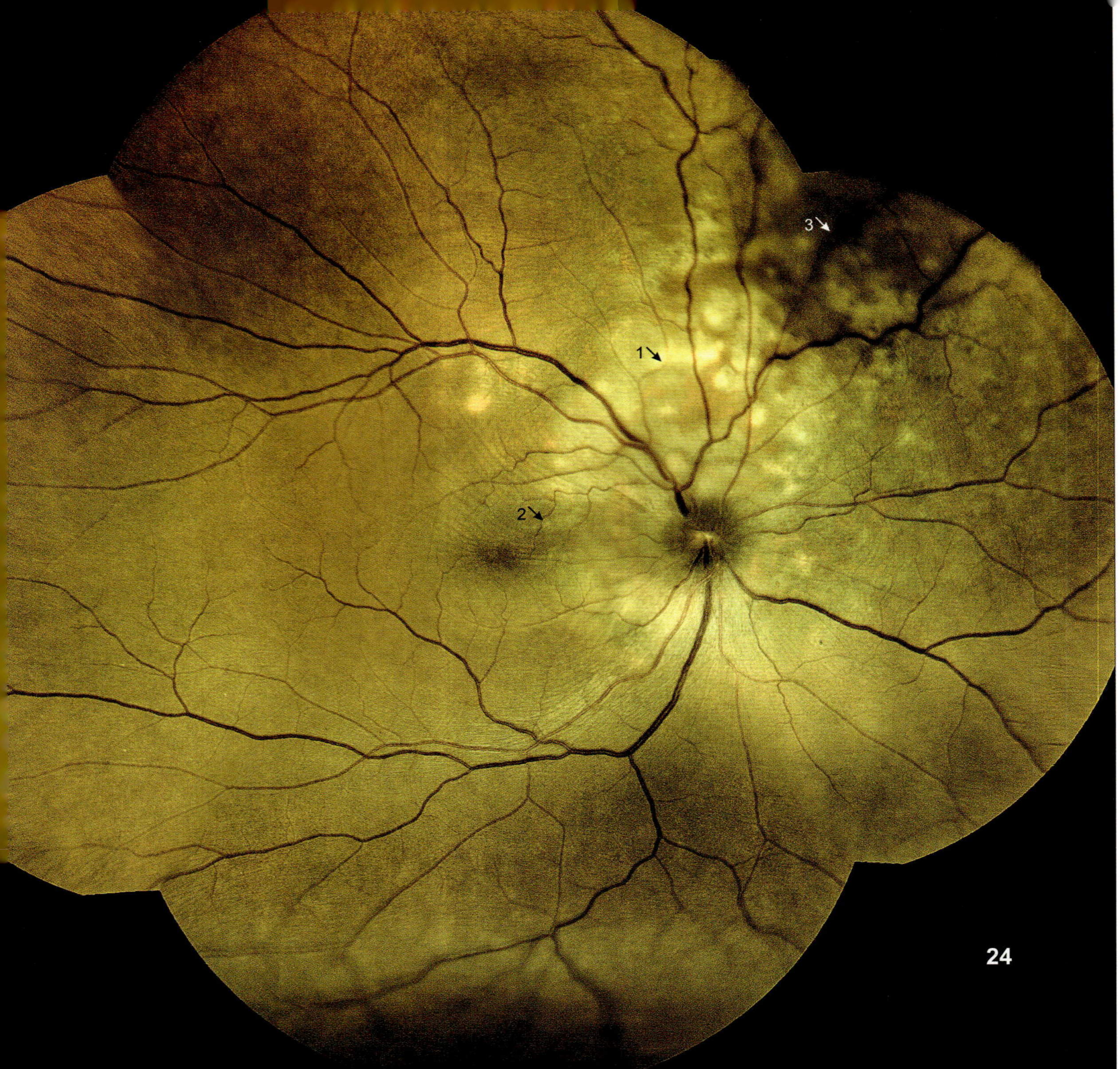

Figure 24

*A case of choroidal metastasis: Yellowish raised mass lesions is seen along the superonasal quadrant with ill-defined borders (1). Note the presence of associated subretinal fluid that has extended to involve the superior macula (2). There are also dark pigmented patches resembling leopard skin at superior edge of lesions (3).*

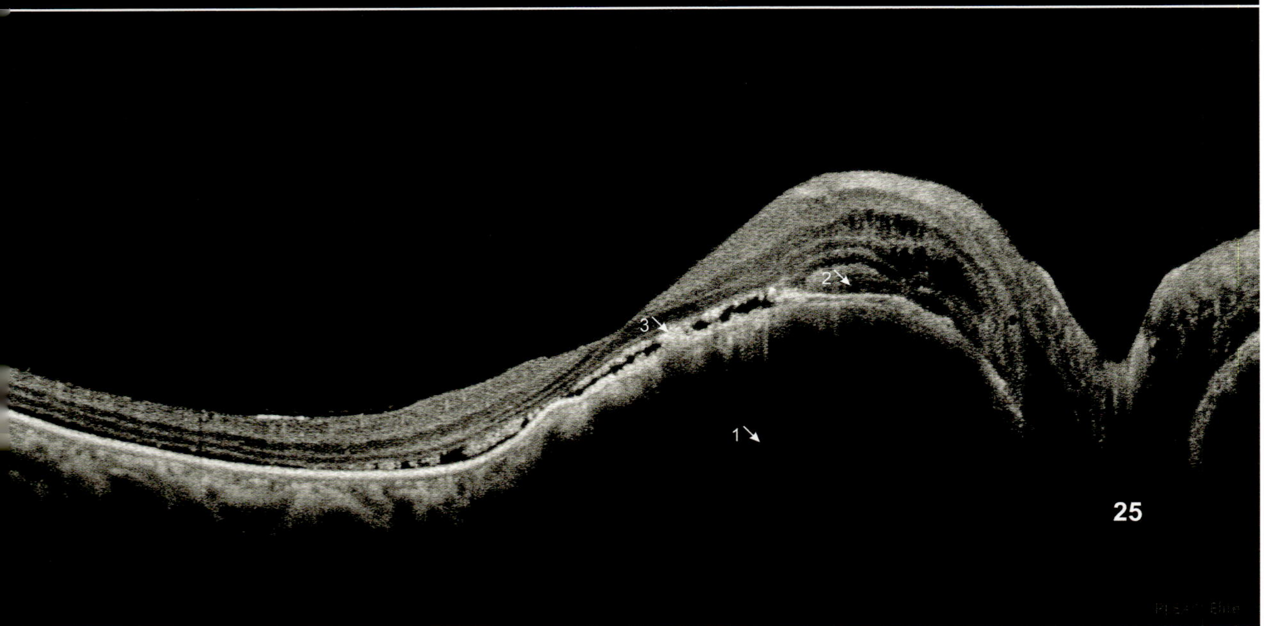

Figure 25

*SS-OCT scan in a case of choroidal metastasis showing extremely raised hypo-reflective choroidal mass lesion (1) with overlying subretinal fluid (2) and retinal pigmented epithelial alterations (3).*

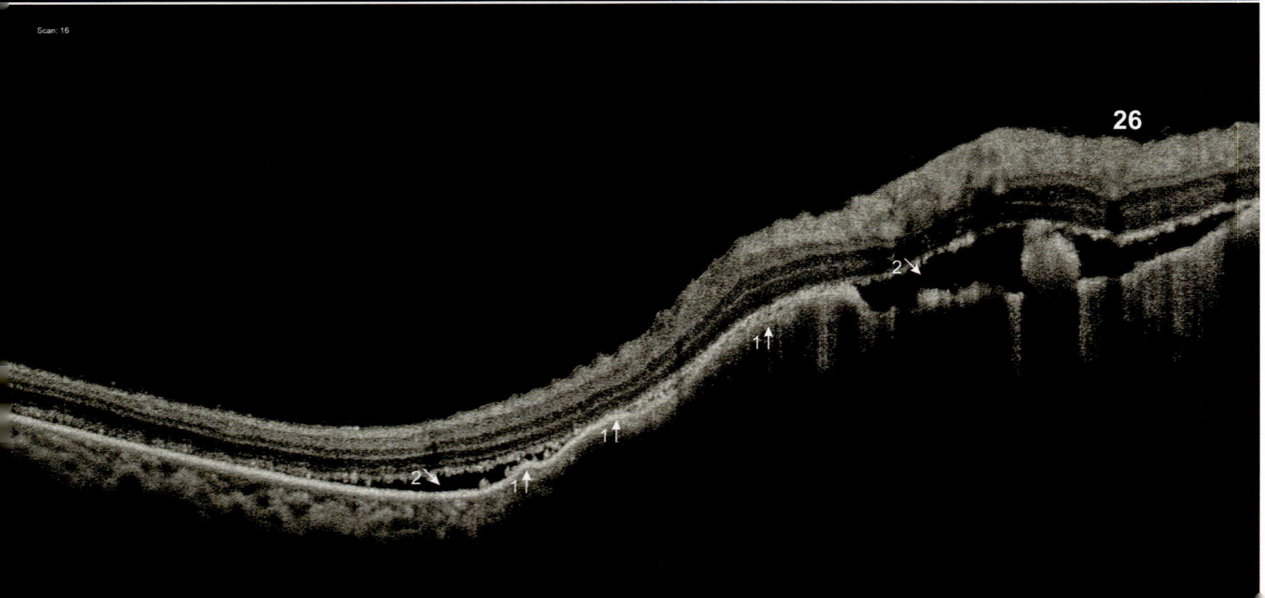

Figure 26

*Swept-source optical coherence tomography scan at the superonasal location showed characteristic lump bumby (1) appearance of metastasis mass lesions associated with subretinal fluid (2).*□

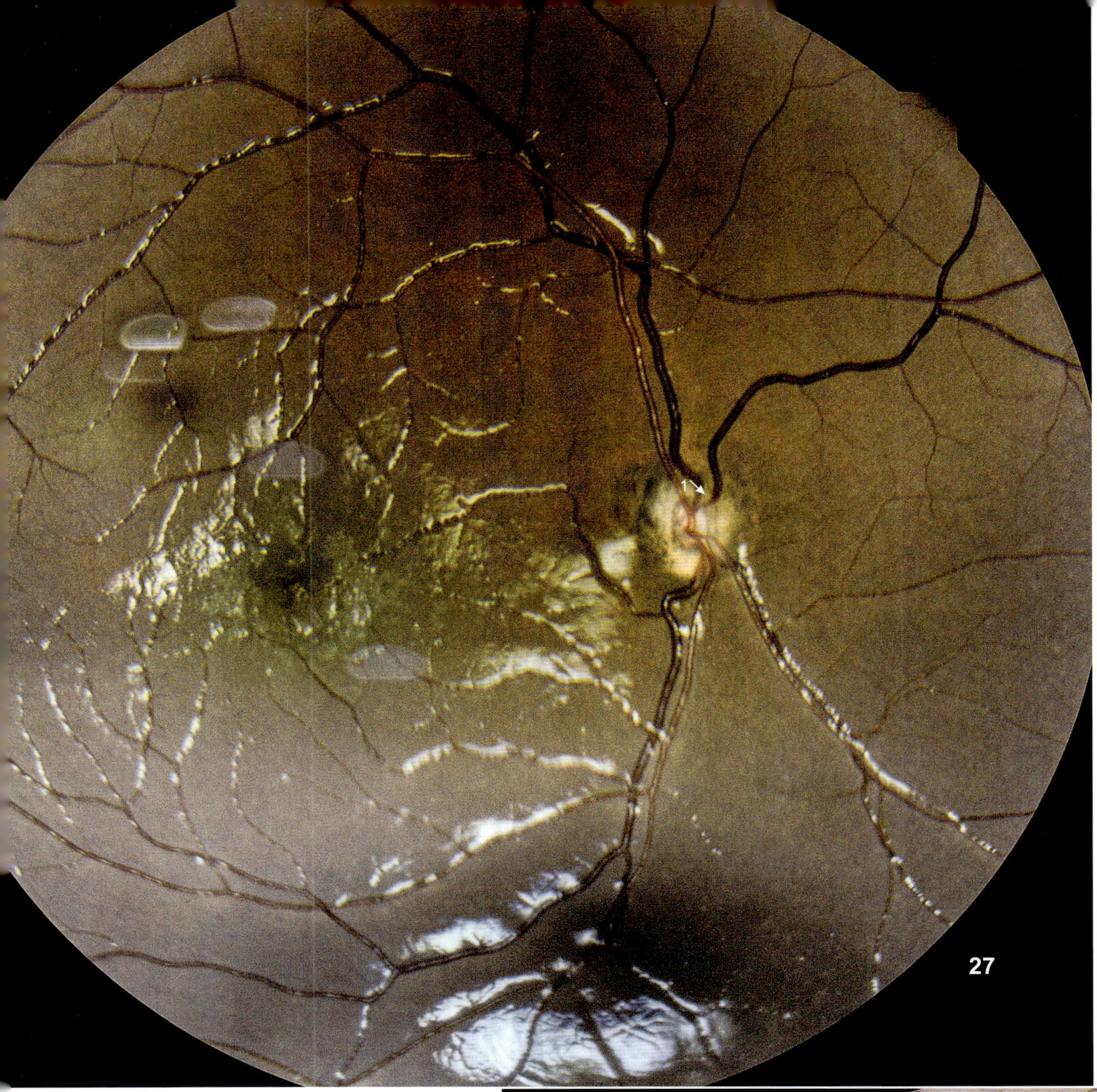


Figure 27

*Optic nerve hypoplasia color fundus montage image of right eye with hypoplastic disk pale colored oval-shaped optic disk smaller in size as compared to optic disk in figure 28 (1). A ring of hyperpigmentation is also seen surrounding hypoplastic disk defining the area of the putative scleral canal.*

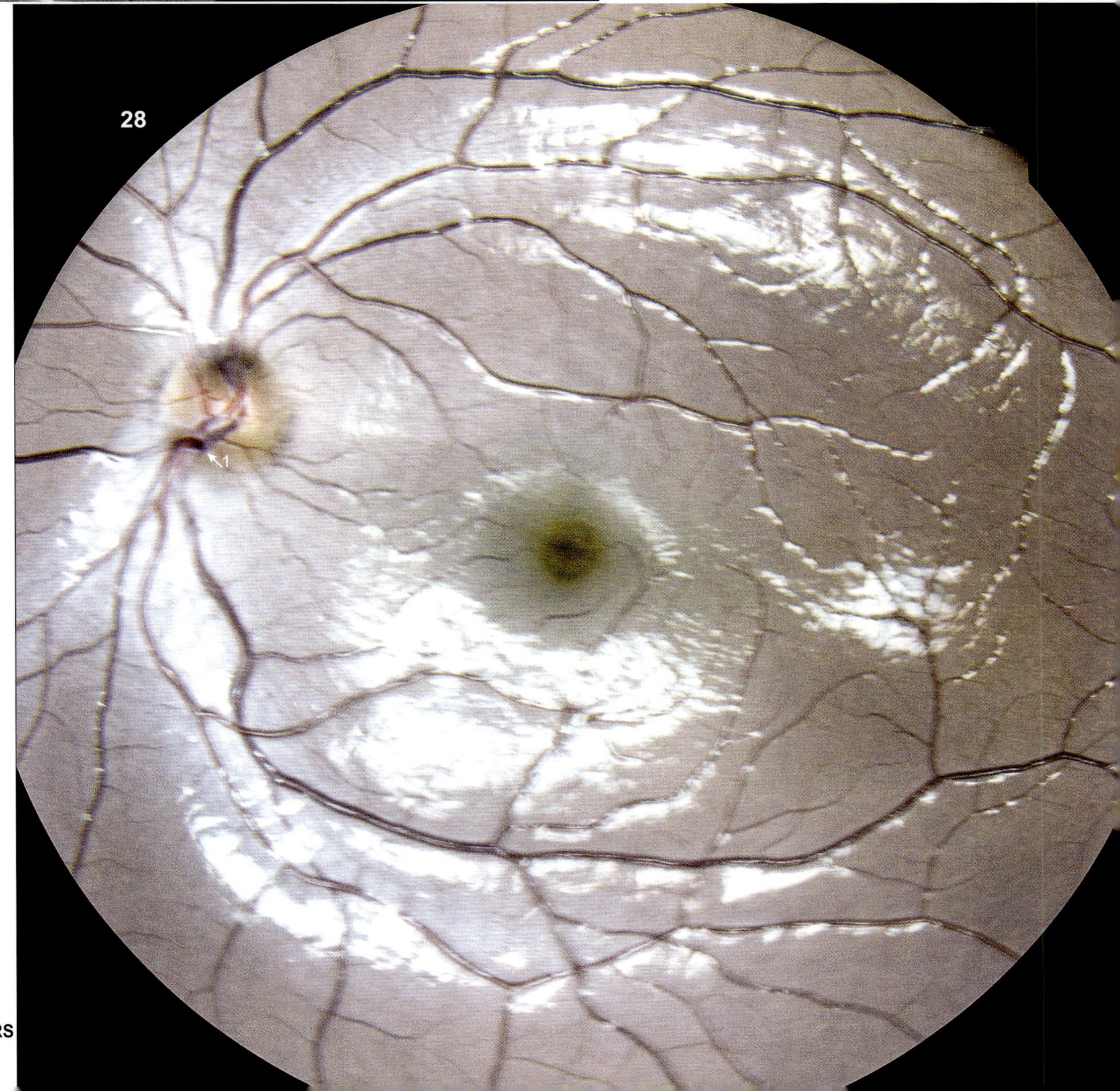


Figure 28

*Color fundus montage image of left eye with round morphological optic disk (1).*

Optic nerve hypoplasia is considered as 3rd most-prevalent cause of visual impairment in children less than 3 years of age.

It is characterized by decreased number of optic nerve axons and it may present either as an isolated abnormally or be associated with CNS abnormality and neurodevelopmental handicaps.

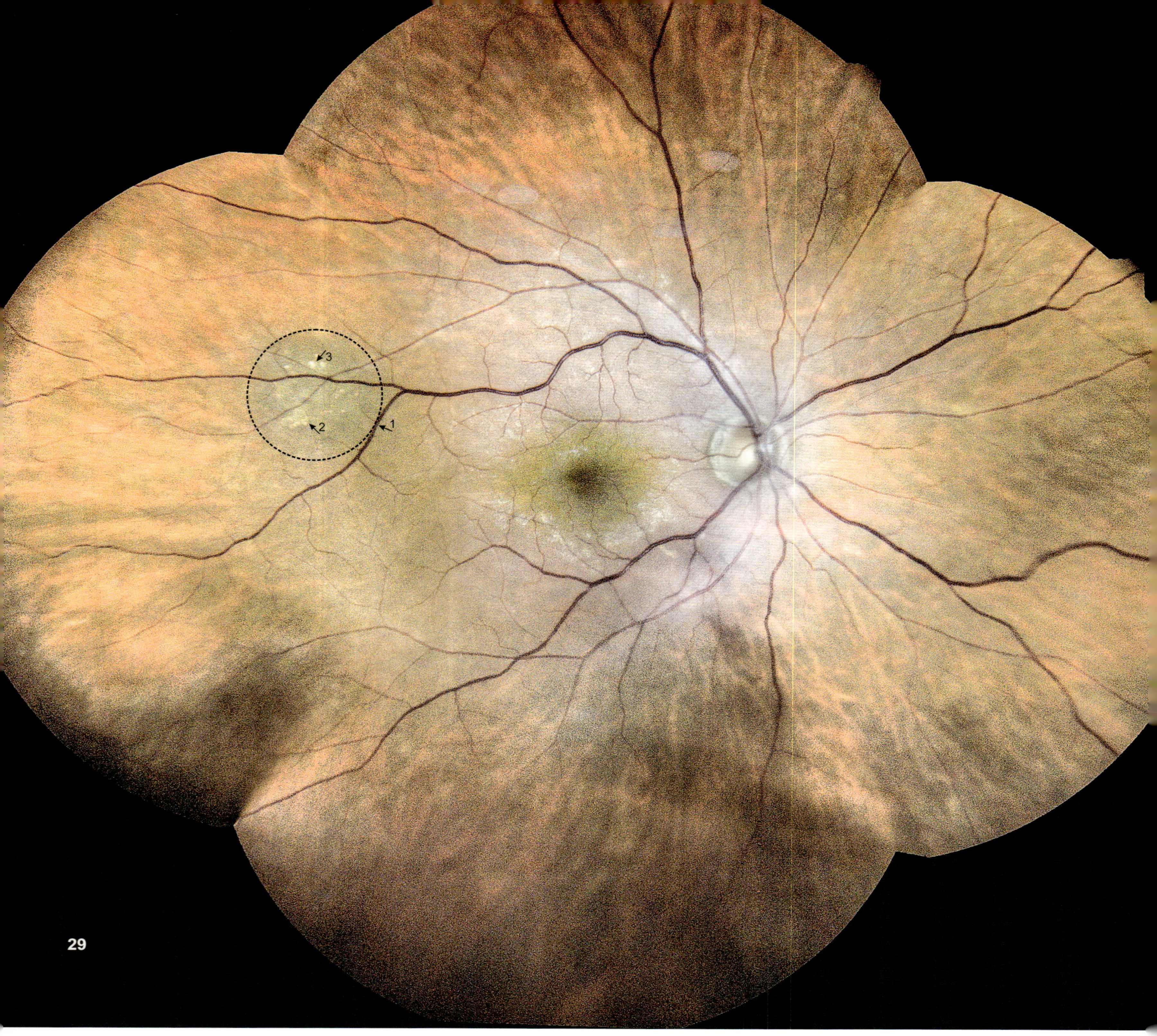


Figure 29 *Color fundus montage of choroidal nevus: Note the presence of brownish round (1) almost flat lesion in superotemporal mid-periphery of retina with associated dot-like whitish opacities (2) representing RPE alterations and a few layer RPE excrescences (3) suggestive of drusen.*

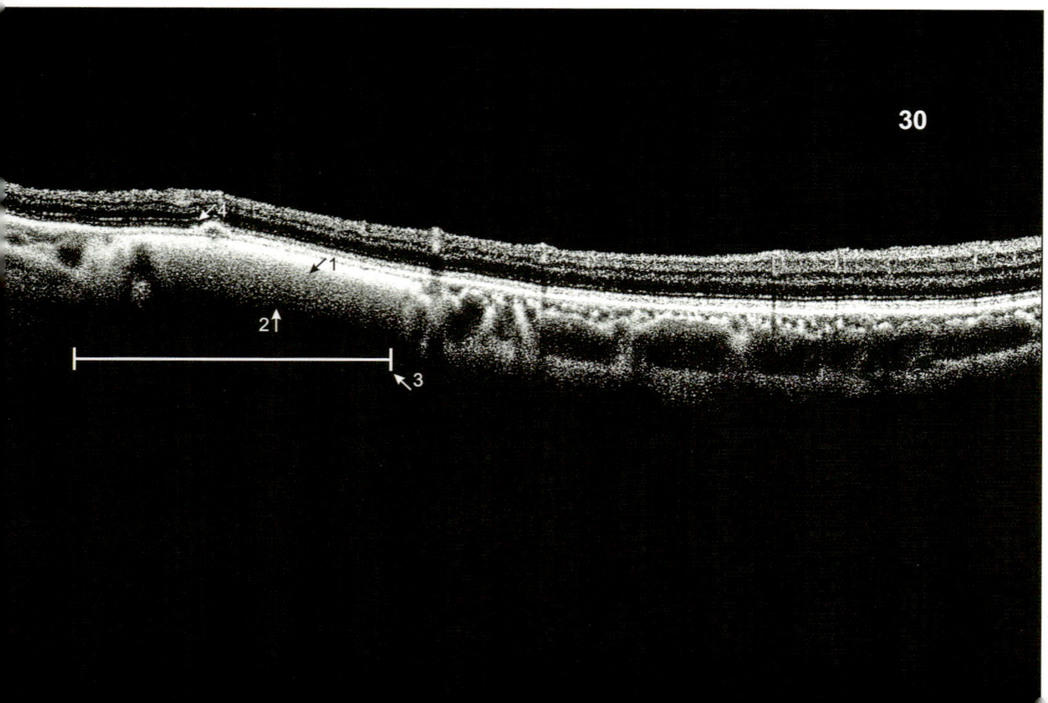


Figure 30 *SS-OCT passing through choroidal nevus demonstrates hyper-reflective inner choroid (1) and hyporeflective outer choroid (2) with loss of normal choriocapillary architecture in area of extent of choroidal nevus (3). Also, note the presence of RPE excrescences suggestive of drusen (4).*

Choroidal nevus is most common intraocular tumor and are generally benign, although malignant transformation into a melanoma has also been reported with an estimated test of 1 in 8000.□

# CHAPTER 9

## MISCELLANEOUS

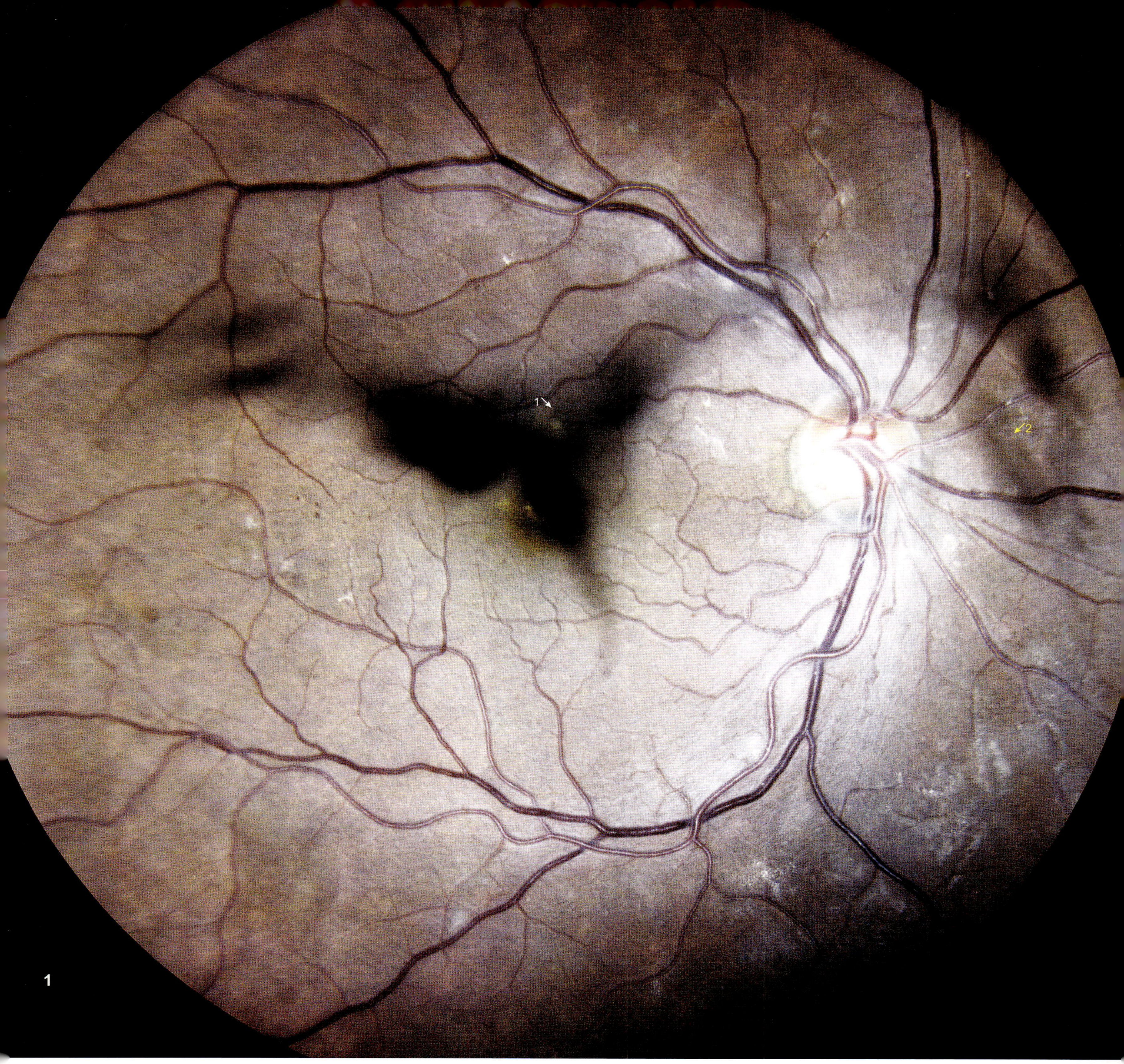


Figure 1 *A case of acute posterior vitreous detachment which happens usually with age, as the posterior hyaloid membrane separates from the retina posterior to the vitreous base.*

A 62-year-old female presented with complaints of sudden onset of flashes and floaters in her right eye since 2 days. Color fundus photo shows dark shadows in the vitreous cavity in front of retina faintly obscuring retinal details (1). A faint Weiss ring (2) can be seen nasal to the disk owing to separation of hyaloid form the optic disk margin suggestive of posterior vitreous detachment (PVD).

The incidence of retinal break formation following acute posterior vitreous detachment is variously reported as occurring in between 8 and 15% of patients. The patient had no evidence of a retinal tear or detachment in either eye on 360 degree scleral depressed examination. This usually occurs in one eye at a time, but a PVD in the contralateral eye often occurs 6–24 months later.

In high myopia, PVD develops increasingly with age and the degree of myopia. Confocal fundus photographs pick-up the vitreous opacities and show them as dark shadows. Routine fundus camera will not pick-up these changes.□

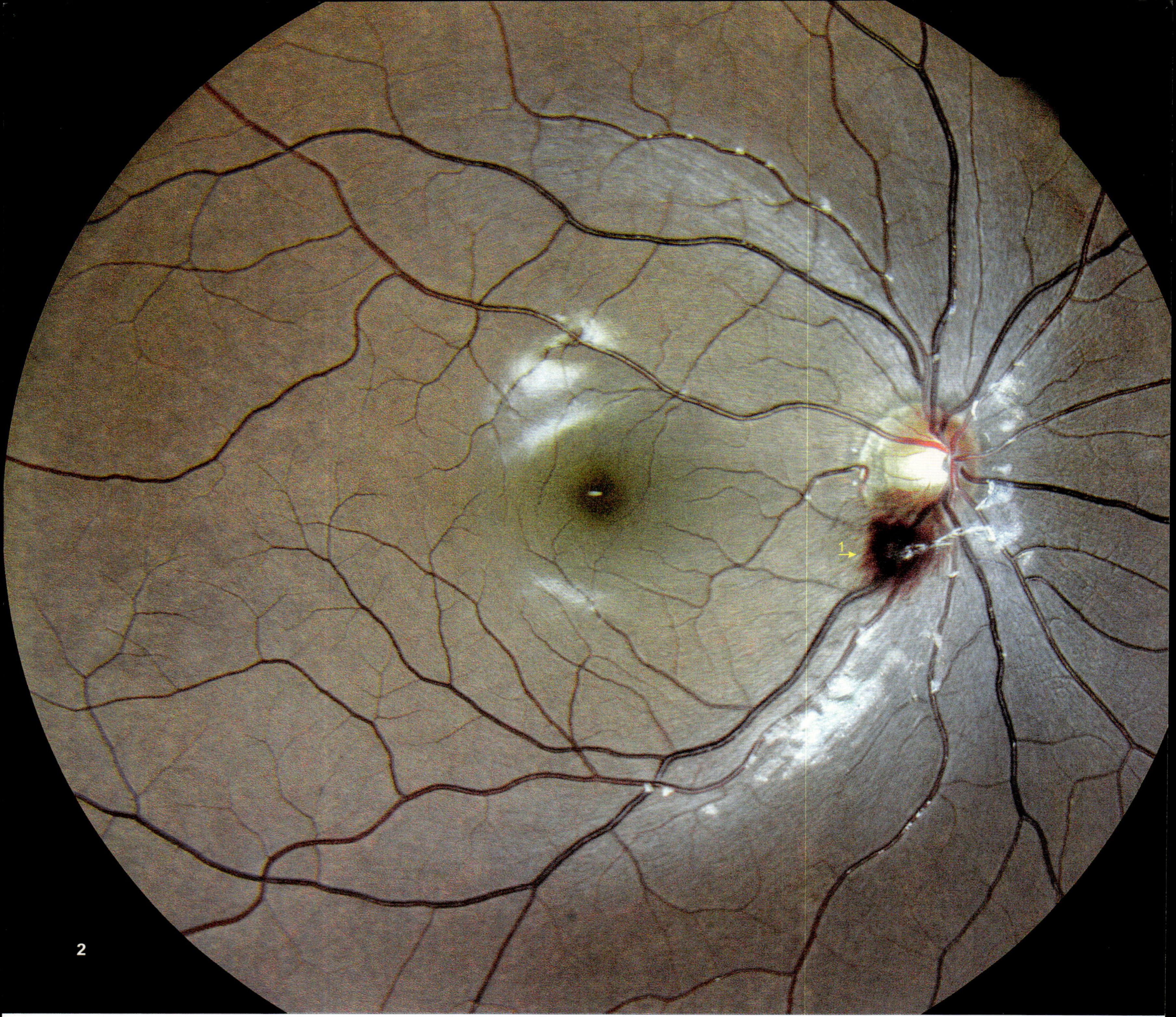


Figure 2 *A 20-year-old female was referred for an eye checkup after suffering from mild altitudinal sickness (breathlessness/headache) due to her recent travel to a high-altitude region (Leh, India). Color fundus photograph done 2 days after her descent shows a splinter hemorrhage (1) at the inferior margin of the optic disk.*

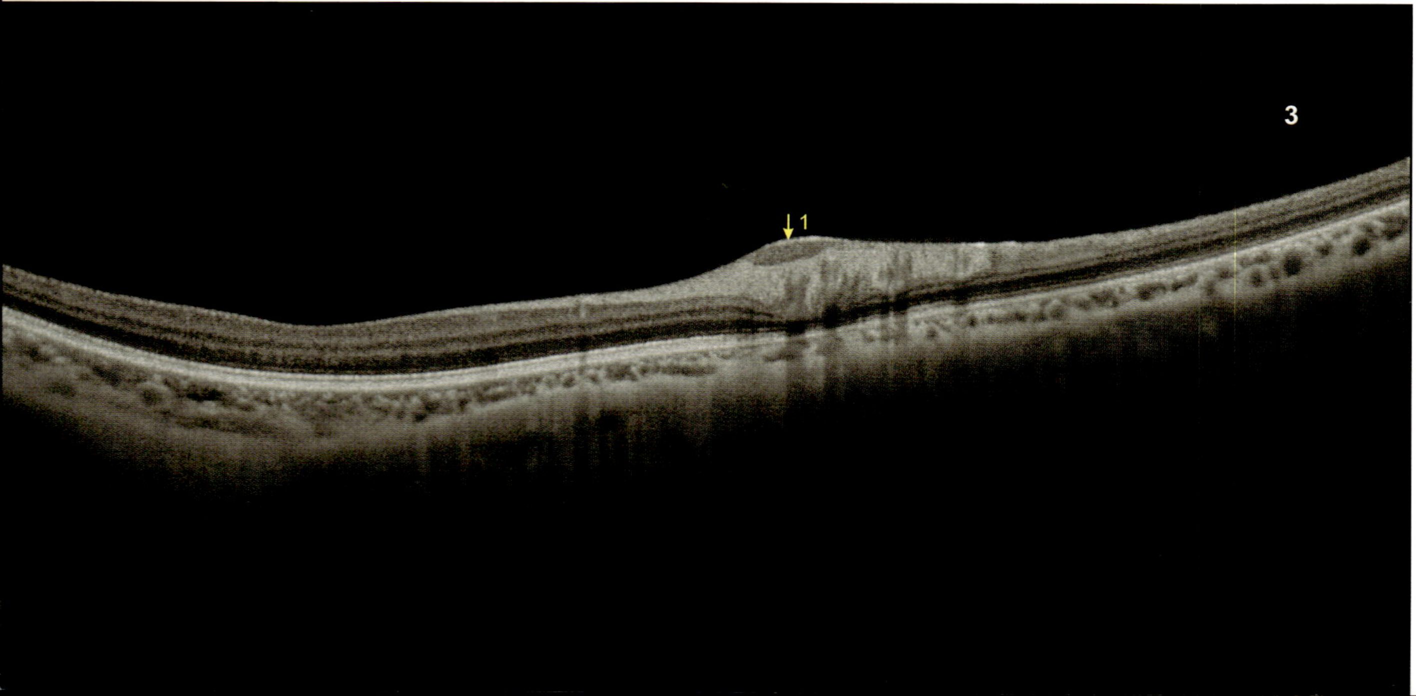


Figure 3

*Swept-source OCT scan taken at the level of optic disk shows hyper-reflective elongated lesions (1) at the nerve fiber layer suggestive of retinal hemorrhage.*

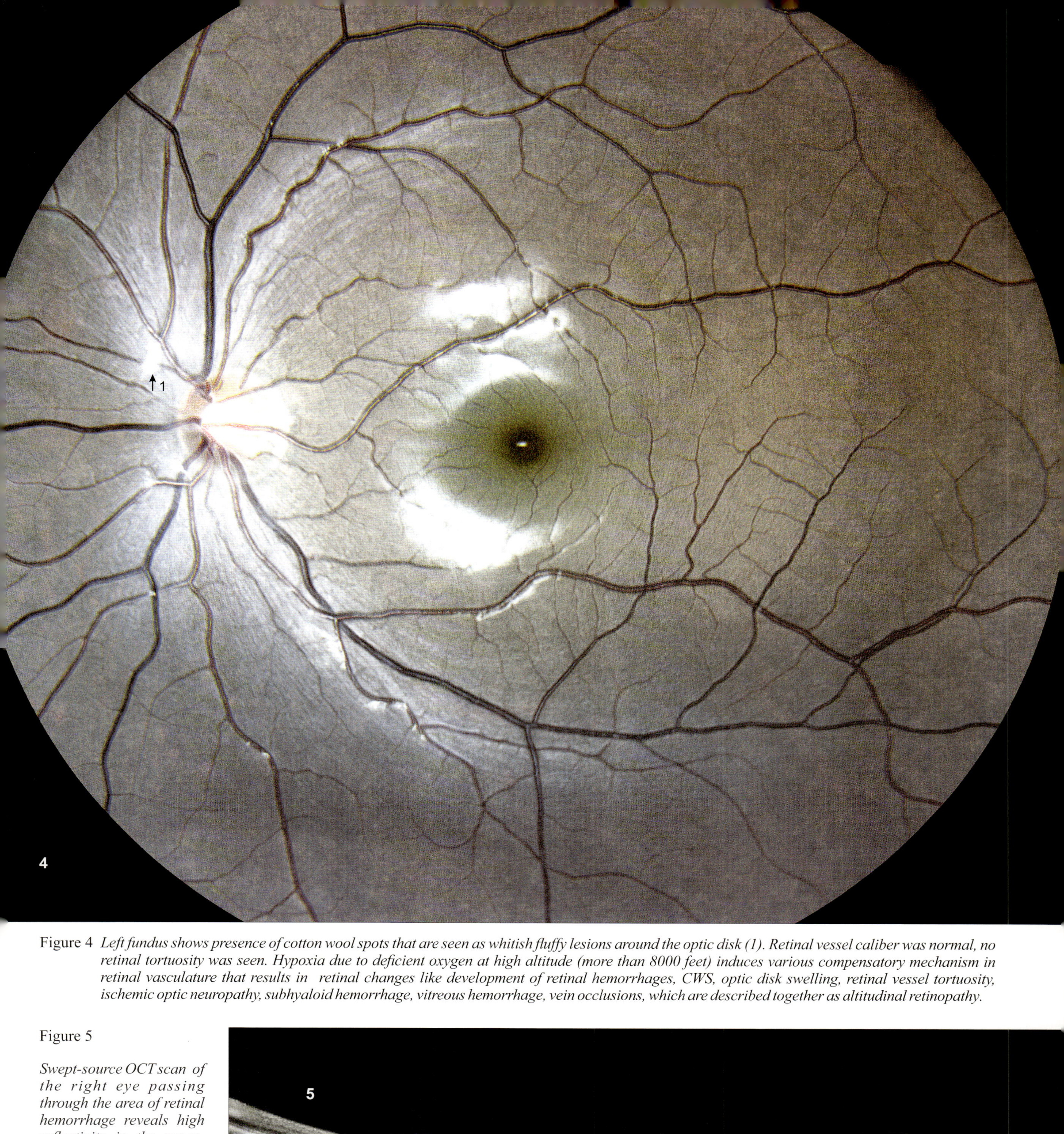


Figure 4 *Left fundus shows presence of cotton wool spots that are seen as whitish fluffy lesions around the optic disk (1). Retinal vessel caliber was normal, no retinal tortuosity was seen. Hypoxia due to deficient oxygen at high altitude (more than 8000 feet) induces various compensatory mechanism in retinal vasculature that results in retinal changes like development of retinal hemorrhages, CWS, optic disk swelling, retinal vessel tortuosity, ischemic optic neuropathy, subhyaloid hemorrhage, vitreous hemorrhage, vein occlusions, which are described together as altitudinal retinopathy.*

Figure 5

*Swept-source OCT scan of the right eye passing through the area of retinal hemorrhage reveals high reflectivity in the superficial retinal layers, with lifting of inner limiting membrane due to underlying hemorrhage (1).* □

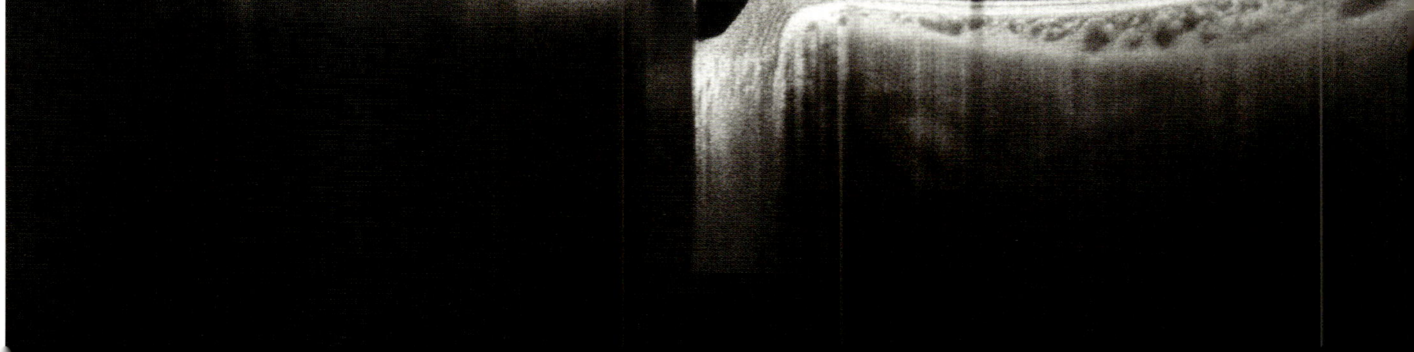

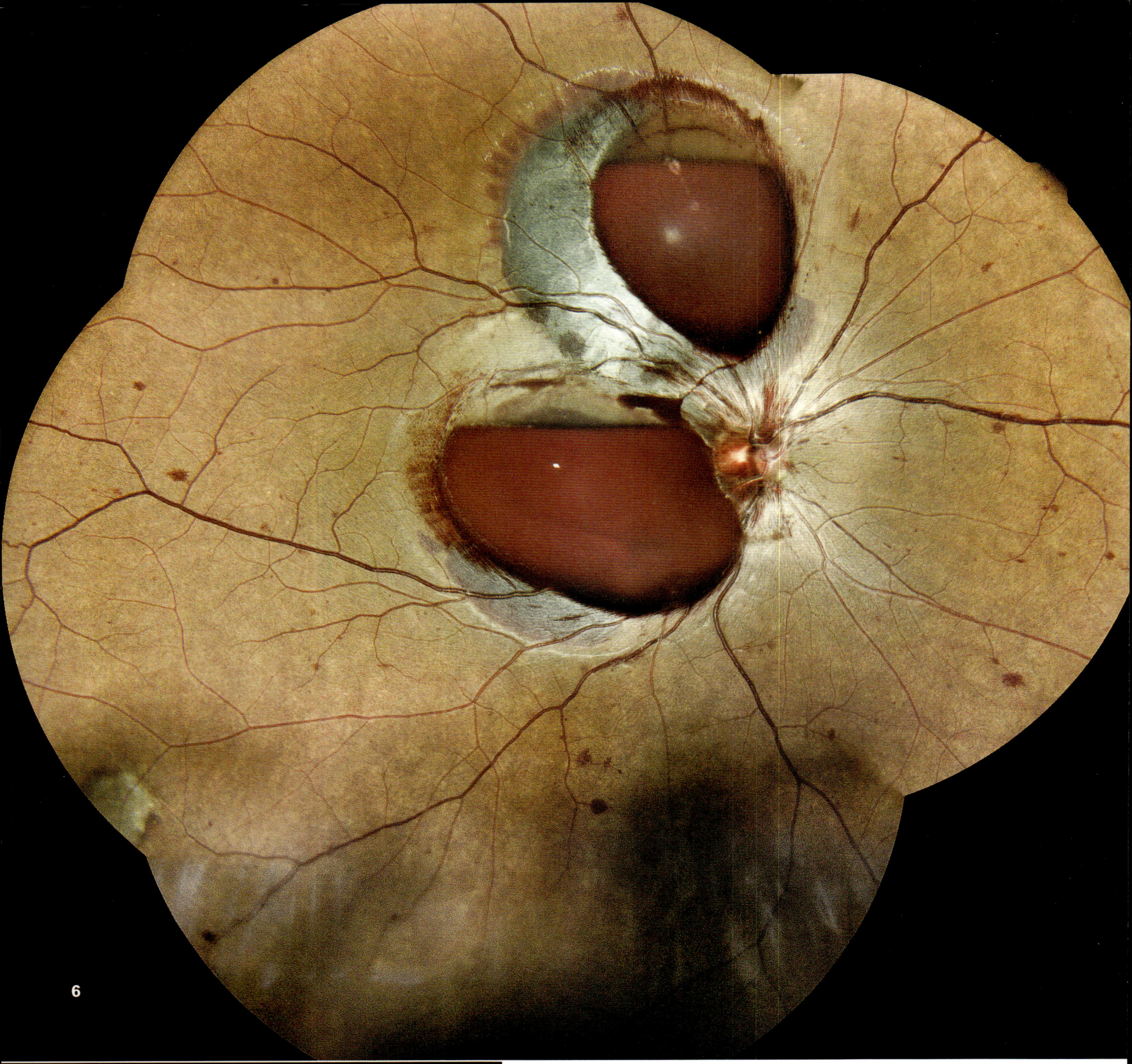

6

7

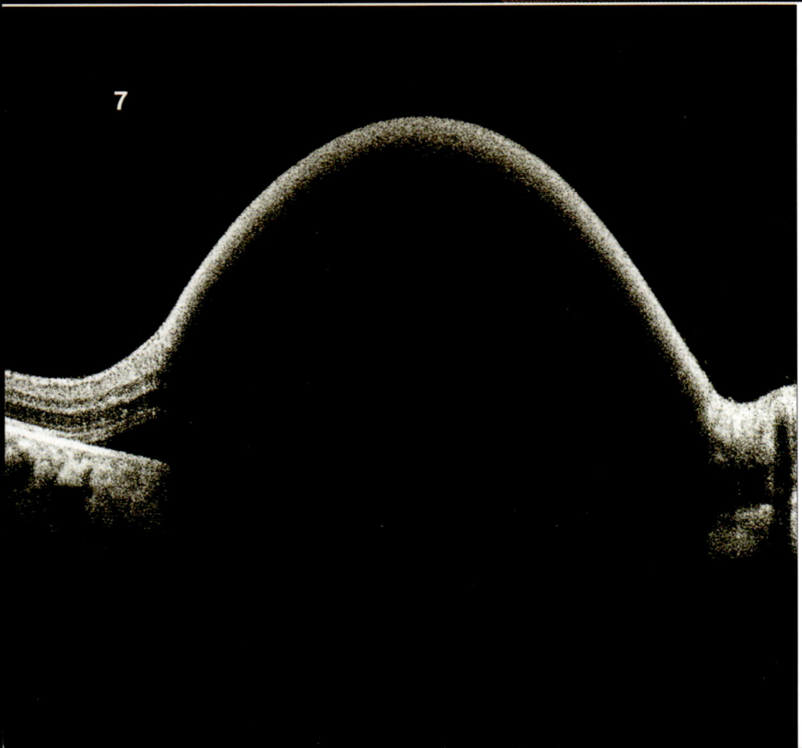

Figure 6 *A case of valsalva retinopathy managed with 25-gauge pars plana vitrectomy with internal limiting membrane peel.*

A 32-year-old male complaints of sudden decrease in vision from his right eye after a bout of severe cough. BCVA was counting finger close to face.

Fundus photo shows dense preretinal bleed located in front of the macula and another located superior to the disk. A rim of dark colored bleed can be seen around the preretinal bleed with retinal vessels crossing over it suggestive of subretinal bleed. Multiple superficial dot like hemorrhage can be seen in the periphery.

Figure 7 *OCT shows dense, dome-shaped subretinal bleed and shadowing of the retinal and choroidal layers beneath it.*

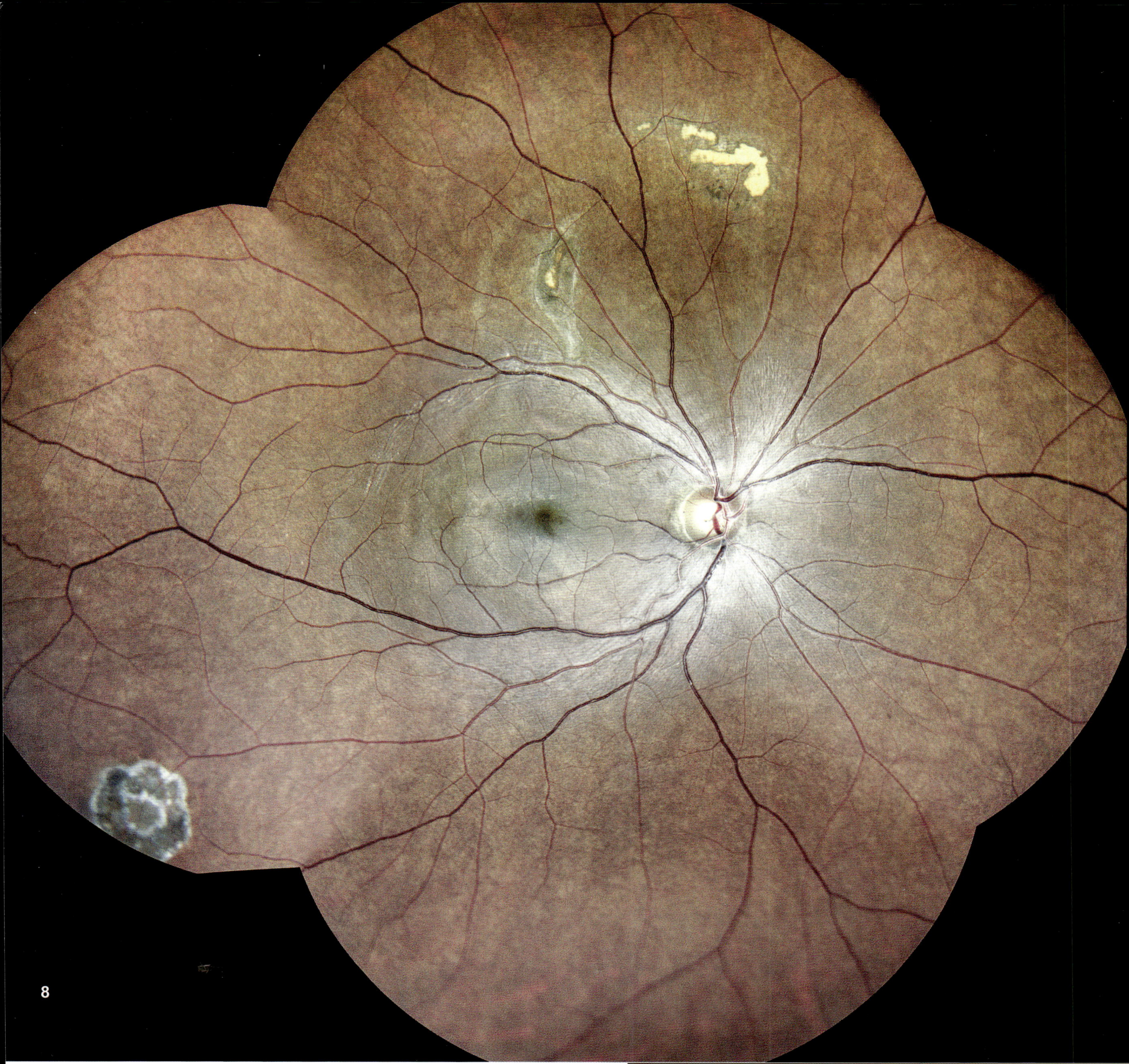

8

9

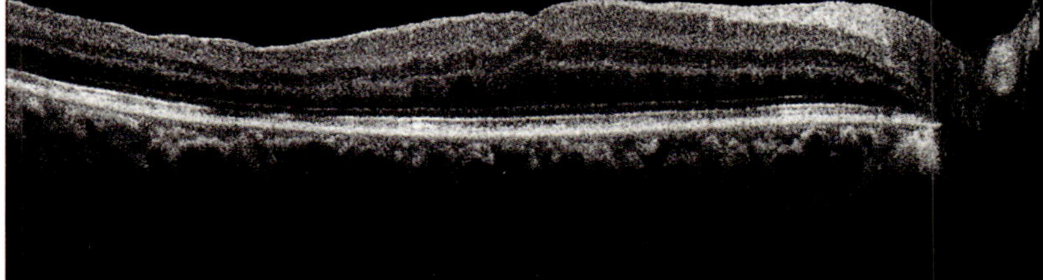

Figure 8 *25-gauge pars plana vitrectomy was done, ILM was stained with brilliant blue G, and peeled using ILM forceps. Retinal bleed was aspirated using silicone soft tip.*
*BCVA improved to 6/6. Fundus photo shows complete resolution of preretinal bleed. Some patches of faint old subretinal bleed can be seen superiorly which eventually resolve with time. Barrage laser was done to an atrophic patch inferotemporally.*

Figure 9 *Postoperative OCT shows complete resolution of preretinal bleed, neurosensory retina is well-attached to underlying retinal pigment epithelium, with intact neurosensory layers.* □

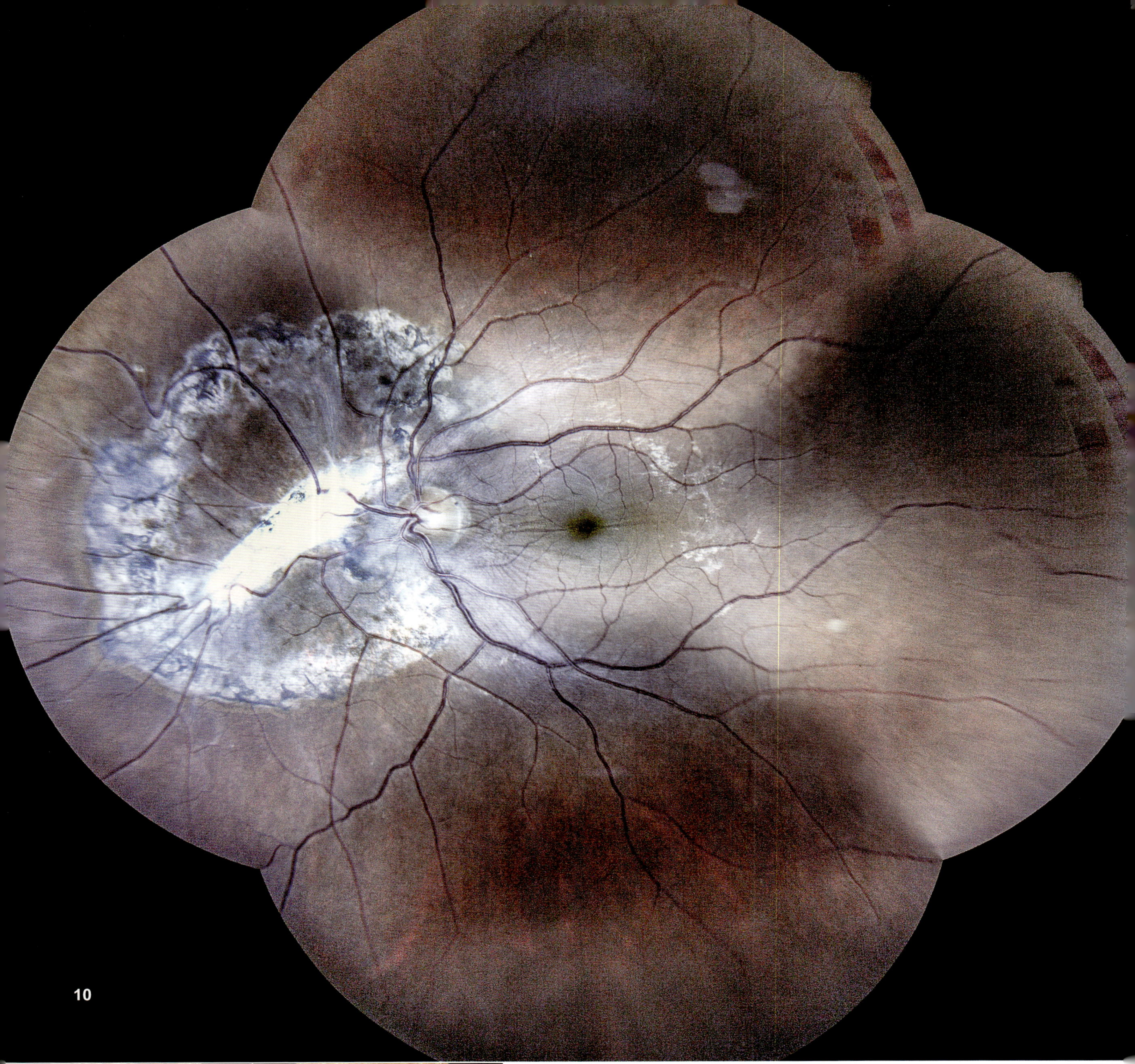

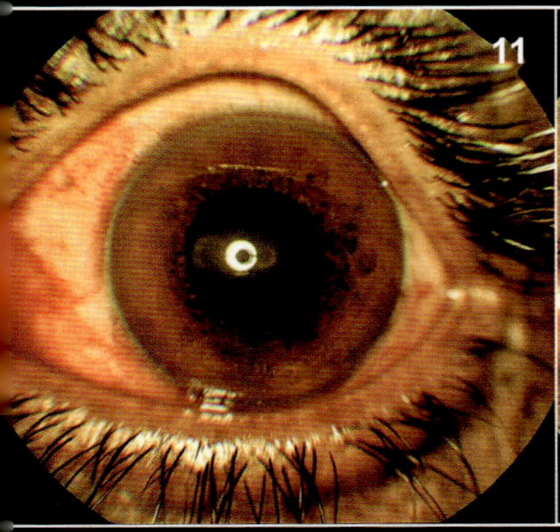

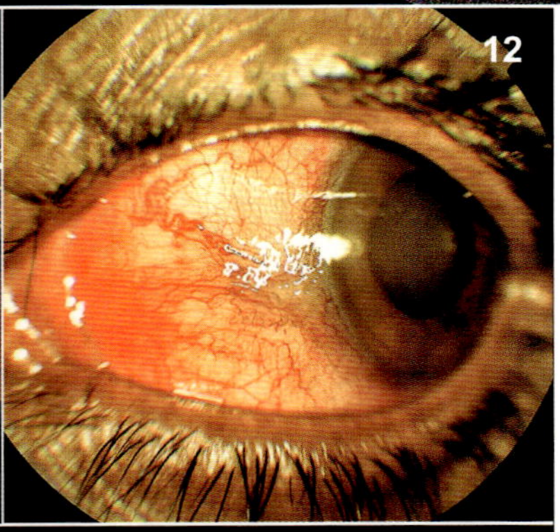

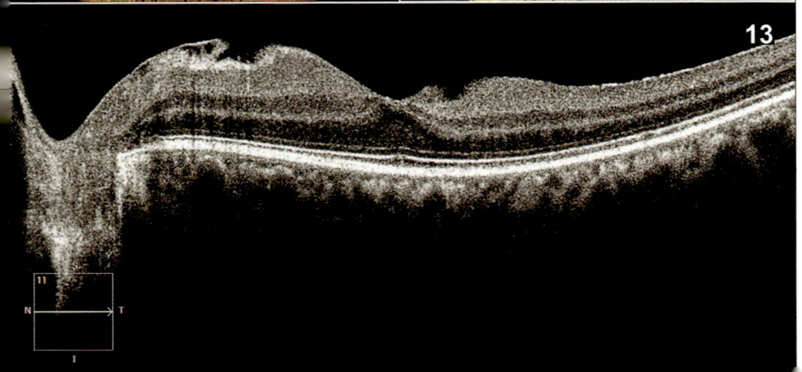

Figure 10 *Twenty-five gauge pars plana vitrectomy was performed with removal of intraocular foreign body using intraocular magnet via a corneal limbal incision and sulcus supported intraocular lens implanted.*

The scar at site of impact is visible nasal to disk. Retina is attached. Macula is spared. Best corrected visual acuity improved to 6/9. Few linear folds can be seen at the macula due to early epiretinal membrane temporal to the disk.

Figure 11 *A 54-year-old male presented with retained intraocular foreign body. Best corrected visual acuity was hand motion close to face. Anterior segment examination shows dense cataract.*

Figure 12 *Anterior segment examination shows dense cataract and the conjunctival laceration at the site of entry of metallic foreign body is clearly visible.*

Figure 13 *OCT confirms the finding of thin hyper-reflective membrane nasal to the disk, suggestive of epiretinal membrane which is commonly seen after trauma.* □

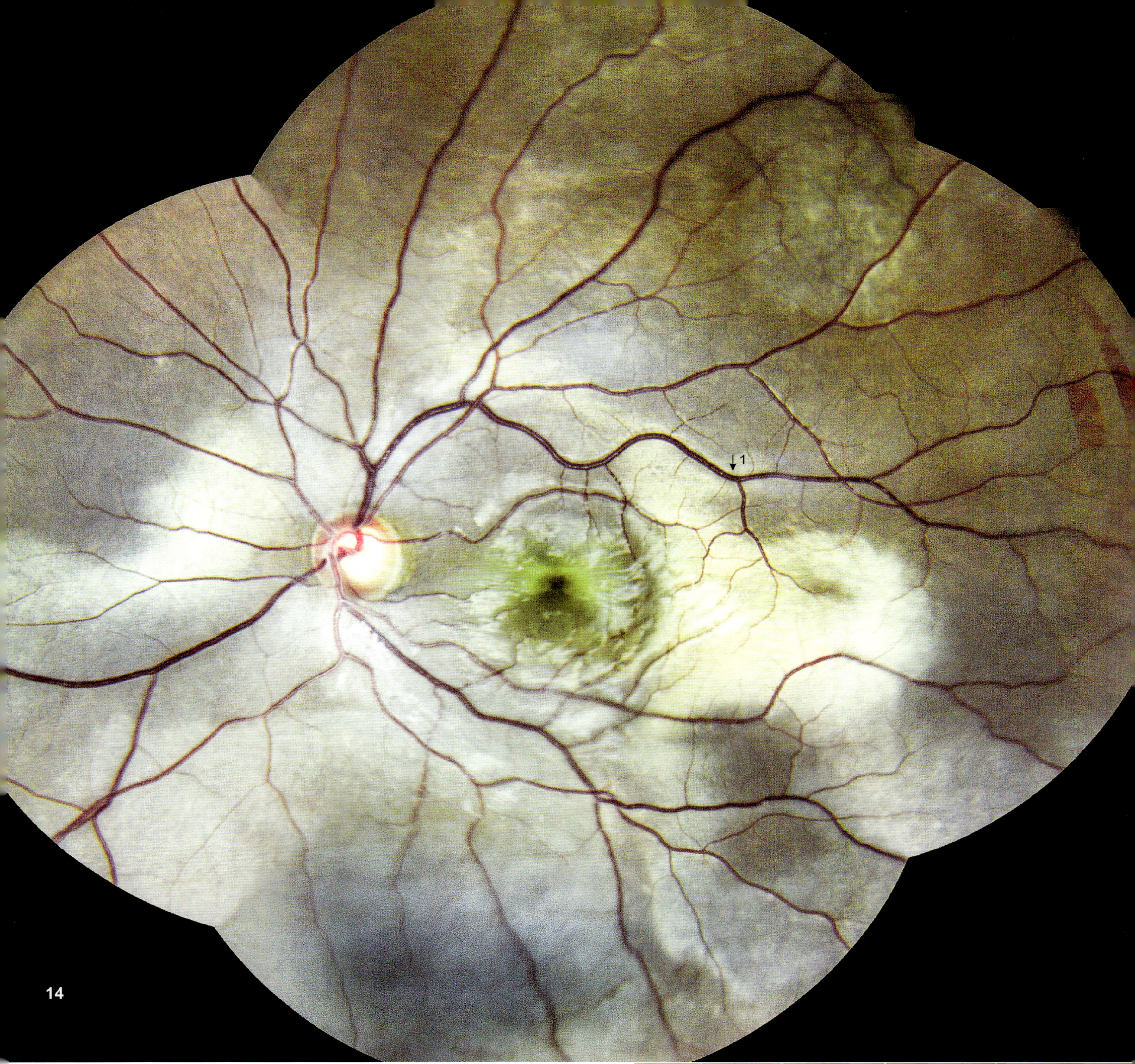


14

Figure 14 *A case of blunt trauma to the globe leading to berlins edema.*

A 24-year-old male presented with history of injury with a cricket ball 1 day ago followed by sudden diminution of vision, BCVA was CF 3 meters. Color fundus photo shows opaque retina (1) which is white in color the blood vessels traversing it are normal in color and caliber.

Figure 15 *Fundus fluorescein angiography shows hyperfluorescent areas corresponding to contrecoup concussive retinopathy.*

Figure 16 *Fundus fluorescein angiography in the late phase shows diffuse hypofluorescence with no leakage reflecting the diffuse photoreceptor damage.*

Figure 17 *OCT shows involvement of outer photoreceptor zone with preservation of inner retinal architecture. Hyper-reflectivity (1) is seen in the outer layers along with shallow neurosensory detachment (2).* □

15

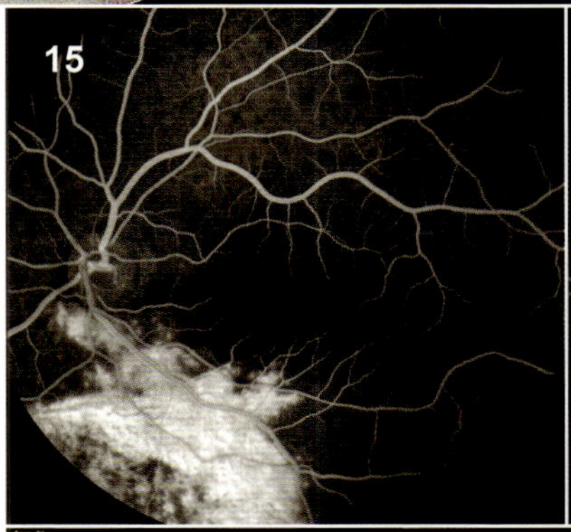

16

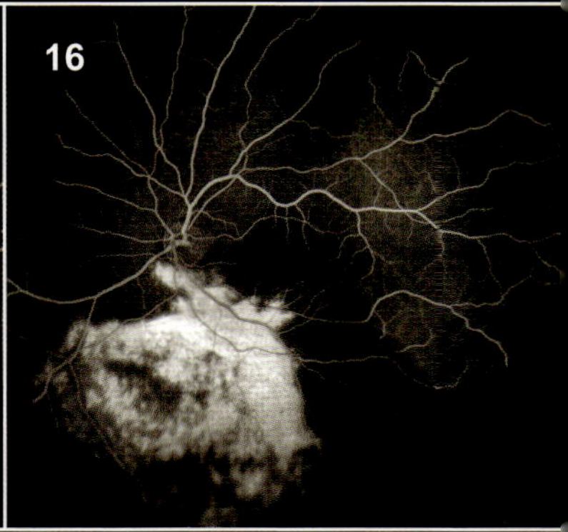

17

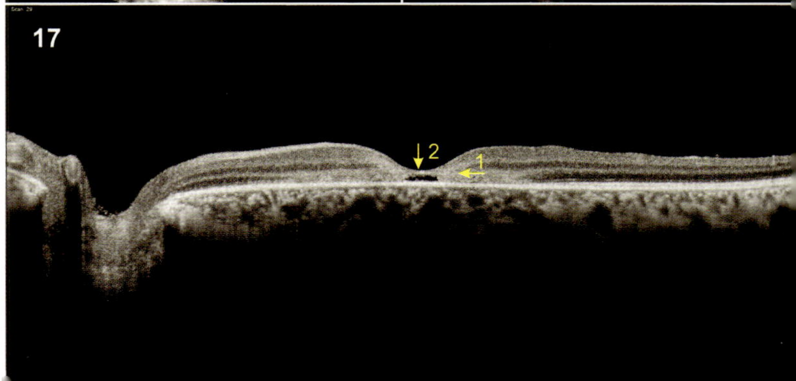

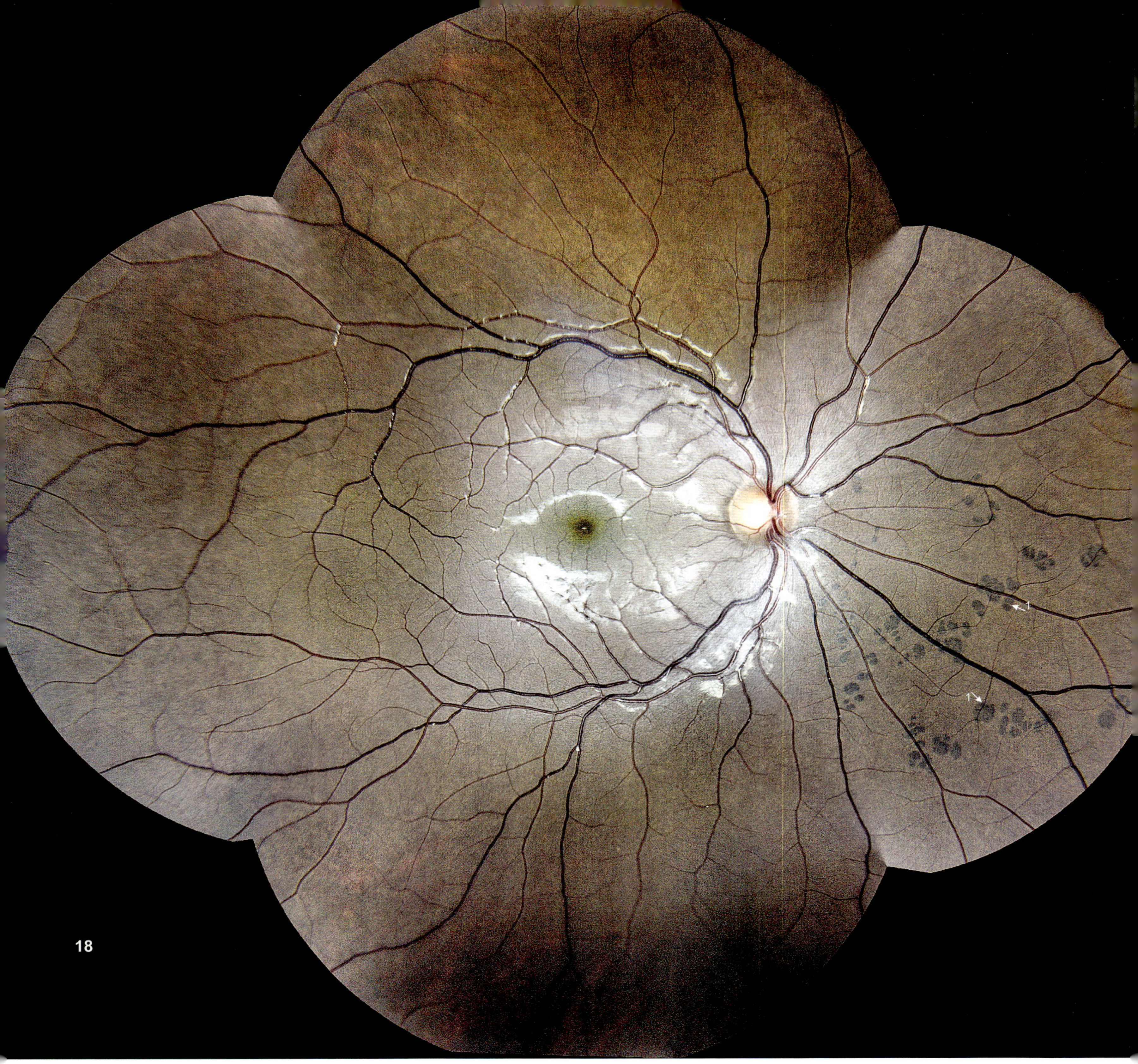


Figure 18 *Color fundus montage image in case of congenital hypertrophy of retinal pigment epithelium (CHRPE). Note the presence of the multiple rounds to oval small, black in color (1) well-demarcated hyperpigmented lesions arranged in configuration resembling the footprint of bear (bear track lesions).*

Congenital hypertrophy of retinal pigment epithelium (CHRPE) is commonly encountered, generally benign non-progressive lesion within RPE cell layer of outer retina. Rarely, such lesions are known to be associated with other systemic findings such as familial adenomatous polyposis and Gardner syndrome.

Complete gastroenterological workup is required only in those CHRPE lesions when they are bilateral, occur in multiple quadrants are pisiform shape and have irregular borders.□

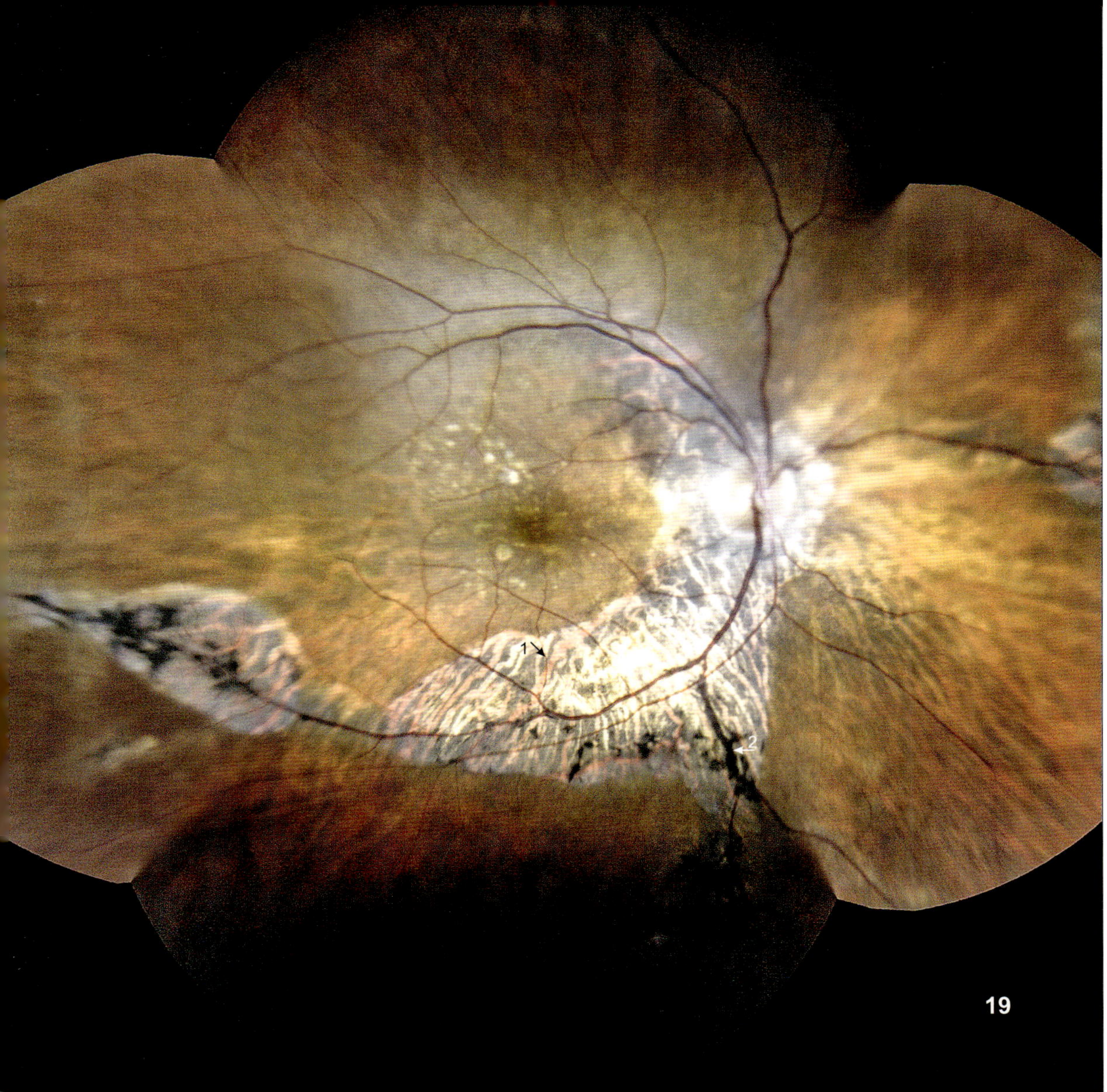


Figure 19

*Right color fundus montage image of a patient with pigmented paravenous retina choroidal atrophy. Generalized pale patches of RPE atrophy could be seen along the inferotemporal vein and underlying choroidal vasculature could be seen due to loss of RPE. (1) Also, note coarse pigment clumping of RPE. (2)*

Figure 20

*Fundus autofluorescence in case of PPRCA demonstrating hypo-AF (1) in majority of lesions due to loss of RPE and hyper-AF (2) margins indicating some level of RPE dysfunction and lipofuscin accumulation in those area.*

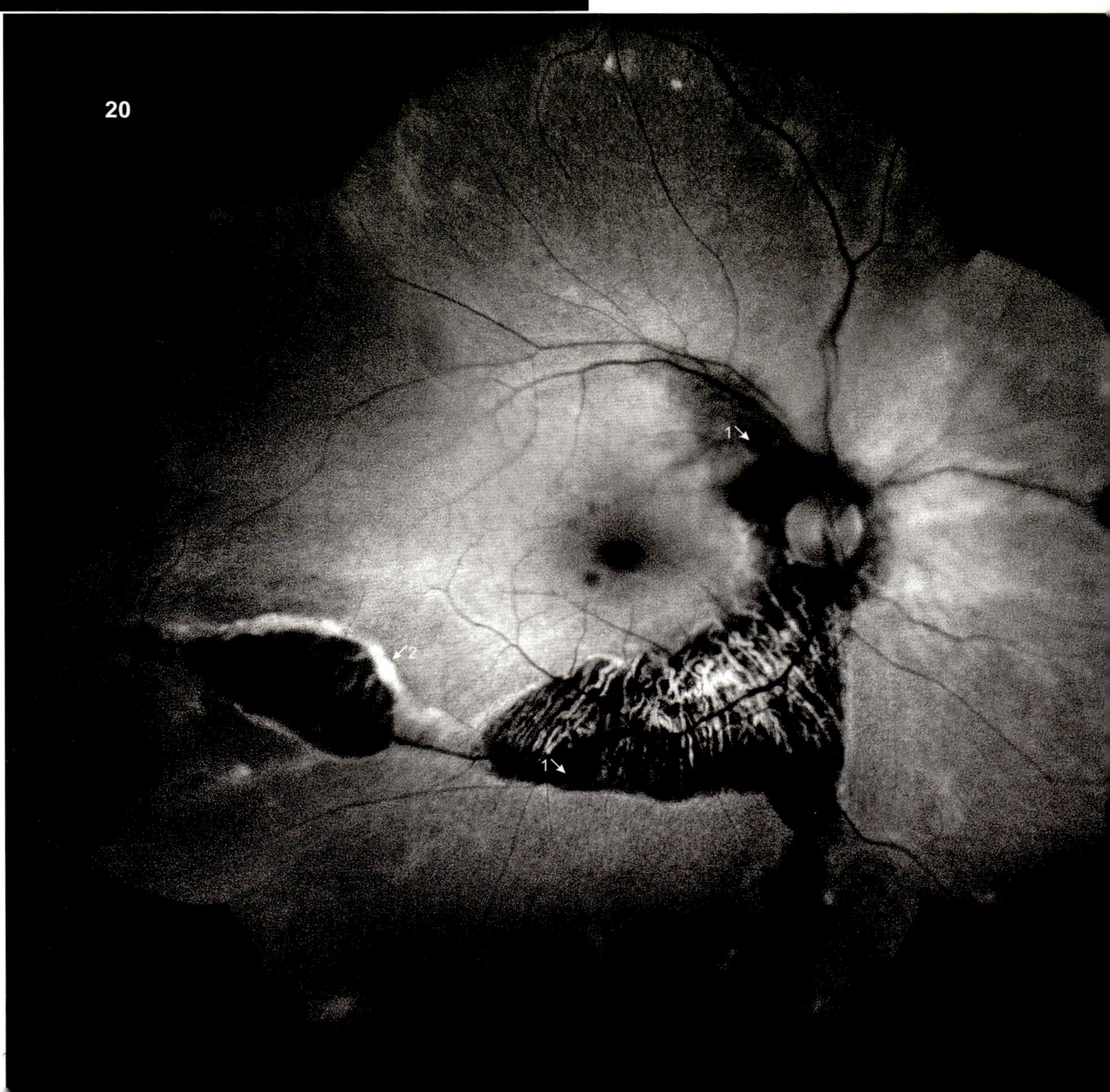


Pigmented paravenous retinochoroidal atrophy (PPRCA) is a rare disorder of vitreous etiology characterize by pigment accumulation along the distribution of retinal veins visual acuity is normally not affected unless there is macular involvement. □

# GLOSSARY

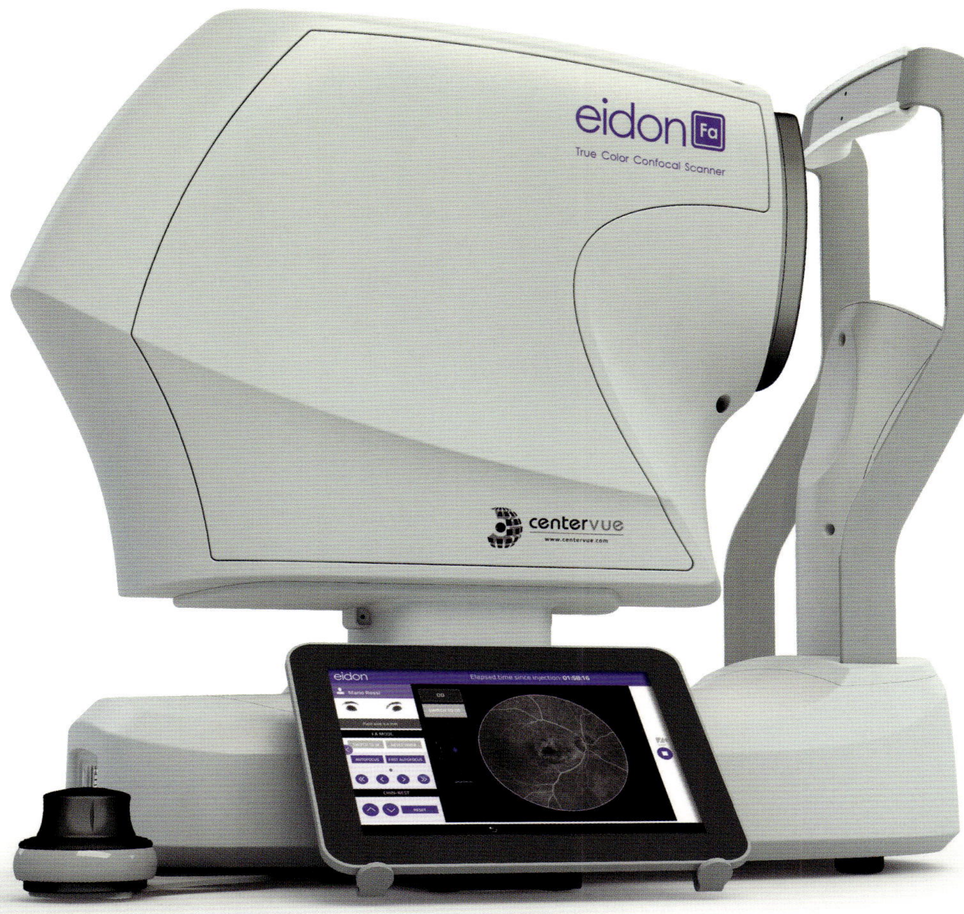
eidon Fa
True Color Confocal Scanner
centervue
www.centervue.com